Nephrology

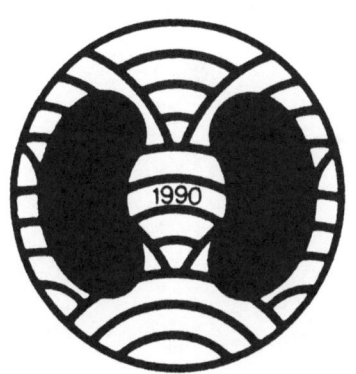

1990

Nephrology VOLUME I

PROCEEDINGS OF THE
XIth INTERNATIONAL CONGRESS OF NEPHROLOGY

Editor
Michinobu Hatano

Associate Editors
Nishio Honda · Hyoe Ishikawa · Kenkichi Koiso
Kiyoshi Kurokawa · Tadao Niijima
Nobuhiro Sugino · Susumu Takahashi

With 253 Figures

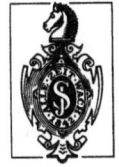

Springer Japan KK

Editor

MICHINOBU HATANO, M.D., Professor of Medicine, Director, Department of Internal Medicine, Nihon University School of Medicine, Tokyo, Japan

Associate Editors

NISHIO HONDA, Tokyo Senbai Hospital, Tokyo
HYOE ISHIKAWA, Nara Medical University, Nara
KENKICHI KOISO, The University of Tsukuba, Ibaraki
KIYOSHI KUROKAWA, University of Tokyo, Tokyo
TADAO NIIJIMA, Tokyo Seamen's Medical College, Tokyo
NOBUHIRO SUGINO, Tokyo Women's Medical College, Tokyo
SUSUMU TAKAHASHI, Nihon University, Tokyo

ISBN 978-3-540-70074-6

Library of Congress Cataloging-in-Publication Data
International Congress on Nephrology (11th: 1990: Tokyo, Japan); Nephrology: proceedings of the XIth International Congress of Nephrology/editors, Michinobu Hatano: associate editors, Nishio Honda...[et al.].
p. cm. Congress held in Tokyo, Japan, July 15-20, 1990. Includes bibliographical references. Includes index.
ISBN 978-3-540-70074-6   ISBN 978-3-662-35158-1 (eBook)
DOI 10.1007/978-3-662-35158-1
1. Kidneys – Diseases – Congresses.
2. Nephrology – Congresses. 3. Kidney Diseases – congresses. 4. Nephrology – congresses. I. Hatano, Michinobu, 1926- . II. Honda, Nishio. III. Title. [DNLM: WJ 300 I59n 1990]. RC902.A2I56 1990. 616.6'1 –dc20. DNLM/DLC. for Library of Congress 91-4651

Typesetting: Publishers Service of Montana, Bozeman, Montana

Foreword

The proceedings of the XIth International Congress of Nephrology held in Tokyo in 1990, form the most international and complete document of the present state of basic and clinical science in nephrology. In addition, they document the progress made in this field during the 3 years since the London Congress. The result is nothing short of impressive. The material presented by the invited lecturers and the participants of the symposia all show a remarkable pattern; not only the "height" of the science, but also the depth of the specialized knowledge, both prerequisites of excellency in science, which do not necessarily imply narrowness of outlook. On the contrary, this written document of the Tokyo Congress is a witness to the enormous progress made over the last few years in communication between basic scientists and clinical scientists.

The International Society of Nephrology is a fine example of how fruitful and productive this interaction can be, if it is conducted with the desire to understand each other. The members of the Scientific Program Committee of the Tokyo Congress are to be congratulated, not only for a thoughtful and well designed program, but also for carefully selecting those speakers who, besides their own contribution to nephrological science, also have the talent of being able to communicate with a large, international audience. In particular, I would like to express my deep appreciation to the editors of the Proceedings for their commitment and industriousness which made it possible for this publication to appear so soon after the Congress.

Since the first Congress of the International Society of Nephrology in Evian in 1960, nephrologists have witnessed a phenomenal increase in knowledge, a progress which still continues and will do so in the future. The present proceedings are a snapshot of this process. The counterpoint to the intellectual challenge of acquiring deeper understanding is the duty and promise to utilize that understanding for the benefit of our patients.

KLAUS THURAU, M.D.
President,
International Society of Nephrology
(1987–1990)

V

Preface

The XIth International Congress of Nephrology was held in Tokyo, Japan from July 15–20, 1990.

Since the first congress in Evian, France in 1960, this is the first time that this prestigious congress has been held in Asia. Therefore, enthusiastic expectations were held by nephrologists not only in Japan but also throughout the world.

In organizing the congress under the estimable guidance of Prof. Klaus Thurau, President of the International Society of Nephrology, the ISN Executive Committee and the International Advisory Committee, Prof. Michinobu Hatano, Chairman of the local organizing committee as well as the organizing committee made every effort to make the congress a success.

Over three thousand participants from 71 countries attended the congress. These included 1,470 participants from Japan, 472 from the United States, 150 from France, and 128 from Italy. We were particularly pleased to welcome eight representatives from Czechoslavakia as well as an increased participation from other eastern European countries, the Soviet Union, and China. Forty-nine delegates from Taiwan were also in attendance.

The opening ceremony was held at the New Takanawa Prince Hotel in the presence of the Crown Prince, whose address noted that progress in nephrology would contribute greatly to the welfare of patients worldwide.

The scientific program consisted of 15 state-of-the-art lectures, 36 symposia, 11 workshops, 256 oral and 1,778 poster presentations. Following the advice of the ISN Executive Committee, the Scientific Program Committee encouraged the presentation of clinical and research papers at the same time in each session. This ensured that throughout the scientific program, discussions were constructive, and this helped to make the congress both stimulating and fruitful.

A total of 12 ISN satellite symposia, 4 overseas and 8 in Japan, were also held. The specific topics discussed at each symposium, combined with sightseeing tours at each site, contributed greatly to exchanges of both friendship and information.

VIII Preface

Finally, we would like to express our sincere thanks and appreciation to the ISN Committee and all the participants of the congress.

KENZO OSHIMA, M.D.
President

YAWARA YOSHITOSHI,
M.D.
Vice-President

YASUSHI UEDA, M.D.
Vice-President

HIROSHI ABE, M.D.
Vice-President

XIth International Congress of Nephrology

ORGANIZED BY: The Organizing Committee of the XIth International
Congress of Nephrology

UNDER THE AUSPICES OF: International Society of Nephrology

SPONSORED BY: Japanese Society of Nephrology
The Kidney Foundation, Japan

IN COOPERATION WITH: The Japanese Association of Medical Science
Japan Medical Association
The Japanese Urological Association
The Japan Society for Transplantation
Japanese Society for Artificial Organs
Japanese Society for Dialysis Therapy
The Japanese Society of Pediatric Nephrology
Japan Incorporated Medical Association for Dialysis

SUPPORTED BY: Ministry of Education, Science and Culture
Ministry of Health and Welfare
Science Council of Japan
Tokyo Metropolitan Government

The International Society of Nephrology

EXECUTIVE COMMITTEE 1987–1990

Klaus Thurau	FRG	President
Donald W. Seldin	USA	Past President
Roscoe R. Robinson	USA	President Elect
John Stewart Cameron	UK	Vice-President
Claude Amiel	France	Secretary-General
Robert W. Schrier	USA	Treasurer
Thomas E. Andreoli	USA	Editor, Kidney International

ADVISORY COMMITTEE FOR THE 1990 CONGRESS

Klaus Thurau	FRG	Chairman
Robert C. Atkins	Australia	
Claude Amiel	France	
John Stewart Cameron	UK	
Jared James Grantham	USA	
Roscoe R. Robinson	USA	

NOMINATING COMMITTEE

Paul Michielsen	Belgium	President
Franklin H. Epstein	USA	
Gerhard Giebisch	USA	
Richard J. Glassock	USA	
Colin I. Johnston	Australia	
Norman F. Jones	UK	
Franciszek Kokot	Poland	
Jean-Philippe Mery	France	
Jose C. Pena	Mexico	
Mordecai M. Popovtzer	Israel	
Yawara Yoshitoshi	Japan	

Management Committee

Klaus Thurau	FRG	President
Roscoe R. Robinson	USA	President Elect
Claude Amiel	France	Secretary-General
Robert W. Schrier	USA	Treasurer
Thomas E. Andreoli	USA	Editor, Kidney International
Saulo Klahr	USA	Councillor
D. Keith Peters	UK	Councillor

Council

Stephen Angielski	Poland
Robert C. Atkins	Australia
Knut Auklund	Norway
Vittorio Bonomini	Italy
Barry M. Brenner	USA
Giuseppe D'Amico	Italy
Vincent W. Dennis	USA
John H. Dirks	Canada
Evert J. Dorhout Mees	The Netherlands
Carl W. Gottschalk	USA
Jean-Pierre Grünfeld	France
Jean Hamburger	France
Klaus Hierholzer	FRG
David N.S. Kerr	UK
Saulo Klahr	USA
Robert T. McCluskey	USA
Gerhard Malnic	Brazil
D. Keith Peters	UK
Hidekazu Shigematsu	Japan
Jay Stein	USA
Nobuhiro Sugino	Japan
Guillermo Whittembury	Venezuela

XIth International Congress Officers

President	Kenzo Oshima
Vice Presidents	Yawara Yoshitoshi
	Yasushi Ueda
	Hiroshi Abe

ORGANIZING COMMITTEE

Chairman	Michinobu Hatano
Secretary-General	Susumu Takahashi

Members

Yoshio Aso	Tadashi Miyahara
Toshiyuki Furukawa	Toshihiko Nagasawa
Kohei Hara	Mitsuharu Narita
Nishio Honda	Hiromi Nihira
Takeshi Hoshi	Tadao Niijima
Kazunari Iidaka	Teruo Omae
Hyoe Ishikawa	Zensuke Ota
Chuichi Kawai	Fuminori Sakai
Teruo Kitagawa	Takao Sonoda
Kenkichi Koiso	Nobuhiro Sugino
Kiyoshi Kurokawa	Shizuo Tojo
Sunao Maki	

SCIENTIFIC PROGRAM COMMITTEE

Chairmen Nobuhiro Sugino
Nishio Honda

Executive Secretary Kiyoshi Kurokawa

Members
Akitoshi Ando Koichi Matsumoto
Kikuo Arakawa Toshihiko Nagasawa
Masaaki Arakawa Mitsumasa Nagase
Hitoshi Endou Yasushi Nakamoto
Mamoru Fujimoto Hiroshi Nihei
Gerhard Giebisch Michio Odaka
Takashi Harada Hiroyuki Ohi
Eiji Higashihara Yoshimasa Orita
Kazunari Iidaka Kazuo Ota
Masashi Imai Hideto Sakai
Hiroshi Kida Osamu Sakai
Hikaru Koide Tadasu Sakai
Kenkichi Koiso Takao Saruta
Shozo Koshikawa Hidekazu Shigematsu
Akio Koyama Kenjiro Yamamoto
Kenji Maeda Nobuyuki Yoshizawa
Sunao Maki

FUND RAISING COMMITTEE

Chairmen Tadao Niijima
Hyoe Ishikawa

Members
Keishi Abe Joichi Kumazawa
Yoshio Aso Yuji Nagura
Tohru Azuma Zensuke Ota
Kohei Hara Tsutomu Sanaka
Yoshihei Hirasawa Takao Sonoda
Hiroshi Kida Naohiko Ueda

FINANCE COMMITTEE

Chairman Kenkichi Koiso

Members
Hiroshi Kawamura Gengo Osawa

Contents of Volume I

State of the Art Lectures

Symposia

Immunological and Cellular Mechanisms of Glomerulonephritis

Role of Potassium in Acid-Base Disturbances

Role of Kidney in the Pathogenesis of Hypertension

Cellular and Integrative Functions of the Juxtaglomerular Apparatus

Systemic Dysfunctions in Renal Failure and Their Management

ATPases of the Kidney

Vitamin D and Uremic Bone Disease

AIDS/AIDS — Nephropathy

Cellular and Integrative Regulation of Renal Circulation

Dietary Factors and Progression of Chronic Renal Failure

Renal Diseases in Asia

Pathobiology of Glomerular and Tubular Basement Membranes

Contents of Volume II

Symposia

Cytokines, Mitogens and Their Receptors on Glomerular Cells

Frontiers of Research on Natriuretic Peptides

Cystic Diseases of the Kidney

Continuous Ambulatory Peritoneal Dialysis (CAPD)

Autacoids and the Kidney

Ion Channels of the Kidney

List of Contributors

For contributors' addresses see chapter opening pages

AIDS/AIDS-Nephropathy

Chair: Gerhard Treser (USA)
Filoteo A. Alano (Philippines)

Highlights of Major Differences Between Children and Adults with HIV-Associated Nephropathy

JOSE STRAUSS, GASTON ZILLERUELO, CAROLYN ABITBOL,
BRENDA MONTANE, GWENDOLYN SCOTT, CHARLES MITCHELL,
ANDREA GRECO,[1] and VICTORIANO PARDO[2]

SUMMARY. Major differences between human immunodeficiency virus (HIV) associated nephropathy (HIVN) in children and HIVN in adults include the following: HIVN occurs in both HIV-1+ and AIDS adults, but apparently only in AIDS children. In HIVN patients, the virus has been transmitted to adult males mostly by intravenous drug use, and to adult females mostly by intercourse with infected males, but the virus has been transmitted to male and female infants and children by the mother. Renal histology changes in HIVN adults are mostly of the focal and segmental sclerosis (FSS) type, but FSS type changes are found in only one-third–one-half of HIVN children. The onset of chronic renal failure in adults heralds a rapid (few weeks) course to death, but in children the course is much slower (several months). Acute renal failure is rarely diagnosed in HIVN children while it is commonly diagnosed in HIVN adults.

Introduction

The clinical and immunologic characteristics of patients with the human immunodeficiency virus (HIV) and the acquired immunodeficiency syndrome (AIDS) sparked our interest in 1981 and we began studying renal involvement in HIV and AIDS pediatric patients at the University of Miami/Jackson Memorial Medical Center. In 1984, urine and renal histology abnormalities in AIDS children were described by our group [1] and were described in AIDS adults by Pardo and Rao [2,3]. Subsequently, we published our updated data on HIV associated nephropathy (HIVN) in children [4]; also available are other investigators' data on children [5–13]

[1]Departments of Pediatrics and [2]Pathology, University of Miami School of Medicine, and Laboratory Services, Veterans Administration Medical Center (V.P.), Miami, FL 33101, USA

and on adults [9,10,12–29]. Based on these data, this paper presents and analyzes some of the differences between HIVN in children and in adults.

Occurrence of HIVN and Clinical Status of the HIV-1 + Patient

In 1984, the severity of renal histologic changes was found to be greater in AIDS adults than in AIDS pediatric patients, and it was concluded that AIDS children do not live long enough for severe changes to develop [1]. Now, however, with a greater number of children studied, more active search for urine changes, and availability of biopsy material, children have been found to have a broad range of renal abnormalities, including severe ones which lead to renal failure [4–13]. A major difference that seems to exist between adults as a group and children as a group is the occurrence of HIVN in HIV-1 + adult patients, without clinical manifestation of the infection. This has been well documented in numerous adults [13–29], while to date no such association has been found in children [4–13]. In adults, HIVN has been reported as being the first manifestation of the HIV-1 infection [21,22]. What could be the cause of this difference? Race can be excluded, since the great majority of children, as well as adult patients, who have HIVN are Black [1–29]. Possible causes are the manner in which the infection was acquired and the characteristics of the host.

Mode of Transmission of the Virus

Mode of transmission may play a role in determining the time of appearance of the nephropathy. Adult males who develop HIVN have acquired the infection almost exclusively through intravenous drug (IVD) use; children who develop HIVN seem to become infected only through their mothers, mostly in utero, but some in the perinatal period or even during lactation. Mothers may be IVD addicts, but most (about two-thirds) seem to have been infected through heterosexual intercourse with bisexual or IVD abuser men [30].

Characteristics of the Host

The difficulties the neonate has in fighting off infections are well known. Even so, only one-third–one-half of the babies born to HIV-1 + mothers are infected; most have maternal anti-HIV-1 + antibodies which have crossed the placenta [30]. What makes so many infants resistant to such a severe infection when for months all of their organs have been perfused by contaminated blood? Determinants may be the time at which the mother acquired the infection, the route by which the mother acquired the infection, and the stage of evolution of her disease. Another host difference is that HIVN children in our group were 2:1 male to female [4] while an overwhelming majority of HIVN adults are males [13–29]. In addition, since only a small percentage of patients infected with HIV-1 develop HIVN, the susceptibility of mesangial cells of glomeruli to the virus may be modified by predisposing agents or conditions [23].

Histologic Renal Changes

It has been amply documented that most adults with HIVN have focal and segmental sclerosis (FSS); this finding is regarded as the characteristic glomerular histologic change in an adult patient with suspected HIV-1 infection [13–29]. Mesangial hyperplasia has been reported in some adult patients [13]. From our data we concluded that a broader spectrum of disease seems to be present in younger patients: in our report five children had FSS, five had mesangial hyperplasia, one had segmental necrotizing glomerulonephritis, and one had minimal changes [4]. Even a rough estimate of the various reports on HIVN in children identified only 30 of 80 patients as evidencing FSS [24]. In addition, we have identified one patient with membranoproliferative changes and another with microangiopathic thromboses. Though an occasional adult patient also has been reported to have changes similar to those found in children, they occur much less frequently [25]. We also have identified the apparent conversion of mesangial hyperplasia (by biopsy) into FSS (by autopsy) in one child; this finding lends support to the belief that mesangial hyperplasia is an early stage of FSS in HIVN [23]. No differences have been identified between children and adults with HIVN in regard to the tubulointerstitial lesions or the tubuloreticular inclusions of glomerular endothelial cells [4,16,21].

HIVN Patients as Percentage of the HIV-1+/AIDS Population

As stated already, HIV-1+ patients with HIVN were found only among adults; HIVN has not been identified in any children who are HIV-1+ but who do not have AIDS [4]. This could be due to incomplete assessment of the population, since not all HIV-1+ children have been checked for urine changes; only those children admitted to our Medical Center for other AIDS-related problems have had their urines evaluated consistently. The only published data on adults have been almost equally biased; still, patients were seen by a nephrologist when a request for consultation was received [23] and a significant number of asymptomatic adults have had HIVN [23,24]. As already mentioned, renal involvement has even been reported as the first manifestation of the infection [21,22]. Requests for Nephrology consultations for patients with HIV-1 infection and with AIDS were received in 7%–12% of the total HIV-1+ and AIDS adult population [23]. In the pediatric AIDS population, a similar percentage of children was found to have HIVN [4]. The true incidence of HIVN in those populations can be identified only when *all* patients (those with only the infection and those with the syndrome) are assessed prospectively and at regular intervals. With the support of the National Institutes of Health, we are currently doing this in infants and children and hope to have meaningful data soon.

Impact of HIVN on Survival

AIDS adults who develop HIVN have a rapidly deteriorating course and die more rapidly than those without HIVN [23,24,27]; children with and without HIVN die at a similar age [4]. Some AIDS children under our care with biopsy-proven renal involvement have survived for up to one year after diagnosis of HIVN, while most AIDS adults who develop HIVN die within weeks [23].

Number of AIDS Children Who Develop HIVN

Between January 1981 and June 1987 (6.5 years) we identified 12 AIDS children who developed HIVN [4]. During the subsequent three years, we have identified 20 additional AIDS children with HIVN. Thus, we have gone from 12 HIVN patients out of 155 AIDS children (7.7%) in the first 6.5 years (1.85 patients/year), to 20 HIVN patients out of 195 AIDS children (10%) in 3.0 years (6.67 patients/year), or a total of 32 HIVN patients out of 350 AIDS patients in 9.5 years.

Other communities with endemic characteristics for HIV-1+ infection also have reported the identification of several children with HIVN. These communities include areas of Newark [7], New York [8,28], and Canada [6]. The reason for this increased occurrence or identification of new HIVN cases remains unknown.

Though in some patients the increase coincided with regular IV administration of gamma globulins [9], most of the patients from our Medical Center did not receive such medication. Increased awareness of the occurrence of proteinuria with or without hematuria among AIDS children may have led to early identification among patients who otherwise might have died before a nephrotic syndrome-like clinical picture was apparent.

Chronic/Renal Failure

As stated above, it was not uncommon for children who were diagnosed as having HIVN to live for a period which lasted several months from the time of diagnosis; this was true even (or particularly) in those who developed chronic renal failure [4]. Although children and adults with HIVN and FSS have in common the development of chronic renal failure, the latter was present in only 6 of 12 HIVN children, while sooner or later, it becomes a regular feature in HIVN adults [23].

Acute Renal Failure

This functional alteration has been diagnosed often in adults with the HIV infection or with AIDS [23,25]. For reasons not clearly understood, such a diagnosis has rarely, if ever, been made in the children admitted to our Medical Center. The difference may be due to a multiplicity of factors, among which repeated insults from allergenic medications, nephrotoxic drugs, x-ray contrast material, certain infections, etc., may play an important etiopathogenic role in adults. Ischemic renal injury also is more likely to occur in adults (often with other organ involvement through atherosclerosis, hypertension, etc.) than in children.

The possible delay in the increase of blood urea nitrogen and serum creatinine, because of severe malnutrition in children, may contribute to the lack of diagnosis of acute renal failure. Our use of radionuclides to assess glomerular filtration rate and renal blood flow prospectively should answer this question.

Summary and Conclusion

The differences between children and adults infected with HIV-1 or suffering from AIDS have been presented and briefly evaluated in terms of the reasons for those differences. It is hoped that in-depth prospective studies will help clarify these perplexing problems. The possibility is that careful follow-up of large numbers of children will eliminate some of the differences now seen between HIV infected or AIDS adults and children with renal involvement.

Acknowledgments. Supported in part by a grant (1R01 DK-40838-02) from the National Institute of Diabetes and Digestive and Kidney Diseases, a grant from Children's Medical Services, Florida Department of Health and Rehabilitative Services, and grants (5R01 AI-20736 and 5R37 AI-23524) from the National Institute of Allergy and Infectious Diseases.

We thank Pearl Seidler for study coordination, LaDemia Albury for typographical assistance, and Mozhe Jalali and Rhonda Davis for computer processing.

References

1. Strauss J, Montane B, Scott G, Freundlich M, Abitbol C, Zilleruelo G, Pardo V (1984) Urinary and renal histological changes in children with acquired immunodeficiency syndrome (AIDS). Pediatr Res 18(Suppl):371A
2. Pardo V, Aldana M, Colton RM, Fischl MA, Jaffe D, Moskowitz L, Hensley GT, Bourgoignie JJ (1984) Glomerular lesions in the acquired immunodeficiency syndrome. Ann Inter Med 101:429–434
3. Rao TK, Filippone EJ, Nicastri AD, Landesman SH, Frean E, Chen CK, Friedman EA (1984) Associated focal and segmental glomerulosclerosis in the acquired immunodeficiency syndrome. N Engl J Med 310:669–673
4. Gardenswartz MH, Lerner CW, Seligson GR, Zabetakis PM, Rotterdam H, Tapper ML, Michelis MF, Bruno MS (1984) Renal disease in patients with AIDS: a clinicopathologic study. Clin Nephrol 21:197–204
5. Strauss J, Abitbol C, Zilleruelo G, Scott G, Paredes A, Malaga S, Montane B, Mitchell C, Parks W, Pardo V (1989) A spectrum of renal disease in children with acquired immunodeficiency syndrome. N Engl J Med 321:625–630
6. Rousseau E, Russo P, Lapointe N, O'Reagan S (1988) Renal complications of acquired immunodeficiency syndrome in children. Am J Kidney Dis 11:48–50
7. Connor E, Gupta S, Joshi V, DiCarlo F, Offenberger J, Minnefor A, Uy C, Oleske J, Ende N (1988) Acquired immunodeficiency syndrome-associated renal disease in children. J Pediatr 113:39–44
8. Chander P, Sagel I, Weiss R, Pimentel C, Gupta A, Bamji M, Treser G (1989) Renal disease in human immunodeficiency virus infected children (abstract). Kidney Int 35:368
9. Ingulli E, Gonzalez R, Rajpoot D, Pomrantz A, Tejani A (1989) Demography, morphology, treatment and outcome of AIDs nephropathy. Pediatr Nephrol 3:C168
10. Kaplan MS, Wechsler M, Benson MC (1987) Urologic manifestations of AIDS. Urology 30:441–443
11. Cohen AH, Nast CC (1988) HIV-associated nephropathy: a unique combined glomerular, tubular, and interstitial lesion. Mod Pathol 1:87–97
12. Horowitz L, Greco MA, Feiner V (1988) Renal pathology in pediatric AIDS. Abstracts 4th international conference on AIDS. Stockholm pp 402

13. Rao TKS, Friedman EA, Nicastri AD (1987) The types of renal disease in the acquired immunodeficiency syndrome. N Engl J Med 316:1062-1068
14. Pardo V, Meneses R, Ossa L, Jaffe DJ, Strauss J, Roth D, Bourgoignie JJ (1987) Aids-related glomerulopathy: Occurrence in specific risk groups. Kidney Int 31:1167-1173
15. Vaziri ND, Barbari A, Licorish K, Cesario T, Gupta S (1985) Spectrum of renal abnormalities in acquired immune-deficiency syndrome. J Natl Med Assoc 77:369-375
16. D'Agati V, Suh JI, Carbone L, Cheng JT, Appel G (1989) Pathology of HIV-associated nephropathy: a detailed morphologic and comparative study. Kidney Int 35:1358-1370
17. Heredia JB, Angeles AA, Gutierrez ER, Correa-Rotter R, Saldiyar S, Pena JC (1987) Nephropatia associada al sindrome de inmunodeficiencia acquirida. Rev Invest Clin 39:105-115
18. Kim KK, Factor SM (1987) Membranoproliferative glomerulonephritis and plexogenic pulmonary arteriopathy in a homosexual man with acquired immunodeficiency syndrome. Hum Pathol 18:1293-1296
19. Cantor ES, Kimmel PK, Bosch JP (1989) Impact of race on renal disease in patients with AIDS (abstract). Kidney Int 35:222
20. Weiss MA, Daquioaq E, Margolin EG, Pollak VE (1986) Nephrotic syndrome, progressive irreversible renal failure, and glomerular "collapse:" A new clinicopathologic entity? Am J Kidney Dis 7:20-28
21. Chander P, Soni A, Suri A, Bhagwat R, Yoo J, Treser G (1987) Renal ultrastructural markers in AIDS-associated nephropathy. Am J Pathol 126:513-526
22. Alpers CE, Harawi S, Rennke HG (1988) Focal glomerulosclerosis with tubuloreticular inclusions: Possible predictive value for acquired immunodeficiency syndrome (AIDS). Am J Kidney Dis 12:240-242
23. Bourgoignie JJ (1990) Renal complications of human immunodeficiency virus type I. Kidney Int 37:1571-1584
24. Rao TKS, Fiedman EA (1989) AIDS (HIV)-associated nephropathy; Does it exist? Am J Nephrol 9:441-453
25. Rao TKS (1988) Renal complications in patients with AIDS. Kidney failure is potentially manageable and reversible. J Crit Illness 3:55-74
26. Chander P, Agarwal A, Soni A, Kim K, Treser G (1988) Renal cytomembranous inclusions in idiopathic renal disease as predictive markers for the acquired immunodeficiency syndrome. Hum Pathol 19:1060-1064
27. Humphreys MH, Schoenfeld PY (1987) Renal complications in patients with the acquired immune deficiency syndrome (AIDS). Am J Nephrol 7:1-7
28. Langs C, Gallo GR, Schacht RG, Sidhu G, Baldwin DS (1990) Rapid renal failure in AIDS-associated focal glomerulosclerosis. Arch Intern Med 150:287-292
29. Glassock RJ, Cohen AH, Danovitch G, Parsa KP (1990) Human immunodeficiency virus (HIV) infection and the kidney. Ann Intern Med 112:35-49
30. Scott GB, Hutto C, Makuch RW, Mastrucci MT, O'Connor T, Mitchell CD, Trapido EJ, Parks WP (1989) Survival in children with perinatally acquired human immunodeficiency virus type I infection. N Engl J Med 321:1791-1796

Human Immunodeficiency Virus Associated Nephropathy (HIVAN)

T.K. Sreepada Rao[1]

SUMMARY. Although human immunodeficiency virus (the causative agent of acquired immunodeficiency syndrome) infection in man leads primarily to multiple infectious complications, it also results in multisystem disorders as well. While coincidental acute renal failure and fluid-electrolyte, acid-base disorders were commonly seen early in the AIDS epidemic, HIV associated nephropathy (HIVAN), an unusual disorder, was recognized only in 1984 in certain geographic areas in the United States. Approximately half the patients with HIVAN are intravenous drug abusers, and those remaining include recent immigrants from Haiti (mostly in Brooklyn and Miami) who deny drug use or homosexuality, gay men, sexual partners of HIV infected persons, contaminated blood/blood product recipients, and children born to infected women. HIVAN is typically a disease of young black men and is characterized by massive proteinuria, hypoalbuminemia, large echogenic kidneys, normotension, and a fulminant progression to end stage renal disease (ESRD) within a few months. The renal histopathology consists of focal and segmental glomerulosclerosis, with deposition of IgM, C3, C1q, and, rarely, other immune globulins. There is disproportionate tubular injury, manifested by microcystic dilatation of renal tubules, and sparse interstitial infiltrates and fibrosis. Ultrastructurally, tubulo-reticular structures and unusual cytoplasmic inclusions, along with peculiar nuclear chromatin changes, are present which suggests a possible viral etiology in the genesis of HIVAN. The pathogenesis of HIVAN is unknown, and no effective treatment exists at present. Patients with clinical AIDS and ESRD do poorly when supported by renal replacement therapy.

Introduction

Acquired immunodeficiency syndrome (AIDS), a disease identified in early 1980, is caused by human immunodeficiency virus (HIV), a retro virus which preferentially

[1]SUNY Health Science Center at Brooklyn, Brooklyn, NY 11203, USA

infects and depletes the T helper lymphocytes (CD4 cells), a key component of the immune system. Our understanding of HIV disease in man has evolved over the past decade, and we now recognize its clinical manifestations, which include various stages from an asymptomatic (HIV antibody seropositive) state, to non specific illnesses such as weight loss, persistent fever/diarrhea, lymphadenopathy (AIDS related complex (ARC)), and finally to the development of opportunistic infections and or unusual malignancies (clinical AIDS). In patients with HIV infection, the duration, and the factors which determine progression from an asymptomatic state to clinical AIDS are unclear. While HIV seropositive individuals survive for long periods, the mortality in patients with AIDS continues to be very high. Persons at risk for acquiring HIV infection include intravenous drug abusers (by needle sharing), homosexual and bisexual men, recipients of contaminated blood products, heterosexual partners of HIV infected persons, and children born to HIV infected mothers. In Miami and Brooklyn, the increased incidence of HIV infection in recent immigrants from Haiti, who deny homosexuality and intravenous drug use, remains unexplained. Although infectious complications dominate the clinical picture in AIDS, signs and symptoms referring to other organs, which contribute greatly to patients' morbidity and mortality, are increasingly being recognized. Renal syndromes encountered in patients with HIV infection include:

1. Coincidental diseases such as a spectrum of fluid-electrolyte, acid-base disorders, renal infections, infiltrations, and potentially reversible acute renal failure.
2. An unusual form of HIV associated nephropathy (HIVAN), possibly related to HIV infection, per se.
3. Various known forms of renal disease in patients already infected with HIV.
4. Patients with prior renal disease who subsequently acquire HIV infection through known modes of viral transmission.

Prior to the introduction of serological studies, such as enzyme-linked immunoadsorbent assay (ELISA) and Western Blot tests, which could detect HIV infection, clinicians followed the criteria established by the Center for Disease Control (CDC) to diagnose AIDS. Consequently, the initial descriptions in 1984 of a renal syndrome in AIDS patients was referred to as AIDS associated nephropathy (AAN). As the experience accumulated, it became evident that nephropathy could be an initial manifestation in asymptomatic HIV seropositive individuals. Hence, the terminology was changed to HIV associated nephropathy, a comprehensive name which included all HIV disease patients with the renal syndrome, irrespective of the clinical stage of their illness. This report will focus on clinical features of patients with HIVAN. The epidemiology and pathological features will be described in greater detail by other workers in this area.

Clinical Features of HIVAN

HIV associated nephropathy is not only a disease of clinically ill AIDS patients, as studies indicate that more than half the patients with nephrotic syndrome may be either asymptomatic seropositive carriers of the virus, or those with ARC. In our experience, about 15%–20% of patients with HIVAN at initial presentation do not have other signs and symptoms of ARC/AIDS. The commonest clinical manifestation is proteinuria, discovered either because of a routine urine examination during a clinic visit, or during investigation of patients with pedal edema. Proteinuria is usually massive and is a component of nephrotic syndrome (greater than 3.5 grams in 24 hour urine collections), along with hypoalbuminemia (serum albumin of less than 2.5 g/dl), and generalized edema. Hyperlipidemia may or may not be present. Nephrotic proteinuria is accompanied by normal glomerular filtration rate (Ccr), or varying degrees of azotemia. An analysis of the first 82 patients at our institutions revealed that 74 (90%) had nephrotic syndrome with normal to impaired Ccr, and only 8 (10%) presented with azotemia, hematuria, and proteinuria of less than 2 grams per day. The onset of edema with massive proteinuria and renal insufficiency can sometimes be abrupt. Many of our patients who have been followed in the HIV clinic, with no evidence of prior renal disease, have had explosive presentations with edema and or severe azotemia during routine follow-up visits. Investigations fail to reveal evidence for collagen vascular disease and other known causes of renal syndrome. The serum complement levels are not depressed, and polyclonal elevations of IgG and IgM levels in the blood are detectable. By definition, all nephropathy patients are HIV seropositive, and in our studies, absolute levels of circulating CD4 cells are low, along with a reversal in the ratio of T4:T8 cells (even in asymptomatic individuals with nephrotic syndrome). Ultrasound studies of the kidney reveal large echogenic kidneys in the nephrotic stage of the illness. When serially followed, despite progression to ESRD, renal size remains large; these findings have been repeatedly observed both in clinical and in autopsy studies. One major clinical finding in HIVAN is the notable absence of hypertension both in the early and in the late stages of the disease. The other distinctive feature in HIVAN is the malignant nature of the syndrome and the rapidity with which renal functional deterioration occurs in the absence of additional insult from anoxic injuries and nephrotoxic agents. In most large series, ESRD has developed in 4–6 months, although wide variations in renal progression have been observed. In our large experience, the mean duration from the discovery of proteinuria to irreversible renal failure was 16 weeks, as compared to several months to years in patients with heroin associated nephropathy (HAN). The reasons for the rapid renal failure in HIVAN are unclear. Some have speculated that HIV infection, per se, is responsible, and that HIVAN is a unique disease of combined glomerular, tubular, and interstitial lesions. The development of ESRD in HIVAN patients (those with clinical AIDS), also marks the beginning of a progressive clinical deterioration, ending in death in most patients in less than a year, despite maintenance dialysis. Some HIVAN patients, who do not manifest signs and symptoms of ARC/AIDS during renal replacement therapy, tolerate dialysis well and survival for prolonged periods has been reported.

The most frequently encountered renal pathology in HIVAN is focal and segmental glomerulosclerosis (FSGS). Other uncommonly reported renal histology in HIVAN includes minimal change disease, glomerular mesangial changes, and membranous and membrano proliferative glomerulonephritis. If the mesangial lesions represent an early change before evolution to focal sclerosis, then about 95% of all renal histological changes described in HIVAN will be comprised of FSGS. In the early stages of the disease, the visceral epithelial cells are enlarged, with coarse cytoplasmic vacuoles and with collapse of underlying capillary walls. In late stages, there is a pronounced obliteration of capillary lumen with increase in mesangial matrix and advanced sclerosis. The proximal renal tubular cells contain numerous protein absorption droplets. But the most striking feature is the dilatation of renal tubular lumen filled with pale staining casts, and hence the term "microcystic dilatation" to describe these changes. The dilated tubules are present throughout the cortex and medulla, although they may be more abundant at the cortico-medullary junction. Interstitial fibrosis, renal tubular atrophy, and vascular changes of arteriolosclerosis are minimally present, or strikingly absent, and there is sparse infiltration of interstitium by lymphocytes and other mononuclear cells. Immunofluorescent studies reveal intraglomerular deposition of IgM, C1q, and C3, and rarely, IgG, in the mesangium and sclerotic areas. The nature of these immune deposits is unknown. They may represent deposited immune complexes, or nonspecific trapping of immunoglobulins in the mesangium or sclerotic areas.

Ultrastructural renal changes consist of fusion of epithelial foot processes, increase in mesangial matrix, and detachment of epithelial cells from the basement membrane. Electron dense deposits may be found in the mesangium. But the most striking feature is the presence of abundant tubuloreticular structures in the endothelium of glomerular and peritubular capillaries, interstitial cells, and leukocytes. Multiple complex (Types III and IV) and budding forms of nuclear bodies are increasingly found in AIDS patients with proteinuria. Other ultrastructural changes, considered by some as distinctive in HIVAN, include peculiar nuclear cell bodies in the tubular and interstitial cells, a granulofibrillary transformation of tubular and interstitial cell chromatin, and the presence of intracytoplasmic and intranuclear inclusions of test tube and ring shaped forms in different cells. Based on these findings, a viral etiology for HIVAN has been strongly suggested. The recent in situ hybridization studies employing cDNA probes, and clearly demonstrating the localization of proviral HIV nucleic acid in the glomerular and renal tubular epithelium offer a strong support for the direct HIV infection theory in the initiation (causation) of HIVAN.

The clinical and pathological features of this renal syndrome, HIVAN, may be confused with those of heroin associated nephropathy (HAN), which is also a disease of young black addicts between the ages of 18 and 45 years. While in some patients this distinction may be impossible, the two diseases can be distinguished by some unusual characteristics, as described below. Although the light microscopic and immunofluorescence glomerular findings in HIV associated FSGS resemble those seen in heroin related, idiopathic variety, or other forms of focal sclerosis, the differentiating features in HIV include a larger percentage of "collapsed" glomeruli, a greater degree of tubular degeneration, and microcystic dilatation of renal tubules. Ultrastructurally, in HIVAN, there is an abundance of tubuloreticular inclusions in the glomerular endothelial cells; inclusions which are distinctively rare or absent in other forms of FSGS. Another major point of distinction between the two entities is that children, Haitian immigrants, and gay men constitute about 50% of patients with HIVAN, while HAN, by definition, includes only intravenous drug addicts. A fulminant clinical course of development of ESRD in 3–4 months, large kidney size, and persistent normotension, despite severe uremia in HIVAN patients contrasts clearly to the clinical course of patients with HAN, a disease marked by severe hypertension and shrunken kidneys, as azotemia progresses with the development of global glomerulosclerosis.

The pathogenesis of HIVAN is poorly understood. As is the case with idiopathic FSGS, in HIV associated glomerulosclerosis evidence is lacking which either supports or disputes the role of immune complexes in the development of the disease.

The significance of IgM, C3, and the occasional IgG, seen on immunofluorescent studies of the glomerulus, is unclear. These immune globulins may represent either localization of immune complexes, or merely a non specific trapping in the injured glomerulus. Attempts to localize HIV antigens in these presumed immune complexes have been uniformly unsuccessful. The electron microscopic features, and the in situ hybridization studies, on the other hand, lend a strong support for a direct role of HIV in the initiation and possibly in the progression of renal disease. An intriguing question, still unanswered, is the mechanism of HIV-induced renal injury, in the absence of CD4 receptors in various target cells in the kidney.

Other than symptomatic treatment of edema and hypoalbuminemia, consisting of salt restriction, diuretics, and protein supplementation, no specific treatment is available for HIV associated nephropathy. Neither short-term nor long-term use of corticosteroids or other immunosuppressive agents has been tested, because of fear of inducing infectious complications. Anecdotal data reportedly showing the efficacy of Zidovudine (AZT) in the treatment of patients with HIVAN needs confirmation by large prospective studies.

At present, the survival and rehabilitation of patients with chronic uremia and AIDS treated by maintenance dialysis can be summarized only as dismal and unsatisfactory. Despite renal replacement therapy, ESRD in AIDS is associated with a patient survival of under one year. During hemodialysis therapy, major problems contributing to a high mortality are unexplained malnutrition and a wasting phenomenon encountered in these patients, whether or not an underlying malignancy and/or opportunistic infection is present. During maintenance hemodialysis, AIDS patients manifest a "failure to thrive" syndrome, which fails to respond to nutritional support by hyperalimentation. Death usually results from a combination of cachexia and superimposed opportunistic and or other intercurrent infections.

References

1. Murray HW, Godbold JH, Jurica KB, Roberts RB (1989) Progression to AIDS in patients with lymphadenopathy or AIDS-related complex: reappraisal of risk and predictive factors. Am J Med 86:533–538
2. Rao TKS, Filippone EJ, Nicastri AD, Landesman SH, Frank E, Chen CK, Friedman EA (1984) Associated focal and segmental glomerulosclerosis in the acquired immunodeficiency syndrome. N Engl J Med 310:669–673
3. Rao TKS, Friedman EA, Nicastri AD (1987) The types of renal disease in the acquired immunodeficiency syndrome. N Engl J Med 316:1062–1068
4. Rao TKS, Friedman EA (1989) AIDS (HIV) associated nephropathy; does it exist?, an in-depth review. Am J Nephrol 9:441–453
5. Bourgoignie JJ, Meneses R, Pardo V (1988) The nephropathy related to acquired immunodeficiency syndrome. Adv Nephrol 17:113–126
6. Bourgoignie JJ, Meneses R, Ortiz C, Jaffe D, Pardo V (1988) The clinical spectrum of renal disease associated with human immunodeficiency virus. Am J Kidney Dis 12(2):131–137
7. Chander P, Soni A, Suri A, Bhagwat R, Yoo J, Treser G (1987) Renal ultrastructural markers in AIDS-associated nephropathy. Am J Pathol 126:513–526
8. Chander P, Agarwal A, Soni A, Kim K, Treser G (1988) Renal cytomembranous inclusions in idiopathic renal disease as predictive markers for the acquired immunodeficiency syndrome. Hum Pathol 19:1060–1064

9. D'Agati V, Suh JI, Carbone L, Cheng JT, Appel G (1989) Pathology of HIV-associated nephropathy: a detailed morphologic and comparative study. Kidney Int 35:1358–1370

10. Glassock RJ, Cohen AH, Danovitch G, Parsa P (1990) Human immunodeficiency virus (HIV) infection and the kidney. Ann Intern Med 112:35–49

11. Cohen AH, Nast CC (1988) HIV-associated nephropathy: a unique combined glomerular, tubular, and interstitial lesion. Mod Pathol 1:87–97

12. Cohen AH, Sun NCJ, Shapshak P, Imagawa DT (1989) Demonstration of human immunodeficiency virus in renal epithelium in HIV-associated nephropathy. Mode Pathol 2:125–128

13. Rao TKS (1988) Maintenance dialysis in patients with human immunodeficiency virus infection. Semin Dialysis 1(4):203–208

14. Ortiz C, Meneses R, Jaffe JA, Fernandez JA, Perez G, Bourgoignie JJ (1988) Outcome of patients with human immunodeficiency virus on maintenance hemodialysis. Kidney Int 34:248–253

15. Bowen II PA, Lobel SA, Caruana RJ, Leffell MS, House MA, Rissing PJ, Humphries AL (1988) Transmission of human immunodeficiency virus (HIV) by transplantation: clinical aspects and time course analysis of viral antigenemia and antibody production. Ann Intern Med 108:46–48

The Epidemiology of Human Immunodeficiency Virus-Associated Nephropathy

JACQUES J. BOURGOIGNIE, CARMEN ORTIZ-INTERIAN, DOLLIE F. GREEN, DAVID JAFFE, DAVID ROTH, and VICTORIANO PARDO[1]

SUMMARY. The data from the literature and our own cumulative experience in Miami indicate differences in the occurrence of HIV-associated nephropathy among different groups at risk. HIV-associated glomerulosclerosis is observed almost exclusively among intravenous drug abusers and in blacks, often presenting with uremia or the nephrotic syndrome associated with rapidly progressive renal failure. In contrast, renal involvement in HIV-infected caucasians who do not use IV drugs is usually limited to diffuse mesangial hyperplasia with modest proteinuria and little progression of renal dysfunction. Socio-ethnic factors likely explain the variable occurrence of HIV-associated nephropathy reported from different geographic areas where HIV is widespread.

Introduction

In 1984, investigators in New York and Miami reported the clinical presentation of nephrotic syndrome accompanied by rapid progression into renal failure among patients with the acquired immunodeficiency syndrome (AIDS) [1–3]. Renal histology most often demonstrated an aggressive focal and segmental glomerulosclerosis (FSGS). These observations were later expanded upon by the original investigators and confirmed by others [4–11]. Since the nephropathy often occurred in asymptomatic carriers of the human immunodeficiency virus Type 1 (HIV) and in patients with AIDS-related complex before the opportunistic infections or the malignancies characteristic of AIDS developed, the syndrome was referred to as HIV- rather than AIDS-associated nephropathy.

These initial observations met with skepticism, largely because they were not confirmed in San Francisco, a center of AIDS [12]. Second, the nephropathy was not

---

[1]Departments of Medicine and Pathology, University of Miami School of Medicine, Miami, FL 33101, USA

Table 1. Glomerulosclerosis in AIDS patients at autopsy

		Non-Blacks %	IVDAs %
North America			
1983 Reichert (Bethesda) [13]	0/10	80	10
1984 Hui (Los Angeles) [14]	0/12	83	33
1984 Welch (San Francisco) [15]	0/34	97	0
1984 Guarda (Houston) [16]	0/13	NA	0
1985 Niedt (New York) [17]	0/56	89	7
1985 Mobley (New York) [18]	1/12	83	25
1986 Balow (Bethesda) [19]	0/50	100	4
1989 Pardo (Miami) [20]	24/240	+	+
1989 D'Agati (New York) [11]	1/30	53	13
1990 Mazbar (San Francisco) [21]	1/91	89	24
1990 Seney (Dallas) [22]	1/50	80	50
Central and South America			
1987 Heredia (Mexico [23]	16/21*	100	0
1990 Marques (Rio de Janeiro) [24]	7/77	NA	NA
Europe			
1988 Dratwa-De Meyer (Brussels)⁺⁺	0/63	43	3
1989 van der Reijden (Amsterdam) [25]	0/47	95	0
1989 Burger (Zurich) [26]	3/210**	100	NA
1989 Giampalmo (Genoa) [27]	6/25	NA	80

IVDA, intravenous drug abuser; NA not available
⁺About 30% Non-Blacks and 40% IVDAs
*Clinically "silent" focal and segmental glomerulosclerosis
⁺⁺Presentation, Societé de Néphrologie, Brussels, 1988
**All 3 with features of idiopathic FSGS

apparent in autopsy series even when it was specifically looked for [13–27] (Table 1). Finally, the same type of nephropathy was known to occur in intravenous drug abusers (IVDAs) irrespective of HIV infection [28]; IVDAs represented 30 to 50 percent of the patients with HIV-associated nephropathy described in New York and Miami.

By 1987, AIDS was recognized to occur in other risk groups besides homosexuals and IVDAs. From Miami, where the population of patients with AIDS is more heterogenous than that in New York or San Francisco, we published a large series of patients, including 8 children infected perinatally, with focal and segmental (or global) glomerulosclerosis or with diffuse mesangial hyperplasia [5]. We then called attention to the apparent preponderance of nephrotic proteinuria and glomerulosclerosis among IVDAs and Haitians, the latter a group in which IV drug use is rare and in which HIV is mostly transmitted heterosexually. In contrast, among homosexuals the incidence of heavy proteinuria and FSGS was low. This variable manifestation of renal disease among different groups at risk suggested the participation of co-factors in the expression of HIV-associated nephropathy. We found no statistically significant differences between the various groups at risk with regard to age, duration of disease, or the incidence and types of major opportunistic infections. Moreover, in many patients the nephrotic syndrome and FSGS preceded any opportunistic infection. The incidence of typical or atypical tuberculosis was greater in Haitians than in IVDAs or in homosexuals, a reflection of an increased exposure of the Haitian community in Miami to tuberculosis. It was not evident, however, whether race or the route of contamination was primarily responsible for the rare occurrence of the nephropathy among homosexuals. Three years later, it is timely to reexamine the epidemiology of HIV-associated nephropathy.

Epidemiology

Glomerulosclerosis is rarely found at autopsy of patients with AIDS, even in recent series aimed at evaluating HIV-associated nephropathy (Table I). In contrast, more than 200 cases of histologically proven (many by biopsy) HIV-associated glomerulo-sclerosis have been formally reported in adults. Half of the cases originated from New York [1,3,7,10,29–31] and 20% were from Miami [2,20], with the balance made up of small series or individual patients from within and outside the United States [6,21–24,26,33–38]. An additional 30 cases have been reported in infants and young children [8,39–43].

Social Factors: Role of IV Drug Use

The use of IV drugs certainly stands out as an important factor in the transmission of HIV. IVDAs represent a large group of patients with HIV-associated nephropathy, with a prevalence varying from 39–84% in the largest series reported [4,10,30,31, 44] from the United States. Of interest, Giampalmo et al [27] from Italy published the only autopsy series made up of a majority of IVDAs (presumably Caucasians) with HIV infection; in this series the prevalence of FSGS was 24% (Table I).

Overall, however, IVDAs represent a minority of patients with glomerulosclerosis and HIV infection. One hundred eighty-eight patients with HIV-associated glomerulosclerosis in whom IV drug use was specifically identified or excluded as a possible risk factor can be recognized in the literature; 50 (27%) were IVDAs and 138 (73%) were not. Thus, IV drug use does not fully explain the clustering of cases of HIV-associated nephropathy among groups living in metropolitan areas where IV drug use is prevalent.

Ethnic Factors

Table 2 is a census, from the literature, of patients with HIV-associated glomerulo-sclerosis for whom race and IV drug use were specifically identified. Whereas HIV-associated glomerulosclerosis was associated with IV drug use in 28% of the patients, the data identify the nephropathy in 113 Blacks (90%) but in only 14 Cauca-sians (10%). The 8:1 ratio of Blacks vs Caucasians with HIV-associated glomerulo-sclerosis increases to 11:1 after exclusion of IV drug users.

Worldwide Experience

In North America, HIV-associated nephropathy has been confined to metropolitan areas of the East Coast of the United States, such as New York, Miami, and Washing-ton D.C. [1,3,4,7,10,29–31,33,44] Small series or individual patients have also

Table 2. Distribution of race and IV drug use in patients with HIV-associated glomerulosclerosis

	Blacks		Caucasians	
	IVDA*	No IVDA	IVDA	No IVDA
Rao (New York) [1]	5	5	–	–
Gardenswartz (New York) [3]	–	–	1	1
Pardo (Miami) [5]	11	16	3	1
Provenzano (Detroit) [6]	–	5	–	–
Cohen (Los Angeles) [8]	1	5	1	2
Alpers (Boston) [9]	1	1	1	–
Soni (New York) [10]	–	–	–	1
Mazbar (San Francisco) [21]	2	2	–	–
Carbone (New York) [30]	11	14	–	–
Weiss (Cincinnati) [32]	–	1	–	–
Cantor (Washington, DC) [33]	–	4	–	–
Patrick (Port of Spain) [34]	–	1	–	–
Dosquet (Paris) [35]	1	10	–	–
Hory (Besancon, France) [36]	–	1	–	–
Babut-Gay (Montfermeil, France) [37]	–	–	–	1
Baumelou (Paris) [38]	–	2	1	1
Connor (Newark) [39]	–	4	–	–
Rousseau (Montreal) [40]	–	4	–	–
Strauss (Miami) [41]	–	5	–	–
Burger (Zurich)**	–	1	–	–
Total	32	81	7	7

Numbers indicate number of patients
*IVDA, intravenous drug abuser
**Personal communication, 1990

been reported from Los Angeles, Dallas, Cincinnati, Boston, Detroit, and San Francisco [6,8,9,21,22,32]. Outside North America, isolated cases have been reported in black natives from the West Indies and Trinidad [34,35].

In Europe, HIV-associated nephropathy was identified in 2 white homosexuals in France (Table 2) and in IVDAs in Italy, but not in Caucasian homosexuals in the Netherlands or in Switzerland (Table I) [25–27,38]. In 1988, 13 cases of FSGS were reported from Brussels and Paris at the Meeting of the Societé de Néphrologie in Brussels in non-IVDAs (D. Kleinknecht, personal communication, 1990).

There are no data directly from Africa. However, several non-IVDA African patients with HIV infection and a nephrotic syndrome and glomerulosclerosis were identified in Belgium, France (Societé de Néphrologie, Brussels, 1988) [35], and Switzerland (HR Burger, German Society of Nephrology, Bern, 1989). These patients were from the Western part of Central Africa [Senegal, Zaire].

In Mexico, FSGS was identified at autopsy in 16 homo- or bisexual men; unlike all other patients reported elsewhere, however, clinically, these patients had minimal renal disease [23]. Seven patients with AIDS and FSGS and three with diffuse mesangial proliferation are reported from Brazil [24]. Cases of HIV-associated nephropathy have not been identified in Chile (A. Valdevieso, Santiago, personal communication, 1990) or in Venezuela (J. Weisinger, Caracas, personal communication, 1990).

There are no data from Asia.

Table 3. Clinical pathology of renal disease identified in Miami in HIV-infected adults who did not use IV drugs

| | | Clinical disease* | |
		Severe	Minimal
Caribbean Blacks			
$n=22$ (9 ♀)	Glomerulosclerosis	12	2
	Diff. mes. hyperplasia	–	6
	Membranous GN	1	–
	Interstitial Nephritis	–	1
American Blacks			
$n=11$ (5 ♀)	Glomerulosclerosis	6	1
	Diff. mes. hyperplasia	–	3
	Membranous GN	–	1
Caucasians			
$n=12$ (1 ♀)	Glomerulosclerosis	–	2
	Diff. mes. hyperplasia	–	9
	Membranoproliferative GN	1	–

*Severe, proteinuria usually > 3.5 g/24 h and serum creatinine > 3 mg/dl; Minimal, proteinuria usually < 2g/24 h and serum creatinine < 2 mg/dl

In Miami

To examine the contribution of race per se, we reviewed our histologic and clinical experience in our adult population with HIV infection and renal disease, after exclusion of IVDAs.

Forty-five patients with abnormal renal biopsy or autopsy specimens were identified, for whom HIV infection was not associated with IV drug use. The patients were divided into Caribbean Blacks, American Blacks, and Caucasians (including Hispanics) (Table 3).

Half of the patients (22 of 45) were Caribbean Blacks (21 Haitians). All denied IV drug use or homosexuality and none had received prior blood transfusions. There were 13 men and 9 women. Fourteen had glomerulosclerosis, 6 had diffuse mesangial hyperplasia (DMH), one had a lupus membranous glomerulonephritis and one had an interstitial nephritis. Eleven American Blacks, 6 homosexual men and 5 women contaminated heterosexually, had a nephropathy characterized as glomerulosclerosis in 7, DMH in 3, and membranous glomerulonephritis in one. In contrast, the nephropathology in 12 Caucasians (11 homosexual men and 1 woman infected by blood transfusion) was limited to early FSGS in 2 patients and DMH in 9. The twelfth patient had a membranoproliferative glomerulonephritis associated with chronic active hepatitis B. Thus, we observed 21 Blacks, but only 2 Caucasians, with HIV infection and glomerulosclerosis in an HIV population where the racial distribution between Blacks and Caucasians was 3:1 [45].

The clinical presentation was also strikingly different, in that 18 Blacks but no Caucasians developed a severe nephropathy (Table 3). Typically, Blacks with advanced glomerulosclerosis presented with nephrotic-range proteinuria (> 3.5 g/24 h) and renal insufficiency (serum creatinine > 3 mg/dl); whereas Caucasians with DMH or FSGS had minimal renal involvement (proteinuria < 2 g/24 h and serum creatinine < 2 mg/dl), although a nephrotic syndrome was the reason for renal biopsy in one Caucasian HIV carrier with DMH.

Separately, we identified 11 additional Blacks (9 Caribbean, of whom 4 were women) and 3 Caucasians (all men) with HIV infection not associated with IV drug use, who developed nephrotic-range proteinuria and a progressive nephropathy. Renal tissue was not available for histologic examination in these patients.

Discussion

The literature and our experience in Miami indicate that factors other than IV drug use may be determinant in allowing the full expression of HIV-associated nephropathy. Race, more than IV drug use, seems to predispose Blacks to the development of progressive HIV-associated nephropathy. In contrast, uremia is rarely observed in Caucasian homosexuals in whom the nephropathology seems to be limited to DMH rather than FSGS. The increased expression of the nephropathy in Blacks infected with HIV may reflect a susceptibility of Blacks to develop FSGS. This is consistent with numerous studies reporting a higher incidence of chronic renal disease occurring in Blacks with hypertension, diabetes, or IV drug use without HIV infection when compared to a cohort of Caucasian patients (see references in [46,47]). In a large series mostly of IVDAs from New York, progression to endstage renal disease was also faster in Blacks than in Hispanics with HIV infection and equivalent proteinuria [10]. In the same context, infants and young children have been identified with HIV-associated glomerulosclerosis [8,39–43]. Of note, all children but one reported so far were Black.

Genetic factors may be involved in the expression of HIV-associated nephropathy. Specific immune response genes may be important in facilitating the expression of FSGS in Blacks or in repressing it in Caucasians. Alternatively, unrecognized environmental factors could be responsible for predisposing Blacks infected with HIV to progressive renal disease. The data indicate that HIV-associated glomerulosclerosis may afflict American Blacks and Caribbean Blacks; preliminary data suggest that West African Blacks may be affected as well. More epidemiologic and histologic data than those presently available are needed to determine whether progressive HIV-associated nephropathy is related to blacks in general or is limited to certain subsets of this population.

The finding of different renal manifestations in different groups at risk for HIV infection is intriguing, particularly since Cohen et al. ([8,48], and personal communication, 1990) have localized the HIV genome in renal glomerular and tubular epithelial cells from IVDAs as well as from Caucasians and Black homosexuals with HIV infection and glomerulosclerosis.

Whatever the reasons for the differences in the expression of HIV-associated nephropathy between Blacks and Caucasians who are not IV drug users, social and ethnic factors likely explain the discrepancies that exist in the literature regarding the occurrence of HIV-associated nephropathy reported from different geographic areas where HIV is widespread.

Acknowledgments. This work was supported by NIH Grant R01-DK 40836. The authors are grateful to Ms. Kim Schauers for expert secretarial assistance.

References

1. Rao TK, Filippone EJ, Nicastri AD, Landesman SH, Frean E, Chen CK, Friedman EA (1984) Associated focal and segmental glomerulosclerosis in the acquired immunodeficiency syndrome. N Engl J Med 310:669-673
2. Pardo V, Aldana M, Colton RM, Fischl MA, Jaffe D, Moskowitz L, Hensley GT, Bourgoignie JJ (1984) Glomerular lesions in the acquired immunodeficiency syndrome. Ann Intern Med 101:429-434
3. Gardenswartz MH, Lerner CW, Seligson GR, Zabetakis PM, Rotterdam H, Tapper ML, Michelis MF, Bruno MS (1984) Renal disease in patients with AIDS: A clinicopathologic study. Clin Nephrol 21:197-204
4. Rao TK, Friedman EA, Nicastri AD (1987) The types of renal disease in the acquired immunodeficiency syndrome. N Engl J Med 316:1062-1068
5. Pardo V, Meneses R, Ossa L, Jaffe DJ, Strauss J, Roth D, Bourgoignie JJ (1987) AIDS-related glomerulopathy: Occurrence in specific risk groups. Kidney Int 31:1167-1173
6. Provenzano R, Kupin W, Santiago GC (1987) Renal involvement in the acquired immunodeficiency syndrome: Presentation, clinical course and therapy. Henry Ford Hosp Med J 35:38-41
7. Kaplan MS, Wechsler M, Benson MC (1987) Urologic manifestations of AIDS. Urology 30:441-443
8. Cohen AH, Nast CC (1988) HIV-associated nephropathy: A unique combined glomerular, tubular and interstitial lesion. Mod Pathol 1:87-97
9. Alpers CE, Harawi S, Rennke (1988) Focal glomerulosclerosis with tubuloreticular inclusions: Possible predictive value for acquired immunodeficiency syndrome (AIDS). Am J Kidney Dis 12:240-242
10. Soni A, Agarwal A, Chander P, Yoo J, Singal D, Salomon N, Robinson B, Treser G (1989) Evidence for an HIV-related nephropathy: A clinicopathological study. Clin Nephrol 31:12-17
11. D'Agati V, Cheng JI, Carbone L, Cheng JT, Appel G (1989) The pathology of HIV-nephropathy: A detailed morphologic and comparative study. Kidney Int 35:1358-1370
12. Humphreys MH, Schoenfeld PY (1988) Renal complications in patients with the acquired immune deficiency syndrome. Am J Nephrol 7:1-7
13. Reichert CM, O'Leary TJ, Levens DL, Simrell CR, Macher A (1983) Autopsy pathology in the acquired immune deficiency syndrome. Am J Pathol 112:357-382
14. Hui AN, Koss MN, Meyer PR (1984) Necropsy findings in acquired immunodeficiency syndrome: A comparison of premortem diagnoses with postmortem findings. Hum Pathol 15:670-676
15. Welch K, Finkbeiner W, Alpers CE, Blumenfeld W, Davis RL, Smuckler EA, Beckstead JH (1984) Autopsy findings in the acquired immune deficiency syndrome. JAMA 252:1152-1159
16. Guarda LA, Luna MA, Smith JL Jr (1984) Acquired immune deficiency syndrome: postmortem findings. Am J Clin Pathol 81:549-557
17. Niedt GW, Schinella RA (1985) Acquired immunodeficiency syndrome. Arch Pathol Lab Med 109:727-734
18. Mobley K, Rotterdam HZ, Lerner CW, Tapper ML (1985) Autopsy findings in the acquired immune deficiency syndrome. Pathol Annu 20:45-65
19. Balow JE, Macher AM, Rook AH (1986) Paucity of glomerular disease in acquired immunodeficiency syndrome (AIDS) (abstract). Kidney Int 29:178
20. Pardo V, Bell M, Ortiz C, Strauss J, Bourgoignie JJ (1989) The spectrum of glomerular lesions in patients with HIV infection (abstract). Fed Proc 3:A1281
21. Mazbar SA, Schoenfeld PY, Humphreys MH (1990) Renal involvement in patients infected with HIV: Experience at San Francisco General Hospital. Kidney Int 37:1325-1332

22. Seney FD Jr, Burns DK, Silva FG (to be published) AIDS and the kidney. Am J Kidney Dis.
23. Heredia JB, Angeles AA, Gutierrez ER, Correa-Rotter R, Saldiyar S, Pena JC (1987) Nephropatia associada al sindrome di immunodeficiencia acquirida. Rev Invest Clin 39:105-115
24. Marques LPJ, Oliveira AV, Basilio de Oliviera CA, Riodja LS, Lopes GS, Santos OR (1990) Renal histologic alterations in AIDS. Abstracts 11th Int Congr Nephrology, 15-20 July, Tokyo, p. 174A
25. van der Reijden HJ, Schipper HE, Danner SA, Arisz L (1989) Glomerular lesions and opportunistic infections of the kidney in AIDS: an autopsy study of 47 cases. Adv Exp Med Biol 252:181-189
26. Burger HR, Kriemler S, Mihatsch M (1989) Gibt es eine AIDS-Nephropathie? Resultate von 210 Autopsiefällen (abstract). Nieren - und Hochdruck -Krankeiten 6:379
27. Giampalmo A, Ardoino S, Borghesi MR, Buffa D, Lapertosa G, Pagano S, Pesce C, Provaggi MA, Ravetti GL, Guaglia AC, Ravetti GL, Terragna A (1989) Anatomo-pathologic findings in 25 autopsy cases of AIDS. Pathologica 81:1-46
28. Rao TKS, Nicastri AD, Friedman EA (1977) Renal consequences of narcotic abuse. Adv Nephrol 7:261-290
29. Chander P, Agarwal A, Soni A, Kim K, Treser G (1988) Renal cytomembranous inclusions in idiopathic renal disease as predictive markers for the acquired immunodeficiency syndrome. Hum Pathol 19:1060-1064
30. Carbone L, D'Agati V, Cheng JT, Appel GB (1989) The course and prognosis of human immunodeficiency virus-associated nephropathy. Am J Med 87:389-395
31. Langs C, Gallo GR, Schacht RG, Sidhu G, Baldwin DF (1990) Rapid renal failure in AIDS-associated focal glomerulosclerosis. Arch Intern Med 150:287-292
32. Weiss MA, Daquioag E, Margolin EG, Pollak VE (1986) Nephrotic syndrome, progressive irreversible renal failure, and glomerular "collapse": A new clinicopathologic entity? Am J Kidney Dis 7:20-28
33. Cantor ES, Kimmel PL, Bosch JP (1989) Impact of race on renal disease in patients with AIDS (abstract). Kidney Int 35:222
34. Patrick AL, Roberts LA, Burton EN, Jankey N, Shah DH (1986) Focal and segmental glomerulosclerosis in the acquired immunodeficiency syndrome. West Indian Med J 35:200-202
35. Dosquet P, Michel C, Elyaszewicz M, Matheron S, Meychas MC, Ronco P, Mignon F (1990) Focal and segmental glomerulosclerosis (FSG) among HIV infected patients: possible favorable effect of treatment with azidothymidine (AZT). Abstracts 11th Int Congr Nephrology, 15-20 July, Tokyo, p 14A
36. Hory B, Bresson C, Lorge JF, Perol C (1988) Associated focal and segmental glomerulo-sclerosis in the acquired immunodeficiency syndrome. Am J Kidney Dis 12:169
37. Babut-Gay ML, Echard M, Kleinknecht D, Meyrier A (1989) Zidovudine and nephropathy with human immunodeficiency virus (HIV) infection. Ann Intern Med 111:856-857
38. Baumelou A, Assogba V, Beaufils H, Hinglais N, Ben Hmida M, Christin S, Eugene M, Deray G, Jacobs C (1989) Pathologie rénale associée à l'infection à virus VIH et au syndrôme d'immunodéficience acquise. In: Chatelain C, Jacobs C (eds) Séminaires d'Uro-Nephrologie. Masson, Paris, pp 42-49
39. Connor E, Gupta S, Joshi V, DiCarlo F, Offenberger J, Minnefor A, Uy C, Oleske J, Ende N (1988) Acquired immunodeficiency syndrome-associated renal disease in children. J Pediatr 113:39-44
40. Rousseau E, Russo P, Lapointe N, O'Regan S (1988) Renal complications of acquired immunodeficiency syndrome in children. Am J Kidney Dis 11:48-50
41. Strauss J, Abitbol C, Zilleruelo G, Scott G, Paredes A, Malaga S, Montane B, Mitchell C, Parks W, Pardo V (1989) A spectrum of renal disease in children with acquired immunodeficiency syndrome. New Engl J Med 321:625-630

42. Chandler P, Sagel I, Weiss R, Pimentel C, Gupta A, Bamji M, Treser G (1989) Renal disease in human immunodeficiency virus (HIV)-infected children (abstract). Kidney Int 35:368

43. Horowitz L, Greco MA, Feiner Y (1988) Renal pathology in pediatric AIDS. Abstracts 4th Int Conf on AIDS, Stockholm, I, 402

44. Bourgoignie JJ, Meneses R, Ortiz-Interian C, Jaffe D, Pardo V (1988) The clinical spectrum of renal disease associated with human immunodeficiency virus. Am J Kidney Dis 12:131–137

45. Bourgoignie JJ, Ortiz-Interian C, Green DF, Roth D (1989) Race, a co-factor in HIV-1 associated nephropathy. Transplant Proc 21:3899–3901

46. Rao TKS, Friedman EA (1989) AIDS (HIV)-associated nephropathy; Does it exist? An in-depth review. Am J Nephrol 9:441–453

47. Stephens GN, Gillaspy JA, Clyne D, Mejia A, Pollak VE (1990) Racial differences in the incidence of end-stage renal disease in types I and II diabetes mellitus. Am J Kidney Dis 15:562–567

48. Cohen AH, Sun NCJ, Shapshak P, Imagana DT (1989) Demonstration of human immunodeficiency virus in renal epithelium in HIV-associated nephropathy. Mod Pathol 2:125–128

Pathology of Human Immunodeficiency Virus (HIV) Associated Nephropathy in Adults and Children

Praveen N. Chander[1], Inge Sagel[2], and Gerhard Treser[3]

SUMMARY. A variety of renal lesions are identified in patients infected with Human Immunodeficiency virus (HIV). A distinctive clinicopathologic entity, termed HIV-associated nephropathy (HIVAN) is noted in 7–10% of the unselected adult and pediatric hospital admissions for Acquired Immunodeficiency Syndrome (AIDS). Adult HIVAN is more common in Blacks and in intravenous (IV) drug users and is characterized clinically by acute onset of severe, often nephrotic range proteinuria with generally rapid and irreversible progression to renal failure. Histologically, focal segmental sclerosis (FGS) is frequently accompanied by a unique globally collapsing glomerulopathy with dilatation of Bowman's space, microcystic ectasia of tubules, scant interstitial cellular infiltrate and fibrosis in the well established lesions. A combination of these distinctive clinical features and histologic findings, along with abundant tubulo-reticular inclusions (TRI) in renal vascular endothelium on electronmicroscopy, distinguishes HIVAN from heroin-associated nephropathy (HAN). A constellation of these clinicopathological findings also allows one to make a presumptive diagnosis of HIV infection with a high degree of accuracy in an asymptomatic HIV carrier. Greater frequency of multiple, budding, and complex nuclear bodies, and various cytomembranous and intranuclear inclusions, presumed to be "viral footprints," suggest a viral etiology for HIVAN.

In children with HIV infection, the commonest lesion is proliferative glomerulonephritis, often present as mesangial hyperplasia, accompanied by a mild degree of focal segmental and global glomerulosclerosis, with clinically modest proteinuria and mild progression to renal insufficiency.

Introduction

A broad spectrum of renal lesions has been observed in patients infected with the Human Immunodeficiency Virus (HIV), ranging from renal infections and tumors to

[1]Departments of Pathology, Pediatrics[2], and Medicine[3], New York Medical College, Valhalla, NY 10595, USA

493

tubulointerstitial lesions and a variety of glomerular pathology [1–4]. The glomerular pathology includes focal segmental sclerosis (FGS), mesangial proliferation, membranoproliferative glomerulonephritis, minimal change disease, postinfectious glomerulonephritis, membranous nephropathy, amyloidosis, hemolytic uremic syndrome, infarcts, and cortical necrosis.

In spite of such a variety of observed "nonspecific" pathology, a more specific and characteristic clinical and pathological entity has been recognized and has been named HIV associated nephropathy (HIVAN). It was first described as a rapidly progressive renal disease accompanied by heavy proteinuria, with FGS as the glomerular lesion [5]. Subsequent investigations have broadened the clinical presentations and defined the structural lesions in the kidney [6–15]. In this report we have summarized our observations of the renal pathology of HIV infected adults and children and included a review of the literature, in an attempt to characterize the specific HIV associated nephropathy.

Renal Pathology in HIV-Associated Nephropathy in Adults

We compared the renal biopsy or autopsy tissues of patients with AIDS and severe proteinuria (> 2g/day) with the renal tissues of other AIDS patients with comparable clinical features, but without proteinuria, and with the renal tissues of patients with heroin associated nephropathy (HAN) [6]. The patients with HAN had a similar degree of proteinuria and were of comparable age. The HAN tissues were from our files and were taken prior to 1982 and the spread of the AIDS epidemic. The following account is a summary based on our cumulative experience and on the consensus of other published reports on this subject [2,6,7,12,15].

Histology

Histologically, nephropathy in patients with AIDS was characterized by segmental glomerulosclerosis which was quantitatively and qualitatively similar to HAN (Fig. 1). The FGS however, was often accompanied by a global collapse of capillary tufts with dilated Bowman Spaces, filled with bright eosinophilic proteinaceous material. Tubules were frequently enormously dilated, sometimes to microcystic proportions, and filled with large hyaline casts and often lined by degenerating and/or simplified flattened epithelium. Retracted glomerular capillary tufts were in general devoid of hyaline deposits, foam cells, and excessive accumulation of mesangial matrix and revealed mesangial hypocellularity in many of the autopsy specimens. Small shrunken capillary tufts retracted towards the vascular pole, giving the appearance of a rapidly progressive event, akin to the rapid progression of renal failure described clinically, due perhaps to the loss of axially supporting mesangial cells. Focal mesangial hyperplasia was observed in other areas of the same tissue. (Mesangial proliferation has also been reported in some patients with HIVAN. Many of these were non-IV-drug-user Caucasian men with mild to moderate proteinuria and slight progression to renal insufficiency.) In addition there was severe hypertrophy and focal hyperplasia of visceral epithelium, containing abundant and massive protein resorption droplets, overlying segmentally sclerotic areas of globally collapsing glomeruli. Interstitial infiltrate could be moderately dense, in the early lesions, particularly in

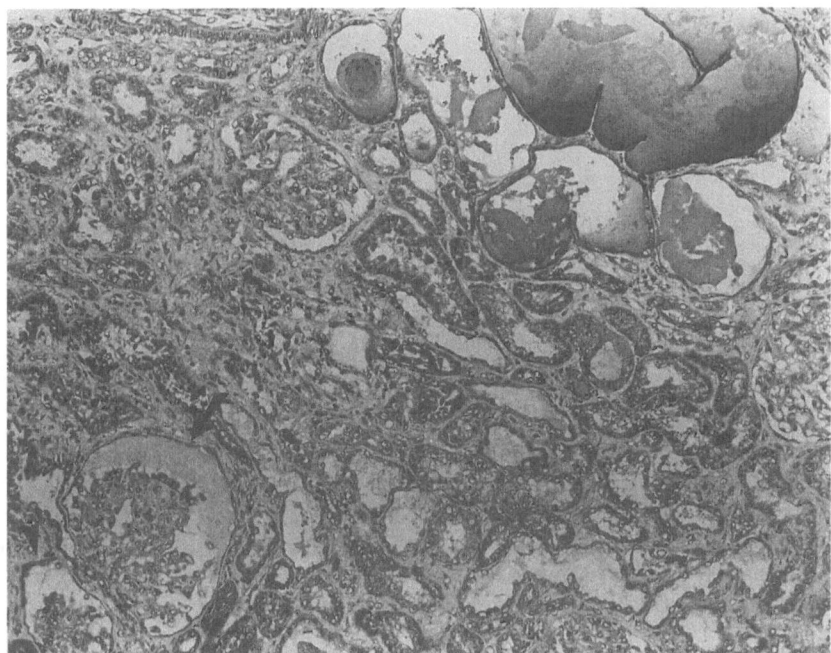

Fig. 1. Segmentally sclerotic glomerulus with global capillary tuft collapse and prominent visceral epithelial cells crowding the sclerotic tuft and dilated Bowman space (*arrow*). Another glomerulus with global capillary tuft retraction without deposits of hyaline, foam cells, or excessive mesangial matrix (*arrow head*). There is tubular degeneration, regeneration and microcystic ectasia. Interstitium is edematous with sparse inflammatory infiltrate. H&E, × 125

biopsy specimens (Chander, unpublished work), [14] but in the later stages, in the autopsy specimens, the infiltrate was invariably scanty in an interstitium that frequently appeared edematous and was sometimes replaced by a homogenous acidophilic substance [6,7]. The paucity of interstitial infiltrate in the autopsy specimens is perhaps related to leucopenia in patients dying of AIDS. Microscopic calcium deposits (nephrocalcinosis) were noted in tubules and interstitium.

In contrast, globally sclerosing glomeruli in HAN and idiopathic FGS appeared as solid mass consisting of excess accumulation of mesangial matrix and focal hyaline deposits. "Capping" by the hypertrophic and proliferated visceral epithelium, dilatation of Bowman's spaces, microcystic ectasia of tubules, and degenerative epithelial changes were not a prominent feature in either. Tubular atrophy and interstitial fibrosis were commensurate with the degree of glomerulosclerosis. The interstitium in HAN frequently contained marked infiltrates of lymphocytes and plasma cells in early, and in the well established late lesions.

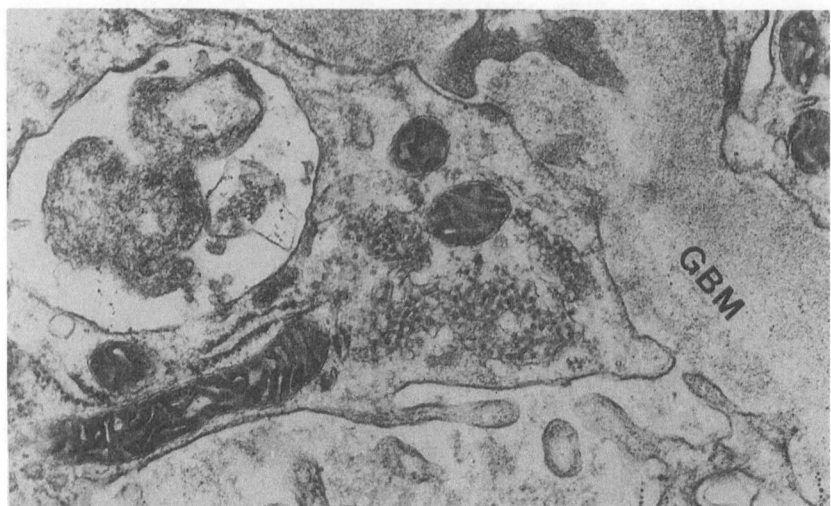

Fig. 2. Tubuloreticular inclusions in the endoplasmic cisternae of a swollen glomerular endothelial cell × 20,000. Glomerular basement membrane (GBM)

Immunofluorescent Findings

No distinctive pattern could be distinguished by immunofluorescence. Segmental coarsely granular deposits of IgM and C_3 were frequently seen in sclerosing glomeruli, similar to those seen in HAN and in idiopathic FGS. In addition, variable scattering of C_1, IgG, and IgA was also present. The same deposits however, could be identified in apparently normal glomeruli, in patients without the nephropathy who were dying of AIDS [2,6,7]. Deposits found by immunofluorescence and electron-microscopy correlated best with chronic infections such as hepatitis B virus infection [6].

Electronmicroscopy

On electron microscopy, in addition to scattered mesangial and, rarely, subendothelial and subepithelial deposits, GBM wrinkling and collapse was noted in the sclerosing glomeruli with, and often without, accumulation of mesangial matrix. Diffuse effacement and focal detachment of foot-processes were seen in such areas. Visceral epithelial cells were markedly swollen and hypertrophic and showed frequent villous transformation. The most notable finding on electron microscopy was the presence of numerous tubuloreticular inclusions (TRI) (Fig. 2) in the glomerular and peritubular capillary endothelium and interstitial leukocytes [6,9,12,15,17]. These TRI are reticular aggregates of apparently branching membranous tubules, measuring approximately 25 nm in diameter. The TRI have been described in association with a variety of different nephritides including HAN, SLE, and other collagen vascular, autoimmune, and viral diseases. Except for lupus nephritis, a persistent and diligent search is needed to document the presence of TRI in the renal parenchyma in most other nephritides. In contrast, in particular to HAN, TRI were in abundance in HIV associated nephropathy; with little experience they were detectable, at the low power scanning magnification, in the often swollen endothelial cells. Frequently, multiple aggregates of TRI were present in a single capillary loop as well as in different parts of the cytoplasm of the same endothelial cell. The clear abundance of TRI has also been documented by D'Agati et al. [15], who, by a semi-quantitative analysis of randomly taken electron-micrographs, arrived at the figure of 0.86 TRI on average per capillary loop in HIVAN. Cylindrical confronting cisternae (CCC), another ultrastructure marker of HIV infection described in peripheral leukocytes, were detected only rarely in the renal tissue, and required a more persistent and diligent search, than was needed for documenting TRI. Possibly derived from endoplasmic reticulum, CCC are parallel, cylindrical, or concentrically arranged cisternae with electron dense material interposed between the two membranous lamellae. They measure approximately 3.5 μm in length with a width of approximately 250 μm. In the kidney, CCC were found mostly in the glomerular endothelial cells, often in association with TRI [6,9,17]. These CCC have never been seen in HAN or in idiopathic FGS.

On comparative renal morphologic analysis of the HIV infected patients, with and without nephropathy, and the HAN patients, a variety of unusual ultrastructural findings were observed in HIVAN, and were observed with lesser frequency in AIDS without nephropathy. These are best described as viral "foot prints" and may suggest a viral etiology for HIVAN [6,17,18]. These findings are summarized as follows: Type I and II nuclear bodies are a ubiquitous feature of normal cells, but are induced in cells activated by viruses, amongst other stimuli. Nuclear bodies (NB) were seen in greater frequency, complexity, size, and budding configuration, and also in increased frequency of multiple NBs per cell, in HIV nephropathy, than in the cells without nephropathy and in the HAN cells.

A peculiar granulofibrillary change of the normal nuclear chromatin was seen with greater frequency in the interstitial and tubular cells in HIVAN. The nature of this transformation is unclear, but greater frequency and complexity of nuclear bodies in the nuclei thus affected, suggests "activated" rather than normally degenerating cells (Fig. 3). These findings were confirmed by D'Agati et al. [15]. In addition, we observed a great variety of other intranuclear inclusions in interstitial fibroblasts of HIV infected patients, with an even greater frequency in HIVAN. These included filamentous crystalline and fibrillary inclusions, membranous lamellae or profiles, vacuolar, lipid, and granular vesicles and, rarely, CCC. None were present in HAN. Some of these inclusions have been described in various human viral diseases. Except for CMV in 2 children with HIVAN, we have been unable, ultrastructurally, to detect other specific viral agents, including HIV-1, in spite of thorough search. A recent report of HIV nucleic acid and p-24 antigen in tubular and visceral epithelial cells, by in-situ hybridization and immunohistochemical techniques, respectively, deserves further study [19].

TRI as Predictive Markers for HIV Disease and HIVAN

In an effort to evaluate the value of TRI in the diagnosis of HIVAN we carefully studied the renal tissue available from 13 patients with risk factors for AIDS, who

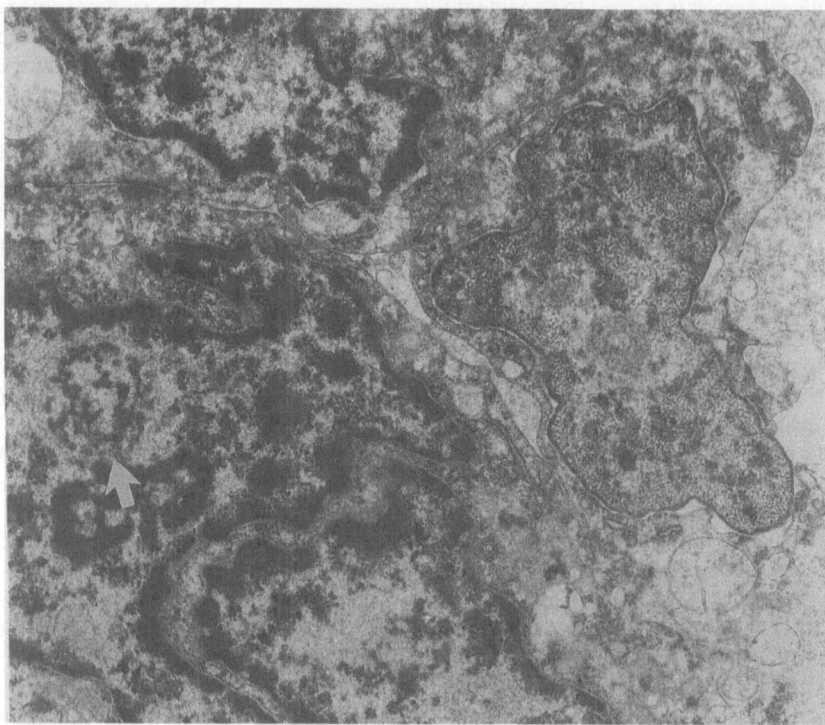

Fig. 3. Distal tubular cell nucleus with two type II nuclear bodies and partial granular fibrillary transformation (*right*). A type IV nuclear body is present in an adjacent cell nucleus (*arrow*) × 15,000

underwent renal biopsy for severe proteinuria. On the basis of the clinical presentation and follow up, these patients could be grouped into 4 categories: A. Two patients who had AIDS at the time of biopsy; B. four patients who had ARC; C. four patients who had risk factors for AIDS but no evidence of AIDS or ARC at the time of biopsy, but developed AIDS subsequently, and D. three patients who were similar to those in group C, except that AIDS did not manifest over a prolonged observation period (Table 1). Our findings and conclusions from this study [9] were: Renal pathology was similar in groups, A, B, and C; nephropathy with severe, often nephrotic range proteinuria, with or without rapid progression to endstage renal disease, can occur in patients with AIDS or with AIDS related complex, but most importantly, also in asymptomatic HIV carriers. Globally collapsing glomerulopathy was seen, frequently associated with focal and segmental glomerulosclerosis, dilated Bowman spaces and microcystic tubular ectasia.

Tubuloreticular inclusions were uniformly present in all biopsies of patients from groups, A, B, and C. They were not seen in the renal tissue of the 3 group D patients who subsequently never developed AIDS, in spite of the fact that one patient was documented to be HIV infected. Therefore, TRI are not uniformly present in

Table 1. Analysis of renal biopsies from patients with HIV risk factors and proteinuria

Groups	Risk factors	Follow-up average months (n)*	Histology				Positive HIV Ab (n tested)
			FGS	GCG	PGN	TRI	
A AIDS(n−2)	IVDA-1 gay-1	14 (2)	1	2	0	2	1 (1)
B ARC(n−4)	IVDA-3 het-1	3 (1)	3	3	1	4	4 (4)
C Prturia to AIDS (n−4)	IVDA-1 gay-1 het -2	11 (4)	4	4	0	4	2 (2)
D Prturia No AIDS (n−3)	IVDA-2 gay-1**	16 (3)	1	0	2	0	1 (3)

FGS, focal and segmental glomerulosclerosis; GCG, globally collapsing glomerulopathy; het, heterosexual transmission in women; PGN, proliferative glomerulonephritis; Ab, antibody; Prturia, proteinuria; *number of patients available for follow-up; **died of lung cancer

glomerular lesions, other than in HIV associated nephropathy in HIV infected patients. We have confirmed these observations in some additional cases (Chander, unpublished work). Combination of the characteristic glomerulo-tubular findings described above and TRI on electron microscopic examination are almost pathognomonic and we suggested that a presumptive diagnosis of HIV infection and/or nephropathy can be made with a high degree of accuracy, in the appropriate clinical setting [9,17]. Similar observations have also been made by other investigators [15,20]. At present, however, it is not clear whether TRI in kidney are simply markers for systemic HIV disease or are specific for HIVAN in HIV infected patients.

Renal Pathology in Perinatally HIV Infected Children

In perinatally HIV-infected children, the occurrence of a nephropathy similar to that seen in adults, supports the existence of a specific HIV-associated nephropathy. Children with HIV infection were analyzed by us and by Strauss et al. [21,22]. Although mild proteinuria was very frequent, ranging from 40–50% of unselected admissions for AIDS, the incidence of heavy proteinuria, defined as >2+ on dipstick examination and/or > 1 g/day per square meter of body surface area, was between 8 and 9%, similar to that reported in adults. Altogether, 29 such cases are reported in the entire literature, all born to HIV infected mothers with IV drug use or heterosexual contact with an IV drug user as the risk factors [12,15,21–24]. Of these, 25 were Black and 4 were Hispanic children. Rapid progression to renal failure was rare and the nephropathy was generally milder than that seen in adults. The renal histology was variable, with several distinctive features different from the adult form of disease. Focal segmental sclerosis was not a dominant lesion, and was seen in only 9 of the 29 reported cases. An associated fulminant globally collapsing glomerulopathy with dilation of Bowman spaces and microcystic ectasia of tubules was infrequent and milder, when present. There were no distinctive histologic tubulo-interstitial findings. Proliferative glomerulonephritis was more prevalent, and was observed in 18 of the 29 reported cases. Mesangial proliferation or hyperplasia constituted the great majority. Although not an exclusive finding, greater than normal prevalence of segmental and often global glomerulosclerosis, (defined as >5% affected glomeruli), was observed frequently in association with proliferative glomerular disease. Deposits of the immune type were frequent on immunofluorescent and electron microscopic studies. These, along with abundant TRI in vascular endothelium and variable immunologic abnormalities suggested a superficial resemblance to lupus nephritis. Diagnosis of lupus nephritis was documented in 2 of the 29 cases in view of highly positive ANA and anti-double stranded DNA [15,22].

Since the children have milder renal disease and shorter survival, proliferative glomerulonephritis, frequently occurring with immune-deposits, may be considered an early mild form of HIV-associated nephropathy. However, a progression of mesangial proliferative lesion to segmentally sclerosing and globally collapsing glomerulopathy has not been documented. Only one case of minimal change disease (MCD) on biopsy that progressed to FGS has been reported [15] amongst several cases of MCD reported in the setting of HIV disease. It has been speculated that lymphokines liberated by T-cells are involved in the etiology of both MCD and HIV nephropathy. Alternatively, mesangial proliferation and FGS may be two separate independent lesions, with the former of post-infectious etiology.

Renal Pathology Other than HIVAN in HIV Infected Patients

The incidence of various renal lesions is different in large series reporting primarily on renal biopsy versus autopsy material [10,11,15]. There is a preponderance of tubulo-interstitial disease, such as acute tubular necrosis, allergic interstitial nephritis, colonization by opportunistic pathogens, nephrocalcinosis etc., in the autopsy series. These are often related to AIDS, its complications, and a variety of necessary therapeutic and diagnostic interventions. Table 2 lists the majority of non-glomerular renal lesions seen in patients with AIDS. Although focal segmental sclerosis was present in 28% and mesangial hyperplasia in 32% of the autopsy results

Table 2. Spectrum of non glomerular renal lesions in human immunodeficiency virus (HIV) infection

1. *Acute tubular necrosis*: toxic ischemic (e.g. sepsis, dehydration, amphotericin, pentamidine)
2. *Drug induced allergic interstitial nephritis* (e.g. trimethoprim-sulfamethoxazole, cephalosporines and other beta-lactam antibiotics)
3. *Renal infections*
   CMV
   Mycobacterium
   Cryptococcus
   Candida
4. *Tumors*
   Kaposi's sarcoma
   lymphomas
   renal cell carcinoma
5. *Vascular* hemolytic uremic syndrome, renal cortical necrosis, vasculitis
6. *Nephrocalcinosis* amphotericin B

Table 3. Glomerular pathology in patients with human immuno-deficiency virus (HIV) infection

1. Focal and segmental glomerulosclerosis with epithelial "capping"
2. Globally sclerosing (collapsing) glomerulopathy
3. Mesangial Proliferation
4. Membranoproliferative glomerulonephritis
5. Acute postinfectious glomerulonephritis
6. Membranous nephropathy
7. Hepatitis B-Virus associated nephropathy
8. Minimal change disease
9. Heroin-associated nephropathy
10. Amyloidosis
11. Hemolytic-uremic syndrome with or without renal cortical necrosis
12. Lupus nephritis
13. ? vasculitis
14. End stage kidney

reported [3], the incidence of clinically evident glomerular disease was rather low [15]. In contrast, glomerular lesions predominate in renal biopsies obtained from HIV infected patients, including AIDS, ARC, and asymptomatic HIV carriers. This is undoubtedly related to selection bias, because renal biopsies were performed mostly in patients with unexplained proteinuria. Focal segmental sclerosis with globally collapsing glomerulopathy accounts for 83% biopsies reported in the literature, mesangial proliferation for 6%, minimal change disease for 3%, and other glomerulonephritides for 6%. The greater frequency of mesangial hyperplasia at autopsy, as compared to biopsy material, is also best explained by the lack of clinically significant proteinuria and progressive renal insufficiency in such cases [7]. Even though HIVAN is the most common lesion in those biopsied, present in 76% of cases in one series [15], not every HIV infected patient with proteinuria can be presumed to have HIVAN. Other glomerular lesions commonly seen in such patients include those associated with IV drug use (such as HAN, amyloidosis), and Hepatitis B Virus associated nephropathies, or perhaps nephropathies which are of post-infectious etiology (immune complex mediated proliferative glomerulonephritides) (Table 3). Rarely, vasculitis, hemolytic-uremic syndrome with or without renal cortical infarcts, and lupus nephritis are reported. These lesions are intriguing in view of the well known autoimmune abnormalities noted in patients with HIV infection [25].

References

1. Gardenswartz MH, Lerner CW, Seligson GR, Zabetakis PM, Rotterdam H, Tapper ML, Michelis MF, Bruno MS (1984) Renal disease in patients with AIDS – A clinicopathologic study. Clin Nephrol 21:197–204
2. Pardo V, Aldana M, Colton RM, Fischl MA, Jaffe D, Moskowitz L, Hensley GT, Bourgoignie JJ (1984) Glomerular lesions in the acquired immunodeficiency syndrome. Ann Intern Med 101:429–434
3. Bourgoignie JJ (1990) Renal complications of human immunodeficiency virus type 1. Kidney Int 37:1571–1584

4. Glassock RJ, Cohen AH, Danovitch G, Parsa P (1990) Human immunodeficiency virus (HIV) infection and the kidney. Ann Intern Med 112:35–49

5. Rao TKS, Filippone EJ, Nicastri AD, Landesman SH, Frank E, Chen CK, Friedman EA (1984) Associated focal and segmental glomerulosclerosis in the acquired immunodeficiency syndrome. N Engl J Med 310:669–673

6. Chander P, Soni A, Suri A, Bhagwat R, Yoo J, Treser G (1987) Renal ultrastructural markers in AIDS-Associated nephropathy. Am J Pathol 126:513–526

7. Pardo V, Meneses R, Ossa L, Jaffe DJ, Strauss J, Roth D, Bourgoignie JJ (1987) Aids-related glomerulopathy: Occurrence in specific risk groups. Kidney Int 31:1167–1173

8. Rao TKS, Friedman EA, Nicastri AD. The types of renal disease in the Acquired Immunodeficiency Syndrome (1987) N Engl J Med 316:1062–1068

9. Chander P, Agarwal A, Soni A, Kim K, Treser G (1988) Renal cytomembranous inclusions in idiopathic renal disease as predictive markers for the acquired immunodeficiency syndrome. Hum Pathol 19:1060–1064

10. Bourgoignie JJ, Meneses R, Pardo V (1988) The nephropathy related to acquired immunodeficiency syndrome. Adv Nephrol 17:113–126

11. Bourgoignie JJ, Meneses R, Ortiz C, Jaffe D, Pardo V (1988) The clinical spectrum of renal disease associated with human immunodeficiency virus. Am J Kidney Dis 12(2):131–137

12. Cohen AH, Nast CC (1988) HIV-associated nephropathy: a unique combined glomerular, tubular, and interstitial lesion. Mod Pathol 1:87–97

13. Soni A, Agarwal A, Chander P, Yoo J, Singal D, Salomon N, Robinson B, Tresser G (1989) Evidence for an HIV-related nephropathy: A clinicopathological study. Clin Nephrol 31:12–17

14. Carbone L, D'Agati V, Cheng JT, Appel GB (1989) The course and prognosis of human immunodeficiency virus-associated nephropathy. Am J Med 87:389–395

15. D'Agati V, Suh JI, Carbone L, Cheng JT, Appel G (1989) Pathology of HIV-associated nephropathy: a detailed morphologic and comparative study. Kidney Int 35:1358–1370

16. Langs C, Gallo GR, Schacht RG, Sidhu G, Baldwin DS (1990) Rapid renal failure in AIDS nephropathy. Arch Intern Med 150:287–292

17. Chander PN, Treser G (1987) Ultrastructural markers of "AIDS nephropathy." Kidney Int 31:335

18. Chander PN, Treser G (1987) Nuclear bodies and ultrastructural markers in "AIDS associated nephropathy." Lab Invest 56:39

19. Cohen AH, Sun NCJ, Shapshak P, Imagawa DT (1989) Demonstration of human immunodeficiency virus in renal epithelium in HIV-associated nephropathy. Mod Pathol 2:125–128

20. Alpers CE, Harawi S, Rennke HG (1988) Focal glomerulosclerosis with tubuloreticular inclusions: Possible predictive value for acquired immunodeficiency syndrome (AIDS). Am J Kidney Dis 12:240–242

21. Chander P, Sagel I, Weiss R, Pimentel C, Gupta A, Bamji M, Treser G (1989) Renal disease in human immunodeficiency virus infected children. Kidney Int 35:368

22. Strauss J, Abitbol C, Zilleruelo G, Scott G, Paredes A, Malaga S, Montane B, Mitchell C, Parks W, Pardo V (1989) A spectrum of renal disease in children with acquired immunodeficiency syndrome. N Engl J Med 321:625–630

23. Connor E, Gupta S, Joshi V, DiCarlo F, Offenberger J, Minnefor A, UyC, Oleske J, Ende N (1988) Acquired immunodeficiency syndrome-associated renal disease in children. J Pediatr 113:39–44

24. Rousseau E, Russo P, Lapointe N, O'Reagan S (1988) Renal complications of acquired immunodeficiency syndrome in children. Am J Kidney Dis 11:48–50

25. Kopelman RG, Zolla-Pazner S (1988) Association of human immunodeficiency virus infection and autoimmune phenomena. Am J Med 84:82–86

HIV-Associated Nephropathy in Children in Spain

SERAFÍN MÁLAGA*, FERNANDO SANTOS, CORSINO REY,
and GONZALO OREJAS[1]

SUMMARY. Although it is well known that children who acquire HIV infection during the perinatal period may develop renal disease, the natural history of HIV-associated nephropathy (HIV-AN) remains to be determined. Although a variety of renal lesions may occur, both focal glomerulosclerosis (FGS) and mesangial hyperplasia are the most common. By the end of March 1990, 160 cases of pediatric AIDS and almost 1400 perinatally HIV-infected children had been reported in Spain, all of them Whites.

In order to identify the prevalence of HIV-AN in children in Spain, a survey of 20 Spanish hospital Divisions of Pediatric Nephrology was undertaken; 18 Divisions responded (90%). Three (3) HIV-infected children with renal disease were identified. Clinically, all three had proteinuria, two had hematuria and none had renal failure. One was found to have FGS. Only one is alive, free of proteinuria, after treatment with prednisone.

These findings provide evidence for the existence of renal disease in HIV-infected children in Spain, but the low incidence suggests that unrecognized co-factors, including race, may be important in the development of renal disease. Further studies are needed to determine the correlations between the clinical and the pathological features of HIV-AN in children.

Introduction

The acquired immunodeficiency syndrome (AIDS) is a lethal multisystemic disease that has become a major public health problem since its recognition in the USA in 1981. The syndrome, caused by the human immunodeficiency virus (HIV) has been described in children as well as in adults.

---
[1]Section of Pediatric Nephrology, Department of Pediatrics, Covadonga Hospital, University School of Medicine, 33006 Oviedo, Asturias, Spain
*Representing the Spanish Society of Pediatric Nephrology

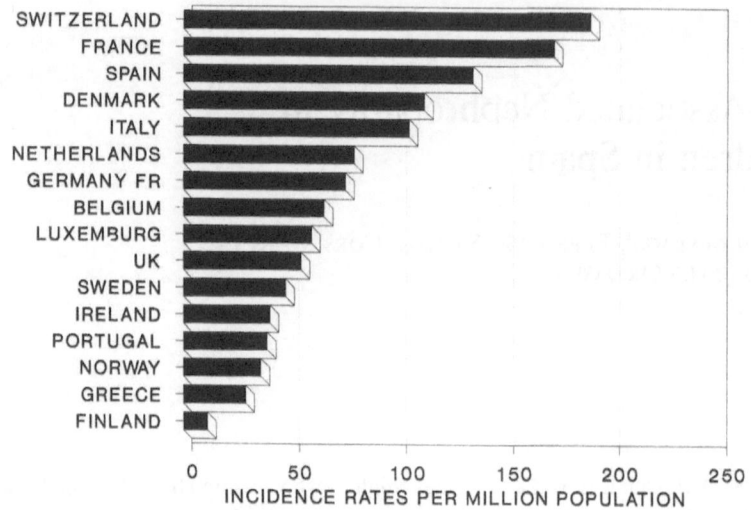

Fig. 1. AIDS cases in European countries. Reported by March 1990

The first cases suggestive of an AIDS-like illness in children were reported by the Center for Disease Control (CDC) in the United States in 1982. From then until June 1989, 1681 cases in patients under 13 years of age were registered [1]. These numbers represent only approximately 2% of all cases of AIDS reported to date in the United States.

Although the AIDS epidemic began in Europe in 1981, the first cases of pediatric AIDS were diagnosed in 1983. Since then the number, both of HIV infected children and of those with AIDS, has markedly increased [2].

According to the CDC definition, pediatric cases are limited to patients under 13 years of age. Thus, we shall discuss the problem only for this group of patients with AIDS. We shall use the current CDC definition of AIDS for this group [3] and we will also use the classification system developed by the CDC [4].

A positive HIV antibody test in a child over 15 months of age, born to an HIV infected mother, indicates that the child is also infected. In children younger than 15 months, HIV genome or HIV antigen has to be demonstrated before HIV infection is proven.

In Europe, the most comprehensive data are available from the World Health Organization Collaborating Center on AIDS, using the standard CDC definition [5].

By March 1990, sixteen participating European countries had reported 34047 cases of AIDS; 5295 (15.5%) of them are from Spain. Our country leads in those cases where intravenous drug abuse (IVDA) is the risk factor. Figure 1 summarizes the situation of AIDS in Europe by the end of March 1990.

Separate analysis of pediatric AIDS surveillance has revealed that until the end of December 1989 135 cases of pediatric AIDS were registered in Spain (Fig. 2) and at the end of March 1990 there were 165 cases [6]. This represents about 3.1% of all cases of AIDS, a percentage higher than the cumulative pediatric percentage observed in the United States and in the rest of Europe, where the incidence is

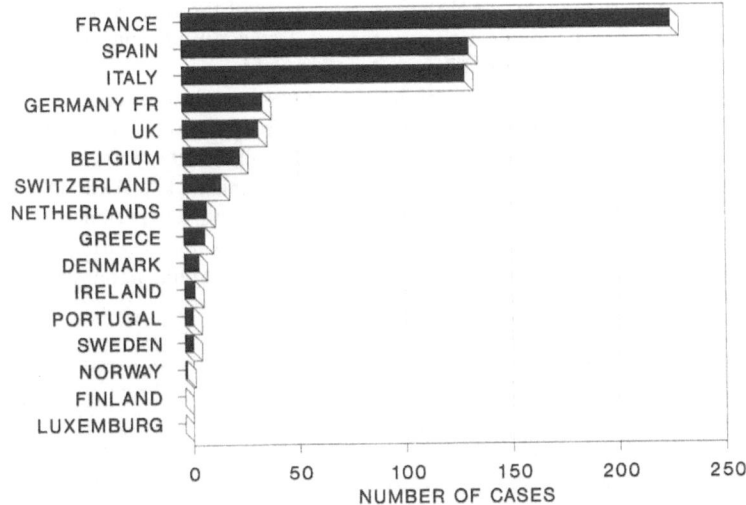

Fig. 2. Pediatric AIDS cases in Europe. Reported by December 1989

approximately 2%. The continuous increase in the relative percentage of these cases in Spain indicates rapid spread of the disease in this group. All cases of pediatric AIDS reported in Spain are in Whites and 60% of them are in males.

In Europe, pediatric AIDS is reported most frequently in France, followed by Spain and Italy. Most cases in Europe (77%) have been acquired vertically (Fig. 3).

Since the first reports of renal disease in patients with AIDS were published in 1984 [7,8], a variety of renal lesions have been described, although focal glomerulosclerosis (FGS) is the most common, and is thought by some authors, to be the true HIV-associated nephropathy (HIV-AN) [9,10].

Although renal disease is not considered a common clinical manifestation of AIDS, approximately 10% of adult and 7% of pediatric AIDS patients are affected (V. Pardo et al., manuscript in preparation). Children may represent a more appropriate

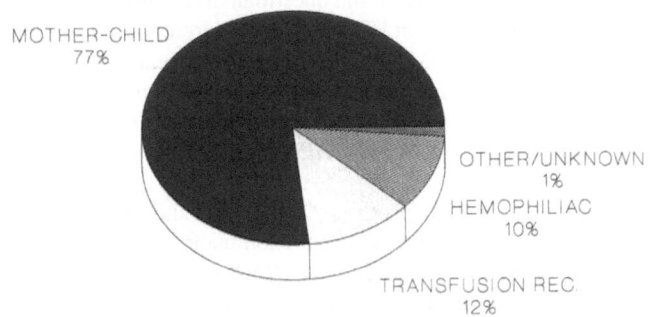

Fig. 3. Pediatric AIDS in Europe: Transmission groups. Reported by December 1989

group than adults for studying HIV-AN, because the onset of the infection may be accurately established, and complicating risk factors, frequently present in adults, such as homosexuality or IVDA, can be excluded.

There have been relatively few descriptions of HIV-AN in children; reports have been primarily from Miami (V. Pardo et al., manuscript in preparation [11]) and New York [12–15] on the East Coast of the United States, although recent reports attest to the presence of the disease in the West Coast [16] and in Canada [17]. Although at present HIV-AN has become a common problem in many hospitals, experience with appropriate diagnostic facilities is still limited to a few centers in the world.

To assess the situation of childhood HIV-AN in Spain, we would like to outline the present magnitude of the problem.

Design of the Study

In order to identify the prevalence of HIV-AN in the pediatric population in Spain, we performed a survey of all Spanish hospitals with Divisions of Pediatric Nephrology. During the period April–June 1990 a total of 20 centers were contacted.

The questionnaire included a retrospective analysis of their experience with HIV infected and HIV-AN infected children. Several aspects of clinical presentation were assessed.

HIV-AN was considered to be present when FGS or some degree of mesangial hyperplasia was confirmed by necropsy or biopsy. Clinical renal disease was considered when one or more of the following were present [11]:

– persistent urinary excretion (found on more than two occasions during a period of at least four weeks) of more than 0.1 g of protein per square meter of body surface area per day, an Albustix reading above 1+, or a urinary protein/creatinine ratio more than 0.1;

– heavy proteinuria, diagnosed when there was persistent excretion of more than 1 g of protein/m2 per 24 h, an Albustix reading above 2+, or a urinary protein/creatinine ratio more than 1.5.

Results

Eighteen centers (90%) responded to the questionnaire. Nine of them had screening programs to detect renal disease in HIV infected children. Of the responders 15 had not treated any patients with HIV-AN or HIV infected patients with clinical renal disease. Only 3 centers, 2 from Madrid and the other from Valencia, had had experience with HIV-AN or HIV infected patients with clinical renal disease. They reported 3 children with clinical manifestations of HIV infection and renal disease (one with FGS at autopsy).

All patients were followed prospectively. The clinical and pathological characteristics are shown in Table 1. There was a male predominance: (2/1), all were White, and all had perinatally acquired HIV infection. None of the children presented with peripheral edema or hypertension. Onset of the nephropathy was taken as the time of detection of persistent proteinuria or hematuria. Microscopic hematuria was seen in two of the children and proteinuria was seen in all of them, but was seen in

Table 1. Clinical and pathologic data of 3 children with HIV infection and renal manifestations

CDC Class	Sex Age[a] Race	Clinical finding			Pathologic data	Outcome (months)
		Proteinuria (mg/dl)	Hematuria	Renal failure		
P_2	M/7/W	300	Not	Not	ND	Dead/8
P_2	F/21/W	300	++	Not	FGS	Dead/22
P_1	M/18/W	Heavy	+	Not	ND	Alive/42

FGS, focal glomerulosclerosis; ND, not done
[a] Age (months) at the time the nephropathy was detected

nephrotic range in only one child. None of the patients developed renal failure. The single child with nephrotic syndrome is alive after treatment with prednisone. The other two children died of infectious complications of AIDS.

Comments

At this time the natural history of HIV-infection in children remains to be determined. Children with HIV infection show both similarities to and differences from adults. The incubation period appears to be shorter in children who have acquired their infection perinatally than it is in adults with sexually or blood product acquired HIV. At the same time there is a spectrum for disease, because some children with perinatally acquired infection have not become symptomatic for 7–8 years, suggesting that genetic factors, virus strains, or cofactors might contribute to this heterogeneity [1].

Since multiorgan involvement, kidney included, is noteworthy in pediatric AIDS, it is possible that more widespread yet subtle deficits may become evident in the long term follow-up of congenitally infected infants who may be clinically free of AIDS in the first years of life.

The review of epidemiological aspects of pediatrics AIDS in Spain raises further questions. In Spain we have a high incidence of IVDA in women, nearly 79% of whom are of reproductive age (15–45 years). Perinatal infection in their infants may be anticipated. In a recent survey, performed in more than 70% of the hospitals in the country by The Spanish Pediatric Association [18], 1416 HIV-infected children were detected. In Spain the number of female HIV positive and AIDS cases is still increasing. Thus, for a significant number of years pediatricians have to expect a slowly increasing number of HIV positive children and children with AIDS.

By March 30, 1990, 165 cases of AIDS in children below 13 years of age had been reported to the *Centro Nacional de Epidemiologia* [16]. These represent 3.1% of all cases of AIDS reported in Spain until that time.

At least two factors account for the emerging impact of HIV as a serious disease among children. First, the criteria used to define AIDS in children have become less stringent and more concordant with the clinical profile of the disease in children. The revision of the CDC criteria [3] in September 1987 provided guidelines more consistent with the disease manifestations in children and offered the opportunity for more accurate reporting.

Most infants and children who have acquired HIV perinatally live in urban areas with a high frequency of IVDA. Among the most prominent of these high frequency IVDA areas are Madrid, Barcelona, Valencia, and Málaga.

Since the first reports of renal disease in patients with AIDS were published in 1984 [7,8], a variety of renal lesions have been described, although FGS is the most common [19–21]. It is characterized clinically by nephrotic range proteinuria and by rapidly advancing renal failure; it has been observed in about 10% of adult patients with AIDS [22].

Most of the cases of HIV-AN in adult patients have been observed in Blacks, with IVDA as the AIDS risk factor, suggesting that the HIV-AN could be a variant of heroin nephropathy, which is also characterized by FGS and is confined largely (90%) to black IVDA patients. However, only 53% of patients with HIV-AN are heroin addicts, so it is clear that IVDA plays a role in the development of renal disease [23].

On the other hand, again for unknown reasons, Blacks have increased risks for renal diseases of all types. While Blacks represent 12% of the United States population, they represent 28% of all end-stage renal disease (ESRD) cases. Adjusted for age and sex differences, Blacks had 3.8 times higher rates of new ESRD cases in 1987 than did Whites [24]. The predilection of HIV-AN for Black people is apparent in the unbalanced distribution of the disease according to race. In a review of the literature we found a 3:1 ration in the number of White vs Black people with AIDS, while HIV-AN has been reported ten times more frequently in Blacks (V. Pardo et al., manuscript in preparation). It seems evident that Black race is a major cofactor in the predisposition of patients with HIV infection to acquire the nephropathy. The reasons why HIV-AN occurs basically in Blacks and in IVDA patients are not well known. Although genetic factors may indeed play some role in the racial differences, both genetic and environmental theories have been proposed, suggesting higher susceptibility of the kidney to immunologic and vascular forms of injury in black people [25,26].

In recent reports, Rao et al. [9] and Mazbar et al. [26] recognize that Blacks with HIV infection are more likely, in general, to suffer from structural renal disease than are Whites. All adult HIV infected patients who develop renal disease share several features in common.

They are mostly young men, likely to be black, who have nephrotic syndrome, azotemia of varying degree, FGS, and IVDA as a risk factor; they have a low incidence of Kaposi's sarcoma.

Since, however, HIV-AN also develops in white homosexuals and in infants with AIDS, neither race nor IVDA is solely responsible.

The natural history of HIV-AN in children is, up to now, poorly understood, because there are only a few published cases (Table 2). In children, the predominant presenting symptoms include the nephrotic syndrome, and although the commonest renal lesions found are those of FGS, some degree of mesangial hyperplasia and the proliferative forms of glomerulonephritis are often observed [11,24]. Strauss et al. [11] found HIV-AN in 12 out of 155 children with perinatal HIV infection (7%). One additional series included 5 patients with FGS and mesangial hyperplasia [14]. A second additional series included two children with FGS and perinatal nephritis [13]. On the other hand, Rousseau et al. [17] studied 17 children with perinatal AIDS and described only one patient, a Haitian, with FGS and renal disease. Another study [15] showed proliferative glomerulonephritis as the predominant lesion.

Table 2. HIV-associated nephropathy in children

Ref.	Year	No. patients	Age (months)	FGS	MH
Kaplan et al. [13]	1987	5	3–36	NR	NR
Rao et al. [10]	1987	4	2–24	2	0
Connor et al. [15]	1988	5	6–108	2	3
Rousseau et al. [18]	1988	4	3–36	4	0
Cohen et al. [17]	1988	1	24	1	0
Horowitz et al. [14]	1988	3	3–60	2	0
Chandler et al. [16]	1989	38	NR	12	0
Strauss et al.[a] [12]	1989	12	7–95	5	5
Spanish serie	1990	3	7–21	1	0
Total		75		29	8

FGS, focal glomerulosclerosis; MH, Mesangial hyperplasia; NR, not reported
[a]Eight cases from Miami, reported previously by Pardo et al. [30] are included

Although various other parenchymal renal lesions have been described in HIV infection, including those of acute glomerulonephritis, membranous glomerulonephritis, etc., in these circumstances HIV infection is more coincidental than causative [27]. The HIV-AN in children has rarely been described in Europe.

Although the incidence of HIV-AN in children is similar to that in adults, the clinical criteria for defining renal disease are different, since only approximately 50% of pediatric patients exhibit FGS. This fact would explain that progression of HIV-AN in children is not as rapid as that in adults since renal failure occurred within a mean period of one year after recognition of the nephropathy (V. Pardo et al., manuscript in preparation). The rapid progression to ESRD which has previously been reported is not the universal outcome [26]. Some authors have recommended that the term HIV-AN should be reserved for those disorders with FGS, tubular and interstitial changes, ultrastructurally defined cytoplasmic and nuclear damage, heavy proteinuria, and renal impairment [9,27], in which mesangial changes represent an early form of the disease and are likely to progress to FGS with time.

Our report drew attention to the fact that the occurrence of HIV-AN in the pediatric population in Spain is extremely rare, but although many centers are only now beginning to detect this disease, we suggest that the occurrence of HIV-AN in children is, as of now, not a nationwide problem, but the problem will become serious if the epidemic continues. On the other hand, the fact that Zidovurine may slow the progression toward ESRD [28] may make early treatment with Zidovurine, as soon as proteinuria is detected in an HIV carrier, worthwhile.

At our present level of knowledge, we conclude that the occurrence of renal disease in children with HIV infection in Spain is not frequent. The reasons for the differences between our study and the experience reported by other centers from Miami or New York City may relate to our study having a lower proportion of black patients, as occurs in centers from the West coast of the United States [26,29]

Careful screening of proteinuria and microscopic hematuria in pediatric patients with HIV infection may lead to the discovery of further cases of HIV-AN. On the other hand, it is necessary to determine clinical criteria, which will be accepted by all centers for indications for renal biopsy only in children who exhibit evident symptoms suggesting HIV-AN.

Acknowledgments. The authors acknowledge the cooperation of the following Centers and physicians that kindly provided information about their patients: Barcelona: Hospital Infantil Vall d'Hebrón. L. Callís, M.D. Hospital Infantil San Juan de Dios. L. García, M.D. Hospital Clínico Universitario. C. Pérez Prado, M.D. Bilbao: Hospital Infantil Cruces. A. Vallo, M.D. Madrid: Hospital Infantil La Paz. M. Navarro, M.D. Hospital Infantil Niño Jesús. M. Vázquez, M.D. Hospital Infantil 12 de Octubre. R. Muley, M.D. Hospital Infantil Gregorio Marañón. A. Luque, M.D. Málaga: Hospital Infantil Carlos Haya. J.M. Millán, M.D. Murcia: Hospital Virgen de la Arritxaca. F. Rodrigo, M.D. Oviedo: Hospital Covadonga. L.M. Rodríguez, M.D. Hospital General de Asturias. M. Roza, M.D. Santander: Centro Médico Marqués de Valdecilla. M. García Fuentes, M.D. Sevilla: Hospital Infantil Virgen del Rocio. J. Martín Govantes, M.D. Valencia: Hospital Infantil La Fe. C. Canosa, M.D. and I. Zamora, M.D. Hospital General Universitario. A. Lurbe, M.D. Valladolid: Hospital Infantil Del Rio Ortega. F. de las Heras, M.D. Zaragoza: Hospital Infantil Miguel Servet. C. Loris, M.D. We also thank Jorge Román (Unidad de estadística e Informática. INSALUD-ASTURIAS), for his professional and technical assistance.

References

1. Pizzo Ph A (1990) Pediatric AIDS: Problems within problems. J Infect Dis 161:316–325
2. Wahn V, Tangermann R (1988) Pediatric AIDS in Europe. Pediatr Eur 2:16–21
3. Centers for Disease Control (1987) Revision of the CDC surveillance case definition for acquired immunodeficiency syndrome. Morb Mort Wkly Rep 36 (Suppl 15):3–15
4. Centers for Disease Control (1987) Classification system for human immunodeficiency virus (HIV) infection in children under 13 years of age. Morb Mort Wkly Rep 36:225–230
5. WHO Collaborating Centre on AIDS: AIDS surveillance in the European Community. (1990) Data reported by December 1989. Paris
6. Centro Nacional de Epidemiología: Registro Nacional del SIDA (1990) Ministerio de Sanidad y Consumo. marzo 1990. Madrid
7. Rao TKS, Filippone EJ, Nicastri AD, Landesman SH, Frank E, Chen CK, Friedman EA (1984) Associated focal and segmental glomerulosclerosis in the acquired immunodeficiency syndrome. N Engl J Med 310:669–673
8. Pardo V, Aldana M, Colton RM, Fischi NA, Jaffe D, Mokowitz L, Hensley GT, Bourgoignie JJ (1984) Glomerular lesions in the acquired immunodeficiency syndrome. Ann Intern Med 101:429–434
9. Rao TKS, Friedman EA (1989) AIDS (HIV)-Associated nephropathy. Does it exist? Am J Nephrol 9:441–453
10. Rao TKS, Friedman EA, Nicastri AD (1987) The types of renal disease in the acquired immunodeficiency syndrome. N Engl J Med 316:1062–1068
11. Strauss J, Abitbol C, Zilleruelo G, Scott G, Paredes A, Málaga S, Montané B, Mitchell C, Parks W, Pardo V (1989) Renal disease in children with the acquired immunodeficiency syndrome. N Engl J Med 321:625–630
12. Kaplan MS, Wechsler M, Benson MC (1987) Urologic manifestations of AIDS. Urology 30:441–443
13. Horowitz I, Greco MA, Feiner V, et al. (1988) Renal pathology in pediatric AIDS (abstract) Lab Invest 58:5
14. Connor E, Gupta S, Joshi V, DiCarlo F, Offenberg J, Minnefor A, Uy C, Oleske J, Ende N (1988) Acquired immunodeficiency syndrome-associated renal disease in children. J Pediatr 113:39–44

15. Chander P, Sagel I, Weis R, Pimentel C, Gupta A, Bamji M, Treser G (1989) Renal disease in human immunodeficiency virus (HIV)-infected children. Kidney Int 35:368
16. Cohen AH, Nast CC (1988) HIV-associated nephropathy: a unique combined glomerular, tubular, and interstitial lesion. Mod Pathol 1:87–97
17. Rousseau F, Russo P, Lapointe M, O'Regan S (1988) Renal complications of acquired immunodeficiency syndrome in children. Am J Kidney Dis 11:48–50
18. Asociación Española de Pediatría.: Registro español de la infección HIV en edad pediátrica. Noviembre 1989. Madrid
19. Soni A, Agarwal A, Chander P, Yoo J, Singal D, Salomon N, Robinson B, Treser G (1989) Evidence for an HIV-related nephropathy: a clinico-pathological study. Clin Nephrol 31:12–17
20. D'Agati V, Suh JI, Carbone L, Cheng JT, Appel (1989) Pathology of HIV-associated nephropathy: a detailed morphologic and comparative study. Kidney Int 35:1358–1370
21. Van der Reijden HJ, Schipper ME, Danner SA, Arisz LU (1989) Glomerular lesions and opportunistic infections of the kidney in AIDS: an autopsy study of 47 cases. Adv Exp Med Biol 252:181–188
22. Carbone L, D'Agati V, Cheng JT, Appel GB (1989) Course and prognosis of human immunodeficiency virus-associated nephropathy. Am J Med 87:389–95
23. Shemin D, Chazan JA (1989) A risk factor for AIDS nephropathy. Nephron 51:558
24. Gordon D (1990) Racial differences in ESRD. Dial Transplant 19:114–116
25. Bourgoignie JJ, Ortín-Interian C, Green DF, Roth D (1989) Race, a cofactor in HIV-1-associated nephropathy. Transplant Proc 21:3899–3901
26. Mazbar SA, Schoenfeld PY, Humphreys MH (1990) Renal involvement in patients infected with HIV: experience at San Francisco General Hospital. Kidney Int 37:1325–1332
27. Cohen AH (1990) Renal pathology of human immunodeficiency virus (HIV) infection. In: Glassock RJ (moderator) Human immunodeficiency virus infection and the kidney. Ann Intern Med 112:37–40
28. Kleinknecht D, Meyrier A, (1989) Zidovurine and nephropathy with human immunodeficiency virus (HIV) infection. Ann Intern Med 111:856–857
29. Humphreys MH (1990) Human immunodeficiency virus-associated nephropathy. East is East and West is West? Arch Intern Med 150:253–255
30. Pardo V, Menseses R, Ossa L (1987) AIDS-related glomerulopathy. Kidney Int 31:1167–1173

Considerations of Pathogenesis of HIV-Associated Nephropathy

ARTHUR H. COHEN[1]

SUMMARY. The structural abnormalities in HIV-associated nephropathy affect cells of all renal components and result in a combination of focal and segmental glomerulosclerosis and acute tubular necrosis. Ultrastructural features of the cellular injury are considered markers associated with viral infection, although not necessarily indicative of viral protein per se. The prominent abnormalities of glomerular visceral and tubular epithelium suggest that a single insult to these cells is responsible for the lesions. This led us to consider the role of HIV infection of renal epithelium; using in situ hybridization, we identified HIV genome in glomerular visceral and tubular epithelium in HIV-associated nephropathy. While these results are promising at elucidating the pathogenesis of this nephropathy, many unanswered questions remain. Are other infectious agents also necessary to produce the structural and functional abnormalities? How does the virus gain access to these cells which lack CD4 receptors? Why is the disorder so common in Blacks? Are other factors, such as heredity or drug use also necessary? What is the role of altered renal hemodynamics? At the present time, further studies, including a valid animal model, are needed to explain adequately these perplexing questions and other features of this renal disorder.

The structural abnormalities in HIV-associated nephropathy have been documented to be diverse and to affect cells of all renal components [1,2,3]. As emphasized in several series, focal and segmental glomerulosclerosis, often in an early stage of evolution, acute tubular cell injury with microcystically dilated tubules often containing precipitates of plasma proteins, and interstitial edema coexist to cause widespread renal structural and functional damage [1,3]. Glomerular visceral and tubular epithelial cells demonstrate a variety of degenerative features; vascular endothelium, among many cell types, contains large and numerous tubulo-reticular structures and cylindrical confronting cisternae, and nuclei from most cells have a

---

[1]Departments of Pathology and Medicine, Harbor-UCLA Medical Center, 1000 W. Carson Street, Torrance, CA 90509, USA

large variety of inclusion bodies and undergo peculiar granular and granulo-fibrillar transformations [4–6]. These and other alterations are considered morphological markers associated with viral infection, although they do not necessarily indicate viral protein per se [4].

Unlike many other glomerular disorders associated with infections, the glomerulopathy of HIV-associated nephropathy is not the result of accumulation of immune deposits. The positive immunofluorescence in HIV-associated nephropathy is on a non-immune basis; segmental IgM and complement deposits in focal and segmental glomerulosclerosis associated with other diseases or as a "primary" process are considered trapped in a nonimmune manner [7]. It is known that immune complex mediated glomerulonephritis occurs in some HIV infected individuals [1,3,8, 9,11,12]; however, it should be appreciated that that broad category of glomerular injury is not an integral part of the lesions of HIV-associated nephropathy [1]. Indeed, the pathological aspects of immune complex mediated glomerulonephritis do not bear any relationship to the types of renal injury encountered in HIV-associated nephropathy. While there is some question whether HIV antigen(s) may be a component of glomerular immune complexes, there is no evidence that HIV antigen is a part of the focal and segmental "deposits" in the glomerular lesion of HIV-associated nephropathy.

The pathogenesis of the lesion of segmental glomerulosclerosis is uncertain, although many theories exist. These include the effects of altered glomerular hemodynamics, glomerular hypertrophy, disordered lipid metabolism, other metabolic factors, persistent proteinuria, genetic factors, and aging, to cite but a few [13]. Regardless of which one or more of these "etiologic" considerations are favored, there is some debate as to the glomerular cell which is initially affected. Strong evidence exists to implicate visceral epithelial cells; perhaps equally compelling evidence favors primary mesangial cell injury. It is beyond the scope of this paper to cite all data favoring one or the other cell; however, persistent and pronounced morphological abnormalities are regularly evident in visceral epithelium early in the development of segmental glomerulosclerosis in all settings [7]. Hence, it seems appropriate to consider visceral epithelial cell injury to be important in the pathogenesis of this form of glomerular disease. The lesions manifested in visceral epithelium at the onset of development of focal and segmental glomerulosclerosis include localized hyperplasia and hypertrophy, coarse cytoplasmic vacuoles, protein reabsorption droplets, detachment of cells from basement membranes, and necrosis [1,2]. The stimulus(i) for these changes is unknown; direct cellular injury, e.g., by drugs such as puromycin of aminonucleoside has been suggested. Is it possible that viruses can infect glomerular visceral epithelium and result in similar cellular injury which may well lead to segmental glomerulosclerosis? Viral infection of glomerular cells has been documented in animal models of cytomegalovirus (CMV) and adenovirus infection [14]. With CMV, experimentally infected mice develop transient proteinuria; mesangial cell hyperplasia and intra-nuclear inclusions are found. Visceral epithelium is not regularly affected [15]. With adenovirus, glomeruli of infected dogs have cytopathic effect in and proliferation of mesangial and endothelial cells [14]. On the other hand, in disseminated human CMV infection, there may be viral inclusions in glomerular visceral epithelium as well as in tubular epithelial cells. Antigens of other viruses in humans, such as Coxsackie B, have also been demonstrated in glomerular and tubular epithelium [16]. It is uncertain whether glomerular epithelial localization of virus in these infections can cause the morphological and functional features of segmental glomerulosclerosis or other manifestations of glomerular injury. Nevertheless, it is important to appreciate that viruses can and do infect human glomerular visceral epithelium.

The other major components of the kidney with prominent cellular lesions are the tubules. It has been well established that tubular cell degeneration and necrosis are integral features of HIV-associated nephropathy; they occur in the absence of known eitologic or pathogenetic mechanisms such as renal ischemia and nephrotoxins [1,3]. Indeed, the tubular changes may be equally as prominent in patients who develop HIV-associated nephropathy prior to any other evidence of HIV infection as in those who already have fully developed acquired immunodeficiency syndrome. In a different setting, clinically relevant polyomavirus-induced tubular necrosis has been adequately documented in a child with immunodeficiency who presented with acute renal failure [17]. These and other data indicate that some viruses can and do directly infect tubular epithelium and, in some instances, produce renal functional impairment.

With the above background, we wondered if the major structural and functional components of the renal injury in HIV-associated nephropathy might well be the result of a single mechanism which simultaneously affected glomerular and tubular cells. It seemed appropriate, therefore, to consider the role of direct HIV infection of renal epithelium in its pathogenesis. We used two techniques—in situ hybridization using a cDNA probe for viral nucleic acid and a peroxidase labeled antibody to p24 core protein—to search for virus in renal tissue [18]. These procedures were performed on fixed paraffin-embedded specimens. We evaluated renal tissues (10 biopsies and one nephrectomy) from eleven patients with HIV-associated nephropathy and compared the results with kidney biopsy specimens from HIV infected patients with immune complex mediated glomerulonephritis, autopsy kidneys from AIDS patients without clinical or morphological evidence of renal disease, and biopsies or nephrectomies from patients with "idiopathic" focal and segmental glomerulosclerosis, heroin-associated nephropathy, and normal kidneys. Specimens from the last three groups were obtained prior to 1980. We found that in HIV-associated nephropathy, numerous tubular and glomerular visceral epithelial cells contained hybridization product (Fig. 1); in contrast, very few glomerular and tubular epithelial cells were positive in HIV-infected patients with glomerulonephritis, and rare tubular cell was positive in normal kidneys of patients with AIDS. In contrast, p24 antigen was localized to very few tubular cells and rare glomerular epithelial cells in HIV-associated nephropathy. We interpreted these findings to indicate that HIV infects renal epithelium and may be pathogenetically important in HIV-associated nephropathy. We also documented that in situ hybridization is a more sensitive technique than immunohistochemistry to detect HIV in cells. Two recent preliminary reports tend to support these conclusions. Cronin et al. [19] noted p24 antigen in some proximal tubular epithelial cells in AIDS patients without renal manifestations; they suggested that "silent" HIV infection of renal epithelium is possible. Genderini et al. were unable to demonstrate core (p18 and p25) and envelope (gp 45 and gp 100) antigens in glomerular and tubular epithelium in biopsies from patients with HIV-associated nephropathy [20]. However, they acknowledged that their results did not necessarily exclude direct viral infection of renal epithelium, because of the relative insensitivity of their methods.

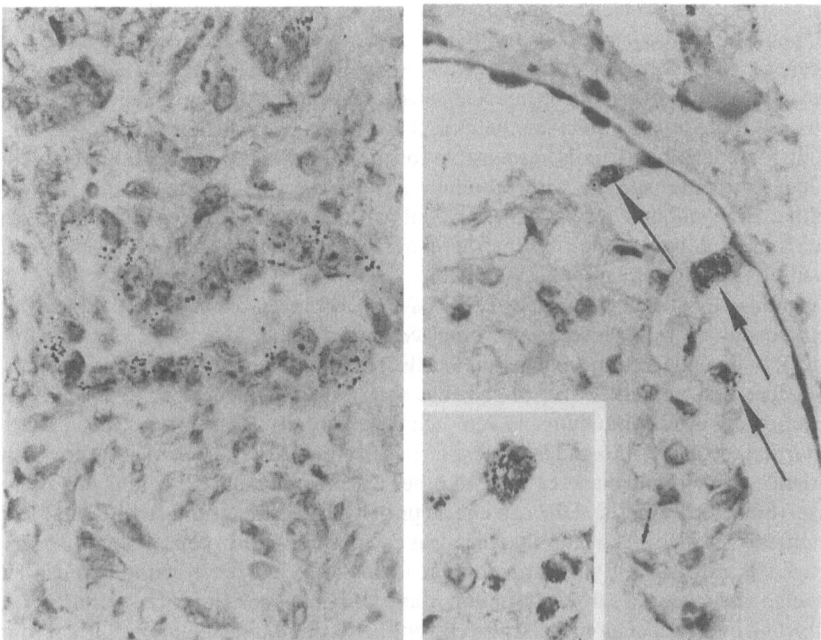

Fig. 1. HIV genome demonstrated in renal epithelium by in situ hybridization. **a** Virtually all cells of a single tubule are positive, ×400. **b** Portion of glomerulus with several positive visceral epithelial cells (*arrows*), ×350. *Inset*, enlarged positive visceral epithelial cell overlying a few patient capillaries, ×480. (Reprinted from [18] with permission]

Our observations actually raise more questions than they answer. How does the virus get to the kidneys? In the absence of CD4 receptors, how does the virus get into glomerular and tubular epithelium? Why is the virus not present in mesangial cells? Three to five percent of these cells are derived from bone marrow and possess CD4 receptors, as suggested by the work of Karlsson-Parra and colleagues [21]. Why has the virus not been identified in renal endothelial or interstitial cells? Is infection by HIV alone responsible for the morphological and functional features? Are other agents also necessary for producing damage? For example, is infection with CMV, hepatitis B, EB virus and/or herpes viruses important in the pathogenesis of HIV-associated nephropathy? What is the role, if any, of *Mycoplasma incognitus*? Why is HIV-associated nephropathy virtually limited to Blacks? What hereditary factors, such as HLA-BW53, influence the development of HIV-associated nephropathy? What is the relationship of HIV-associated nephropathy to heroin-associated nephropathy? What is the role of altered renal hemodynamics in the genesis of some features of the glomerular abnormalities and acute renal failure with tubular cell necrosis?

It is likely that HIV spreads to the kidneys in infected lymphocytes and monocytes [9]. Although the sequence of events following arrival in the kidneys has not been studied yet, certain suppositions are possible. The infected cells may infiltrate the interstitium; from this location, virus can migrate to and infect tubular cells. Either lymphocytes or monocytes can infiltrate into glomeruli; monocytes can extend into the mesangium. The exact route to visceral epithelium is clearly not known; however, passage of either free virus or infected cells across glomerular basement membrane is necessary to infect visceral epithelium. It is remotely possible that monocytes containing HIV can be partially responsible for mesangial hypercellularity observed in kidneys of some patients with proteinuria [9]. However, it should be noted that neither HIV genome, nor antigen, nor viral particles have been identified in cells in the glomerular mesangium. Furthermore, our study did not identify viral genome in interstitial mononuclear leukocytes [18].

Although most cells infected by HIV possess CD4 receptors and are, therefore, of hematopoietic origin, infection of brain cells (microglia, astrocytes, oligodendrocytes), brain endothelium, Langerhans' cells, perhaps myocardial cells, endothelium of endocervix, and other diverse cells has been well documented [22]. In addition, infection of bowel epithelium and enterochromaffin cells has been described in duodenal and rectal biopsies and in these cells in culture; the tissue specimens were from patients with chronic diarrhea with no other discernible cause [23]. This important observation indicates that HIV can infect epithelial cells and result in their functional derangement; it also indicates that the virus can and does infect cells which lack CD4 antigen expression. By direct analogy, it is possible that renal epithelium can be infected and that this can result in important functional consequences – proteinuria following infection of glomerular visceral epithelium and renal failure resulting from tubular cell injury.

No information is available on the possible role of other viral agents in the pathogenesis of HIV-associated nephropathy. However, because of the multiple infections which may be present in HIV infected individuals, other viruses may also infect renal epithelium and play a role in the pathogenesis. Some agents which should be considered include EB virus, hepatitis B virus, herpes virus and cytomegalovirus. We plan to search for these viruses using in situ hybridization and immunohistochemistry on renal specimens.

Although some investigators have postulated that simultaneous infection with HIV and a newly described microorganism, *Mycoplasma incognitus*, is necessary to produce the many and varied aspects of AIDS, there is little evidence that this combination is necessary to cause HIV-associated nephropathy. A single preliminary report has described immunohistochemical and ultrastructural localization of *Mycoplasma incognitus* in glomerular epithelium and endothelium, tubular epithelium and casts, interstitial mononuclear cells, and glomerular basement membrane in what was termed AIDS-associated nephropathy [24]. However, neither we nor others who have performed detailed ultrastructural studies of the kidneys have noted similar organisms. Clearly this observation needs confirmation.

There is some morphological similarity between heroin-associated nephropathy and HIV-associated nephropathy; this is mainly in the glomerular abnormalities, for both lesions are characterized by focal and segmental glomerulopathies; most investigators can distinguish one from the other [1,2,3,4]. However, both have epidemiological similarities in that they are disorders with an extraordinarily high prevalence in Blacks; in excess of 95% of reported cases of HIV-associated nephropathy are in Blacks, a disproportionate representation of HIV infected patients in the United States [25]. Furthermore, approximately 50% of reported patients with HIV-associated nephropathy are intravenous drug users [3,9]. A study by Haskell and colleagues [26] described an increased frequency of HLA-BW53 in patients with heroin-associated nephropathy, suggesting a genetic predisposition to this renal disorder. Similar studies have not yet been directed at patients with HIV-associated nephropathy. The close relationship between clinical and epidemiologic features of heroin-associated nephropathy and HIV-associated nephropathy has suggested to some investigators that HIV-infected patients who develop HIV-associated nephropathy are overt or covert intravenous drug abusers; hence, they consider the renal lesion to be heroin-associated nephropathy and, therefore, not related to HIV infection [27]. Unfortunately, this postulate does not explain the appearance of HIV-associated nephropathy in infants and children and in the many adults who clearly do not use intravenous drugs [1,3,10].

An alternative suggestion for an explanation for the rapidly developing renal failure which characterizes HIV-associated nephropathy was recently offered by Langs and coworkers [28]. They suggested that, rather than viral induced tubular necrosis, altered renal hemodynamics with profound renal ischemia would result in tubular necrosis and progressive renal failure and also in glomerular capillary collapse. No functional data were provided to support this thesis.

At the present time there are no adequate animal models of HIV-associated nephropathy. Focal and segmental glomerulosclerosis has been briefly described in a single rhesus monkey infected with simian AIDS virus [29]. Also briefly reported has been the development of focal and segmental glomerulosclerosis, heavy proteinuria, and renal failure with greatly diminished survival in transgenic mice bearing chromosomally integrated HIV-1 proviral DNA. The morphology of the renal damage is similar to human HIV-associated nephropathy. HIV-1 RNA expression has been documented in the kidneys; the study suggested that HIV-1 gene expression in glomerular epithelium may be responsible for the observed lesions [30]. This preliminary work serves to support our original thesis.

It is clear from the above that continued work on the role of infection, hereditary factors and race, renal hemodynamics, drugs and toxins, and other mechanisms of cell and tissue injury, is necessary before a better understanding of the pathogenesis of HIV-associated nephropathy is realized.

References

1. Cohen AH, Nast CC (1988) HIV-associated nephropathy: a unique combined glomerular, tubular and interstitial lesion. Mod Pathol 1:87–97
2. D'Agati V, Suh J-I, Carbone L, Cheng J-T, Appel G (1989) Pathology of HIV-associated nephropathy: a detailed morphologic and comparative study. Kidney Int 35:1358–1370
3. Glassock RJ, Cohen AH, Danovitch G, Parsa KP (1990) Human immunodeficiency virus (HIV) infection and the kidney. Ann Intern Med 112:35–49
4. Chander P, Soni A, Suri A, Bhagwat R, Yoo J, Treser G (1987) Renal ultrastructural markers in AIDS-associated nephropathy. Am J Pathol 126:513–526
5. Chander P, Agarwal A, Soni A, Kim K, Treser G (1988) Renal cytomembranous inclusions in idiopathic renal disease as predictive markers for the acquired immunodeficiency syndrome. Hum Pathol 19:1060–1064

6. Soni A, Agarwal A, Chander P, Yoo J, Singal D, Salomon N, Robinson B, Treser G (1989) Evidence for an HIV-related nephropathy: a clinico-pathological study. Clin Nephrol 31:12–17

7. Glassock RJ, Adler SG, Ward HJ, Cohen AH (1986) Primary glomerular disease. In: Brenner BM, Rector FC Jr (eds) The kidney. WB Saunders, Philadelphia, pp 929–1013

8. Cohen AH, Sun NCJ, Shapshak P, Imagawa D (1989) Immune complex (IC) glomerulonephritis (GN) in HIV infected patients: lack of HIV antigens in immune complexes (abstract). Lab Invest 60:18A

9. Bourgoignie JJ (1990) Renal complications of human immunodeficiency virus type I. Kidney Int 37:1571–1584

10. Strauss J, Abitbol C, Zilleruelo G, Scott G, Paredes A, Malaga S, Montane B, Mitchell C, Parks W, Pardo V (1989) Renal disease in children with the acquired immunodeficiency syndrome. N Engl J Med 321:625–630

11. Rao TKS, Friedman EA (1989) AIDS (HIV)-associated nephropathy: does it exist? Am J Nephrol 9:441–453

12. Mazbar SA, Schoenfeld PY, Humphreys MH (1990) Renal involvement in patients infected with HIV: experience at San Francisco General Hospital. Kidney Int 37:1325–1332

13. Silva FG, Hogg RJ (1989) Minimal change nephrotic syndrome – focal sclerosis complex (including IgM nephropathy and diffuse mesangial hypercellularity) In: Tisher CC, Brenner BM (eds) Renal pathology with clinical and functional correlations. JB Lippincott, Philadelphia, pp 265–339

14. Ronco P, Verroust P, Morel-Maroger L (1982) Viruses and glomerulonephritis. Nephron 31:97–102

15. Smith RD, Wehner RW (1983) Progressive cytomegalovirus glomerulonephritis: an experimental model. Am J Pathol 112:313–325

16. Burch GE, Chu KC, Colcolough HL, Sohal RS (1969) Immunofluorescent localization of Coxsackie B antigen in the kidney observed at routine autopsy. Am J Med 47:36–42

17. Rosen S, Harmon W, Krensky AM, Edelson PJ, Padgett BL, Grinnell BW, Rubino MJ, Walker DL (1983) Tubulointerstitial nephritis associated with polyomavirus (BK type) infection. N Engl J Med 308:1192–1196

18. Cohen AH, Sun NCJ, Shapshak P, Imagawa DT (1989) Demonstration of human immunodeficiency virus in renal epithelium in HIV-associated nephropathy. Mod Pathol 2:125–128

19. Cronin W, Sevchuck M, daSilva M, Bagchi S (1990) The prevalence of HIV positivity in kidneys of AIDS patients (abstract). Abstracts Sixth International Conference on AIDS 2:212

20. Genderini A, Vago L, Bertoli S, Scorza D, Barone MT, Landriani N, Milani S, Barbiano di Belgiojoso G (1990) HIV-associated-nephropathy: absence of HIV-antigens (abstract). Abstracts Sixth International Conference on AIDS 2:208

21. Karlsson-Parra A, Dimeny E, Fellstrom B, Klareskog L (1989) HIV receptors (CD4 antigen) in normal human glomerular cells. N Engl J Med 320:741

22. Levy JA (1989) The human immunodeficiency viruses. Detection and pathogenesis. In: Levy JA (ed) AIDS, pathogenesis and treatment. Marcel Decker, New York, pp 159–229

23. Nelson JA, Wiley CA, Reynolds-Kohler C, Reese CE, Margaretten W, Levy JA (1988) Human immunodeficiency virus detected in bowel epithelium from patients with gastrointestinal symptoms. Lancet I:259–262

24. Bauer FA, Wear DJ, Angritt P, Lo S-C (1990) *Mycoplasma incognitus* infection in kidneys of AIDS patients with AIDS-associated nephropathy (abstract). Abstracts Sixth International Conference on AIDS 1:255

25. Bourgoignie JJ, Ortiz-Interian C, Green DF, Roth D (1989) Race, a cofactor in HIV-1-associated nephropathy. Transplant Proc 21:3899–3901

26. Haskell LP, Glicklich D, Senitzer D (1988) HLA associations in heroin-associated nephropathy. Am J Kidney Dis 12:45–50

27. Balow JE, Macher AM, Rook AH (1986) Paucity of glomerular disease in acquired immunodeficiency syndrome (abstract). Kidney Int 29:178
28. Langs C, Gallo GR, Schacht RG, Sidhu G, Baldwin DS (1990) Rapid renal failure in AIDS-associated focal glomerulosclerosis. Arch Intern Med 150:287–292
29. Alpers CE, Baskin GB (1989) Sclerosing glomerulopathy in Rhesus monkeys with Simian AIDS (abstract). Kidney Int 35:339
30. Dickie P, Bryant J, Notkins AL, Silver J, Felser JM (1990) Glomerulosclerosis in transgenic mice expressing HIV-1 genes (abstract). Abstracts Sixth International Conference on AIDS 1:192

Cyclosporine Nephrotoxicity: From Experimental Animal to Clinical Practice

Chair: William M. Bennett (USA)
Michael J. Mihatsch (Switzerland)

Cellular Mechanisms of Cyclosporin Nephrotoxicity

Robert James Walker[1]

SUMMARY. Cyclosporin A (CsA) is a neutral lipophilic cyclic undecapeptide used extensively in transplantation. Cyclosporin A accumulates rapidly in renal tubular segments due to a partitioning process of the drug into the lipid components of the cellular membranes. Cyclosporin has been shown to inhibit protein kinase C and peptidyl-propyl *cis-trans* isomerase (identical to cyclophilin, an intracellular CsA-binding protein), as well as other intracellular enzymes. Inhibition of these intracellular regulatory enzymes, along with inhibition of intracellular Ca^{2+} flux, will significantly alter renal cellular function, including contractile activity, DNA and protein synthesis, and synthesis of prostaglandins. Inhibition of renal metabolic enzymes and alterations in renal glutathione content, in a hypoxic milieu, would enhance the toxic effects of cyclosporin.

Cellular toxicity probably has a multifactorial etiology which is related to alterations in renal vascular cells, modifying renal hemodynamics, and the relative ischemia induced by vasoconstriction potentiating sublethal changes in renal tubular epithelial cells. Histological evidence of cell damage will be apparent only if the toxic injury exceeds the capacity of the cellular mechanisms to respond to the toxic insult.

Introduction

Cyclosporin A (CsA) is a unique neutral lipophilic cyclical undecapeptide of fungal origin with potent immune-modulating properties, properties which have enabled dramatic improvements in solid organ transplantation to occur. However, the therapeutic window between immunosuppression and nephrotoxicity is very narrow with considerable overlap. Cyclosporin A-induced nephrotoxicity occurs in all forms of solid organ transplantation [1,2], as well as in bone marrow transplantation [3]. The

[1]Department of Medicine, Otago University Medical School, PO Box 913, Dunedin, New Zealand

clinical manifestations of cyclosporin A nephrotoxicity can be classified into two groups that are not necessarily exclusive. Cyclosporin A has been shown to modify renal tubular function with impaired distal tubular excretion of potassium and hydrogen ions, consistent with a voltage-dependent distal renal tubular acidosis [4,5], increased proximal tubular sodium reabsorption with decreased delivery of solute to the distal tubule [6], and impairment of urinary concentrating ability [6]. Cyclosporin A induces a marked increase in renal vascular resistance, associated with a fall in renal blood flow and a decrease in glomerular filtration rate. These changes are often associated with the development of de-novo hypertension [2,4,5].

Renal histological changes associated with CsA administration suggest injury to the proximal tubules, with foci of tubular dilatation, epithelial cell degeneration, fine reticulin deposition in the interstitium, and the presence of giant mitochondria [7,8]. Cyclosporin A may induce an arteriopathy with the development of constrictive intimal thickening together with mucoid thickening and arteriolar hyalinosis [7,8]. The development of diffuse interstitial fibrosis or striped interstitial fibrosis with tubular atrophy, an obliterative arteriolopathy and ischemic changes in some glomeruli are seen in chronic CsA nephrotoxicity [7-9].

It is difficult to correlate the histological changes and functional changes observed following the exposure to CsA [10,11]. Experimental studies have shown that there is considerable variation between species, strains, and sex of animals in their response to CsA and the development of nephrotoxicity [11]. Hence, there is no suitable experimental model that accurately reflects all the alterations seen in the human kidney.

Rats exposed to CsA will develop evidence of structural damage to the S_3 segment (straight segment) of the proximal tubule within four days [11]. Cellular damage includes vacuolation and dilatation of the endoplasmic reticulum (may also be a non-specific cellular response), tubular inclusion bodies, tubular microcalcification, tubular regeneration, and loss of brush border membranes [10-12]. Jackson and colleagues [13] found that cyclosporin induced focal areas of tubular atrophy and interstitial fibrosis in the outer cortex, and an increase in cell proliferation, the majority of which was located in the interstitium and not in the renal tubules. More recently, chronic CsA administration (12.5mg/kg per day for ten weeks) to rats was shown to produce histological injury to the inner stripe of the outer medulla and the medullary ray of the kidneys [14], similar to that seen in the striped interstitial fibrosis which is associated with chronic CsA administration in humans [8]. The features seen in the medullary ray included S_2-S_3 degenerative changes as well as tubulointerstitial fibrosis [14]. Of significance is that these morphological changes were demonstrated in nephron segments particularly sensitive to limited oxygen availability [14], thus, hypoxia secondary to vasoconstriction may further potentiate cellular injury.

Cyclosporin A has a high lipid solubility and is extensively distributed to extravascular tissues, with the highest concentrations found in fat, liver, and kidney. There is marked variation among individuals in its absorption, metabolism, and elimination [15]. Cyclosporin A has been shown to accumulate rapidly in renal segments in vitro; this accumulation being related to the lipid solubility of CsA and a partitioning process of the lipophilic drug into the lipid components of cellular membranes, which occurs in a saturable fashion. There is no evidence to suggest that CsA binds to a specific cell membrane receptor [16]. Metabolism of CsA is via the

Table 1. NADPH Cytochrome C reductase activity in renal cortical and hepatic microsomal enzymes from vehicle alone and CSA fed rats

	NADPH cytochrome C reductase enzyme activity		
	Specific activity[a]	Km[b]	Vmax[c]
	Hepatic microsomes		
Vehicle	237.2(6.4)	0.85(0.29)	300(29.5)
CSA	150.4(3.5)*	0.86(0.13)	204(8.45)
	Renal microsomes		
Vehicle	34.0(0.5)	1.78(0.08)	59.3(0.16)
CSA	31.1(0.9)*	1.51(0.24)	49.9(2.52)

[a]Specific enzyme activity expressed as nmol cytochrome C reduced/min per mg protein for cytochrome C [2mM] and NADPH [5mM]

[b]Km expressed in uM. (K^m, substrate concentration of half maximum velocity)

[c]Vmax expressed as nmol/min. (V_{max}, maximum enzyme velocity; substrate concentration not rate limiting)

Vehicle microsomes were obtained from pooled microsomes from 7 rats fed olive oil +0.1% ethanol for 4 days. CSA microsomes were obtained from pooled microsomes from 6 rats fed CSA 50mg/kg per day for 4 days. The microsomal protein concentration was kept constant for all reactions. Results are the mean±SE of 6 assays at each substrate concentrations. *$P<0.01$. (From [19] with permission)

cytochrome P-450-dependent mixed function oxidases, predominantly in the liver, with the generation of hydroxylated and N-demethylated metabolites [15].

Experimentally, CsA has been shown to significantly inhibit hepatic mixed function oxidases by uncompetitive inhibition [17,18]. The renal cortex contains similar cytochrome P-450-dependent mixed function oxidases located predominantly in the S_3 segment of the proximal tubules, a major site of histological injury produced by CsA, suggestive of a cause and effect relationship. Walker and colleagues [19] have demonstrated that CsA produces a significant uncompetitive inhibition of renal cortical NADPH cytochrome C reductase, an essential component of the mixed function oxidase enzyme complex (Table 1). Compared to the hepatic enzymes the specific activities of the renal enzymes were of a much lower order of magnitude. Despite similar tissue concentrations of cyclosporin A in the liver and kidney, the propensity for renal tubular damage is increased as compared to hepatic cellular damage. The combined effect of lower enzyme activity, together with a greater degree of uncompetitive inhibition and lower enzyme concentrations probably acting as a rate limiting step, may, in part, explain this propensity [19].

Ischemic damage to the kidney associated with transplantation, coupled with cyclosporin A-induced reduction in renal blood flow, would alter oxygen availability and metabolic requirements in the S_3 segment of the nephron. This reduced oxygen gradient would further limit the activity of the renal mixed function oxidases already compromised by the inhibitory effects of cyclosporin A.

In addition to alterations in metabolism, the hypoxic environment may also significantly impair cellular mechanisms essential for maintaining cell integrity. Cyclosporin A has been shown to reduce renal glutathione content [19] and to produce a small but significant increase in lipid peroxidation, in vitro, in renal cortical microsomes, mitochondria, and membrane fractions [19]. A reduced availability of glutathione (GSH) could impair the ability of glutathione peroxidases to metabolize fatty acid peroxides generated by lipid peroxidation. The net effect could be an increase in oxidant injury to renal tubular cells exposed to a hypoxic environment [19].

There is considerable debate over what influence CsA has on renal cell mitochondrial function and the subsequent development of nephrotoxicity. It has been suggested that decreased mitochondrial function in isolated renal cortical mitochondria following exposure to CsA in vivo and in vitro may contribute to renal tubulotoxicity [20]. Other workers have demonstrated that CsA administered to rats in nephrotoxic doses produced little or no change in mitochondrial function [21] and that these changes are probably in response to the renal hypoxia rather than a direct effect on mitochondrial function [21,22]. It is possible that the alterations in mitochondrial function may be due to alterations in the synthesis and activity of cellular protein components, including mitochondrial proteins, as discussed below [23].

Cyclosporin A has been demonstrated to alter cellular macromolecular synthesis in various cell lines [24]. Cyclosporin A and the immunologically inert cyclosporin, cyclosporin H (CsH), at concentrations comparable to those achieved in vivo, have been demonstrated to alter cellular DNA (^{3}H-thymidine incorporation) and protein synthesis (^{3}H-leucine incorporation) in renal tubular epithelial cells in culture, within two hours of exposure to cyclosporin, suggesting that cyclosporin might be altering the normal regulatory mechanisms that control the cellular enzyme systems [24]. Alterations in cellular synthesis were detected long before there were any substantial effects on cell growth or cell morphology [24]. Early sublethal damage, with altered membrane permeability, has been demonstrated in vascular endothelial cells after six hours exposure to CsA, measured by lactate dehydrogenase (LDH) and ^{51}Cr release [25]. Incubation at 4° prevented these changes, suggesting that CsA toxicity initially requires intact cellular metabolism [25].

Buss and colleagues [23] have demonstrated that a cyclosporin metabolite or a product induced by renal cells in response to CsA, directly interferes with renal microsomal protein translation or the regulation of translation. In vivo administration of CsA was required to produce inhibition of protein translocation. Renal cell sap from CsA-treated rats inhibited protein synthesis (^{3}H-leucine incorporation) in microsomes from control animals, demonstrating that a translocation inhibitor was present in the cell sap of CsA-treated rats (Fig. 1) [23]. Buss & colleagues postulate that this may be due to cyclosporin-induced inhibition of microsomal peptidyl-prolyl cis-trans isomerase [23], an enzyme that facilitates protein folding during synthesis and possibly may modulate some intracellular signal pathways [26]. Furthermore, CsA has been shown to inhibit peptidyl-prolyl cis-trans isomerase (PPI) activity in vitro [26,27], supporting the hypothesis that CsA may mediate some of its effects through alterations in protein synthesis and/or changes in protein configuration [26,27]. This enzyme has recently been demonstrated to be identical to cyclophilin (an intracellular cyclosporin binding protein, M_r 17000) [26,27], which is present in most cells and thought to be important in the intracellular transport of CsA. It has been suggested that CsA-induced inhibition of the Ca^{2+}-dependent Na^+/H^+ antiport (in lymphocytes) might be mediated through CsA binding to cyclophilin [28]. Changes in protein confirmation and possible phosphorylation or dephosphorylation would alter enzyme activity. The exact role that CsA binding to and/or inhibition of cyclophilin (PPI) activity may play in renal toxicity requires further elucidation.

Ziegler and colleagues [29] have demonstrated selective binding of CsA to a M_r 75000 polypeptide component of the renal Na^+-D-glucose cotransporter, with a prob-

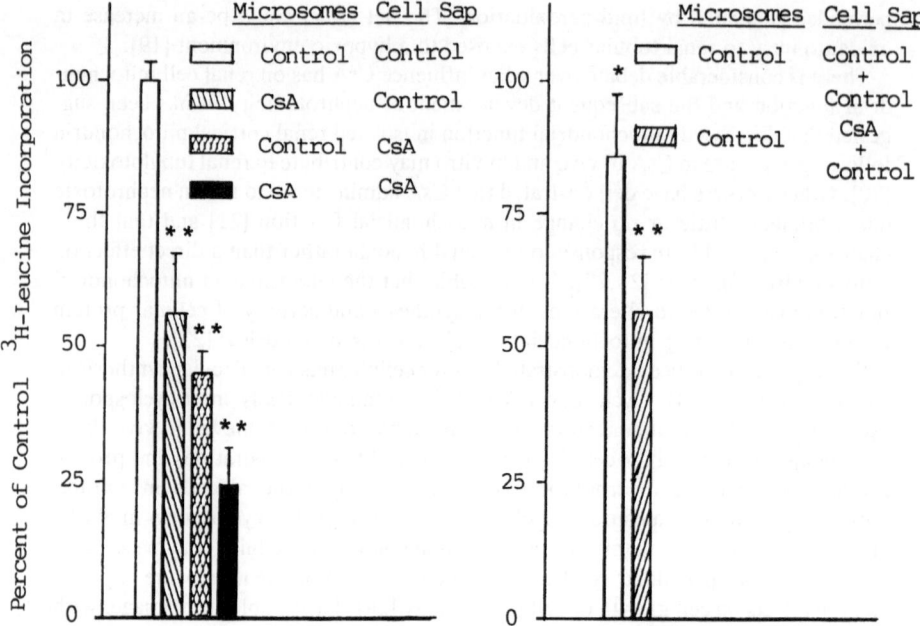

Fig. 1. Cyclosporin-induced inhibition of microsomal translocation in cross-over experiments using renal microsomes and cell saps. Microsomes and cell saps were prepared from CsA-fed (50mg/kg per day for 6 days) or vehicle-fed animals. Protein synthesis was measured as a percentage of control ^{3}H-leucine incorporation. *$P<0.02$; **$P<0.001$ compared to controls. (Reproduced with permission from Pergamon Press PLC 1989 [23])

able allosteric interaction between the binding sites for cyclosporin, D-glucose, and Na$^+$. Cyclosporin did not inhibit Na$^+$ D-glucose cotransport in isolated brush-border vesicles, suggesting that a direct effect of cyclosporin on Na$^+$ D-glucose cotransport across the brush-border membrane is not involved in nephrotoxicity. Rather, cyclosporin may modify the cellular turnover of the transporter protein [29]. Utilizing monoclonal antibodies directed against the cotransporter, increased localization of the antibody to the dilated endoplasmic reticulum following cyclosporin treatment was demonstrated. These authors postulate that cyclosporin, binding to a freshly synthesized component of the Na$^+$ D-glucose cotransporter, may inhibit the assembly of the intact transporter, with subsequent intracellular accumulation of the transport components [29]. The effect that this may have on renal tubular cellular function remains unknown, but it could play a significant role in mediating some of the cellular changes seen with cyclosporin.

Walker and colleagues [30], using partially purified protein kinase C extracts, have demonstrated that cyclosporin A significantly inhibits renal cellular protein kinase C activity both in vivo and in vitro (Fig. 2). Protein kinase C is a ubiquitous enzyme important in regulating a variety of intracellular functions by phosphorylating target proteins and enzymes [31]. It is interesting to speculate what regulatory mechanisms, such as protein phosphorylation, might be involved in regulating PPI (cyclophi-

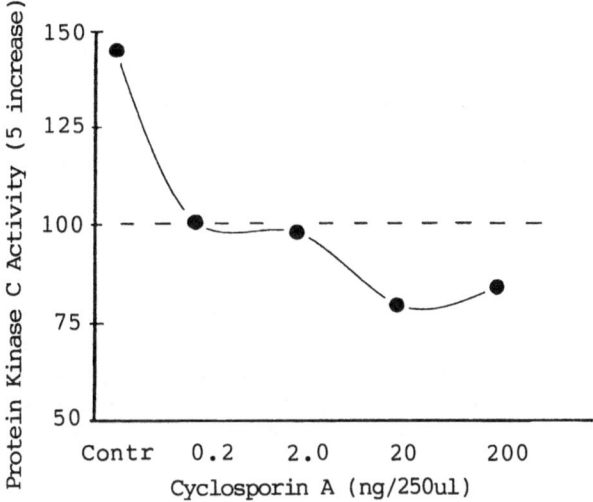

Fig. 2. Cyclosporin A inhibition of partially purified protein kinase C activity. Cytosolic protein kinase C was partially purified from pooled cytosol obtained from renal tubular epithelial cells in culture, using DEAE ion-exchange chromatography. Enzyme activity was measured as the increase in radioactivity (^{32}P) by the phosphorylation of histone. (From [30] with permission)

lin) activity and the synthesis of proteins related to the Na$^+$-D-glucose cotransporter. The net effect of the inhibition of various intracellular enzymes would be to impair the ability of renal cells to maintain their function and integrity in response to the toxic insult. Histological evidence of cell damage will be apparent only if the toxic injury exceeds the capacity of the cellular mechanisms to respond to the damage.

Within the literature there is controversy over the role of CsA as compared to the roles of cyclosporin metabolites or analogues in the generation of nephrotoxicity. Earlier studies, utilizing histological criteria for toxicity, suggested that it was the parent molecule of CsA, with its associated immunosuppressive properties, that was responsible for generating nephrotoxicity and that metabolites produced only minimal changes [10]. More recent studies (described below) suggest that toxicity, although variable in extent, is related to the unique cyclic ring structure of cyclosporin.

CsA has been shown to be rapidly metabolized by hepatocytes in culture, and, by 30 minutes, intracellular concentrations of metabolites were greater than the parent CsA [32]. Indirect evidence suggests that similar changes occur within renal tubular epithelial cells in culture, with an excess of metabolites present by two hours (RJ Walker, unpublished work). Renal clearance of CsA and metabolites is very low and it has been suggested that the high molecular weight of CsA and the metabolites would prevent the secretion of the drug. This would allow accumulation of both drug and metabolites in renal tubular cells which may then contribute to the development of nephrotoxicity [33,34].

As described above, CsH, an immunologically inert cyclosporin, produced changes similar to those induced by CsA in renal tubular cell DNA and protein synthesis [22].

Cyclosporin H (D N-MeVal [11]-cyclosporin) differs from CsA only by the substitution of the L-methyl valine at position 11 with its D-isomer. The primary and secondary structure of the molecule is preserved, with only a change in its tertiary structure rendering the molecule immunologically inert [35]. Cyclosporin H also has been demonstrated to inhibit glomerular mesangial cell prostaglandin synthesis to an extent similar to that seen with CsA [36]. Cyclosporin G (Nva[2]-Cs) has been demonstrated to produce hemodynamic changes in vivo similar to those produced by CsA [37] (see subsequent sections). This would suggest that the mechanism by which renal cellular function is altered is common to all cyclosporins and is related to the basic molecular structure of cyclosporin.

Further supportive evidence is provided by Gschwendt and colleagues [38], who demonstrated that CsA, CsD, and CsH significantly inhibited phorbol ester-stimulated protein kinase C phosphorylation as well as Ca^{2+}/calmodulin-dependent phosphylation in vitro. This was associated with inhibition of protein and DNA synthesis, as well as with phorbol ester-induced tumor promotion in a mouse skin graft model. These actions were independent of the immunosuppressive actions of CsA [38].

The acute administration of cyclosporin A causes a dose-dependent increase in renal vascular resistance and a reduction in renal blood flow and glomerular filtration rate [39]. These early changes are functional, with no structural damage evident, and are reversible on withdrawal of the drug [39]. In the renal microcirculation similar reductions were observed. The reduction in single nephron glomerular filtration rate was associated with an increase in afferent and efferent arteriolar resistances and a fall in glomerular plasma flow. The mean glomerular capillary hydraulic pressure increased and the glomerular ultrafiltration coefficient decreased significantly [40].

The glomerular mesangial cells with their diverse roles of providing structural support for the capillary loops; modulation of the glomerular surface area and hence glomerular filtration by their smooth muscle activity, which is in turn regulated by vasoactive agents; and the ability of these mesangial cells to synthesize vasoconstrictor and vasodilatory hormones [41]; probably play a critical role in mediating the reductions in glomerular filtration rate produced by CsA administration.

Baxter and colleagues [42] have shown that cyclosporin A activates the renin angiotensin system in vivo and in vitro and that this is not accompanied by an appropriate release of the vasodilatory prostaglandins [42]. Similarly, cyclosporin A has been shown to stimulate and enhance the release of renin from juxtaglomerular cells in culture [43]. Cyclosporin A has been demonstrated to enhance arginine vasopressin stimulated mesangial cell and vascular smooth muscle cell contractility in vitro [44]. Stimulation of mesangial cells by cyclosporin A alone does not modify the release of the vasodilatory prostaglandin PGE_2, or produce an increase in the vasoconstricting prostaglandin thromboxane A_2 (TXA_2). However, CsA inhibited angiotensin II (AII)-stimulated prostaglandin release from mesangial cells (Fig. 3) [36], as well as in vascular smooth muscle cells in culture [45]. This was not associated with an increase in mesangial cell thromboxane A_2 release [36]. Alteration of mesangial cell phospholipid content, by substituting omega 3 fatty acids for omega 6 fatty acids, did not alter CsA-induced inhibition of AII-stimulated mesangial cell prostaglandin synthesis in vitro [46]. Cyclosporin H produced a similar degree of inhibition of AII-stimulated PGE_2 release [36]. Therefore, it would seem probable that cyclosporin-induced alterations in the concentrations of vasoactive hormones

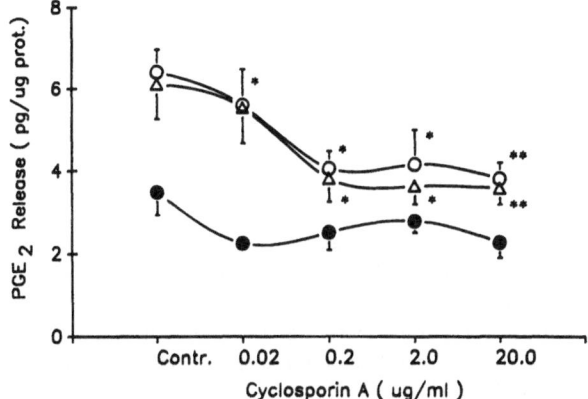

Fig. 3. Effects of CsA on Angiotensin II (*AII*)-stimulated PGE$_2$ release from rat mesangial cells. Following a 5 min pre-incubation with CsA, AII (0.1uM) was added to the culture media. PGE$_2$ release following 5 min and 15 min stimulation with AII was measured by radioimmunoassay (*RIA*). •–•, CsA alone; ∘–∘, CsA + AII 5min; ▲–▲, CsA + AII 15 min *$P<0.01$; **$P<0.001$ compared to control + AII. (From [36] with permission)

would allow mesangial cell contraction to predominate [36]. The net effect would be a reduction in the glomerular ultrafiltration coefficient, with an associated reduction in glomerular filtration rate, as seen both clinically and experimentally.

Exaggerated glomerular thromboxane synthesis has been suggested as a potential mechanism in producing the cyclosporin A-induced reductions in glomerular filtration rate. Perico and colleagues [47] have shown, in vivo, that glomerular synthesis and urinary excretion of thromboxane progressively increase with cyclosporin A therapy. Other studies have demonstrated that the increase in urinary thromboxane excretion is a consequence of intrarenal platelet and macrophage activation, probably triggered by cyclosporin-induced endothelial damage [48,49], rather than arising from glomerular mesangial cells [36,47]. The increased release of the vasoconstricting thromboxane from these non-renal sources could potentiate the reduction in glomerular filtration rate associated with cyclosporin A.

Cyclosporin A has been shown to enhance the transmembrane Ca^{2+} flux and to increase intracellular Ca^{2+} stores, which, in response to agonist stimulation, leads to enhanced contractility [44]. This effect on calcium flux appears to be dissociated from cyclosporin's immunosuppressive potential, as CsG and CsH, as well as CsA, have been demonstrated to significantly increase vasopressin-stimulated intracellular free calcium release from cultured rat mesangial cells [50]. Cyclosporin A inhibits protein kinase C activation [30] which also requires Ca^{2+} for its activity. Therefore, it is reasonable to assume that cyclosporin A is modulating the hormone receptor activated pathway, at several different points at least, with subsequent impairment of cellular function.

An alternative, but not necessarily opposing, hypothesis proposes that cyclosporin A nephrotoxicity, like its immunosuppressive action, is mediated by inhibition of gene transcription of critical humoral regulators of mesangial cell or vascular endothelial and/or vascular smooth muscle cell activity, particularly locally active vasodilatory agents [51]. As suggested above, this may be due to phosphorylation of critical regulatory cellular enzymes, including those responsible for transcription and translocation.

Cyclosporin has been shown to directly induce tension development in isolated rat aortic rings [52] and to augment the contractile response of arterial strips in vitro to endogenously released and exogenous norepinephrine [53]. It was suggested that CsA was acting at the level of the plasma membrane, decreasing the membrane potential, which would augment adrenergic neurotransmission and/or the response of the vascular smooth muscle cells to contractile stimuli [53]. One could speculate that the alterations in membrane potential could be mediated by CsA-induced changes in the membrane Na^+/ATPase pump [54], Na^+/H^+ antiport and intracellular pH [28], and intracellular Ca^{2+} flux [44].

Cyclosporin appears to affect many facets of renal function, from changes in whole kidney function in vivo, to alterations at a subcellular level demonstrated in cell culture models. Cyclosporin-induced changes in the renal vascular cells mediate changes in renal hemodynamics. As a consequence, the reduced oxygen availability must then influence the subsequent ability of the renal tubular epithelial cells to maintain their cellular integrity in response to cyclosporin-induced changes in cellular metabolism. The hypoxic milieu induced by CsA may be sufficient to allow potentially lethal changes in cellular function to occur, with the development of cell death and interstitial fibrosis as seen clinically. Despite the large number of studies investigating cyclosporin nephrotoxicity, there are still many unanswered questions as to how this unique agent produces the various changes that are manifested in the development of nephrotoxicity.

Acknowledgments. The expert technical assistance of Miss Vicki Lazzaro in all the studies carried out by the author is gratefully acknowledged. These studies were undertaken in, and with the valuable support of, the Department of Renal Medicine, Royal Prince Alfred Hospital, Sydney, Australia. Dr RJ Walker was the recipient of a National Health and Medical Research Council (Aust) Postgraduate Research Scholarship.

References

1. Klintmaln GBG, Iwatsuki S, Stazel TE (1981) Nephrotoxicity of cyclosporin A in liver and kidney transplantation patients. Lancet II:470–471
2. Hall BM, Tiller DJ, Duggin GG, Horvath JS, Farnsworth A, May J, Johnson JR, Shiel AGR (1985) Post-transplant acute renal failure in cadaver renal recipients treated with cyclosporine. Kidney Int 28:178–186
3. Atkinson K, Biggs JC, Hayes J, Ralston M, Dodds AJ, Concannon AJ, Naidoo D (1983) Cyclosporin associated nephrotoxicity in the first 100 days after allogenic bone marrow transplantation: 3 distinct syndromes. Br J Haematol 54:59–67
4. The Canadian Multicenter Transplantation Study Group (1986) A randomized clinical trial of cyclosporine in cadaveric renal transplantation: analysis at three years. N Engl J Med 314:1219–1225
5. Myers BD (1986) Cyclosporine nephrotoxicity. Kidney Int 30:964–974

6. Dieperink H, Leysacc PP, Kemp E, Starklint H, Frandsen NE, Tvede N, Moller J, Buchler Fredericksen P, Rossing N (1987) Nephrotoxicity of cyclosporine A in humans: effects on glomerular filtration and tubular reabsorption rates. Eur J Clin Invest 17:493–496
7. Fainsworth A, Hall BM, Ng ABP, Duggin GG, Horvath JS, Shiel AGR, Tiller DJ (1984) Renal biopsy morphology in renal transplantation: a comparative study of the light microscopic appearances of biopsies from patients treated with cyclosporine A or azathioprine prednisone and anti lymphocyte globulin. Am J Surg Pathol 8:243–252
8. Mihatsch MJ, Thiel G, Basler V, Ryffel B, Landmann J, van Overbeck J, Zollinger HU (1985) Morphological patterns in cyclosporine-treated renal transplant recipients. Transplant Proc 17(Suppl 1):101–116
9. Myers BD, Sibley R, Newton L, Tomlanovich SJ, Boshokos C, Stinson E, Luetscher JA, Whitney DJ, Kransey D, Coplaon NS, Perloth MG (1988) The long term course of cyclosporine-associated chronic nephropathy. Kidney Int 35:590–600
10. Ryffel B, Hiestand P, Foxwell B, Donatsch P, Boelsterli HJ, Maurer G, Mihatsch MJ (1986) Nephrotoxic and immunosuppressive potentials of cyclosporine metabolites in rats. Transplant Proc 18(Suppl 5):41–45
11. Duncan JI, Thomson AW, Aldridge RD, Simpson JG, Whiting PH (1986) Cyclosporine-induced renal structural damage: influence of dosage, strain, age and sex with reference to the rat and guinea pig. Clin Nephrol 25(Suppl 1):S14–S17
12. Bertani T, Perico N, Abbate M, Battaglia C, Remuzzi G (1987) Renal injury induced by long term administration of cyclosporin A to rats. Am J Pathol 127:569–579
13. Jackson NM, Hsu CH, Visccher E, Vankatachalam MA, Humes HD (1987) Alterations in renal structure and function in the rat model of cyclosporine nephrotoxicity. J Pharmacol Exp Ther 242:749–756
14. Rosen G, Greenfeld Z, Brezis M (1990) Chronic cyclosporine-induced nephropathy in the rat. Transplantation 49:445–452
15. Wood AJ, Lemaire M (1985) Pharmacologic aspects of cyclosporine therapy: pharmacokinetics. Transplant Proc 17(Suppl 1):27–32
16. Jackson NM, O'Conner RP, Humes HD (1988) Interactions of cyclosporine with renal proximal tubule cells and cellular membranes. Transplantation 46:109–114
17. Augustine JA, Zemaitis MA (1986) The effects of cyclosporin A on hepatic microsomal drug metabolism in the rat. Drug Metab Dispos 14:73–78
18. Cunningham C, Gavin MP, Whiting PH, Burke MD, MacIntyre F, Thomson AW, Simpson JG (1984) Serum cyclosporin levels, hepatic drug metabolism and renal tubulotoxicity. Biochem Pharmacol 33:2857–2861
19. Walker RJ, Lazzaro VA, Duggin GG, Horvath JS, Tiller DJ (1990) Cyclosporin-induced alterations in renal metabolism: The role of lipid peroxidation and enzyme inhibition in cyclosporin nephrotoxicity. Transplantation 50:487–492
20. Jung K, Reinholdt C, Scholz D (1987) Inhibited efficiency of kidney mitochondria isolated from rats treated with cyclosporin A. Nephron 45:43–45
21. Elzinga LW, Mela-Riker LM, Widener LL, Bennett WM (1989) Renal cortical mitochondrial integrity in experimental cyclosporine nephrotoxicity. Transplantation 48:102–106
22. Lemmi CAE, Pelikan PCD, Sikka SC, Hirschberg R, Geesaman B, Miller RL, Park KS, Liu SC, Koyle M, Rajfer J (1989) Cyclosporine augments renal mitochondrial function in vivo and reduces renal blood flow. Am J Physiol 257:F837–F841
23. Buss WC, Stepanek J, Bennett WM (1989) A new proposal for the mechanism of cyclosporine nephrotoxicity: Inhibition of renal microsomal protein chain elongation following in vivo cyclosporine A. Biochem Pharmacol 38:4085–4093
24. White DJG, Plumb AM, Pawlee G, Brons G (1979) Cyclosporin A: An immunosuppressive agent preferentially active against proliferating T cells. Transplantation 27:55–58
25. Zoja C, Furci L, Ghilardi F, Zilio P, Benigni A, Remuzzi G (1986) Cyclosporin-induced endothelial cell injury. Lab Invest 55:455–462

26. Takahashi N, Hayano T, Suzuki M (1989) Peptidyl-prolyl *cis-trans* isomerase is the cyclosporin A-binding protein cyclophilin. Nature 337:473–475
27. Fischer G, Wittman-Liebold B, Lang K, Kiefhaber T, Schmid FX (1989) Cyclophilin and peptidyl-prolyl *cis-trans* isomerase are probably identical proteins. Nature 377:476–478
28. Rosoff PM, Terres G (1986) Cyclosporine A inhibits Ca^{2+} dependent stimulation of the Na^+/H^+ antiport in human T cells. J Cell Biol 103:457–463
29. Ziegler K, Frimmer M, Fritzsch G, Koepsell H (1990) Cyclosporin binding to a protein component of the renal Na^+-D-glucose cotransporter. J Biol Chem 265:3270–3277
30. Walker RJ, Lazzaro VA, Duggin GG, Horvath JS, Tiller DJ (1989) Cyclosporin A inhibits protein kinase C activity: A contributing mechanism in the development of nephrotoxicity? Biochem Biophys Res Commun 160:409–415
31. Nishizuka Y (1988) The molecular heterogeneity of protein kinase C and its implication for cellular regulation. Nature 334:661–665
32. Fabre G, Bertault-Peres P, Fabre I, Maurel P, Just S, Cano JP (1987) Metabolism of cyclosporin A. 1. A study in isolated fresh rabbit hepatocytes. Drug Metab Dispos 15:384–390
33. Caterson RJ, Duggin GG, Critchley L, Baxter C, Horvath JS, Hall BM, Tiller DJ (1986) Renal tubular transport of cyclosporin A and associated changes in renal function. Clin Nephrol 25(Suppl 1):S30–S35
34. Burke MD, Whiting PH (1986) The role of drug metabolism in cyclosporine A nephrotoxicity. Clin Nephrol 25(Suppl 1):S111–116
35. Walkinshaw MD, Weber HP, Widmir A (1986) Molecular recognition in biological systems: Models for rational drug design. Sandoz J Med 25:131–142
36. Walker RJ, Lazzaro VA, Duggin GG, Horvath JS, Tiller DJ (1990) Structure activity relationships of cyclosporins (II): Inhibition of angiotensin II stimulated prostaglandin release in rat mesangial cells. Transplantation 50:343–345
37. Pallor MS, Ferris TF (1987) Effects of Nva²-cyclosporine on glomerular filtration rate and renal blood flow in rats. Transplantation 43:893–895
38. Gschwendt M, Kittstein W, Marks F (1988) The weak immunosuppressant cyclosporin D as well as the immunologically inert cyclosporin H are potent inhibitors in vivo of phorbol ester TPA-induced biological effect in mouse skin and of Ca^{2+}/calmodulin dependent EF-2 phosphorylation in vitro. Biochem Biophys Res Commun 150:545–551
39. Murray MS, Pallor MS (1985) Effect of cyclosporine administration on renal hemodynamics in conscious rats. Kidney Int 28:767–774
40. Barros ESG, Boim MA, Ajzen H, Ramos OL, Schor N (1985) Glomerular hemodynamics and hormonal participation in cyclosporine nephrotoxicity. Kidney Int 32:19–25
41. Schlondorff D (1987) The glomerular mesangial cell: an expanding role for a specialized pericyte. FASEB J 1:272–281
42. Baxter CR, Duggin GG, Hall BM, Horvath JS, Tiller DJ (1984) Cyclosporin A and renal prostaglandin biosynthesis. Res Commun Chem Pathol Pharmacol 45:69–80
43. Kurtz A, Bruna RB, Kuhn KW (1988) Cyclosporine A enhances renin secretion and production in isolated juxtaglomerular cells. Kidney Int 33:947–953
44. Meyer-Lehnert H, Schrier RW (1988) Cyclosporine A enhances vasopressin-induced Ca^{2+} mobilization and contraction in mesangial cells. Kidney Int 34:89–97
45. Kurtz A, Pfeilschifter J, Kuhn K, Koch KW (1987) Cyclosporin A inhibits PGE_2 release from vascular smooth muscle cells. Biochem Biophys Res Commun 147:542–549
46. Walker RJ, Lazzaro VA, Duggin GG, Horvath JS, Tiller DJ (1989) Dietary eicosapentaenoic acid does not modify cyclosporin-induced inhibition of angiotensin II stimulated prostaglandin synthesis in mesangial cells. Renal Failure 11:125–132
47. Perico N, Zoja C, Benigni A, Ghilardi F, Gualandris L, Remuzzi G (1986) Effect of short term cyclosporine administration in rats on renin-angiotensin and thromboxane A_2: possi-

ble relevance to the reduction in glomerular filtration rate. J Pharmacol Exp Ther 239:229–235

48. Benigni A, Chiabrandio C, Piccinelli A, Perico N, Gavinelli M, Furci L, Patino O, Abbate M, Bertani T, Remuzzi G (1988) Increased urinary excretion of thromboxane B_2 and 2,3-dinor TXB_2 in cyclosporin A nephrotoxicity. Kidney Int 34:164–174
49. Rogers TS, Elzinga L, Bennett WM, Kelley VE (1988) Selective enhancement of thromboxane in macrophages and kidneys in cyclosporine-induced nephrotoxicity. Transplantation 45:153–156
50. Goldberg HJ, Wong PY, Cole EH, Levey GA, Skorecki KL (1989) Dissociation between the immunosuppressive activity of cyclosporine derivatives and their effects on intracellular calcium signaling in mesangial cells. Transplantation 47:731–733
51. Kahan BD (1989) Cyclosporine. N Engl J Med 321:1725–1738
52. Xue H, Bukoski RD, McCarron DA, Bennett WM (1987) Induction of contraction in isolated rat aorta by cyclosporine. Transplantation 43:715–718
53. Lamb FS, Webb RC (1987) Cyclosporine augments reactivity of isolated blood vessels. Life Sci 40:2571–2578
54. Suzuki S, Oka T, Ohkuma S, Kuriyama K (1987) Biochemical mechanisms underlying cyclosporine A-induced nephrotoxicity. Effect of concurrent administration of prednisolone. Transplantation 44:363–368

Glomerular Hemodynamic Effects of Cyclosporine

NESTOR SCHOR, MIRIAN A. ROIM, ELVINO J.G. BARROS,
and OSCAR F.P. SANTOS[1]

SUMMARY. We evaluated the effects of acute and chronic Cyclosporine (CsA) administration on renal microcirculation, as well as the role of hormonal systems in this nephrotoxicity. Studies were performed in euvolemic Munich-Wistar rats by using a micropuncture technique. Acute CsA infusion caused a decline in single nephron (SN) glomerular filtration rate (GFR) due to a decrease in glomerular plasma flow (Q_A) and a decrease in the glomerular ultrafiltration coefficient (K_f), despite an increase in transcapillary hydraulic pressure difference (ΔP). Both captopril and verapamil partially prevented the decrease in whole kidney function altered by acute CsA infusion. Conversely, indomethacin did not modify these parameters, suggesting that the renin-angiotensin system and calcium play a role in CsA nephrotoxicity, while the prostaglandin system participated in this event by a direct blocking of CsA. The platelet activating factor (PAF) antagonist, (BN 52 021), blunted CsA effects on superficial nephron function. Since dazmegrel, a thromboxane synthetase inhibitor, did not change the SNGFR already altered by CsA, the beneficial effects of BN 52 021 would appear to be related to a direct blocking of PAF actions. Acute CsA nephrotoxicity was not fully demonstrated in Brattleboro rats, who present a hereditary absence of antidiuretic hormone (ADH), thus suggesting that the absence of ADH can be a protective factor in CsA nephrotoxicity. Short-term chronic infusion of CsA provoked a decline in SNGFR due to a decrease in Q_A and ΔP, while K_f remained unaltered. Glomerular hemodynamic patterns in acute and chronic CsA administration were different, suggesting that distinct pathophysiological mechanisms were involved and that distinct pathophysiological approaches would be required to improve knowledge of CsA nephrotoxicity.

[1]Nephrology Division, Escola Paulista de Medicina, Rua Botucatu no. 740, 04023-Sao Paulo, SP-Brazil

Introduction

Cyclosporine A (CsA) is a potent immunosuppressor drug that has been successfully used to prevent rejection of kidney, heart, bone marrow, and other organ transplants [1]. However, a number of side effects are known, the most common and important one being its nephrotoxicity [2].

It has been suggested that hormonal factors might take part in this acute renal failure, since no significant glomerular lesions have been found by light, immuno-fluorescence, or electron microscopy [3]. Indeed, there is evidence of pronounced renal vasoconstriction after acute and chronic CsA administration [4].

In order to evaluate renal microcirculation and glomerular hemodynamics during acute or chronic CsA administration, as well as the role of some hormonal systems in these events, Munich-Wistar rats were submitted to micropuncture studies.

Material and Methods

Adult male euvolemic Munich-Wistar rats were submitted to a general protocol consisting of two study periods (Groups 1-7). In the first period, saline administration was followed by clearance and micropuncture evaluation, after that, CsA (50 mg/Kg BW, iv, in bolus) was infused and a second study was performed (Group 1, $n=10$). In Group 2 ($n=7$), indomethacin (INDO, 2 mg/Kg, iv, in bolus) was given in the first period and the same dose of CsA was infused. Group 3 ($n=8$) and Group 4 ($n=7$) were treated in the same way as Group 2, but captopril (CAPT, 2 mg/Kg per h, i.v.) and verapamil (VERA, 20 ug/Kg per min, i.v.), respectively, were infused throughout both periods; CsA was also simultaneously administered in the second study period. Group 5 ($n=7$), animals were treated with BN 52 021 (5 mg/Kg, i.v., in bolus), a platelet activating factor (PAF) antagonist, in the first period and with CsA in the second period. Group 6 ($n=7$) were given a thromboxane synthetase inhibitor, dazmegrel (DAZ, 5 mg/Kg, i.v., in bolus), in the first period and CsA in the second period. In order to evaluate the role of ADH in CsA nephrotoxicity, Brattleboro homozygote rats, with genetic diabetes insipidus, were studied before and after CsA administration (Group 8, Homo BB, $n=9$). Heterozygote rats (Group 9, Hetero BB, $n=7$) served as controls for Group 8. Finally, short-term CsA administration (Group 10, $n=9$, 25 mg/Kg, i.p., per day) during 9 days was also evaluated.

In all rats, glomerular filtration rate (GFR) and total renal plasma flow (RPF) were analyzed by inulin and p-amminohippuric acid clearance, respectively.

The total renal vascular resistance (TRVR) was calculated as the quotient between mean arterial pressure (MAP) and RPF. Groups 1, 5, 6, and 10 were submitted to micropuncture studies following the usual routine fashion [5]. Statistical analyses were performed by Student's paired and unpaired two-tailed t test, and by the Mann-Whitney test when appropriate. Statistical significance was defined as $P<0.05$. Data were presented as mean (X±SEM).

Results

Although not shown, when a CsA vehicle, cremophor, was acutely or chronically administered, no change in global or superficial renal function was observed.

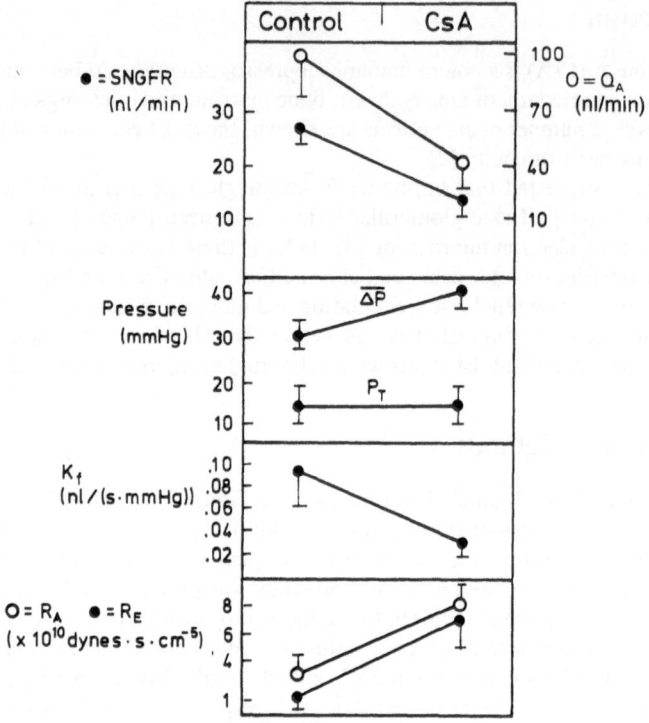

Fig. 1. Summary of CsA acute infusion.

Conversely, acute infusion of CsA induced an important decline in GFR and RPF, from 0.96 ± 0.04 to 0.47 ± 0.07 ml/min and from 2.91 ± 0.19 to 1.30 ± 0.23 ml/min ($P<0.05$), respectively. The TRVR was elevated three times (39 ± 3 vs 129 ± 40 mmHg/min per ml, $P<0.05$). As shown in Fig. 1, CsA, with results similar to those observed for global renal function, provoked a decline in single nephron GFR (SNGFR). A proportional decrease in glomerular plasma flow rate (Q_A) and in the glomerular ultrafiltration coefficient, K_f, were observed. The decline in Q_A was due to a great elevation in both afferent (R_A) and efferent (R_E) arteriolar resistances, mainly in R_E. Thus, this pattern of modification of arteriolar resistances provoked an increase in the mean transcapillary hydraulic pressure difference (ΔP). However, the increase in ΔP was not large enough to compensate for the decline in Q_A and K_f, and so, the SNGFR decreased.

Figure 2 shows the percentage changes from control values of GFR, first bar, renal plasma flow, second bar, and total renal vascular resistance, third bar. The decline of GFR and RPF and the increase in TRVR were not affected by indomethacin infusion when compared with the results for animals receiving CsA alone. On the other hand, both captopril and verapamil improved global renal function when CsA had been given previously. The decline in GFR and RPF, as well as the increase in TRVR, were partially prevented by these two drugs, suggesting that the renin angiotensin system and calcium participate in this model of nephrotoxicity.

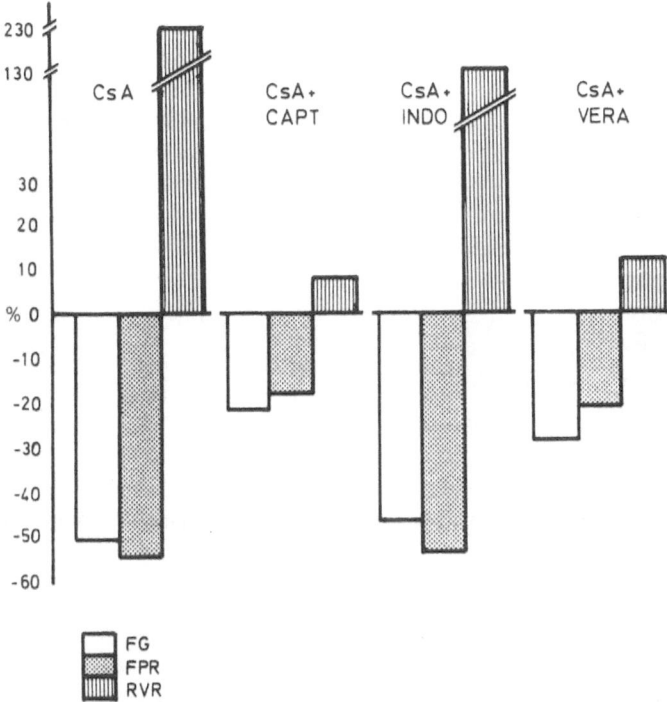

Fig. 2. Effects of CsA during captopril CAPT, Indomethacin (*INDO*), and Verapamil (*VERA*) administration

Simultaneous treatment with BN 52 021 and CsA provoked an improvement in SNGFR due to a normalization in glomerular plasma flow (Q_A) and glomerular capillary hydraulic pressure, P_{GC}. The K_f remained unchanged and the arteriolar resistances were not modified, suggesting that PAF could be one of the mediators involved in CsA nephrotoxicity (Fig. 3). In contrast, despite preventing the glomerular hypertension induced by CsA, DAZ did not modify the reduced SNGFR, Q_A and K_f, suggesting that thromboxane A_2 was not involved in the acute renal failure (ARF) induced by acute infusion of CsA.

As shown in Fig. 4, when renal function in Homo BB was compared with that in Hetero BB rats, it was observed that the declines in GFR and RPF were lower in rats without ADH than the declines in rats with ADH, and as well, the increase in TRVR was blunted in Homo BB rats. These data suggest that the absence of ADH appears to be a protective factor in the ARF induced by CsA.

In contrast to the results observed for acute CsA infusion, short-term CsA treatment provoked a decline in SNGFR with a decrease in Q_A. The reduction in Q_A occurred as a result of an elevation in both arteriolar resistances R_A and R_E, mainly in the afferent arteriolar resistance. This fact caused a decline in ΔP, while the K_f remained unaltered (Fig. 5).

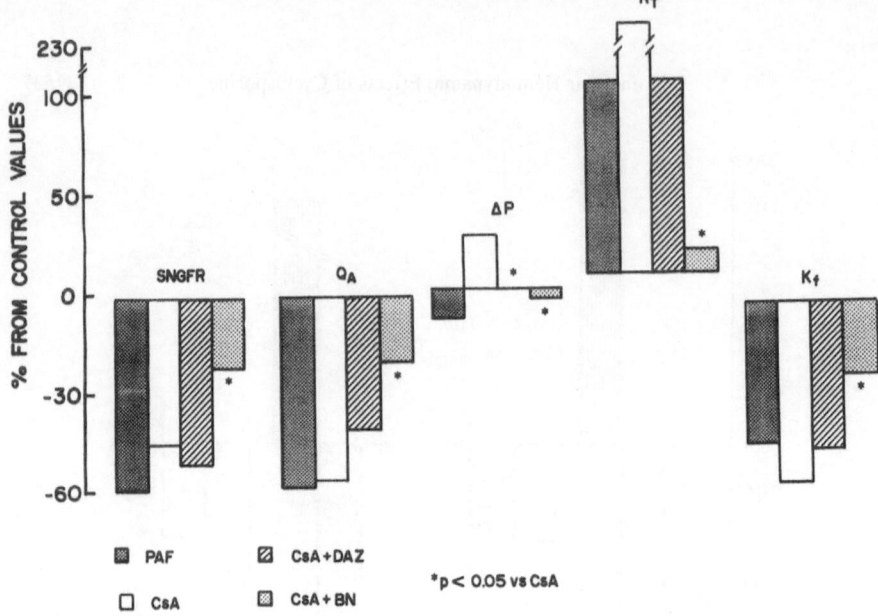

Fig. 3. Effects of PAF, CsA, CsA plus dazmegrel (*DAZ*), and CsA plus BN52 021 on glomerular hemodynamics

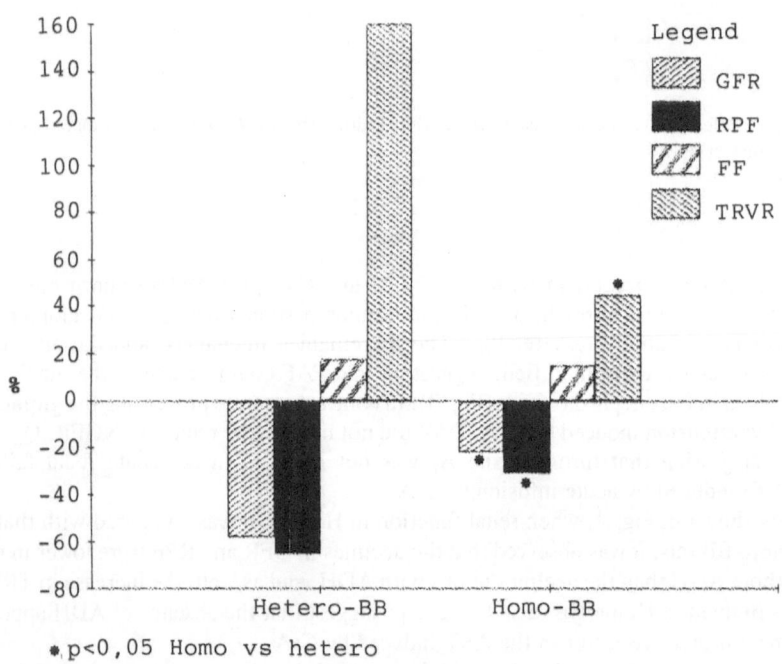

Fig. 4. Acute CsA administration in homozygote (*Homo-BB*) and heterozygote (*Hetero-BB*) Brattleboro rats

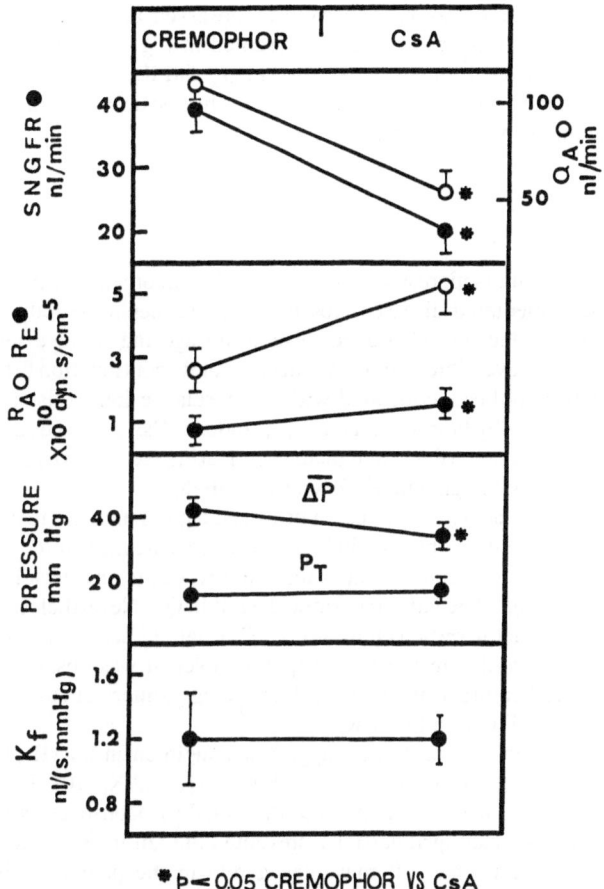

Fig. 5. Summary of CsA chronic treatment

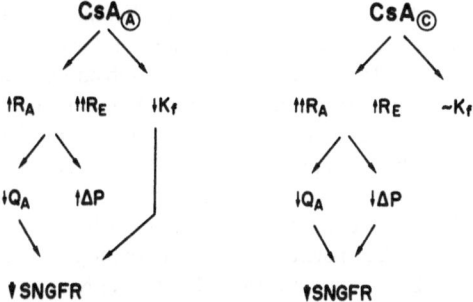

Fig. 6. Glomerular hemodynamic patterns after acute and chronic CsA administration

Thus, the glomerular hemodynamic patterns observed after acute and chronic administration of CsA were different. As presented in Fig. 6, acute CsA infusion caused a decline in SNGFR due to a decrease in Q_A and K_f, despite an increase in ΔP. On the other hand, chronic CsA nephrotoxicity showed decreases in SNGFR and Q_A, but with maintenance of K_f and decline in ΔP.

Discussion

Cyclosporine, an immunosuppressive agent used widely in organ transplantation and in several immune-mediated diseases presents potential nephrotoxicity. The acute renal failure (ARF) induced by CsA depends on its dosage and on the extent of treatment and is generally reversible after CsA reduction or discontinuation [2]. Since the toxicity of CsA has not been associated with glomerular lesions, this suggests that ARF might be mediated by hormonal factors [6]. Indeed, CsA produces activation of the renin angiotensin system (RAS) and platelet activating factor (PAF) and produces direct suppression of prostaglandin (PG) synthesis [6–8].

In this study (Fig. 1), acute CsA infusion provoked a great increase in both R_A and R_E, but the higher increment obtained in R_E determined a significant increase in ΔP. Despite the increase in ΔP, reduced values for SNGFR, due to an arteriolar vasoconstriction, were observed. The latter determined a fall in Q_A. Nevertheless, the fall in Q_A was not the only factor responsible for this. Our data indicate that SNGFR was also decreased by a significant fall in K_f [9]. Moreover, it was observed that CsA caused mesangial cell contraction in vitro [7], reducing glomerular surface available for filtration, thus leading to a lower K_f.

The data from micropuncture studies suggest that angiotensin II (AII), by increasing arteriolar resistance, has a role in the decline in Q_A and K_f [10]. In the animal group treated with captopril, it was observed that renal vasoconstriction induced by CsA was abolished. So, captopril partially prevented the fall in GFR and RPF (Fig. 2). This finding suggests that AII may play a role in the pathogenesis of renal vasoconstriction produced by CsA. Its participation could be mediated by a stimulation of the tubuloglomerular feedback mechanism or by a decrease in K_f [10,11].

Conversely, the use of indomethacin produced essentially the same results as those found with CsA alone (Fig. 2). This indicates that the PG system has a minor effect or that CsA directly decreases prostaglandin production [8].

Once CsA had caused an increase in total renal resistance, it became important to evaluate the observed Ca-channel blocker drug effect. Verapamil attenuated the CsA effects on TRVR and RPF, leading to an improvement in GFR (Fig. 2).

Antidiuretic hormone (ADH) is another vasoactive substance which is capable of influencing the process of glomerular ultrafiltration, mainly by reducing K_f [10]. In the present study, acute CsA administration in Homo BB rats produced only a slight decline in GFR and RPF when compared with both Hetero BB and Munich-Wistar rats (Fig. 4). Therefore, it can be postulated that the presence of ADH, in some way, is necessary for the full range of CsA nephrotoxic action which is observed in the rat kidney. It is possible that ADH participates in this pathophysiology either by its vasoconstrictor effects or by its known action of reducing K_f.

Continuous intravenous infusion of PAF provoked a decline in SNGFR due to a decrease in Q_A, K_f, and ΔP [12]. Thus, the pattern of glomerular hemodynamics induced by PAF and acute CsA was very similar. Moreover, it was observed that a PAF antagonist blunted the mesangial cell contraction induced by CsA [7]. Thus, PAF could be a mediator in this nephrotoxicity. Actually, acute treatment with BN 52 021, a PAF antagonist, before infusion of CsA prevented SNGFR, Q_A, ΔP, and K_f alterations. Thus, these protective actions could be due to an effect on mesangial cell contraction or an effect on minimizing the arteriolar vasoconstriction (Fig. 3). However, it has been shown that PAF can induce release of secondary mediators, including TxA$_2$, from various cell types and organs [13]. Indeed, increased production of renal thromboxane under chronic CsA treatment has been demonstrated [14]. Thus, the protective effects of BN 52 021 could be mediated by blunting the release of TxA$_2$ or by a direct action on PAF responses. In order to separate these two possible mechanisms, dazmegrel (DAZ), a thromboxane synthetase inhibitor, was employed. This inhibitor did not protect against the acute nephrotoxicity induced by CsA, since the SNGFR, Q_A, and K_f remained decreased, despite the decline in ΔP (Fig. 3). These data suggest that the improvement in SNGFR caused by BN 52 021 was mediated by a direct effect on PAF action and not by a blocker of TxA$_2$ release [15].

It was observed that the glomerular hemodynamic alterations induced by acute [9] or chronic [16] CsA administration were different. It is possible that the roles of vasoactive systems were modified during these two models of CsA nephrotoxicity. As chronic CsA toxicity is closer to clinical situations, we also decided to evaluate short-term CsA administration effects on renal function and glomerular hemodynamics in Munich-Wistar rats.

When CsA was given chronically, it was observed that great vasoconstriction, with increases in pre and post glomerular resistances occurred. However, the predominant rise in afferent arteriolar resistance produced a fall in Q_A and ΔP, both being responsible for the decrease in SNGFR.

In contrast with the results observed with acute CsA, K_f presented no significant change after chronic treatment (Fig. 5), despite multiple hormonal interactions.

In summary (Fig. 6), the glomerular hemodynamic patterns observed after acute and after chronic administration of CsA were different. As shown, acute CsA infusion caused a decline in SNGFR due to a decrease in Q_A and K_f, despite the increase in ΔP. On the other hand, chronic CsA nephrotoxicity showed decreases in SNGFR and Q_A, but with maintenance of mean K_f and decline of mean ΔP. These aspects of renal microcirculation, observed for both acute and chronic CsA administration, imply distinct pathophysiological mechanisms; in order to understand and, perhaps, to modify the nephrotoxicity of cyclosporine, distinct pathophysiological approaches will also be required. Also, the hormonal participation in chronic CsA treatment appears to be different from that in the acute model.

References

1. Kahan BD (1985) Cyclosporine: The agent and its actions. Transplant Proc 17:5–18
2. Flechner SM, Van Buren G, Herman RH, Kahan BD (1983) The nephrotoxicity of cyclosporine in renal transplant recipients. Transplant Proc 15:2689–2694
3. Mihatsch MJ, Ryffel B, Hermle M, Brunner FP, Thiel G (1986) Morphology of cyclosporine nephrotoxicity in the rat. Clin Nephrol 25:S2–S8

4. Murray BM, Paller MS, Ferris TF (1985) Effect of cyclosporine administration on renal hemodynamics in conscious rats. Kidney Int 28:767–774
5. Lugon JR, Boim MA, Ramos OL, Ajzen H, Schor N (1989) Renal function and glomerular hemodynamics in male endotoxemic rats. Kidney Int 36:570–575
6. Perilo N, Benigni C, Bosco E, Rossini M, Orisio S, Ghilardi E, Piccinilli A, Remuzzi G (1986) Acute cyclosporine A nephrotoxicity in rats: which role for renin-angiotensin system and glomerular prostaglandins? Clin Nephrol 25:583–588
7. Lama S, Oliveira A, Lopez-Novoa JM, Ortega G, Lopez-Forre A, Rodrigues-Puyol D (1988) El factor activador de las plaquetas (PAF) como mediador de la nefrotoxicidad inducida por ciclosporina A: estudios en glomerulos aislados humanos y de ratos. Nefrologia 7 (Suppl 1):24–29
8. Persan L, Kaskuel F, Barnett R, Wilson T, Moore L, Arbeit L, Schlondorff D (1989) Altered renal prostaglandin and thromboxane production in cyclosporine nephrotoxicity (abstract). Kidney Int 35:508
9. Barros EJG, Boim MA, Ajzen H, Ramos OL, Schor N (1987) Glomerular hemodynamics and hormonal participation in cyclosporine nephrotoxicity. Kidney Int 32:19–25
10. Schor N, Ichikawa I, Brenner BM (1981) Mechanisms of action of various hormones and vasoactive substances on glomerular ultrafiltration in the rat. Kidney Int 208:442–451
11. Siegl H, Ryffel B, Petric P, et al. (1983) Cyclosporine, the renin-angiotensin-aldosterone system, and renal adverse reactions. Transplant Proc 15:2719–2725
12. Badr KF, DeBoer DK, Takahashi K, Harris FC, Fogo A, Jacobson HR (1989) Glomerular responses to platelet-activating factor in the rat: role of thromboxane A_2. Am J Physiol 256:F35–F43
13. Weisman SM, Felsen D, Darracott Vaughan E Jr (1985) Platelet activating factor is a potent stimulus for renal prostaglandin synthesis: possible significance in unilateral ureteral obstruction. J Pharmacol Exp Ther 30:10–15
14. Perico N, Benigni A, Zoja C, Delaini F, Remuzzi G (1986) Functional significance of exaggerated renal thromboxane A_2 synthesis induced by cyclosporine A. Am J Physiol 251:F581–F587
15. Santos OFP, Boim MA, Bregman R, Draibe SA, Barros EJG, Pirotzky E, Schor N, Braquet P (1989) Effect of platelet-activating factor on cyclosporine nephrotoxicity: glomerular hemodynamics evaluation. Transplantation 47:592–595
16. Thomson SC, Tucker BJ, Gabba F, Blantz RC (1989) Functional effects on glomerular hemodynamics of short-term chronic cyclosporine in male rats. J Clin Invest 83:960–969

Mechanisms and Mediators of Cyclosporine-Induced Renal Vascular Changes

NORBERTO PERICO and GIUSEPPE REMUZZI[1]

Cyclosporines are a family of structurally related endecapeptides isolated as metabolites during fermentation of the soil fungi *Trichoderma polysporum Rifae* and *Cylindrocarpon lucidum Booth* [1]. Cyclosporin A (CyA), the clinically active compound, is a hydrophobic cyclic peptide containing a unique, nine-carbon amino acid bearing an ethylene band, which is essential for its biological activity. In contrast with the conventional immunosuppressive drugs, azathioprine and adrenal corticosteroids, CyA selectively inhibits adaptive immune responses, primarily through the inhibition of interleukin-2 gene translocation to mRNA and reduction of interleukin-2 production at T-cell level, while other events of T-cell activation continue unabated [2]. By virtue of its peculiar and selective activity on the immune system, CyA has improved the management of patients with organ transplantation by increasing graft and patient survival rates [3,4]. Moreover, the use of CyA has recently been advocated for the prevention of graft-versus-host disease in bone marrow transplantation [5] and for the treatment of autoimmune diseases such as uveitis [6], systemic lupus erythematosus [7], rheumatoid arthritis [8], and various forms of glomerulonephritis [9]. However, the major concern regarding CyA therapy has focused upon its association with an array of side-effects, the most serious of which is nephrotoxicity [10,11]. Thus, acute reversible dose-related decreases in renal function have been observed in over 50% of cases in some series [12]. Persistent increase in serum creatinine has prompted discontinuation or reduction of the CyA dose in a large number of patients, with subsequent improvement in renal function [13]. In addition, the potential long-term nephrotoxicity of this drug has been suggested by the progressive decline in glomerular filtration rate associated with tubulo-interstitial scarring and the obliterative arteriolopathy and glomerular sclerosis seen in cardiac allograft recipients with excellent cardiac function [14] and in liver allograft recipients [15]. Despite the fact that the clinical and pathological features

[1]Mario Negri Institute for Pharmacological Research, Via Gavazzeni 11, 24100 Bergamo, Italy

of these syndromes differ, all these manifestations of nephrotoxicity are consistent with the changes induced by CyA in the renal vessels, in which elevation in renal vascular resistance is manifested. Extensive investigations have been performed in this area, but the cause of CyA-induced renal vascular damage and the reason for the peculiar susceptibility of renal vessels to CyA-induced injury remain ill defined.

Here we will describe the vascular effects of CyA, comparing the results of human data with experimental studies, and we will analyze the possible pathogenetic mechanism(s) underlying these lesions.

Acute Reversible Renal Vasoconstriction

The administration of CyA is complicated in most renal transplant recipients by the occurrence of one or more episodes of acute renal insufficiency [13,16], usually rapidly reversible after the daily dose of CyA is reduced [17]. Moreover, liver transplant recipients receiving intravenous CyA may develop a syndrome characterized by oliguria and low fractional excretion of sodium [18]. The acute effect of CyA on renal function in animal models varies with respect to species or strain of animal as well as dose, mode of administration, and duration of treatment with CyA [19]. Several investigators have reported elevated reno-vascular resistance, diminished renal blood flow, and functional renal impairment in the rat [19–21]. Because these studies were carried out in vivo, it is difficult to separate the direct acute effects of CyA on the kidney from the indirect effects caused by systemic CyA toxicity. This issue has been addressed, using an isolated perfused rat kidney model, a preparation in which systemic influences on renal function can be eliminated [22]. With this technique we have recently shown that CyA, but not vehicle, caused a dose-dependent fall in renal perfusate flow associated with a concomitant increase in renal vascular resistance [23]. These findings are in line with those of Rossi et al. [24] who found a concentration-dependent increase in perfusion pressure in isolated rat kidneys perfused at constant flow and exposed to CyA. Recently English and coworkers [25], in rat experiments, provided the morphological counterpart of CyA-induced vasoconstriction, showing by scanning electron microscopy a disproportionate and progressive narrowing of the diameter of afferent arterioles which paralleled the decrease in inulin clearance.

CyA-induced renal vasoconstriction has been studied extensively, yet the mechanism of the drug's renovascular activity is still not clearly understood. Because in several studies CyA administration was followed by activation of the renin-angiotensin system, it has been postulated that CyA-induced arteriolar vasoconstriction is mediated by angiotensin II. However, there is no definitive evidence of this. Thus, in animals, renin secretion and plasma renin are increased with CyA treatment, which suggests that angiotensin II might be a mediator [26–28]. In contrast, plasma renin is decreased significantly in some humans with CyA-induced renal failure [14]. Moreover, improvements in renal hemodynamics have not been uniformly observed following converting enzyme inhibition in rats given CyA [21,29–31]. The possible role of activation of the sympathetic nervous system as a cause of CyA-induced vasoconstriction has also been considered. The observation that denervated kidneys fail to constrict in response to CyA in vivo [21], together with findings that α-adrenergic inhibitors antagonize CyA-induced renal vasoconstriction in innervated kidneys [21] and findings that renal sympathetic nerve activity is augmented in CyA-treated rats [32], support the contention that the renal sympathetic nerves mediate CyA-induced renal vasoconstriction, at least in part. Regardless of the validity of these observations, such a mechanism cannot readily account for the acute decline in renal blood flow and glomerular filtration rate (GFR) seen early in transplanted, and therefore denervated, kidneys [33]. CyA has been reported to alter arachidonic acid metabolism in peripheral blood monocytes [34] and in smooth muscle cells in culture [35]. Since arachidonate metabolites generated via cyclooxygenase and lipoxygenase enzymes have been found to play an important role in regulating glomerular function [36,37], one would expect that these compounds may contribute to the renal vasoconstriction induced by acute CyA administration.

Among the arachidonate metabolites formed via cyclooxygenase enzyme, TxA_2, a potent vasoconstrictor, has been shown to reduce GFR in normal rats by increasing glomerular afferent and efferent arteriolar resistances [38] and it has been shown to contract cultured rat mesangial cells through an elevation of free cytosolic calcium [39], reducing the glomerular filtration surface area. To test the possibility that TxA_2 may participate in acute CyA nephrotoxicity we exposed bovine aortic endothelial cells in culture to different concentrations of CyA, and TxA_2 generation was evaluated. In contrast with vehicle only results, incubation of confluent monolayer endothelial cells with CyA caused a time- and concentration-dependent increase in TxA_2 production, measured as its stable breakdown product TxB_2 [40]. To further investigate, in more physiologic conditions, the potential role of TxA_2 in the renal function deterioration induced by CyA, we evaluated the effects of pharmacological inhibition of endogenous TxA_2 activity in an experimental model of acute CyA nephrotoxicity. A specific TxA_2 receptor antagonist, GR32191, but not its vehicle, partially prevented the decline in GFR and renal plasma flow induced by acute CyA administration [41], pointing out a major role for TxA_2 in mediating the acute renal vasoconstriction induced by CyA in the rat. The fact that after GR32191 administration, renal function increased, but did not reach control values suggests that in addition to TxA_2 other factor(s) might be involved in the reduction of GFR induced by CyA.

Sulfidopeptide leukotrienes LTC_4 and LTD_4, derived from the 5-lipoxygenase pathway of the oxidative metabolism of arachidonic acid [42], have recently received considerable attention as modulators of glomerular function, on the basis of the observation that they increase renal vascular resistance and reduce GFR when infused in the intact animal [37] as well as in the isolated perfused rat kidney [43]. That these eicosanoids may play an intermediary role in the renal functional impairment following CyA treatment has been recently documented by the demonstration that a specific LTC_4/D_4 receptor antagonist, L-649923, also partially prevented the fall in GFR and in renal plasma flow (RPF) caused by acute i.v. CyA administration to rats [41]. Of interest, the combined administration of the TxA_2 receptor antagonist, GR32191, and the LTC_4/D_4 receptor antagonist, L-649,923, completely abolished CyA-induced decline in GFR and RPF [41], indicating an additive contribution of TxA_2 and LTC_4/D_4 to the acute renal vasoconstriction caused by CyA, at least in rats. Whether the effect of TxA_2 and/or LTC_4/D_4 on renal vascular resistance is direct or is mediated, at least in part, by their capability of releasing other vasoactive substances from endothelial cells is a matter of debate. The recent isolation and identification of a novel constrictor peptide derived from vessel endothelial cells, termed endothelin [44], and the cloning and sequence analysis of the complementary DNA of its precursor, preproendothelin [44], has aroused interest in its potential physiologic/pathophysiologic significance. Thus in rats, endothelin infusion elicits a concentration-dependent increase in renal vascular resistance and reduction in GFR [45]. Similarly, in isolated perfused rat kidneys, proportional changes in GFR and RPF have been reported over a wide range of endothelin doses [46]. Preliminary experiments in our laboratories have shown that exposure of bovine aortic endothelial cells in culture to the TxA_2 analogue U-46619 increased the expression of preproendothelin mRNA associated with the synthesis and release of the corresponding peptide in the cell supernatant (C. Zoja, personal communication).

That TxA_2 may modulate endothelin gene expression and synthesis is further supported by the recent observation that the TxA_2 mimetic, U-46619, stimulates preproendothelin mRNA expression and endothelin production also in human glomerular mesangial cells in culture [47]. The demonstration that endothelin gene expression and production in endothelial and mesangial cells is regulated by molecules potentially released at glomerular level during CyA administration, may suggest that endothelin participates in the increased renal vascular resistance caused by the drug. This possibility also rests on the fact that if one compares the effect of endothelin on glomerular hemodynamics [48,49] with the effects reported for CyA [30], the two are very similar. We have recently addressed this issue.

In isolated perfused rat kidneys exposed to a specific anti-endothelin antibody, but not to a non-immunized rabbit serum, CyA-induced fall in renal perfusate flow and GFR were markedly prevented [23]. The role of endogenous endothelin in acute CyA nephrotoxicity has been documented in vivo by studies showing that the infusion of specific endothelin antiserum partially, but significantly, prevented the reduction of GFR and RPF induced by intravenous CyA administration [23]. The micropuncture studies of Kon and coworkers [50] also found that in glomeruli infused with anti-endothelin antibody the vasoconstriction induced by CyA was markedly attenuated. The same authors also reported that in rats serum levels of endothelin studied 20 minutes after the acute injection of CyA were elevated as compared to values in identically instrumented rats not given CyA [50]. Altogether, these data support the notion that increased levels of endothelin and intense microvascular constriction following CyA may reflect a perturbed endothelin synthesis and/or metabolism in the kidney. Since CyA nephrotoxicity encompasses a spectrum of renal damage, which also depends upon the length of treatment, it remains to be determined whether the mediator(s) potentially responsible for the acute vasoconstriction also play a role in the chronic form of renal damage associated with CyA.

Persistent Vasoconstriction as a Cause of Progressive Renal Damage in Chronic CyA Treatment

The chronic renal failure which develops after long-term exposure to the drug [14,51,52] is one of the main clinical problems associated with the administration of CyA to human beings. However, any attempt to define the nature and extent of CyA-associated chronic nephropathy in renal transplants is hampered by the contribution of concomitant chronic rejection. No such difficulties are encountered, however, in cardiac or liver transplant recipients who have healthy native kidneys and are also on long-term CyA treatment. Analysis of the available studies [14,15,51] clearly points to an impairment of renal function in patients chronically treated with CyA, which becomes manifest by the development of persistent azotemia and hypertension.

So far, no clear-cut evidence has been provided as to whether chronic exposure to CyA determines a progressive form of renal damage [53,54]. Heart transplant recipients on CyA for more than 1 year have renal vascular damage, the so-called CyA-associated arteriolopathy, associated segmental or global sclerosis of some glomeruli, and a patchy collagenization of the interstitial compartment [53]. Similar pathological changes except for the severe vascular lesions, have been reported in liver allograft recipients followed for up to 4 years [15]. That persistent renal vasoconstriction plays a central role in chronic CyA nephropathy has been suspected on the basis of elevated renal vascular resistance in cardiac transplant recipients treated with CyA for one year or more [53]. Moreover, since determination of renal arcuate vein occlusion pressure revealed an increasing renal artery-to-peritubular capillary pressure gradient occurring between 1 and 12 months of CyA therapy [53], a predilection for a preglomerular site of increased renovascular resistance in CyA-treated humans has been pointed out.

That the afferent arteriole is indeed the predominant site of increased renovascular resistance in CyA-treated heart transplant recipients was also suggested by the striking elevation of transglomerular dextran transport after both 1–4 weeks and 12 months of therapy [53]. However, in the absence of an experimental model, the precise cause of renal vasoconstriction associated with long-term CyA administration remains speculative. We have recently reported that rats given CyA for 5 months, at the dose of 40 mg/kg on alternate days, had a progressive decrease in GFR associated with pathological changes characterized by glomerular endothelial damage, intracapillary hypercellularity, increased mesangial matrix, diffuse isometric vacuolization in the proximal tubules, and interstitial fibrosis with tubular atrophy [55]. Similarly, other investigators have shown that CyA, at doses of 10 and 20 mg/kg [56] or 12.5 and 25 mg/kg [57], given daily to rats for a long-term period caused renal function deterioration with striped interstitial fibrosis. Of interest, the lack of correlation between the reduction in GFR and proximal tubule abnormalities that we found in our model [55] supports the notion that renal vasoconstriction, rather than tubular injury, is a major factor in chronic experimental CyA nephrotoxicity, as it is in humans.

In order to evaluate whether vasoactive substances previously recognized as participating in the acute form of CyA nephrotoxicity may also play a role in chronic renal vasoconstriction, we have recently measured the urinary excretion of endothelin, taken as a marker of intrarenal synthesis of the peptide [58], in rats chronically given CyA. In contrast to results obtained with vehicle, 30-day CyA administration resulted in significant increase in the urinary excretion of endothelin, measured by radioimmunoassay, as compared to pre-treatment values [59]. Since, in these animals, we found a significant correlation between the urinary excretion of endothelin and the serum creatinine concentration [59], a possible contribution of this vasoactive peptide, also, to chronic CyA nephrotoxicity has been postulated. In addition to being a vasoconstrictor, endothelin has been shown to stimulate 15-lipoxygenase activity leading to 15-hydroxyeicosatetraenoic acid (15-HETE) formation [60]. This compound, 15-HETE, is chemotactic for inflammatory cells [61], and may represent the signal for circulating inflammatory cells and platelets to accumulate within glomerular capillaries, such accumulation being a typical feature of rats chronically given CyA [55]. Activation of inflammatory cells and platelets entrapped within the glomerular tuft could explain the increased levels of urinary TxA_2 metabolites that negatively correlated with GFR values in our model [62].

Since a selective thromboxane synthase inhibitor ameliorated GFR in these animals [62] it has been suggested that TxA_2 plays a role in CyA associated chronic nephropathy. In order to discriminate between the relative contribution of extrarenal versus renal TxA_2 to the observed phenomenon we performed experiments with iso-lated perfused kidneys prepared from animals previously treated with CyA (30 days). The perfusion procedure removed virtually all the circulating inflammatory cells entrapped within glomerular capillaries [63]. In such conditions the ratio of 2,3-dinor-TxB_2/TxB_2 urinary excretion markedly decreased as compared to the values found in vivo [63]. Since urinary 2,3-dinor-TxB_2 is derived mainly from inflammatory cells and platelets, while urinary TxB_2 is a likely marker of renal TxA_2 synthesis [64], we concluded for an extrarenal source for urinary thromboxane in CyA-treated animals. The observation that chronic CyA administration to rats enhances urinary excretion of TxB_2 has been confirmed by Coffman et al. [65], who found, in a post-ischemic, denervated rat model, a decline in renal function associated with an increase in urinary excretion of 2,3-dinor-TxB_2 and TxB_2. Recently, Kuhn et al. [66], studying 40 patients with multiple sclerosis who received a two-year treatment with CyA (5 mg/kg per day), found an increased urinary excre-tion of 2,3-dinor-TxB_2 which was accompanied by a significant increase in serum creatinine. Of note, withdrawal of CyA was followed by return of renal function to normal and by a reduction in 2,3-dinor-TxB_2 excretion.

The persistent renal vasoconstriction caused by the increased generation of endothelin and TxA_2 may promote ischemic parenchymal injury associated with structural alteration and eventual obliteration of the renal vessels, which ultimately causes downstream, possibly irreversible, glomerular damage. This natural history of chronic CyA nephrotoxicity has been clearly defined by Myers and coworkers [53] in heart transplant recipients followed up for 48 months. Myers and coworkers found that, despite a stable GFR in the last 2 years, some glomeruli had collapsed and become sclerotic, probably as an effect of ischemia. Moreover, morphometric analy-sis showed that glomerular ischemic changes were associated with the appearance of small size glomeruli, together with a subset of remaining glomeruli larger than nor-mal, probably compensating in this fashion for the loss of surface area in the damaged glomeruli [53] and contributing to the relative stability of the GFR. Similar findings have recently been reproduced in normal rats during long-term exposure to CyA [67]. Thus, CyA administration for 3 months resulted in a marked reduction of GFR and ischemic glomerular lesions. A complete reconstruction of the glomerular corpuscle, used to evaluate the consequences of CyA-induced renal ischemia on capil-lary tuft volume, showed that in these rats glomerular volume distribution was shifted toward small glomeruli. Prolongation of CyA administration for 5 months did not result in a further decrease in GFR, and was associated with the appearance of a subpopulation of glomeruli which became larger than normal.

Besides its potent vasoconstrictor activity, evidence now emerges for TxA_2 partici-pation in the development of glomerulosclerosis. Thus, in differentiated teratocarci-noma (F9+) cells in culture, the TxA_2 analog, U46619, induced a dose-dependent increase in several components of the extracellular matrix, including laminin A, B1, and B2 chains [68]. Similarly, U46619 increased type IV collagen (α1 and α2) gene expression in mesangial cells in culture [69]. This is in line with the notion that spatial and temporal expression of specific proteins which constitute the glomerular basement membrane is altered in many forms of glomerular disease, as it can be in chronic CyA glomerulopathy. Indeed, in mice given CyA for 4 weeks, a dose-dependent increase in mRNA expression for protocollagens type I and IV has recently been reported in kidney fibroblasts [70]. In addition to increasing expression of basement membrane components, the TxA_2 mimetic, U-46619, stimulates [^{3}H]-thymidine uptake in quiescent human mesangial cells in culture [71], suggesting that TxA_2 could contribute to glomerulosclerosis, also inducing the proliferation of mesangial cells.

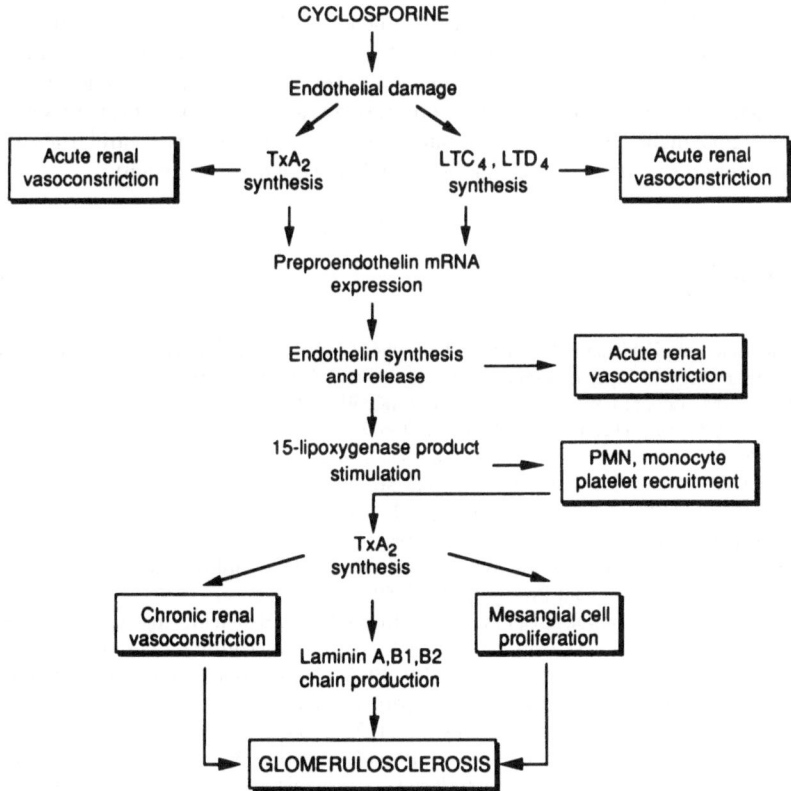

Fig. 1. Proposed mechanisms and mediators of cyclosporine A-induced renal vascular changes: possible link between clinical findings and experimental data. PMN, polymorphonuclear neutrophils

Conclusions

Because of its superior immunosuppressive properties, CyA has become the drug of choice for allograft rejection, and its use in suppressing immune inflammation associated with autoimmune diseases is rapidly increasing. Whereas bone marrow suppression or infections represent limitations to the use of conventional immunosuppressive agents, therapy with CyA is constrained chiefly by the development of protracted acute or progressive chronic renal insufficiency. The initiating event of CyA-induced decline in renal function is probably an intense vasoconstriction as documented by several recent studies that also tried to identify the responsible mechanisms(s) (Fig. 1). Among the potential vasoconstrictors, endothelin and TxA_2 have recently been shown to have pivotal roles in the pathophysiology of both acute and sustained renal vasoconstriction and glomerular dysfunction associated with CyA administration. Drugs that limit the functional consequences of excessive renal generation of endothelin and/or TxA_2 may become effective tools in the future treatment of CyA nephropathy.

Before a method of reducing CyA-induced renal vascular damage becomes available, the theoretical benefits of CyA should be weighed against its adverse effects on the kidney. While the risk of CyA nephropathy might be acceptable for patients with cardiac transplant, as long as no alternative immunosuppressive therapy is practicable, we argue against the use of this molecule in preventing rejection of isolated pancreas graft in non-uremic diabetics [72] and in autoimmune diseases [73] before control trials will convincingly document that the expected benefits overwhelm its toxicity.

References

1. Thomson AW, Whiting PH, Simpson JG (1984) Cyclosporine: immunology, toxicity and pharmacology in experimental animals. Agents and Actions 15:306–327
2. Kronke M, Leonard WJ, Depper JM Arya SK, Wong-Staal F, Gallo RC, Waldmann TA, Greene WC (1984) Cyclosporin A inhibits T-cell growth factor gene expression at level of m-RNA transcription. Proc Natl Acad Sci USA 81:5214–5218
3. Starzl TE, Hakala TR, Rosenthal JT, Arya SK, Wong-Stall F, Gallo RC, Waldmann TA, Greene WC (1983) The Colorado-Pittsburgh cadaveric renal transplantation study with cyclosporine. Transplant Proc 15:2463–2468
4. Oyer PE, Stinson EB, Jamieson SW (1983) Cyclosporine in cardiac transplantation: a 2½ year follow-up. Transplant Proc 15:2546–2549
5. Deeg HJ, Storb R, Thomas ED, Flournoy N, Kennedy MS, Banaji M, Appelbaum FR, Bensinger WI, Bunckner CD, Clift RA, Doney K, Fefer A, McGuffin R, Sanders JE, Singer J, Stewart P, Sullivan KM, Witherspoon RP (1985) Cyclosporine as prophylaxis for graft-versus-host disease: a randomized study in patients undergoing marrow transplantation for acute nonlymphoblastic leukemia. Blood 65:1325–1334
6. Nussenblatt RB, Palestine AG, Chan CC (1983) Cyclosporin A therapy in the treatment of intraocular inflammatory disease resistant to systemic corticosteroids and cytotoxic agents. Am J Ophthalmol 96:275–282
7. Feutren G, Querin S, Chatenoud L, Noel LH, Beaurain G, Tron F, Lesavre P, Bach JF (1985) The effects of cyclosporin in twelve patients with severe systemic lupus. In: Schindler R (ed) Cyclosporin in autoimmune diseases. Springer, New York, pp 366–372

8. Forre O, Bjerkhoel F, Salvesan CF, Berg KJ, Rugstad HE, Saelig G, Mellbye OJ, Kass E (1987) An open, controlled, randomized comparison of cyclosporine azathioprine in the treatment of rheumatoid arthritis: a preliminary report. Arthritis Rheum 30: 88–92

9. Lai KN, Mac-Moune Lai F, Vallance-Owen J (1988) A short-term controlled trial of cyclosporine A in IgA nephropathy. Transplant Proc 20 (Suppl 4):297–303

10. Myers BD (1986) Cyclosporine nephrotoxicity. Kidney Int 30:964–974

11. Kahan BD (1989) Cyclosporine. N Engl J Med 321:1725–1738

12. Salaman JR (1984) Cyclosporine in a renal transplantation: a guide to management. Lancet II:269–271

13. Cohen DJ, Loertscher R, Rubin MF, Tilney NL, Carpenter CB, Strom TB (1984) Cyclosporine: A new immunosuppressive agent for organ transplantation. Ann Intern Med 101:667–682

14. Myers BD, Ross J, Newton L, Leutscher J, Perloth M (1984) Cyclosporine-associated chronic nephropathy. N Engl J Med 311:699–705

15. Dische FE, Neuberger J, Keating J, Parsons V, Calne RY, Williams R (1988) Kidney pathology in liver allograft recipients after long-term treatment with cyclosporin A. Lab Invest 58:395–402

16. Calne RY, White DJG, Thiru S, Evans DB, McMaster P, Dunn DC, Craddock GN, Pentlow BD, Rolles K (1978) Cyclosporin A in patients receiving renal allografts from cadaver donors. Lancet II:1323–1327

17. Flechner SM, van Buren C, Kerman RH, Kahan DB (1983) The nephrotoxicity of cyclosporine in renal transplant recipients. Transplant Proc 15 (Suppl 1):2689–2694

18. Powell-Jackson PR, Young B, Calne RY, Williams R (1983) Nephrotoxicity of parenterally administered cyclosporine after orthotopic liver transplantation. Transplantation 36:505–508

19. Sullivan BA, Hak LJ, Finn WF (1985) Cyclosporine nephrotoxicity: studies in laboratory animals. Transplant Proc 17 (Suppl 1):145–154

20. Humes HD, Jackson NM, O'Connor RP, Hunt DA, White MD (1985) Pathogenetic mechanisms of nephrotoxicity: insights into cyclosporine nephrotoxicity. Transplant Proc 17 (Suppl 1):51–62

21. Murray BM, Paller MS, Ferris TF (1985) Effect of cyclosporine administration on renal hemodynamics in conscious rat. Kidney Int 28:767–774

22. Maack T (1980) Physiological evaluation of the isolated perfused rat kidney. Am J Physiol 238:F71–F78

23. Perico N, Dadan J, Remuzzi G (1990) Endothelin mediates the renal vasoconstriction induced by cyclosporine in the rat. JASN 1:76–83

24. Rossi NF, Churchill PC, McDonald FD, Ellis VR (1989) Mechanism of cyclosporine A-induced renal vasoconstriction in the rat. J Pharmacol Exp Ther 250:896–901

25. English J, Evan A, Houghton DC, Bennett WM (1987) Cyclosporine-induced acute renal dysfunction in the rat. Evidence of arteriolar vasoconstriction with preservation of tubular function. Transplantation 44:135–141

26. Siegl H, Ryffel B, Petric R, Shoemaker P, Muller A, Donatsch P, Mihatsch M (1983) Cyclosporine, the renin-angiotensin-aldosterone system, and renal adverse reactions. Transplant Proc 15 (Suppl 1):2719–2725

27. Baxter CR, Duggin GG, Hall BM, Horvath JS, Tiller DJ (1984) Stimulation of renin release from rat renal cortical slices by cyclosporin A. Res Commun Chem Pathol Pharmacol 43:417–423

28. Perico N, Zoja C, Benigni A, Ghilardi F, Gualandris L, Remuzzi G (1986) Effect of short-term cyclosporine administration in rats on renin-angiotensin and thromboxane A_2: Possible relevance to the reduction in glomerular filtration rate. J Pharmacol Exp Ther 239:229–235

29. Dieperink H, Leyssac PP, Kemp E, Steinbruchel D, Starklint H (1986) Glomerulotubular function in cyclosporine A treated rats. Clin Nephrol 25 (Suppl 1):S70–S74

30. Barros EJG, Boim MA, Ajzen H, Ramos OL, Schor N (1987) Glomerular hemodynamics and hormonal participation in cyclosporine nephrotoxicity. Kidney Int 3:219–225

31. Jao S, Waltzer W, Arbeit LA (1986) Acute cyclosporine induced decrease in GFR is mediated by changes in renal blood flow and renal vascular resistance. Kidney Int 29:431

32. Moss NG, Powell SL, Falk RJ (1985) Intravenous cyclosporine activates afferent and efferent renal nerves and causes sodium retention in innervated kidneys in rats. Proc Natl Acad Sci USA 82:8222–8226

33. Gazdar AF, Dammin GJ (1970) Neural degeneration and regeneration in human renal transplants. N Engl J Med 283:222–224

34. Whisler RL, Lindsey JA, Proctor KVM, Morisaki N, Cornwell DG (1984) Characteristics of cyclosporine induction of increased prostaglandin levels from human peripheral blood monocytes. Transplantation 38:377–381

35. Lindsey JA, Morisaki N, Stitts JM, Zager RA, Cornwell DG (1983) Fatty acid metabolism and cell proliferation. IV. Effect of prostanoid biosynthesis from endogenous fatty acid release with cyclosporin A. Lipids 18:566–569

36. Scharschmidt LA, Lianos E, Dunn MJ (1983) Arachidonate metabolites and the control of glomerular function. Fed Proc 42:3058–3063

37. Badr KF, Baylis C, Pfeffer JM, Pfeffer MA, Soberman RJ, Lewis RA, Austen KF, Corey EJ, Brenner BM (1984) Renal and systemic hemodynamic responses to intravenous infusion of leukotriene C_4 in the rat. Circ Res 54:492–499

38. Baylis C (1987) Effects of administered thromboxanes on the intact, normal rat kidney. Renal Physiol 10:110–121

39. Menè P, Dunn MJ (1986) Contractile effects of TxA_2 and endoperoxide analogues on cultured rat glomerular mesangial cells. Am J Physiol 251:F1029–F1035

40. Zoja C, Furci L, Ghilardi F, Zilio P, Benigni A, Remuzzi G (1986) Cyclosporin-induced endothelial cell injury. Lab Invest 55:455–462

41. Pasini M, Perico N, Remuzzi G (1990) Roles for thromboxane (Tx)A_2 and sulfidopeptide leukotrienes (LT) in cyclosporine (CsA)-induced acute renal failure. Kidney Int 37:350

42. Schlondorff D, Ardaillou R (1986) Prostaglandins and other arachidonic acid metabolites in the kidney. Kidney Int 29:108–119

43. Rosenthal A, Pace-Asciak CR (1983) Potent vasoconstriction of the isolated perfused rat kidney by leukotrienes C_4 and D_4. Can J Physiol Pharmacol 61:325–328

44. Yanagisawa M, Kurihara H, Kimura S, Tombe Y, Kobayashi M, Mitsui Y, Yazaki Y, Goto K, Masaki T (1988) A novel potent vasoconstrictor peptide produced by vascular endothelial cells. Nature 332:411–415

45. King AJ, Brenner BM, Anderson S (1989) Endothelin: a potent renal and systemic vasoconstrictor peptide. Am J Physiol 256:F1051–F1058

46. Perico N, Dadan J, Gabanelli M, Remuzzi G (1990) Cyclooxygenase products and atrial natriuretic peptide modulate renal response to endothelin. J Pharmacol Exp Ther 252:1213–1220

47. Zoja C, Orisio S, Perico N, Benigni A, Morigi M, Benatti L, Rambaldi A, Remuzzi G (to be published) Constitutive expression of endothelin gene in cultured human mesangial cells and its modulation by transforming growth factor β, thrombin and a thromboxane A_2 analogue. Lab Invest

48. Badr KF, Murray JJ, Breyer MD, Takahashi K, Inagami T, Harris RC (1989) Mesangial cell, glomerular and renal vascular responses to endothelin in the rat kidney. J Clin Invest 83:336–342

49. Kon V, Yoshioka T, Fogo A, Ichikawa I (1989) Glomerular actions of endothelin in vivo. J Clin Invest 83:1762–1767

50. Kon V, Sugiura M, Inagami T, Harvie R, Ichikawa I, Hoover RL (1990) Role of endothelin in cyclosporine-induced glomerular dysfunction. Kidney Int 37:1487–1491
51. Moran M, Tomlanovich S, Myers BD (1985) Cyclosporine-induced chronic nephropathy in human recipients of cardiac allografts. Transplant Proc 17 (Suppl 1):185–190
52. Remuzzi G, Bertani T (1989) Renal vascular and thrombotic effects of cyclosporine. Am J Kidney Dis 13:261–272
53. Myers BD, Newton L, Boshkos C, Macoviak JA, Frist WH, Derby GC, Perlroth MG, Sibley RK (1988) Chronic injury of human renal microvessels with low-dose cyclosporine therapy. Transplantation 46:694–703
54. Bantle JP, Paller MS, Boudreau RJ, Olivari MT, Ferris TF (1990) Long-term effects of cyclosporine on renal function in organ transplant recipients. J Lab Clin Med 115:233–240
55. Bertani T, Perico N, Abbate M, Battaglia C, Remuzzi G (1987) Renal injury induced by long-term administration of cyclosporin A to rats. Am J Pathol 127:569–579
56. Simpson JG, Saunders NJ, Thompson KJ, Whiting PH (1988) Chronic renal damage caused by cyclosporine. Transplant Proc 20 (Suppl 3):792–799
57. Dieperink H, Leyssac PP, Starklint H, Kemp E (1988) Long-term cyclosporin nephrotoxicity in the rat: Effect on renal function and morphology. Nephrol Dial Transpl 3:317–326
58. Benigni A, Perico N, Gaspari F, Zoja C, Bellizzi L, Gabanelli M, Remuzzi G (to be published) Increased renal endothelin production in rats with reduced renal mass. Am J Physiol
59. Perico N, Benigni A, Ladny R, Imberti O, Bellizzi L, Remuzzi G (1990) Chronic cyclosporine A (CyA) administration to rats increases urinary excretion of big-endothelin and endothelin. American Society of Nephrology Conference 1990
60. Nagase T, Fukuchi Y, Jo C, Teramoto S, Uejima Y, Ishida K, Shimizu T, Orimo H (1990) Endothelin-1 stimulates arachidonate 15-lipoxygenase activity and oxygen radical formation in the rat distal lung. Biochem Biophys Res Commun 168:485–489
61. Goetzl EJ, Pickett WC (1980) The human PMN leukocyte chemotactic activity of complex hydroxy-eicosatetraenoic acids (HETEs). J Immunol 125:1789–1791
62. Perico N, Benigni A, Zoja C, Delaini F, Remuzzi G (1986) Functional significance of exaggerated renal thromboxane A_2 synthesis induced by cyclosporin A. Am J Physiol 251: F581–F587
63. Benigni A, Chiabrando C, Piccinelli A, Perico N, Gavinelli M, Furci L, Patino O, Abbate M, Bertani T, Remuzzi G (1988) Increased urinary excretion of thromboxane B_2 in cyclosporin A nephrotoxicity. Kidney Int 34:164–174
64. FitzGerald GA, Pedersen AK, Patrono C (1983) Analysis of prostacyclin and thromboxane biosynthesis in cardiovascular disease. Circulation 67:1174–1177
65. Coffman TM, Carr DR, Varger WE, Klotman PE (1987) Evidence that renal prostaglandin and thromboxane production is stimulated in chronic cyclosporine nephrotoxicity. Transplantation 43:282–285
66. Kuhn K, Forstermann U, Frolich JC, Verterqvist O, Green K, Brunkhorst R, Koch KM, Haas J (1987) Effect of cyclosporine A (CyA) on blood pressure and prostacyclin and thromboxane A_2 production. Xth International congress of nephrology, July 26–31 1987. London, United Kingdom p 231
67. Perico N, Imberti O, Remuzzi A, Cavallotti D, Bertani T, Remuzzi G (1990) Distribution of glomerular capillary tuft volume in rats chronically treated with cyclosporine (CsA). Proceedings of the XIth international congress of nephrology, July 15–20 1990. Tokyo, Japan pp 438A
68. Klotmann P, Bruggeman L, Hassell J, Horigan E, Martin G, Yamada Y (1989) Regulation of extracellular matrix by thromboxane. Kidney Int 35:294
69. Bruggeman LA, Burbelo PD, Yamada Y, Klotman PE (1990) Regulation of renal transcriptional factors for type IV collagen gene expression by thromboxane. Proceedings of the XIth international congress of nephrology, July 15–20 1990. Tokyo, Japan pp 30A

70. Wolf G, Neilson EG (1990) Cyclosporine A (CyA) stimulates secretion of collagen IV in murine proximal tubular cells and of collagen I in kidney fibroblasts. Proceedings of the XIth international congress of nephrology, July 15–20 1990. Tokyo, Japan pp 50A
71. Menè P, Dubyak GR, Abboud HE, Scarpa A, Dunn MJ (1988) Mitogenic activity and intracellular signals for thromboxane A_2 in cultured human mesangial cells. Clin Res 36:627A
72. Sutherland DER, Kendall DM, Moudry KC (1988) Pancreas transplantation in non-uremic type I diabetic recipients. Surgery 104:453–464
73. Tegzess AM, Doornbos BM, Minderhound JM, Donker AJ (1988) Prospective serial function studies in patients with nonrenal disease treated with cyclosporine A. Transplant Proc 20 (Suppl 2):390–393

Animal Models of Cyclosporine Nephrotoxicity

THOMAS M. COFFMAN[1]

Introduction

Cyclosporine nephrotoxicity is a significant clinical problem which has limited the therapeutic applications of this potent immunosuppressive agent. Most of the clinical experience defining cyclosporine nephrotoxicity has been in heart, liver and kidney transplant recipients. Since there are a number of factors which influence renal hemodynamics in these patients which are independent of cyclosporine, it has been difficult to isolate specific renal effects attributable to cyclosporine in these patient groups. Thus, much of what is known about the mechanisms of cyclosporine toxicity has been contributed through the development of animal models. The large number of potential cellular and molecular mechanisms of cyclosporine toxicity have been exhaustively reviewed recently [1,2]. In this paper, I will focus on animal models of cyclosporine nephrotoxicity and highlight similarities and differences between these animal models and cyclosporine toxicity in humans.

Clinical Syndromes of Cyclosporine A (CyA) Nephrotoxicity

The two most common clinical syndromes of cyclosporine nephrotoxicity can be broadly divided into acute reversible renal vasoconstriction and chronic irreversible nephropathy. Acute cyclosporine nephrotoxicity is most commonly observed within the first six to twelve months of initiating therapy and is characterized by acute or sub-acute reduction in renal function that is often dose dependent. Generally, this renal dysfunction is non-progressive and reverses with dose reduction or discontinuation of the drug. In renal allograft recipients, it is often difficult to differentiate acute cyclosporine nephrotoxicity from acute rejection. Renal biopsy can be helpful in this setting since aggressive inflammatory cell infiltrates are usually absent in

[1]RM. B3002-Nephrology (111I), VA Medical Center, Durham, NC 27705, USA

acute cyclosporine nephrotoxicity. Further, even stable allograft recipients who have been taking cyclosporine for periods exceeding twelve months will almost invariably manifest some reversible renal dysfunction which is apparent when cyclosporine is discontinued.

Chronic cyclosporine nephropathy is defined by the development of interstitial fibrosis and irreversible reduction in renal function. This form of nephrotoxicity is more ominous than the acute form and is most commonly observed after six to twelve months of therapy [3]. Morphologically, chronic cyclosporine nephropathy is characterized by focal or striped interstitial fibrosis with tubular atrophy [4a]. Often these changes are accompanied by obliterative arteriolar lesions. In more advanced cases, diffuse interstitial fibrosis accompanied by focal and segmental glomerular sclerosis may be seen. In some patients, renal fibrosis and loss of renal function may be progressive [5]. In renal allograft recipients, both the clinical presentation as well as histomorphologic findings in chronic cyclosporine nephropathy are similar to those of chronic rejection. These similarities have made it difficult to identify the role of cyclosporine in producing progressive renal injury in these patients.

While at the extremes these two clinical syndromes are distinct, there is significant overlap of features of both acute and chronic cyclosporine nephrotoxicity in individual patients. Furthermore, the causal relationship between the two syndromes is not clear. Although it has been suggested that chronic renal vasoconstriction and ischemia may produce fibrosis and irreversible renal injury in cyclosporine nephrotoxicity, this has not been proven and would be difficult to establish in clinical trials. Thus, animal models have been developed to attempt to uncover the mechanisms underlying cyclosporine's toxic effects in the kidney. Generally, it has been much easier to reproduce acute reversible renal vasoconstriction in animals than chronic nephropathy. However, several recent reports describe animal models which resemble chronic cyclosporine toxicity in humans [6–10].

Animal Models of Acute and Chronic Cyclosporine Nephrotoxicity

The effects of cyclosporine on the kidney have been evaluated in a number of species including rats, mice, dogs, goats, pigs, and sheep. However, the vast majority of published studies have used rat models and no other species studied present any particular advantage in terms of similarities to the human system. Although CyA pharmacokinetics are very similar in rats and humans [11], the doses of cyclosporine that are required to produce renal dysfunction in rats are generally much higher than those used in patients. The reasons for the rat's resistance to the nephrotoxic effects of CyA have been related to the increased ratio of kidney weight to body weight and increased GFR per kidney weight in rats compared to humans [11]. Despite the difference in dose required to produce nephrotoxicity, there are a number of qualitative similarities in cyclosporine's effects on renal hemodynamics in rats and humans.

As mentioned above, the acute effects of cyclosporine on renal function have been fairly easy to reproduce in animal models. For example, Murray and associates showed that intravenous infusion of cyclosporine to rats produced rapid reduction in renal blood flow and glomerular filtration rate associated with an increase in renal

Table 1. Rat models of chronic cyclosporine nephrotoxicity

Author	CyA dose	Description
Gillum et al.	25 mg/kg per day IP for 28 days	Focal interstitial fibrosis and tubular atrophy, interstitial inflammation and JG hypertrophy
Dieperink et al.	14 mg/kg per day PO for 26 weeks	40% of CyA treated rats developed striped IF
Simpson et al.	20 mg/kg per day for 28–84 days	Striped IF
Rosen et al.	12.5 mg/kg per day SQ for 3–10 weeks	Striped medullary fibrosis in salt depleted animals
Elzinga et al.	15 mg/kg per day SQ for 14–28 days	Tubulointerstitial nephropathy with striped IF in salt depleted animals; progression of IF after CyA withdrawn

vascular resistance [12]. A number of investigators subsequently showed that more prolonged oral or parenteral administration of cyclosporine to rats also caused renal dysfunction. Friedman and associates have shown that CyA has a similar effect on renal hemodynamics in sheep [13]. In studies by Perico et al., rats developed progressive deterioration in renal function over three months when cyclosporine was administered 40 mg/kg every other day [14]. After three months, the cyclosporine was discontinued and GFR rapidly returned to baseline levels. Thus, as in humans, the effects of CyA on renal hemodynamics in rats are reversible when the drug is discontinued.

Early studies of the effects of cyclosporine on the rat kidney focused on the observation of structural abnormalities in the proximal tubule, which included vacuolization and the development of giant mitochondria in proximal tubule cells [15]. Therefore, it was hypothesized that the primary effects of cyclosporine on renal function occurred as a result of this apparent tubular toxicity. However, English et al. subsequently showed that the effect of cyclosporine on renal function in rats was mediated primarily by hemodynamic factors [16]. These authors found that 50 mg/kg per day of cyclosporine caused a progressive fall in glomerular filtration rate without any change in fractional lithium excretion or development of enzymuria which might indicate ongoing tubular injury. In addition, casts made of the renal microvasculature showed a progressive reduction in the diameter of afferent arterioles to less than 50% of control after 14 days of treatment. Studies in humans have also failed to support a significant role for tubular toxicity in CyA associated renal dysfunction.

Although cyclosporine-induced renal vasoconstriction has been relatively easy to reproduce in animals, development of models of chronic cyclosporine nephropathy has been more difficult. Several groups have reported chronic treatment of rats with toxic doses of cyclosporine and have observed only minimal histomorphologic abnormalities [14,17,18]. More recently, several reports have appeared which describe the development of renal fibrosis in rats treated with cyclosporine [6–10]. These papers are summarized in Table 1. In several of these studies rats developed striped interstitial fibrosis which was similar to that described in patients with chronic cyclosporine nephropathy. While these papers have been largely descriptive, the existence of rat models of chronic cyclosporine injury may provide avenues for unravelling the mechanisms of this clinically devastating syndrome. Of particular interest are the

Table 2. Potential mediators of CyA-associated renal vasoconstriction

Sympathetic nervous system
Renin-angiotensin system
Reduced production of vasodilator prostanoids
Increased production of thromboxane A_2
Platelet activating factor
Sulfidopeptide leukotrienes
Endothelin

CyA, cyclosporine A

studies of Rosen et al. [9] and Elzinga et al. [10] which suggest that the development of fibrosis is accelerated by sodium depletion. Furthermore, in the model described by Elzinga, renal fibrosis did not remit when cyclosporine was discontinued. This phenomenon has also been observed in humans.

Mechanisms of Renal Vasoconstriction

Some of the proposed mechanisms of renal vasoconstriction caused by cyclosporine are shown in Table 2. A role for increased activity of the sympathetic nervous system was suggested by Moss et al. [19] who demonstrated increased activity of both efferent and afferent renal nerves in rats receiving intravenous infusions of cyclosporine. Murray and associates showed that renal denervation or treatment with the alpha sympathetic antagonists phenoxybenzamine and prazosin could lessen the degree of renal dysfunction caused by intravenous infusions of cyclosporine in rats [12,20]. Evidence for a role of the sympathetic nervous system in cyclosporine nephrotoxicity in humans is not as compelling. Clearly, cyclosporine nephrotoxicity can occur very soon after renal transplantation before re-innervation of the allograft would be expected to occur. In addition, clinical studies have failed to demonstrate beneficial effects of alpha sympathetic antagonists on renal function in cyclosporine treated renal allograft recipients [21].

There is evidence in both rat and human systems to support a role for altered arachidonic acid metabolism in cyclosporine toxicity. For example, in vitro studies have suggested that cyclosporine may inhibit prostaglandin production [22] and it was hypothesized that this reduced production of vasodilator prostanoids might lead to renal dysfunction. A physiologic role for vasodilator prostanoids was also suggested by the observation that cyclo-oxygenase inhibition exacerbated renal vasoconstriction caused by cyclosporine [12]. However, in vivo inhibition of vasodilator prostaglandins in rats treated with cyclosporine has not been observed [12,17]. Alternatively, pharmacologic doses of stable prostaglandin analogues ameliorate cyclosporine nephrotoxicity in rats [23,24]. For example, Paller showed that 100 µg/kg of the PGE1 analogue misoprostol increased GFR and renal blood flow and reduced renal vascular resistance in cyclosporine treated rats [23]. Kobayashi et al. demonstrated a similar beneficial effect of a stable prostacyclin analogue in another rat model of cyclosporine nephrotoxicity [24]. Efficacy of prostaglandin analogues has also been demonstrated in human renal allograft recipients. Moran et al. showed that renal function in cyclosporine treated renal allograft recipients was improved significantly in patients who also received misoprostol 200 μg four times per day compared to patients who received placebo [25]. In this study, there were no differences in the number of "acute" episodes of cyclosporine nephrotoxicity between the groups. However, the observed differences in long term graft function may reflect a beneficial effect of misoprostol to lessen renal vasoconstriction.

In addition to the potential role of perturbations in the production of vasodilator prostanoids, a number of groups have demonstrated increased production of the vasoconstrictor eicosanoid thromboxane A2 in rats with cyclosporine toxicity [14,17,26,27]. Perico et al. first showed that this increase in thromboxane production is physiologically important by demonstrating an improvement in renal function in cyclosporine toxic rats treated with a thromboxane synthase inhibitor [14]. Several other groups have confirmed this finding. In addition, our group has shown that a thromboxane receptor antagonist had a similar beneficial effect [27]. In our study, intravenous administration of the thromboxane receptor antagonist GR32191 increased GFR and renal blood flow and reduced renal vascular resistance to control levels. We have recently completed a study which suggests that thromboxane may also be important in patients with cyclosporine nephrotoxicity [28]. In this study of cyclosporine-treated renal allograft recipients, we found that urinary excretion of the thromboxane metabolites TXB2 and 2,3 dinor TXB2 were significantly increased in cyclosporine treated patients compared to controls. Intravenous infusions of the thromboxane synthase inhibitor CGS 13080 increased renal plasma flow in eight of the ten patients.

Fish oil supplementation, a non-pharmacologic intervention which also alters arachidonic acid metabolism, has been similarly effective in ameliorating cyclosporine nephrotoxicity. Elzinga et al. have shown in a rat model that by using fish oil as the vehicle for cyclosporine, nephrotoxicity was dramatically reduced [29]. This improvement in renal function was associated with reduced renal cortical thromboxane production. A similar beneficial effect of fish oil in humans was shown by van der Heide [30]. This group found that dietary fish oil supplements improved GFR and renal plasma flow in cyclosporine treated renal allograft recipients. Corn oil supplements had no effect in these patients.

A role for the renin-angiotensin system in cyclosporine mediated renal vasoconstriction has also been postulated [1]. Several groups have reported increased plasma renin activity in rats treated with cyclosporine [12]. Cyclosporine has also been found to stimulate renin release from renal cortical slices [31] and isolated juxtaglomerular cells [32]. However, there have been conflicting reports regarding the efficacy of angiotensin converting enzyme inhibitors in rat models of cyclosporine nephrotoxicity. In addition, plasma renin activity is suppressed in cardiac and renal transplant patients treated with cyclosporine [33]. In renal allograft recipients, the renin-angiotensin system has also been shown to be relatively unresponsive to stimulatory maneuvers such as captopril and diuretics, or changes in posture [34]. Thus, support for a significant role of the renin-angiotensin system is uncertain.

Other isolated reports have suggested the potential involvement of other vasoactive compounds in cyclosporine nephrotoxicity. Santos et al. have demonstrated a beneficial effect of platelet activating factor antagonist on glomerular hemodynamics in rats given cyclosporine [35]. Pasini et al. have shown that a petidoleukotriene antagonist blunts the fall in GFR and renal blood flow caused by 50 mg/kg of cyclosporine given by IV injection [36]. Circulating levels of endothelin have been found to be elevated in rats treated with cyclosporine [37]. In addition, anti-endothelin antibodies given to rats in vivo or in isolated perfused rat kidneys prevent cyclosporine induced renal dysfunction [38]. The relevance of these observations to cyclosporine nephrotoxicity in humans remains to be explored.

Potential Role for Cyclophilin in Nephrotoxicity

Although the molecular mechanisms of cyclosporine's immunosuppressive properties have not been completely defined, recent studies have implicated a 17 kD cyclosporine binding protein as being important in this process [39]. This protein, which has been named cyclophilin, binds avidly and specifically to cyclosporine. It also has peptidyl-prolyl-cis-trans isomerase (PPIase) activity which is inhibited by cyclosporine binding [40]. This PPIase activity is thought to be important in the refolding of proteins. It has been suggested that inhibition of cyclophilin's PPIase activity by cyclosporine may be a mechanism of its immunosuppressive effects. For example, PPIase inhibition may interfere with the conformational assembly of DNA binding proteins which are involved in the transcriptional regulation of genes that are important in generating immune responses, such as interleukin-2.

A role for cyclophilin in animal models of cyclosporine nephrotoxicity has not been explored. However, there are at least three lines of indirect evidence that suggest that cyclophilin and inhibition of its PPIase activity might play a role in cyclosporine nephrotoxicity. Although cyclophilin is present in highest quantities in immune cells, kidney, brain, and liver all contain significant amounts of cyclophilin as well [41]. These organs also represent the three major targets for clinically important toxicities. In addition, the immunosuppressive properties of cyclosporine analogues correlate with cyclophilin binding and, thus far, the major immunosuppressive cyclosporine analogues also appear to be nephrotoxic. Finally, the activity of the new and very potent immunosuppressive agent FK506 also appears to depend on binding to its own specific binding protein which is also a PPIase [42]. The new agent FK506 also causes nephrotoxicity [43,44]. Studies in a rat model showed that renal dysfunction produced by the combination of low doses of cyclosporine and FK506 was greater than that produced by either agent alone [43]. Furthermore, this synergistic nephrotoxicity was also observed in liver transplant patients who were given FK506 as rescue therapy [44]. When FK506 and cyclosporine were being administered simultaneously, patients uniformly developed severe renal toxicities. While the information suggesting that inhibition of certain PPIase enzymes might produce renal toxicity is circumstantial, this area certainly deserves further consideration and study.

Conclusions

Animal models have been useful in defining the mechanisms of cyclosporine induced renal vasoconstriction. These studies suggest that there are similarities in renal hemodynamic responses to cyclosporine in rats compared to humans. Interventions such as treatment with prostaglandin analogues, thromboxane inhibition, and fish oil supplementation are effective in reversing renal hemodynamic abnormalities in both rats and humans treated with cyclosporine. Recent development of models of chronic cyclosporine nephropathy may allow for the definition of the events which lead to this most serious clinical manifestation of cyclosporine renal toxicity. The role of PPIase inhibition in cyclosporine nephrotoxicity is not known; however, there is indirect evidence suggesting its involvement in producing renal dysfunction in this setting.

References

1. Remuzzi G, Bertani T (1989) Renal vascular and thrombotic effects of cyclosporine. Am J Kidney Dis 13:261-272
2. Kopp JB, Klotman PE (1990) Cellular and molecular mechanisms of cyclosporin nephrotoxicity. JASN 1:162-179
3. Ruiz P, Kolbeck PC, Scroggs MW, Sanfilippo F (1988) Associations between cyclosporine therapy and interstitial fibrosis in renal allograft biopsies. Transplantation 45:91-95
4. Myers BD, Sibley R, Newton L, Tomlanovich SJ, Boshkos C, Stinson E, Luetscher JA, Whitney DJ, Krasny D, Coplon NS, Perlroth MG (1988) Kidney Int 33:590-600
4a. Mihatsch MJ, Thiel G, Ryffel B (1988) Histopathology of cyclosporine nephrotoxicity. Transplant Proc 20:759-771
5. Myers BD, Ross J, Newton L, Luetscher J, Perlroth M (1984) Cyclosporine-associated chronic nephropathy. N Engl J Med 311:699-705
6. Gillum DM, Truong L, Tasby J, Migliore P, Suki WN (1988) Chronic cyclosporine nephrotoxicity. Transplantation 46:285-292
7. Dieperink H, Kemp E, Starklint H (1988) Cyclosporine A in high dosages induces renal interstitial fibrosis in the rat. Transplant Proc 20:525-527
8. Simpson JG, Saunders NJ, Thompson KJ, Whiting PH (1988) Chronic renal damage caused by cyclosporine. Transplant Proc 20:792-799
9. Rosen S, Greenfeld Z, Brezis M (1990) Chronic cyclosporine-induced nephropathy in the rat. Transplantation 49:445-452
10. Elzinga LW, Rosen S, Porter GA, Bennett WM (1990) Progression of chronic cyclosporine tubulointerstitial nephropathy despite functional improvement by CSA withdrawal (abstract). Proc XIth Int Congress Nephrol, July 15-20 1990. Tokyo, Japan.
11. Sullivan BA, Hak LJ, Finn WF (1985) Cyclosporine nephrotoxicity: studies in laboratory animals. Transplant Proc 17:145-154
12. Murray BM, Paller MS, Ferris TF (1985) Effect of cyclosporine administration on renal hemodynamics in conscious rats. Kidney Int 28:767-774
13. Friedman AL, Kahng KU, Monaco DO, Rosen BD, Wait RB (1988) Cyclosporine nephrotoxicity in conscious sheep. Transplant Proc 20:595-602
14. Perico N, Benigni A, Zoja C, Delaini F, Remuzzi G (1986) Functional significance of exaggerated renal thromboxane A_2 synthesis induced by cyclosporin A. Am J Physiol 20:F581-F587
15. Thomson AW, Whiting PH, Simpson JG (1984) Cyclosporine: immunology, toxicity and pharmacology in experimental animals. Agents Actions 15:306-327
16. English J, Andrew E, Houghton DC, Bennett WM (1987) Cyclosporine-induced acute renal dysfunction in the rat. Transplantation 44:135-141
17. Coffman TM, Carr DR, Yarger WE, Klotman PE (1987) Evidence that renal prostaglandin and thromboxane production is stimulated in chronic cyclosporine nephrotoxicity. Transplantation 43:282-285
18. Jackson NM, Hsu C-H, Visscher GE, Venkatachalam MA, Humes HD (1987) Alterations in renal structure and function in a rat model of cyclosporine nephrotoxicity. J Pharmacol Exp Ther 242:749-756

19. Moss NG, Powell SL, Falk RJ (1985) Intravenous cyclosporine activates afferent and efferent renal nerves and causes sodium retention in innervated kidneys in rats. Proc Natl Acad Sci USA 82:8222–8226

20. Murray BM, Paller MS (1986) Beneficial effects of renal denervation and prazosin on GFR and renal blood flow after cyclosporine in rats. Clin Nephrol 25:S37–S39

22. Neild GH, Rocchi G, Imaberti L, Fumagalli F, Brown Z, Remuzzi G, Williams DG (1983) Effect of cyclosporine on prostacyclin synthesis by vascular tissue in rabbits. Transplant Proc 4:2398–2400

23. Paller MS (1988) Effects of the prostaglandin E₁ analog misoprostol on cyclosporine nephrotoxicity. Transplantation 45:1126–1131

24. Kobayashi M, Takaya S, Koie H (1988) Effect of a stable analogue of prostacyclin on cyclosporine A-induced nephrotoxicity: morphological qualitative and quantitative studies. Transplant Proc 20:183–186

25. Moran M, Mozes MF, Maddus MS, Veremis S, Bartkus C, Ketel B, Pollak R, Wallemark C, Jonasson O (1990) Prevention of acute graft rejection by the prostaglandin E₁ analogue misoprostol in renal-transplant recipients treated with cyclosporine and prednisone. N Engl J Med 322:1183–1188

25a. Pirotzky E, Colliez P, Guilmard C, Schaeverbeke J, Braquet P (1988) Cyclosporine-induced nephrotoxicity: preventive effect of a PAF-acether antagonist, BN52063. Transplant Proc 20:665–669

26. Petric R, Freeman D, Wallace C, McDonald J, Stiller C, Keown P (1988) Effect of cyclosporine on urinary prostanoid excretion, renal blood flow, and glomerulotubular function. Transplantation 45:883–889

27. Spurney RF, Mavros SD, Collins D, Ruiz P, Klotman PE, Coffman T (1990) Thromboxane receptor blockade improves cyclosporine nephrotoxicity in rats. Prostaglandins 39:135–146

28. Coffman TM, Smith SR, Creech EA, Schaffer AV, Martin LL, Rakhit A, Douglas FL, Klotman PE (1989) The thromboxane synthetase inhibitor CGS13080 improves renal allograft function in patients taking cyclosporine. Kidney Int 37:604A

29. Elzinga L, Kelley VE, Houghton DC, Bennett WM (1987) Modification of experimental nephrotoxicity with fish oil as the vehicle for cyclosporine. Transplantation 43:271–274

30. van der Heide JJH, Bilo HJG, Tegzess AM, Donker AJM (1990) The effects of dietary supplementation with fish oil on renal function in cyclosporine-treated renal transplant recipients. Transplantation 49:523–527

31. Baxter CR, Duggin GG, Hall BM, et al. (1984) Stimulation of renin release from rat renal cortical slices by cyclosporin A. Res Commun Chem Pathol Pharmacol 43:417–423

32. Kurtz A, Della Bruna R, Kuhn K (1988) Cyclosporine A enhances renin secretion and production in isolated juxtaglomerular cells. Kidney Int 33:947–953

33. Schuler S, Thomas D, Hetzer R (1987) Cyclosporine A-related nephrotoxicity after cardiac transplantation: the role of plasma renin activity. Transplant Proc 29:3998–4001

34. Curtis JJ, Luke RG, Jones P, et al. (1988) Hypertension in cyclosporine-treated renal transplant recipients is sodium dependent. Am J Med 85:134–138

35. Santos OFPD, Boim MA, Bregman R, Draibe SA, Barros EJG, Pirotzky E, Schor N, Braquet P (1998) Effect of platelet-activating factor antagonist on cyclosporine nephrotoxicity. Transplantation 47:592–595

36. Pasini M, Perico N, Remuzzi G (1989) Roles for thromboxane and sulfidopeptide leukotrienes in cyclosporine-induced acute renal failure. Kidney Int 37:350A

37. Dadan J, Perico N, Remuzzi G (1989) Role of endothelin in cyclosporine-induced renal vasoconstriction. Kidney Int 37:479A

38. Kon V, Sugiura M, Inagami T, Hoover RL, Fogo A, Harvie BR, Ichikawa I (1989) Cyclosporine causes endothelin-dependent acute renal failure. Kidney Int 37:486A
39. Harding MW, Handschumacher RE (1988) Cyclophilin, a primary molecular target for cyclosporine (1988) Transplantation 46:29S-35S
40. Takahashi N, Hyano T, Suzuki M (1989) Peptidyl-prolyl cis-trans isomerase is the cyclosporin A-binding protein cyclophilin. Nature 337:473-475
41. Koletsky AJ, Harding MW, Handschumacher RE (1986) Cyclophilin: distribution and variant properties in normal and neoplastic tissues. J Immunol 137:1054-1059
42. Harding MW, Galat A, Uehling DE, Schreiber SL (1989) A receptor for the immunosuppressant FK506 is a cis-trans peptidyl-prolyl isomerase. Nature 341:758-760
43. Nalesnik MA, Lai HS, Murase N, Todo S, Starzl TE (1990) The effect of FK 506 and CyA on the Lewis rat renal ischemia model. Transplant Proc 22:87-89
44. McCauley J, Fung J, Jain A, Todo S, Starzl TE (1990) The effects of FK 506 on renal function after liver transplantation. Transplant Proc 22:17-20

Clinical Aspects of Cyclosporine Nephrotoxicity

WILLIAM M. BENNETT[1]

SUMMARY. Nephrotoxicity is the major adverse effect of the valuable immunosuppressive drug cyclosporine. The pharmacology and pharmacokinetic behavior of cyclosporine is complex; clinically relevant considerations, including drug interactions, are covered in this paper. In addition, the major clinical syndromes associated with cyclosporine nephrotoxicity are discussed. These include initial oligoanuria after renal transplant, acute reversible episodes of renal dysfunction, chronic nephrotoxicity with tubulointerstitial fibrosis, hemolytic-uremic syndrome, hypertension, and electrolyte disturbances. An algorithm for distinguishing renal dysfunction due to allograft rejection from acute cyclosporine nephrotoxicity is proposed, since this distinction continues to be a difficult problem for nephrologists. Although therapeutic drug monitoring using blood or plasma cyclosporine levels has not fulfilled its promise, practical guidelines for the use of these studies are presented.

Cyclosporine has emerged has emerged as the mainstay of most transplant immunosuppressive protocols over the past five years. This unique cyclic peptide, containing eleven amino acids, has become the primary immunosuppressive agent in recipients of heart, kidney, liver, heart-lung, and bone marrow allografts. In addition, there are expanding indications for cyclosporine in a wide variety of diseases thought to have an autoimmune or immunologic pathogenesis. This paper will review clinical aspects of cyclosporine nephrotoxicity, the most important adverse reaction observed with this valuable drug. The use of therapeutic drug monitoring as well as important drug interactions will be covered.

Clinically Relevant Pharmacology

Cyclosporine is a neutral hydrophobic compound which selectively inhibits activated lymphocyte function and interleukin-2 mediated events. It is a cyclic undecapeptide

---

[1]Division of Nephrology and Hypertension L463, Oregon Health Sciences University, 3181 S.W. Sam Jackson Park Road, Portland, OR 97201, USA

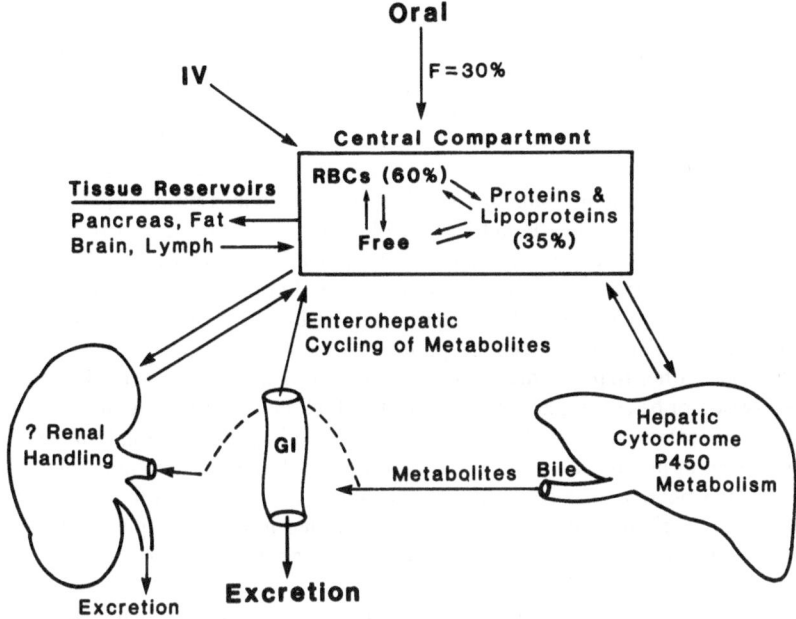

Fig. 1. Cyclosporine pharmacokinetics

produced in cultures as a metabolite of the fungal species *Tolypocladium inflatum gams*. Molecular weight is 1202 Daltons.

Cyclosporine pharmacokinetics are schematically shown in Fig. 1. The prescribing physician should realize that interindividual and intraindividual differences make average kinetic parameters of limited value in the individual complicated transplant recipient. Thus, in the clinical transplant setting, allowance for individual patient factors is necessary for the optimum use of cyclosporine [1].

Cyclosporine is poorly and variably absorbed from the upper part of the small intestine after oral administration. Peak blood concentrations are observed 1 to 8 hours after a given dose, and the extent of absorption varies from 20% to 60%. The extent of absorption and absorption half-life can vary in the same patient over time and differ widely between patients receiving identical doses of cyclosporine on a body weight basis. Time-dependent improvement of absorption is regularly seen in patients treated chronically with cyclosporine, who may increase absorption three- to five-fold over a few months.

Physiologic and pathologic conditions frequently present in transplant recipients may considerably modify cyclosporine absorption. Liver disease and cholestasis can markedly reduce cyclosporine absorption, particularly when there is impairment of bile delivery to the gastrointestinal tract. During the immediate postoperative period in liver transplant recipients, cyclosporine absorption may be less than 5 percent of an administered dose, due to external biliary drainage through a T-tube. When the external drainage of bile is discontinued, drug absorption may increase markedly [1]. Gastrointestinal mucosal disease resulting in diarrhea or poor gastric emptying, as in

Gastrointestinal mucosal disease resulting in diarrhea or poor gastric emptying, as in diabetes mellitus, may also decrease cyclosporine absorption. In liver and gastrointestinal diseases the use of intravenous cyclosporine may be needed in the early post-transplant period to provide consistent immunosuppression.

In whole blood, 55–60% of cyclosporine is bound to red cells, and an additional 30%–35% is bound to lipoproteins. Thus the distribution of cyclosporine in blood is dependent on the patient's hematocrit and lipoprotein concentration [2]. The blood cyclosporine increases linearly until whole blood concentrations reach 1000 ng/ml, after which red blood cells are substantially saturated. When cyclosporine blood concentrations drawn from patients are allowed to stand at room temperature, there is redistribution of cyclosporine from plasma into red cells, falsely lowering plasma concentrations. Thus, many centers prefer to monitor cyclosporine therapy with whole blood rather than plasma levels, particularly in situations where plasma and red cells cannot be separated immediately. The high-density lipoprotein, very low-density lipoprotein and low-density lipoprotein fractions bind virtually all of the cyclosporine in plasma [2]. In transplant patients with plasma lipid abnormalities, free and thus pharmacologically active cyclosporine concentrations may be altered. For example, serious neurotoxicity has been reported in liver transplant recipients with low total cholesterol concentrations and relatively increased concentrations of "free" cyclosporine [3].

Cyclosporine is extensively metabolized by hepatic P450 microsomal mixed function oxidase enzymes, with metabolites and unchanged parent compound appearing primarily in bile. Metabolites probably undergo enterohepatic recycling, resulting in small secondary and tertiary peak blood concentrations in some patients. The predominant metabolites result from demethylation and hydroxylation reactions, leaving the ring structure of the parent cyclosporine molecule intact. In normal volunteers, the elimination half-life of the parent compound is 6–8 h with a slightly longer value (8–9 h) for metabolites [1]. The metabolites of cyclosporine have less immunosuppressive effect than the parent cyclosporine molecule, although some metabolites demonstrate in vitro effects which decrease interleukin-2 production [4]. Since experimental nephrotoxicity can be reduced by hepatic microsomal enzyme inducers such as phenobarbital, it is presumed that the parent cyclosporine molecule, rather than a nephrotoxic metabolite, is the major cause of renal dysfunction. However, the activation of cyclosporine to a nephrotoxic metabolite, by renal tubular drug metabolizing enzymes, has been suggested by recent experimental data [5]. The presence of documented nephrotoxicity with "therapeutic" parent cyclosporine concentrations, as measured by HPLC, is consistent with a role for renally generated metabolites in cyclosporine nephrotoxicity.

Table 1. Clinical presentations of cyclosporine nephrotoxicity

1. Delayed initial function, oligoanuria and acute renal failure
2. Episodes of acute renal dysfunction
3. Chronic cyclosporine-associated nephropathy
   Reversible depression of glomerular filtration rate
   Progressive renal insufficiency
4. Hemolytic-uremic syndrome; thrombotic microangiopathy
5. Hypertension-*de novo* or aggravating pre-existing hypertension
6. Electrolyte disturbances: hyperkalemia, metabolic acidosis, Hypomagnesemia

Pediatric transplant recipients rapidly metabolize cyclosporine, necessitating larger doses on a weight basis to achieve any given cyclosporine blood concentration. Renal excretion plays a limited role in overall cyclosporine elimination, with small amounts of radiolabeled drug appearing in the urine within four days of drug administration. Thus the presence of renal failure does not influence cyclosporine pharmacokinetics, and no adjustment of dosage is required. Due to its high molecular weight and relatively avid binding to blood components, little cyclosporine is lost during hemodialysis or peritoneal dialysis, and no dosage adjustments are necessary.

Nephrotoxicity

Although the most frequent and potentially limiting consequence of cyclosporine immunosuppression is nephrotoxicity, the clinical presentations of these adverse effects are diverse [6] (Table 1). Each of these syndromes will be briefly summarized.

Oligoanuria and Acute Renal Failure

Lack of initial function of renal transplants, necessitating dialysis, is more frequent with cyclosporine immunosuppression than with azathioprine. This has been attributed to high initial cyclosporine doses (> 15 mg/kg) or introduction of the drug prior to onset of urine flow. Ischemic injury to the kidney due to adverse procurement conditions potentiates this problem [7]. Cyclosporine-treated patients, even when function ultimately improves, have approximately twice as long a period of oligoanuria as azathioprine-treated patients [8]. There is evidence that cadaver kidneys experiencing prolonged oligoanuria have inferior one- and two-year survival despite the fact that serum creatinine often returns to normal following the oliguric period. There is an analogous period of acute renal failure following heart transplantation, presumably due to high initial cyclosporine doses interacting with the ischemic renal injury produced by heart bypass.

Reduction of initial cyclosporine doses to 5–8 mg/kg in renal transplantation and 8–10 mg/kg in cardiac transplantation has minimized the problem of poor initial renal function. Some centers prefer to withhold cyclosporine until serum creatinine falls below 2–3 mg/dl and urine output is well established. There is increasing use of induction immunosuppression with monoclonal antibodies or antilymphocyte globulin to prevent early rejection, prior to beginning cyclosporine.

Monitoring of cyclosporine blood levels and percutaneous allograft biopsy during the period of oligoanuria is crucial for minimization of this problem. In patients with non-function for more than 7–10 days, percutaneous biopsy of the allograft is very helpful in excluding clinically silent rejection so that anti-rejection treatment can be instituted.

Episodes of Acute Renal Dysfunction

Many renal transplant patients treated with cyclosporine develop episodes of acute renal insufficiency. Since these episodes improve rapidly within a few days if cyclosporine dosage is reduced, and since similar episodes are common in recipients of

Table 2. Renal histopathology in cyclosporine-treated allograft recipients[9]

Clinical condition	Finding	Comment
Acute renal dysfunction	Proximal tubular cell vacuolization Microcalcification in tubular cells	Nonspecific, probably a marker of cyclosporine treatment since tubular function preserved. Cell necrosis absent
	Glomerular capillary thrombi	Associated with a poor graft outcome; can be noted in grafts without cyclosporine and in grafts with stable function
	Obliterative arteriopathy of varying severity in interlobar and arcuate vessels; patchy cell necrosis	May produce microangiopathic hemolytic anemia and thrombocytopenia; results in graft loss; found in approximately 10 percent of cases
Initial oligoanuria with acute renal failure	Arteriolar wall hyalinosis	Present with prolonged renal failure; may be permanent; infrequently found
	Diffuse interstitial fibrosis	Renal failure may be partially reversible; seen primarily in nonbeating heart cadaver donors
	Normal post-transplant biopsy	Most frequent finding in first 3–4 post-transplant weeks
Chronic renal dysfunction	Striped pattern of tubulointerstitial fibrosis, glomerulosclerosis	Irreversible changes; frequently associated with hypertension
	Hyalinosis and sclerosis of arterioles and small arteries	May be observed in normotensive patients

non-renal allografts, they have been attributed to cyclosporine nephrotoxicity. In the renal transplant recipient these episodes are difficult to distinguish from rejection, particularly in the absence of fever, allograft tenderness, and oliguria. Both rejection and cyclosporine nephrotoxicity may be associated with decreased fractional sodium excretion and isosthenuria. Often the correct diagnosis of these episodes can be made only after observing the patient's response to a therapeutic maneuver such as anti-rejection therapy or cyclosporine dose reduction. Although trough cyclosporine levels may be high in patients subsequently proven to have acute cyclosporine nephrotoxicity, a normal or low level does not exclude the diagnosis. In some circumstances, cyclosporine can act synergistically with rejection to produce renal dysfunction.

Biopsy of the easily accessible renal allograft during episodes of acute renal dysfunction is often critical to exclude treatable rejection. The histopathologic features observed in patients treated with cyclosporine (summarized in Table 2) are largely markers of therapy with this agent, not necessarily indicative of toxicity.

The management of acute renal dysfunction can be difficult, particularly in renal transplant recipients, since rejection is often impossible to exclude confidently. Table 3 compares features of rejection to acute cyclosporine nephrotoxicity. Since rejection is still the most likely reason for renal dysfunction, especially in the first six months after transplant, this possibility needs to be actively excluded in order for the patient to receive appropriate therapy. An elevation of trough cyclosporine blood concentrations is helpful if present, but cyclosporine-induced renal dysfunction is frequently present despite "therapeutic" levels. Signs suggesting rejection include

Table 3. Comparison of acute rejection and cyclosporine-associated renal allograft dysfunction

Signs or symptoms	CSA	Rejection
Fever, graft tenderness	Absent	Present in 25%
Oliguria	Absent	Present in 50%
Graft swelling (clinical ultrasound, NMR, fine needle manometry)	Absent	Present in 50%
Hypertension	75%	50%
Blood CSA concentration	Normal or High	Normal
Renal perfusion by isotope scan	Decreased in 75%	Decreased in virtually all
Hyperkalemic metabolic acidosis with hyperchloremia	15%	5%
Factional excretion of sodium	Low	Low in first 2 days, then increased
Biopsy; fine needle aspirates	Subtle features; absence of rejection	Usually diagnostic

increase in graft size found by ultrasound, elevations of intra-renal hydrostatic pressure found by thin needle manometry, or tubular cell changes in fine needle aspirates. Most centers prefer to perform a core biopsy on the allograft to diagnose and treat subtle rejection, if present. If steroid or monoclonal antibody treatment for rejection is unsuccessful in effecting an improvement in renal function, reduction in cyclosporine dosage by 0.5–1.0 mg/kg every 5–7 days may be beneficial. Rejection can be diagnosed with confidence if a diffuse interstitial infiltrate or arteritis is present. Focal mononuclear infiltrates can be present with proven cyclosporine nephrotoxicity and thus are not specific for rejection. Arteriolar hyalinosis is more frequently observed in patients with cyclosporine nephrotoxicity [10]. If the transplant biopsy fails to show acute rejection, particularly if arteriolar hyalinosis is present, empiric dose reduction is indicated in an attempt to avoid chronic tubulointerstitial fibrosis, which has been noted in many patients with frequent episodes of reversible cyclosporine-induced creatinine rises. An algorithm which can be used for this differential diagnosis is shown in Table 4.

Chronic Cyclosporine-Associated Nephropathy

Progressive renal insufficiency is well documented in transplant recipients receiving cyclosporine for over 12 months. While this process can be attributed to chronic allograft rejection in renal transplant recipients, in non-renal recipients and in patients with autoimmune disease, it is most certainly due to a nephrotoxic effect of cyclosporine. Long-term cyclosporine treated recipients, as a group, have lower glomerular filtration rates than comparable patients immunosuppressed with azathioprine [11]. In a series of heart transplant recipients the decline in renal function could not be attributed to cardiac dysfunction since cardiac performance was normal and similar to that in azathioprine-treated heart recipients [12]. Similar chronic renal dysfunction has been described in long-term liver transplant recipients and patients receiving long-term cyclosporine therapy for autoimmune uveitis [13,14]. While excessive initial doses of cyclosporine may play a role in chronic nephrotoxicity, the condition may be progressive, despite dose reduction. In some patients, however, stopping cyclosporine altogether after a year of treatment results

Table 4. Algorithm for management of acute renal dysfunction in renal transplantation

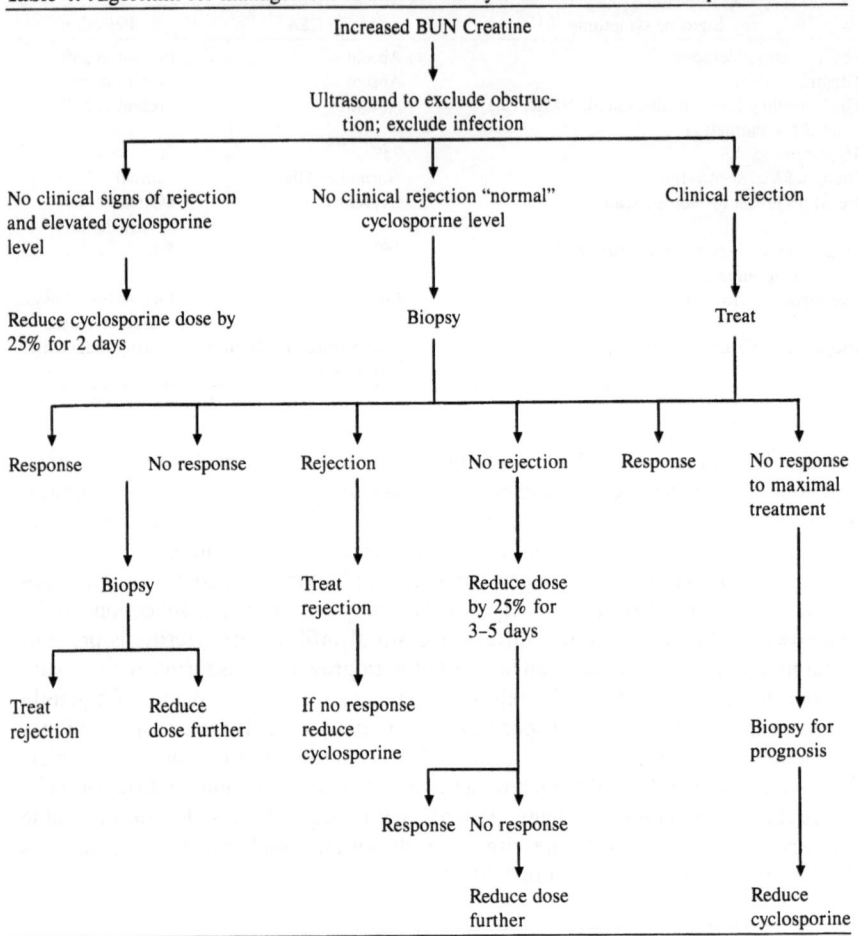

in rapid improvement in renal hemodynamics and function [15]. Whether permanent structural damage remains is unknown. Several patients have required dialysis for end-stage renal disease due to chronic cyclosporine nephrotoxicity [12]. Clinically, hypertension and proteinuria are noted even in non-renal recipients, excluding rejection as an explanation for the findings. Biopsy findings in renal and non-renal recipients show chronic tubulointerstitial fibrosis with focal and segmental glomerulosclerosis [12].

Patients treated with cyclosporine may have very subtle changes in renal function. In patients with autoimmune disease, for example, creatinine clearance commonly falls gradually. When the drug is withdrawn, renal function returns to baseline even after one year of treatment. Some, but not all, of these patients develop *de novo* hypertension, and most have rises in mean arterial pressure even though values remain less than 140/90. These patients generally have no other reason for the decline in renal function and maintain stable but elevated serum creatinine values during the entire treatment period. Reduction of dose and combination therapy with other immunosuppressive drugs may minimize the decline in creatinine clearance. The lack of sensitivity of the serum creatinine and creatinine clearance in discerning progressive tubulointerstitial renal disease make it difficult to dismiss this result of cyclosporine therapy as harmless and "reversible" until long-term follow-up is available. The number of cases of chronic nephrotoxicity evolving within the group thought to have stable but reversible renal dysfunction described above is unknown.

Gradual withdrawal of cyclosporine or triple-therapy regimens using low-dose cyclosporine with azathioprine and prednisone may reduce the severity and frequency of chronic cyclosporine nephrotoxicity [16,17].

Hemolytic-Uremic Syndrome: Thrombotic Microangiopathy

Rises in direct bilirubin without other liver function abnormalities have been reported with cyclosporine immunosuppression. In some patients this is associated with fulminant acute renal failure and thrombocytopenia [18]. This syndrome, reported primarily in bone marrow transplant recipients, also occurs *de novo* in renal transplantation [19]. In renal transplantation, this vasculopathy confers a poor prognosis on the allograft despite absence of pathologic changes of acute rejection. Histological examination of the kidneys reveals arteriolar lesions similar to the hemolytic-uremic syndrome, with thrombotic microangiopathy and occasionally afferent arteriolar thrombosis. Plasmapheresis has been used to induce hematological remission and renal recovery [20]. The causative role of the nodular hyalinotic vascular lesions, without obvious clinical rejection, seen in some renal transplant biopsies in this rare manifestation of cyclosporine nephrotoxicity is unclear, since a minority of patients develop clinical symptoms. However, thrombotic microangiopathy may occur in transplants not treated with cyclosporine, as recurrence of original disease or as a rare manifestation of allograft rejection.

During periods of renal dysfunction related to cyclosporine, high concentrations of factor VIII related antigen have been noted; these fall to normal as the dose of the drug is decreased [21]. This phenomenon has been interpreted as additional evidence that vascular injury is a major component of cyclosporine nephrotoxicity.

Hypertension

Increases of blood pressure, either *de novo* or from previously hypertensive levels, are frequently seen in cyclosporine treated patients [22]. In cardiac transplantation where renal rejection is not present, the majority of cyclosporine-treated patients are hypertensive, compared to historical data from azathioprine-treated patients [23]. Although renal function is usually also decreased, this is not uniformly true. Conventional approaches to antihypertensive therapy are often ineffective, necessitating multiple drug regimens. When measured, plasma volume is increased, plasma renin activity is low, and the renin-angiotensin axis is relatively unresponsive to stimulatory maneuvers such as upright posture and diuretics [24]. Increases in plasma renin activity in response to converting enzyme inhibition by captopril is blunted, compared to the usual hypertensive subject.

Despite this indirect evidence for volume expansion, diuretics may actually aggravate the pressure elevation. There is emerging evidence that calcium entry blockers are useful as monotherapy. Poor therapeutic results are often obtained with vasodilators, beta blockers, and converting enzyme inhibitors.

Electrolyte Disturbances

Hyperkalemia, with mild hyperchloremic metabolic acidosis, has been reported with cyclosporine therapy in patients with relatively well-preserved glomerular filtration rates [25]. Anion gaps are normal, and virtually all patients reported have urine pH values less than 6. Plasma renin activities are low or normal and plasma aldosterone levels are normal. When cyclosporine dosage is reduced, the electrolyte patterns return towards normal. Whether this is a primary renal effect of the drug or, more likely, the result of chronic tubulointerstitial fibrosis and hyporeninemic hypoaldosteronism is unclear. Detailed studies of the renin-angiotensin system correlated with renal histopathology are unavailable.

Hypomagnesemia is common during cyclosporine therapy, especially in bone marrow recipients. Accompanying tubular toxins such as aminoglycosides and amphotericin are often present. Occasionally serum magnesium concentrations fall to less than 1 mEq/l in conjunction with inappropriate urinary magnesium wasting [26]. Magnesium deficiency could partially explain some of the seizures which can occur in patients as an adverse effect of cyclosporine.

Drug Interactions

Drugs which influence hepatic drug metabolizing enzymes may cause clinically significant changes in cyclosporine pharmacokinetics. Drugs which interact with cyclosporine are listed in Table 5. Some of these interactions have been reported only in anecdotal case reports, and their clinical importance is unclear. Corticosteroids used in most transplant recipients have complex effects on cyclosporine metabolism. High doses of methylprednisolone used for treatment of rejection crises, as well as long-term steroid therapy, may increase cyclosporine biotransformation to inactive metabolites [27]. Any potential loss of immunosuppressive effect may be counterbalanced by an independent effect in which cyclosporine decreases prednisone metabolism [27,28].

Monitoring of Cyclosporine Blood Concentrations

Because of the multiple clinical and pharmacological variables present in any individual allograft recipient, therapeutic drug monitoring is practiced in some form by most transplant units. Whether such monitoring justifies its expense and inconvenience is still not clear after a decade of wide therapeutic use of cyclosporine. By monitoring blood concentrations, problems in patient compliance and/or drug absorption can be discovered. However, as a goal for therapy in individual patients, blood level monitoring may be disappointing. Rejection of an allograft frequently occurs with "therapeutic" blood levels, and reversible nephrotoxicity can be documented in patients when decreases in "nontoxic" blood concentrations result in

Table 5. Clinically relevant drug interactions with cyclosporine

Increased metabolism: Decreased blood levels, loss of immunosuppression
  Anticonvulsants
    Carbamazepine
    Phenytoin
    Phenobarbital
  Antituberculous Drugs
    Rifampicin
    Isoniazid

Decreased metabolism: Increased blood levels, increased risk of nephrotoxicity
  Antimicrobial Agents
    Erythromycin
    Fluconazole
    Ketoconazole
  Miscellaneous
    Androgens, oral contraceptives[a]
    Cimetidine
    Calcium blockers – nicardipine, diltiazem, verapamil

Potentiated or Additive Nephrotoxicity
  Aminoglycoside antibiotics
  Amphotericin B
  Cephalosporin antibiotics (cefotaxime, cefuroxime)[b]
  Digoxin[d]
  Etoposide[c]
  Mannitol[b 7.5]
  Furosemide[b]
  Melphelan
  Nonsteroidal anti-inflammatory drugs
  Trimethoprim-sulfamethoxazole

[a]Hepatotoxicity reported
[b]Documented only in experimental animals
[c]Enhanced CNS and hepatotoxicity
[d]Reduced volume of distribution of digoxin

improved kidney function. Whenever a major change, such as a concomitant illness or a new therapeutic agent, occurs in the patient's condition it may be prudent to measure a cyclosporine level after two to three days to be assured that no major change in cyclosporine kinetics has occurred.

Because of the differences in absolute drug concentrations between individuals on given doses and the confounding effects of dose regimen (once versus twice daily dosing), food, age, meals, and even time of day, generalizations are difficult. These factors must constantly be considered before making changes in an effective therapeutic program simply because of a change in blood concentration. Most transplant programs monitor blood levels two to three times per week in the perioperative period, followed by a period of weekly surveillance for several months, and then checks at monthly or quarterly intervals. It should also be remembered that higher doses are required shortly after transplant and that target concentrations can be reduced at later time periods. Most transplant centers monitor the cyclosporine level prior to the next scheduled dose because of the marked variability in the time and height of peak concentrations.

References

1. Ptachcinski RJ, Venkataramanan R, Burckart GJ (1986) Clinical pharmacokinetics of cyclosporine. Clin Pharmacokinet 11:107-132
2. Sgoutas D, MacMahon W, Love A, Jerkunica I (1986) Interaction of cyclosporin A with human lipoproteins. J Pharm Pharmacol 38:583-588
3. de Groen PC, Aksamit AJ, Rakela J, Forbes GS, Krom RAF (1987) Central nervous system toxicity after liver transplantation: the role of cyclosporine and cholesterol. N Engl J Med 317:861-866
4. Freed BM, Rosano TG, Lempert N (1987) In vitro immunosuppressive properties of cyclosporine metabolites. Transplantation 43:123-127
5. Buss WC, Stepanek J, Bennett WM (1989) A new proposal for the mechanism of cyclosporine A nephrotoxicity: inhibition of renal microsomal chain elongation following *in vivo* cyclosporine A. Biochem Pharmacol 38:4085-4093
6. Von Graffenried B, Krupp P (1986) Side effects of cyclosporine (Sandimmun) in renal transplant recipients and in patients with autoimmune diseases. Transplant Proc 18:876-883
7. Canadian Multicentre Trial Group (1983) A randomized clinical trial of cyclosporine in cadaveric renal transplantation. N Engl J Med 309:809-815
8. Hall BM, Tiller DJ, Duggin GG, Horvath JS, Farnsworth A, May J, Johnson JR, Shiel AGR (1985) Post-transplant acute renal failure in cadaver renal recipients treated with cyclosporine. Kidney Int 28:178-186
9. Mihatsch MJ, Thiel G, Spichtin HP (1983) Morphological findings in kidney transplants after treatment with cyclosporine. Transplant Proc 15:2821-2835
10. Nield GH, Taube DH, Hartley RB, Bignardi L, Cameron JS, Williams DG, Ogg CS, Rudge CJ (1986) Morphological differentiation between rejection and cyclosporin nephrotoxicity in renal allografts. J Clin Pathol 39:152-159
11. Myers BD (1986) Cyclosporine nephrotoxicity. Kidney Int 30:964-974
12. Myers BD, Sibley R, Newton L, Tomlanovich SJ, Boshkos C, Stinson E, Luetscher JA, Whitney DJ, Krasney D, Coplon NS, and Perlroth M (1988) The long term course of cyclosporine-associated chronic nephropathy. Kidney Int 33:590-600
13. Dische FE, Neuberger J, Keating J, Parsons V, Calne RY, Williams R (1988) Kidney pathology in liver allograft recipients after long-term treatment with cyclosporin A. Lab Invest 58:395-402
14. Palestine AG, Austin HA, Balow JE, Antonovych TT, Sabnis SG, Preuss HG, Nussenblatt RB (1986) Renal histopathologic alterations in patients treated with cyclosporine for uveitis. N Engl J Med 314:1293-1298
15. Curtis JJ, Luke RG, Jones P, Dubovsky EV, Whelchel JD, Diethelm AG (1986) Cyclosporine in therapeutic doses increases renal allograft resistance. Lancet II:477-479
16. Kahan BD (1989) Cyclosporine. N Engl J Med 321:1725-1738
17. Bennett WM, Normal DJ (1986) Action and toxicity of cyclosporine. Ann Rev Med 37:215-224
18. Shulman H, Striker G, Deeg HJ, Kennedy M, Storb R, Thomas EG (1981) Nephrotoxicity of cyclosporin A after allogeneic marrow transplantation: Glomerular thromboses and tubular injury. N Engl J Med 305:1392-1395
19. Van Buren D, Van Buren CT, Flechner SM, Maddox AM, Verani R, Kahan BD (1985) *De novo* hemolytic uremic syndrome in renal transplant recipients immunosuppressed with cyclosporine. Surgery 98:54-62
20. Keusch G, Gmür J, Baumgartner D, Burger HR, Largiader F, Binswanger V (1986) *De novo* hemolytic uremic syndrome in two renal allograft recipients treated with cyclosporine: Successful therapy with plasmapheresis. Transplant Proc 18:1097-1098

21. Braun Z, Neild GH, Willougby JJ, Somia NV, Cameron SJ (1986) Increased Factor VIII as an index of vascular injury in cyclosporine nephrotoxicity. Transplantation 42:150–153
22. Luke RG (1987) Hypertension in renal transplant recipients. Kidney Int 31:1024–1037
23. Bellet M, Cabrol C, Sassano P, Leger P, Corvol P, Menard J (1985) Systemic hypertension after cardiac transplantation: Effect of cyclosporine on the renin-angiotensin-aldosterone system. Am J Cardiol 56:927–931
24. Bantle JP, Nath KA, Sutherland DE, Najarian JS, Ferris TF (1985) Effects of cyclosporine on the renin-angiotensin-aldosterone system and potassium excretion in renal transplant patients. Arch Intern Med 145:505–508
25. Stahl R, Kanz L, Maier B, Schollmeyer P (1986) Hyperchloremic metabolic acidosis with high serum potassium in renal transplant recipients: A cyclosporine A associated side· effect. Clin Nephrol 25:245–248
26. June CH, Thompson CB, Kennedy MS, Nims J, Thomas ED (1985) Profound hypomagnesemia and renal magnesium wasting associated with the use of cyclosporine for marrow transplantation. Transplantation 39:620–624
27. Ost L, Klintmalm G, Ringden O (1985) Mutual interaction between prednisolone and cyclosporine in renal transplant patients. Transplant Proc 17:1252–1255
28. Burckart GJ, Canafax DM, Yee GC (1986) Cyclosporine monitoring. Drug Intell Clin Pharm 20:649–652

Evolution of Cyclosporin Nephrotoxicity

Michael J. Mihatsch and Bernhard Ryffel[1]

Summary. Cyclosporine (CsA) nephrotoxicity is reviewed with special emphasis on the development of the morphological lesion. Renal lesions are essentially confined to the proximal tubules and arterioles. At both sites cellular degenerative changes develop, which consist of vacuolization, inclusion bodies, mitochondrial abnormalities, and single cell necroses. Similar morphological changes, which indicate a direct effect of the drug, are inducible in experimental animals and in cell culture.

In contrast to the occurrence of functional nephrotoxicity (reduction of glomerular filtration rate) the morphological changes essentially occur after high CsA exposure. Whereas tubular lesions are generally reversible, the arteriolar alterations may progress and cause irreversible ischemic tissue damage. From repeat biopsies in single patients the evolution, especially of the arteriolar lesions, was followed. Endothelial cell and myocyte degeneration with platelet deposition and protein extravasation was followed by tissue repair, resulting in luminal obliteration and downstream ischemic fibrosis.

Studies with radiolabelled CsA on cells from different sources revealed that CsA is concentrated intracellularly by the specific binding protein cyclophilin. Analyses of the radioligand data revealed two binding components: a saturable cytosolic binding and a non-saturable membrane binding. It is speculated that immunosuppression is mediated by cyclophilin, whereas morphological renal changes which occur at high drug levels are due to binding and probably disintegration of the cell membranes.

Introduction

Recently, there has been discussion of a variety of factors which may mediate Cyclosporin (CsA) toxicity [1,2], e.g., disturbed prostaglandin metabolism, release of endothelin, reduction of endothelium-derived relaxing factor, activation of the

---

[1]Institute of pathology, Schönbeinstrasse 40, CH-4003 Basel, Switzerland

renin-angiotensin system, and stimulation of the autonomous nervous system. However, changes of many of these factors are secondary rather than causative of CsA toxicity. This hypothesis is supported by experimental studies in rats in which glomerular filtration and prostaglandin metabolism was investigated. Whereas CsA caused immediate reduction in glomerular filtration rates, renal urinary prostaglandin excretion occurred at least 6 days after commencement of CsA treatment. Thus, alterations in prostaglandin metabolism are unlikely to be the cause of renal vasoconstriction. As a second example, the possible role of an activated renin-angiotensin system in CsA toxicity has been investigated. An immunohistochemical study of the juxtaglomerular apparatus was performed on kidney biopsies from patients before and after CsA therapy [3]. The CsA treatment group consisted of patients with kidney transplants, bone marrow transplants, heart transplants, and juvenile diabetes. The size of the juxtaglomerular apparatus did not differ in patients with either short or long term drug administration. This finding, however, does not invalidate the functional findings reported by Myers [4], who showed increased prorenin levels, but it does refute consistent hypertrophy of the juxtaglomerular apparatus. Without reviewing all the experimental evidence, the proposed pathogenic factors mentioned above cannot explain the morphologic lesions which possibly are the key to the understanding of CsA toxicity. The following overview, therefore, focuses on factors responsible for the development of morphologic lesions and addresses the question whether CsA has a direct toxic effect on target cells.

The concept of CsA nephrotoxicity was developed on the basis of morphological findings in man. Therefore, in the first part of this review, CsA toxicity found in man and duplicated in animal and cell culture is presented; with emphasis being placed on the development of the structural lesions. In the second part of this review, the role of cellular drug uptake, intracellular concentration, and binding to the cell membrane for the development of morphologic lesions is discussed.

Overview of CsA-Toxicity in Man

Based on morphological criteria, CsA toxicity can be divided into functional toxicity and morphological toxicity [1,2,5]. Functional and morphological toxicity occur in the renal tubule and in the vascular system, as shown in Fig. 1. Morphological lesions, which will be discussed here, may also be a key for understanding functional toxicity.

The morphological changes seen in *tubular toxicity* (Fig. 2) comprise inclusion bodies in tubular epithelial cells (corresponding to giant mitochrondria), isometric tubular vacuolization, and microcalcification. These different lesions of tubular toxicity are most often found in one and the same biopsy. They may occur, however, in any combination and even giant mitochondria or isometric vacuolization or microcalcification may be found alone. Vascular lesions (see below) may be present or absent. Tubular changes are found in kidney transplants as well as in bone marrow and heart transplant recipients and in patients with autoimmune diseases.

Giant mitochondria, usually one per cell, occur predominantly in the convoluted part (S 1,2 segment) of the proximal tubule. The morphology of giant mitochondria lacks any specificity. Isometric vacuolization is almost exclusively found in the straight part of the proximal tubule (S 3 segment) of a few nephrons. The light microscopic picture is identical to that of osmotic nephrosis. All or most of the

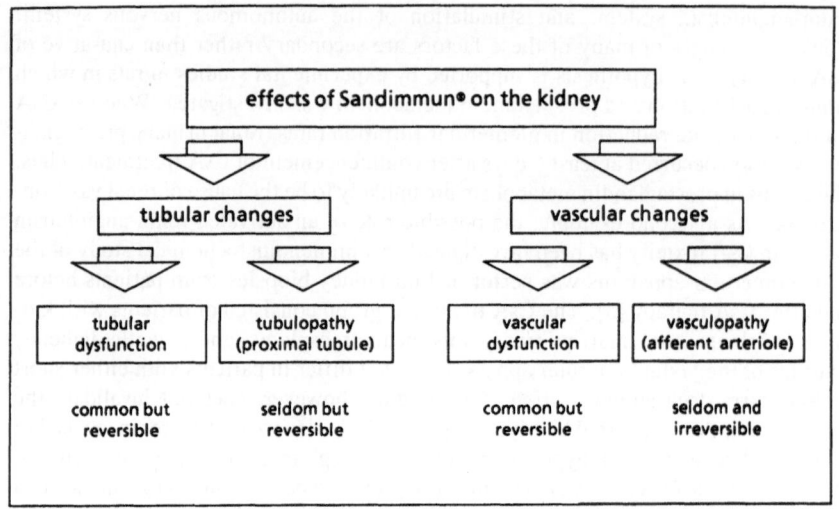

Fig. 1. Classification of CsA (Sandimmun)-toxicity

tubular cells in a cross-section contain densely packed empty vacuoles (free of lipids) of equal size. Vacuolization is at least partly due to a dilatation of the smooth endoplasmatic reticulum. Giant mitochondria and isometric vacuolization were never observed in one and the same cell. Sometimes the nuclei of the cells affected by isometric vacuolization are pycnotic, and the brush border of the cells may be missing. Single cell necroses are rare. Microcalcifications of a single cell or groups of tubular cells are found in various parts of the nephron. They are round, crescent,

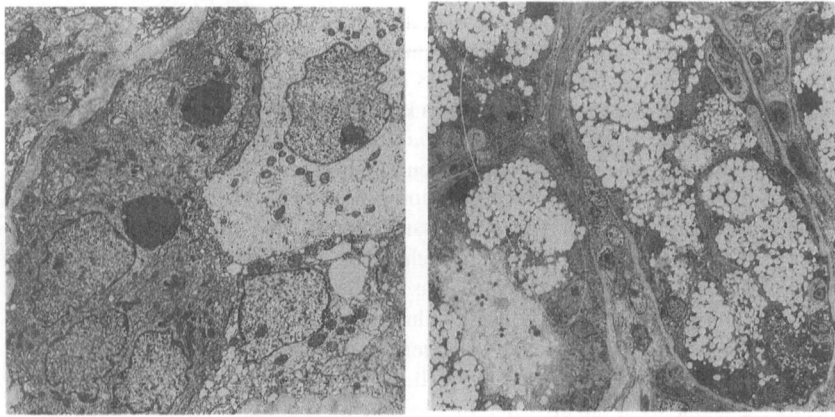

Fig. 2. Tubular toxicity: tubular cross-sections with inclusion bodies (giant mitochondria (*left*) or isometric vacuolization (*right*))

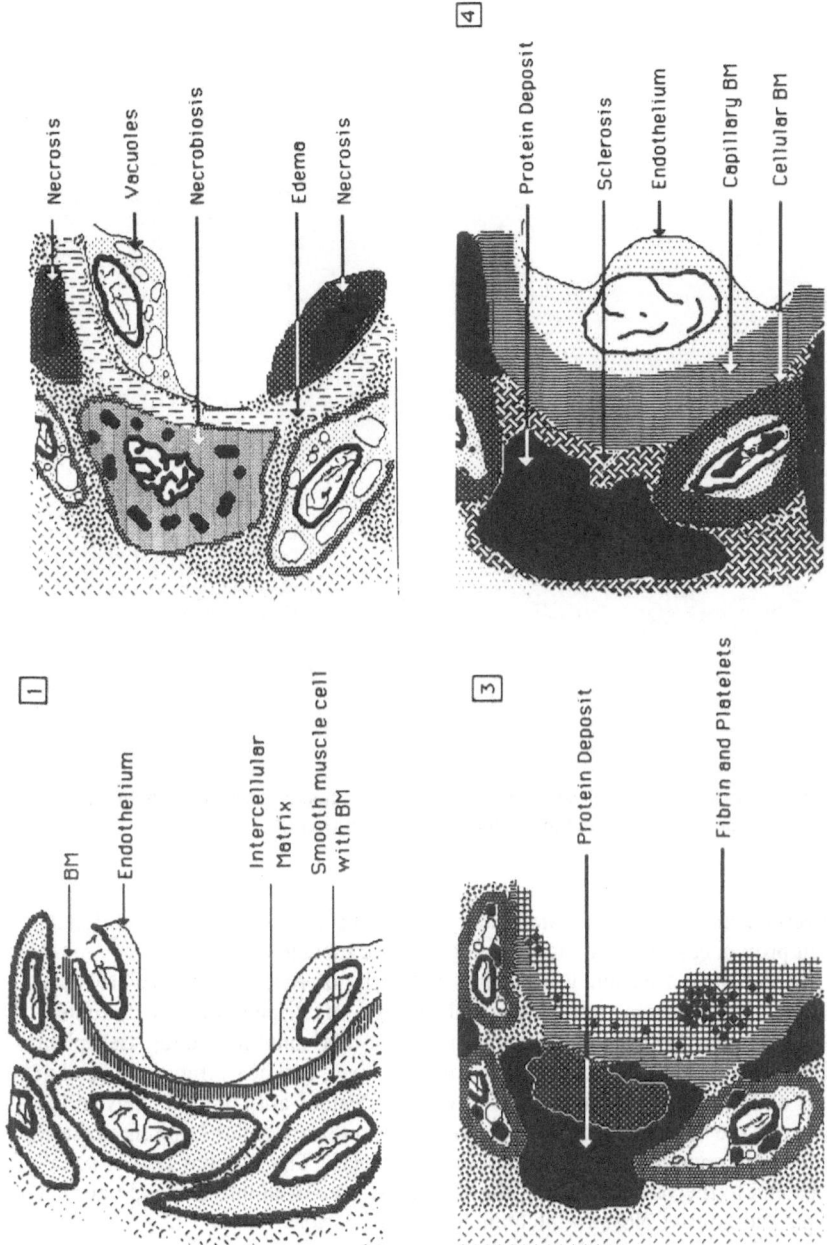

Fig. 3. Morphogenesis of CsA-associated arteriolopathy (see text)

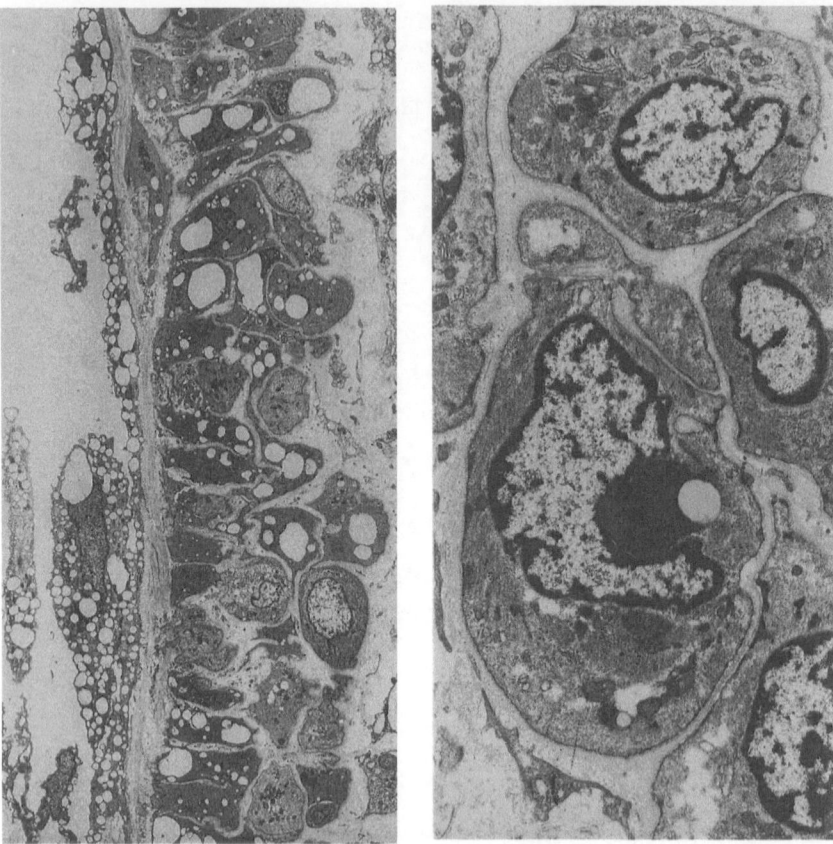

Fig. 4. Vascular toxicity: vacuolization of endothelial and smooth muscle cells of an arteriole (*left*) or inclusion body (*lysosome*) in a smooth muscle cell (*right*)

or polycyclic in shape. Microcalcification is the result of calcification of Tamm-Horsfall protein casts and possibly also of necrotic tubular cells.

By far the most frequent lesions and hallmarks of *vascular toxicity* are CsA-associated arteriolopathy and interstitial fibrosis of striped form with tubular atrophy. Vascular (interstitial) toxicity is found not only in kidney transplant recipients, but also in patients with bone marrow, liver, and heart transplants and in patients with autoimmune diseases. The vascular lesions are predominately in the periphery of the vascular tree. They are confined to the arterioles (afferent vessels) and arteries in up to two layers of smooth muscle cells. The vascular lesions sometimes extend to the vascular pole of the glomerulus and even into some glomerular segments and arteries close to the branching into arterioles.

The morphogenesis [6] is deduced from observations of the various stages occurring concurrently or in serial biopsies (Fig. 3). The earliest lesions visible by light microscopy, and seen even more clearly by electron microscopy, are endothelial or

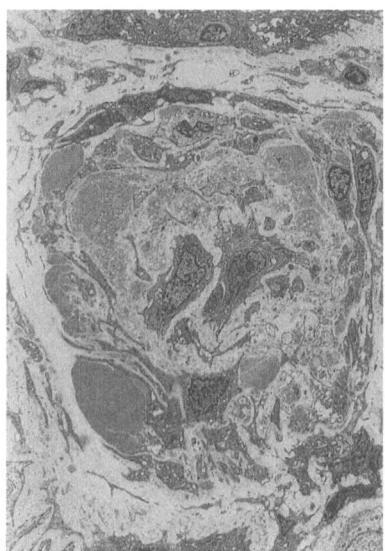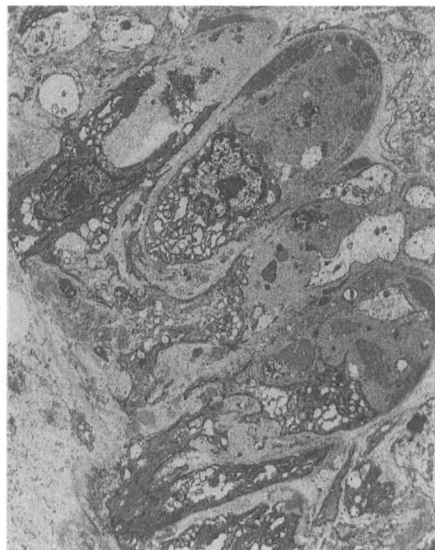

Fig. 5. Vascular toxicity: Nodular protein deposits in necrotic smooth muscle cells and complete occlusion of the arteriolar lumen (*left*). Higher magnification showing necrotic smooth muscle cells replaced by protein insudates (*right*)

myocyte damage with vacuolization, inclusion bodies (lysosomes), and single cell necrosis (Fig. 4). These lesions are followed by fibrin and platelet deposition in arterioles and/or in glomeruli. The full picture of CsA-associated arteriolopathy results from the insudation of plasma proteins into the damaged vessel wall giving rise to nodular and circular protein deposits, often at sites of necrotic myocytes (Fig. 5). The protein deposits give positive immunohistological reactions for complement components and also for IgM. If the arteriole is not completely occluded, the endothelium regenerates and rests upon a thickened basement membrane. In the arteriolar tunica media the nodular protein deposits persist and the remaining myocytes are surrounded by thickened basement membranes and embedded in a sclerotic matrix. If the arterioles are completely occluded, the glomeruli become obsolescent, but if the vascular lumen is only narrowed the glomerulus may collapse. Since the blood supply of the tubular-interstitial space depends on the integrity of the preglomerular vessels, narrowing of the arterioles results in the ischemic damage of these structures. Thus, tubular atrophy and interstitial fibrosis (Fig. 6) are the consequences of the arteriolar changes.

In summary, the primary morphological lesions seen in man are confined to the proximal tubules and the arterioles. They consist of mitochondrial abnormalities, vacuolization, and occasional single cell necrosis. All other lesions, e.g., fibrin or platelet thrombi, protein insudation in the vascular wall, and interstitial fibrosis with tubular atrophy—must be considered as sequelae of the primary lesions.

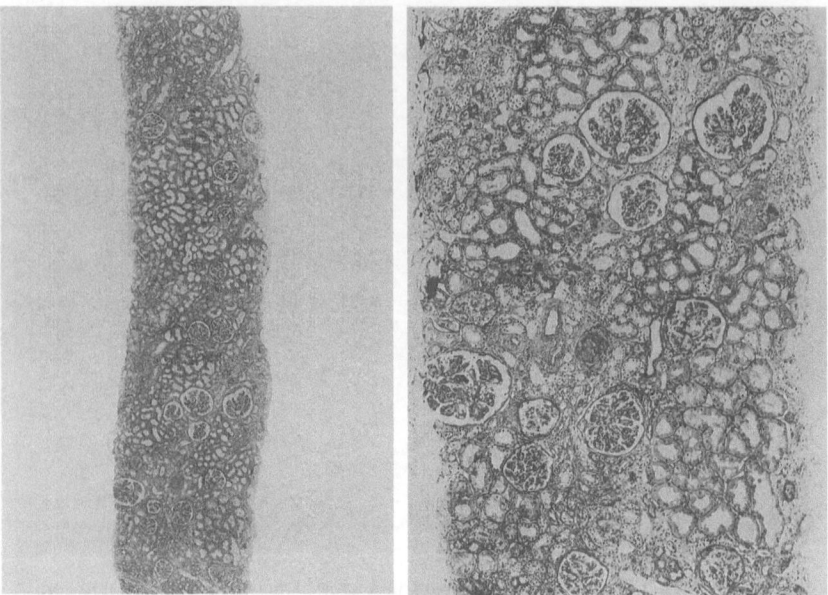

Fig. 6. Striped form of interstitial fibrosis and tubular atrophy as seen by lower and higher magnification

CsA-Toxicity in Animal Experiments and Cell Culture

To define the primary lesions described in man as specific for CsA toxicity and independent of species, animal experiments and cell culture studies were performed. Toxic tubulopathy (Fig. 7) can easily be reproduced in all commonly used animals and the morphology has been described identically by many investigators [7]. There are only minor differences in comparison with tubular toxicity in man. Tubular inclusion bodies in the rat correspond mainly to giant autophagolysosomes containing fragments of degenerate mitochondria; more rarely, typical giant mitochondria are present. Tubular vacuolization is more irregular in the rat than in man, i.e., the vacuoles are more variable in size and clearly due to dilatation of the endoplasmatic reticulum. After long-term treatment tubular microcalcifications are more widespread in the rat than in man and are found mainly along the cortical-medullary junction.

It is far more difficult to reproduce vascular toxicity in experimental animals. In normotensive animals single cell necrosis of vascular smooth muscle cells is seen rarely, but vacuolization of endothelial and smooth muscle cells is never observed [8]. In spontaneously hypertensive rats (SH), however, there is a significantly more pronounced vasculopathy than in the control animals, despite concommitant reduction of blood pressure, heart rate, and plasma renin activity [7] (Fig. 8). Electron microscopy shows the typical picture of necrotising hypertensive vasculopathy, similar to the spontaneously occurring vasculopathy seen in this rat strain without CsA treatment.

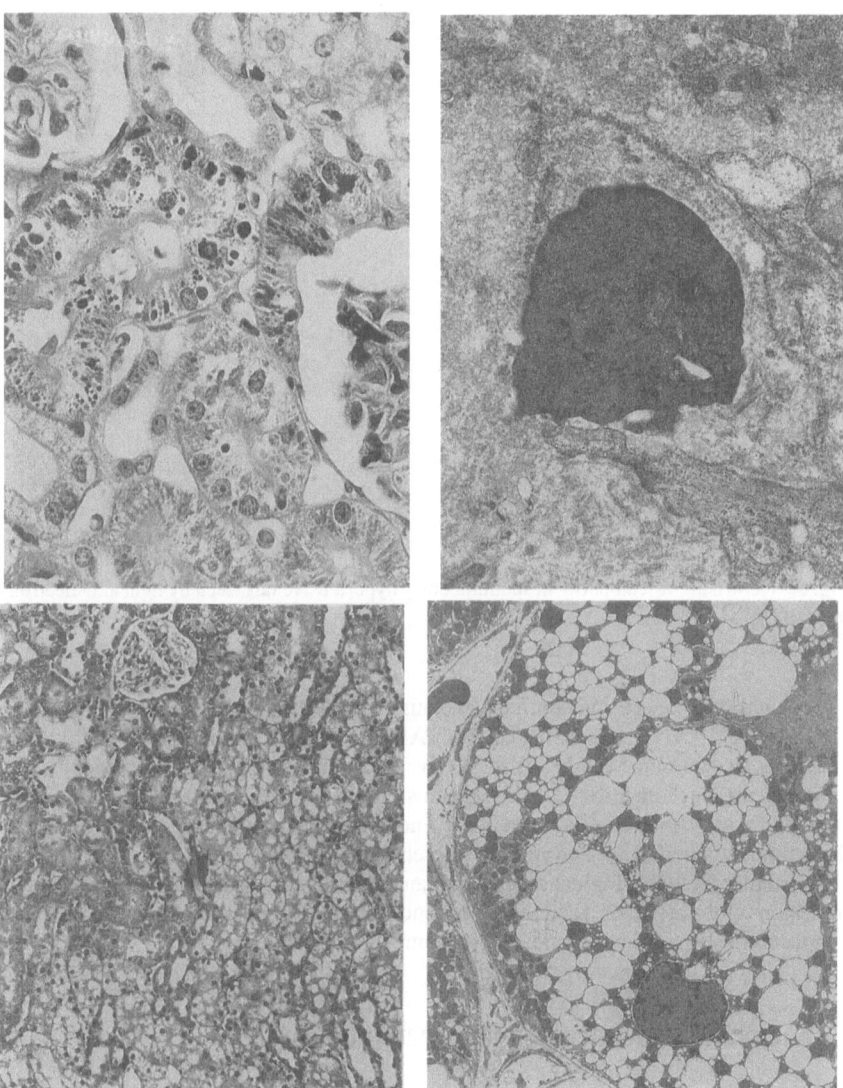

Fig. 7. Tubular toxicity in the rat: Cytoplasmatic inclusion bodies (*giant mitochondria*) in the convoluted part (*top*) and vacuolization (*dilatation of the endoplasmatic reticulum*) (*bottom*) in the straight part of the proximal tubule, by light and electron microscopy

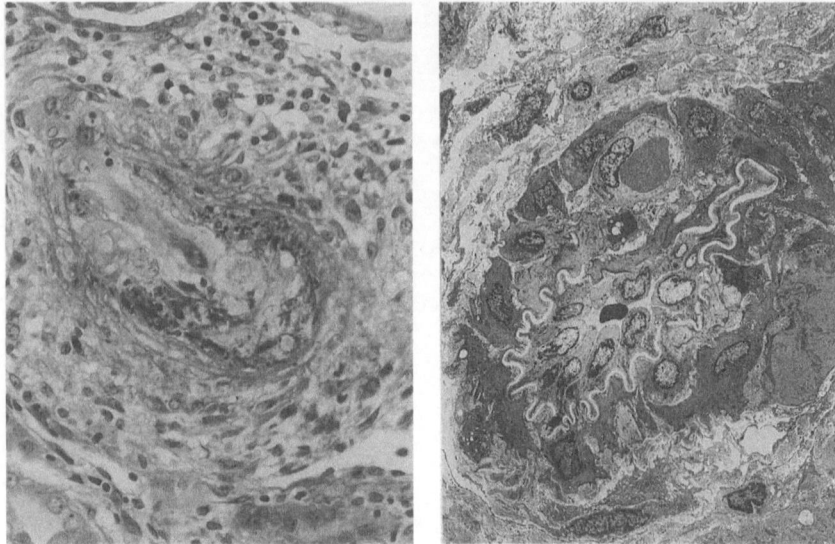

Fig. 8. Necrotising vasculopathy in spontaneously hypertensive rats, seen by light and electron microscopy

Cell culture studies using porcine and canine tubular cells (LICK-PK1 and MDCK, respectively), bovine endothelial cells (CPAE and FBHE), and human and gibbon T cell lines (Jurkat and MLA 144, respectively) exhibited, by light microscopy, cell enlargement, vacuolization, and lipid inclusions, as well as necrotic cells [9]. Electron microscopy showed dilatation of the endoplasmatic reticulum, giant mitochondria, lipid accumulation, and necrobiotic changes (Fig. 9).

In summary, morphological studies in man, animals, and cell culture show a group of lesions consisting of vacuolization (endoplasmatic reticulum), mitochondrial abnormalities (giant mitochondria, lysosomes), and cell necrosis.

CsA Uptake and Intracellular Accumulation

Cellular uptake was investigated by the use of radiolabelled CsA [10]. The cell membrane allows free permeability of CSA; there is no evidence of active or receptor mediated transport. It has recently been shown that the drug binds to specific membrane proteins, such as p-glycoprotein in liver and kidney apical membranes. Furthermore, binding to the Na^+-glucose co-transporter in the kidney and bile acid transporter in the liver were shown. The functional relevance of CsA binding to these proteins is not yet clear; however, these transporters are unlikely to be necessary for CsA transport.

Studies with radiolabelled CsA revealed intracellular accumulation of the drug, suggesting an intracellular binding protein. Two CsA binding proteins have been described, calmodulin and cyclophilin. Whereas the former's role in calcium-

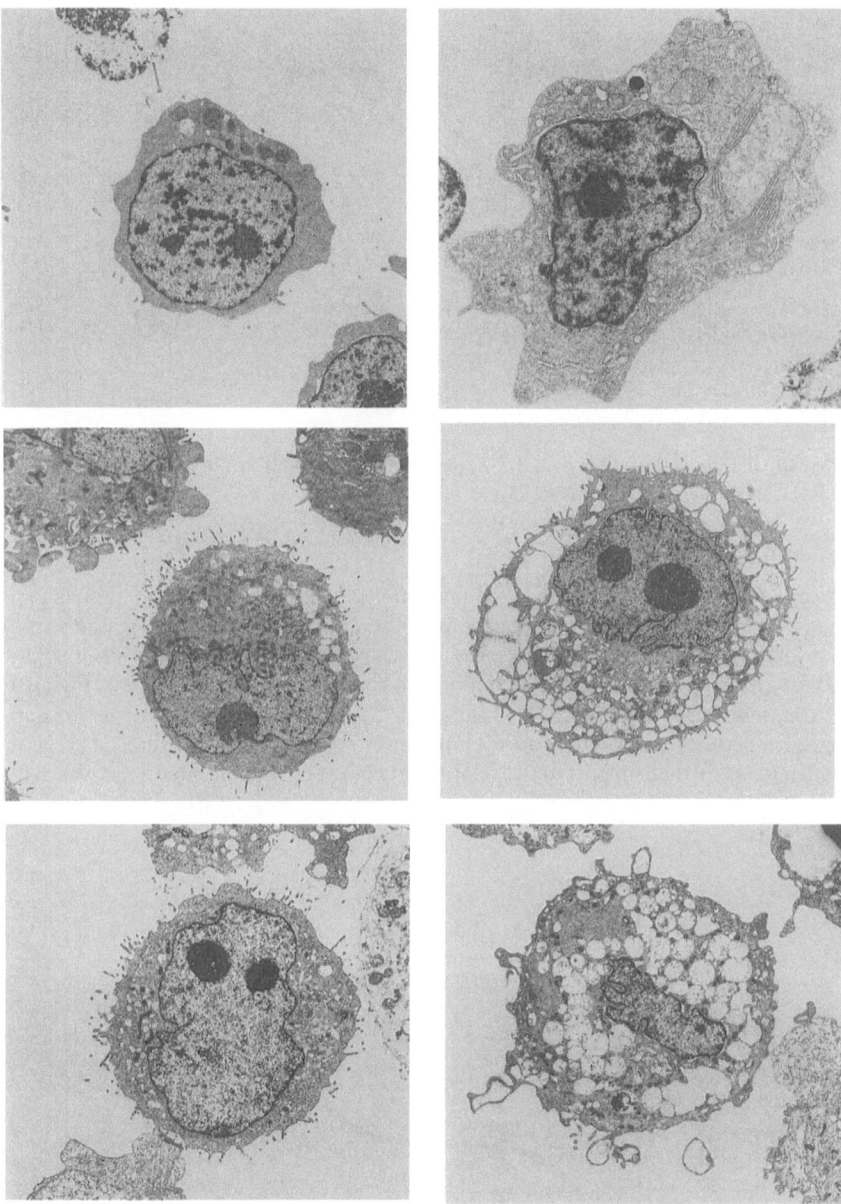

Fig. 9. Ultrastructural changes of Jurkat, FBHE, and PK1 cells after 24-h culture in the presence (*right*) or absence, of CsA (*left*). Cellular swelling and giant mitochondrion is noted in Jurkat cells (*top*), swelling and vacuolization are present in FBHE (*endothelial*) and PK1 (*tubular*) cells (*bottom*)

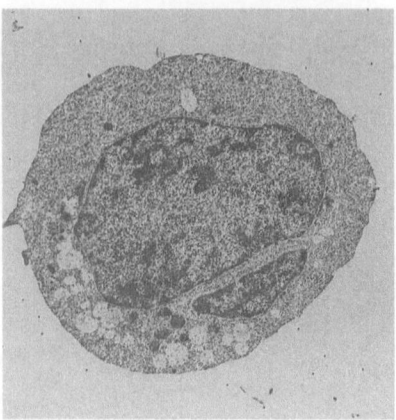 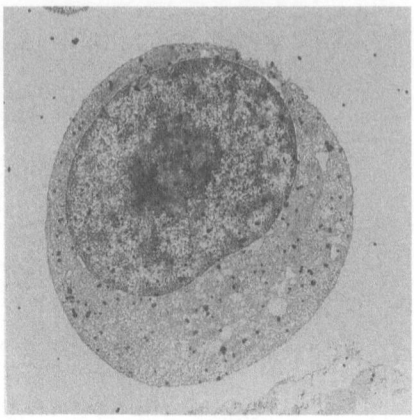

Fig. 10. Immunogold staining with anti-cyclophilin antiserum at the electron microscopic level. Control (*left*) with rabbit serum

dependent enzyme activation is well known, cyclophilin is another ubiquitous peptide which is present in all tissues at comparable concentrations. Investigations from our laboratory, as well as others, have suggested that calmodulin has little, if any, affinity for CsA. In contrast, cyclophilin has high affinity binding to CsA (Fig. 10). Furthermore, Quesniaux et al. [11] showed a good correlation between immunosuppressive activity and binding to cyclophilin of various CsA structural analogues, which lends further support to the relationship between immunosuppressive activity

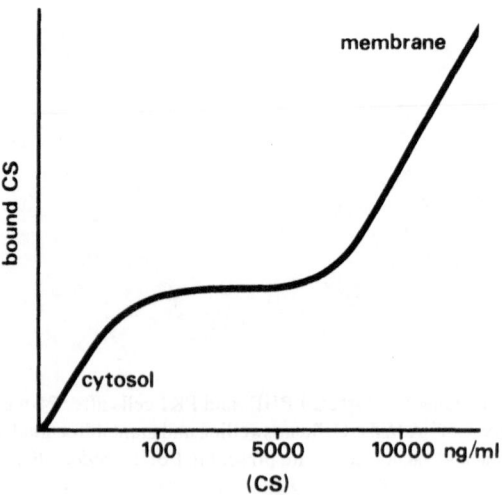

Fig. 11. CsA-binding characteristics: Cytosolic binding saturated below 1 µM, and non-saturable membrane binding

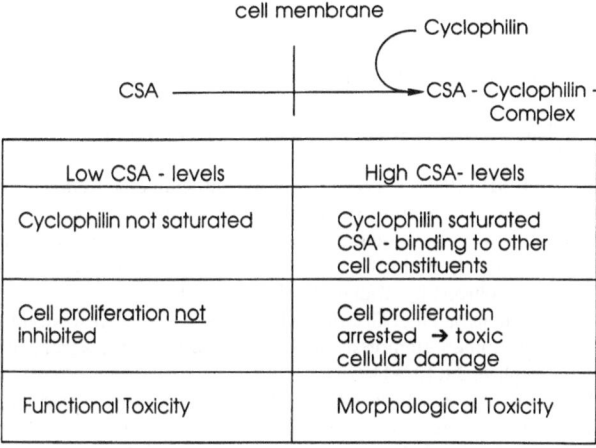

Fig. 12. Hypothesis of cellular mechanisms responsible for CsA toxicity

and toxicity. Furthermore, the cloned protein has a cis-trans-isomerase activity, which may be necessary to the proper folding of regulatory proteins and which is inhibited by CsA. Based on present knowledge, it is assumed that binding to cyclophilin and inhibition of its enzymatic activity is in some way connected to immunosuppression. However, the specific substrate for this enzyme is presently unknown.

Analyzing the CsA binding properties of whole cells over a broad range of concentrations revealed two components: a] a saturable, cytosolic binding, which is most likely due to cyclophilin at concentrations below 1 μM and b] a non-saturable membrane associated binding (Fig. 11) [12]. Since CsA toxicity occurs only at concentrations above 1 μM, i.e., at concentrations which have already saturated cytosolic cyclophilin pools, we presently assume that its toxicity is related to non-specific insertion of the drug into cell membranes, disrupting their integrity. This accumulation of CsA occurs not only in the surface membrane but also intracellularly, e.g., in the endoplasmic reticulum, mitochondria, and Golgi apparatus.

Hypothesis for the Pathogenesis of CsA Toxicity

At pharmacological concentrations, i.e., below 1 μM, CsA binds to cyclophilin and inhibits specifically induced gene transcription in lymphoid cells (Fig. 12). At these concentrations there is no general inhibition of cell proliferation and protein synthesis. At higher concentrations CsA accumulates in the membranes and disrupts membrane functions. Concomitantly, cell proliferation and protein synthesis are inhibited and overt toxic changes are apparent. This may be the basis of the observed morphological toxicity which occurs in the tubular and vascular systems in man and animals as well as in cell culture. This hypothesis does not explain why the kidney is the main target of toxicity. Since CsA is not accumulated in renal tissue, other factors unique to the tubular, endothelial, and smooth muscle cells of the kidney must be involved.

References

1. Mihatsch MJ, Ryffel B, Gudat F, Thiel G (1988) Cyclosporin nephropathy. JB Lippincott. Philadelphia, 1555-1586
2. Mihatsch MJ, Thiel G, Ryffel B (1986) Morphology of Cyclosporin nephropathy. Prog Allergy 38:447-465
3. Nizze H, Mihatsch MJ (1989) Führt die diclosporintherapie zu Veränderungen des juxtaglomerulären Apparates? Nieren- Hochdruck. krankheiten 18:418
4. Myers B, Sibley R, Newton L, Tomlanovich S, Boshkos C, Stinson F, Leutscher J, Whitney D, Krasny D, Coplon N, Perlrothj M (1988) The long-term course of Cyclosporin-associated chronic nephropathy. Kidney Int 33:590-600
5. Bergstrand A, Bohmann S, Thiel G, Mihatsch MJ (1985) Renal histopathology in kidney transplant recipients immunosuppressed with Cyclosporin A: results from an international workshop. Clin Nephrol 24:107-119
6. Nizze H, Mihatsch MJ, Zollinger HU (1988) Cyclosporin-associated nephropathy in patients with heart and bone marrow transplants. Clin Nephrol 30:248-260
7. Thile G (1985) Experimental Cyclosporin A nephrotoxicity: a summary of the international workshop. Clin Nephrol 25:205-210
8. Fasel J, Kaissling B, Ludwig K, Ryffel B, Mihatsch MJ (1987) Light- and electron microscopic changes in the kidney of Wistar rats following treatment with Cyclosporine A. Ultrastruct Pathol 11:435-448
9. Ryffel B, Foxwell B, Gee A, Greiner B, Woerly G, Mihatsch MJ (1988) Cyclosporin-relationship of side effects to mode of action. Transplantation 46:90s-96s
10. Ryffel B (1989) Cellular activation: regulation of intracellular events by Cyclosporin. Pharmacol Rev 41:407-422
11. Quesniaux V, Schreier M, Wenger R, Hiestand PC, Haveling MW, van Regenmortel MHV (1987) Cyclophilin binds to the region of Cyclosporin involved in its immunosuppressive activity. Eur J Immunol 17:1359-1365
12. Foxwell B, Frazer G, Winters M, Hiestand PC, Wenger R, Ryffel B (1988) Identification of Cyclophilin as the erythrocyte Cyclosporin-binding-protein. Biochim Biophys Acta 938:447-455

Cell Volume Regulation
in Health and Disease

Chair: Guillermo Whittembury (Venezuela)
Walter G. Guder (FRG)

Water Permeability, Reflection Coefficients, and Cell Volume Regulation

LARRY W. WELLING and DAN J. WELLING[1]

SUMMARY. Isolated, lumen collapsed, proximally and distally occluded segments of rabbit proximal tubule were equilibrated in isotonic medium and then exposed acutely to a medium identical to the first, except for the deletion or addition of a single test solute. The result was a water flux across the basolateral membrane and a swelling or shrinking of the tubule that could be measured within the first 0.1 s or less following a change from steady state. Tubule volume change was proportional to applied osmotic difference and differed consistently with the solute employed. By use of the impermeant solute raffinose, the membrane hydraulic conductivity was found to be 300 $\mu m \cdot s^{-1}$. By comparing their effects to that of raffinose, NaCl and KCl were found to have reflection coefficients of 0.56 and 0.70, respectively. Other considerations indicate that the reflection coefficients of Na^+, Cl^-, and K^+ are approximately 0.68, 0.50, and 0.94, respectively. The implications of these findings are considered in the context of cell volume maintenance and regulation.

Introduction

When challenged by an acute reduction in bathing osmolality, most tissues undergo a very rapid increase in volume and then, over a much longer period of time, recover toward their original volume. Dellesaga and Grantham observed these events in isolated renal tubules nearly 20 years ago [1]. They used the term "osmometric phase," to describe the very rapid initial increase in volume and the term "volume regulatory phase," to describe the subsequent volume decrease toward normal.

In this symposium, as in the recent literature, the main emphasis in this area of cell volume control is on the second, volume regulatory phase of the osmotic response,

---

[1]Research Service, Veterans Administration Medical Center, Kansas City, MO 64128, USA and Departments of Pathology and Physiology, University of Kansas Medical Center, Kansas City, KS 66103, USA

and on how cell membranes can accommodate the water and solute fluxes necessary to accomplish the regulatory task. However, since research in our laboratory touches more directly on the earlier events, the emphasis here will be on the osmometric phase and the information about cell membrane characteristics that can be gained from the study of such events. It will be assumed that membrane properties in the first instant after change from steady state will carry into and set a baseline for properties in the subsequent time periods. The membrane properties of principal interest will be hydraulic conductivity and solute reflection coefficients.

Experimental Method

The techniques we use are designed to evaluate rabbit, proximal renal tubule, basolateral cell membranes in the first instant after a change from steady state osmotic conditions, as close as possible to time t = 0 and before major fluxes of water or solutes dissipate the osmotic difference imposed by the anisotonic test medium [2–4].

Individual tubules are isolated, transferred to a long, narrow bathing chamber, and viewed through an inverted microscope. A 0.15 mm segment is then occluded at both ends by holding pipettes, oriented transverse to the long axis of the chamber, and positioned about 0.1 mm above a cover slip that forms the bottom of the chamber. All studies are performed at 37°C.

The volume of the bathing medium usually is 0.5 ml and is limited by the height of a suction drain. Immediately before a medium exchange, however, it is reduced to about 20 µl and to a hemispheric droplet covering only the tubule and pipette tips. Immediately thereafter, a large bolus of new medium is rapidly injected down the length of the bathing chamber. It is estimated that the original medium is displaced within 4 ms and that the unstirred layers at the tubule surface are less than 2.6 µm in thickness and 7 ms in duration [3,5].

The osmotic events are observed by video camera and recorder with 17 ms, field-by-field replay. Figure 1 shows a typical recorded image, along with an oscilloscopic display of the light intensity across a single raster line parallel to the tubule diameter. Diameter measurements are taken directly from the monitor screen and involve the eclipsing of the bright highlights at each tubule edge by the opaque jaws of a caliper. In our hands, a given tubule can be measured repeatedly with a standard deviation of ± 0.03 µm. These measurements are not limited by, nor are they closely related to, the Rayleigh criteria for estimating optical resolution.

The tubules are first equilibrated in an isotonic medium and then, to produce a rapid swelling or shrinkage, are exposed acutely to a medium identical to the first, except for the deletion or addition of a single test solute. The result is a water flow, into or out of the tubule, that can be described by the equation

$$J_{V_0} = (L_p A)\,(\sigma \Delta \pi)$$

in which J_{V_0} is the water flow per mm tubule length (nl·min⁻¹·mm⁻¹) at time t = 0, $L_p A$ is the basolateral membrane hydraulic conductivity per mm tubule length (nl·min⁻¹·mm⁻¹·mOsm⁻¹), σ is the reflection coefficient of the test solute used, and

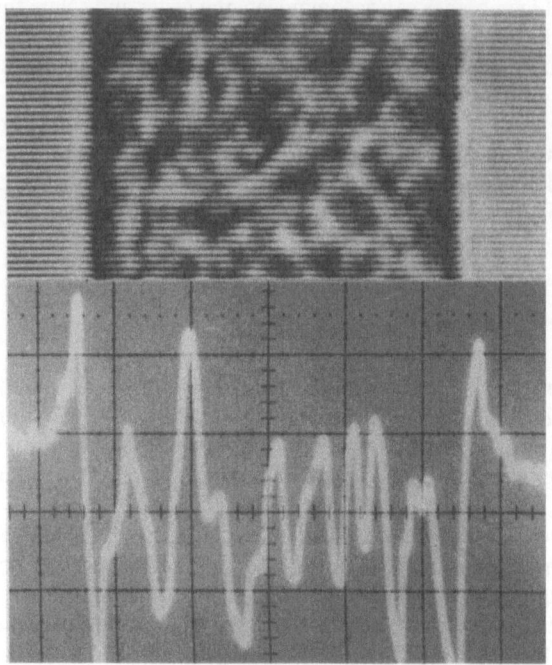

Fig. 1. *Top* Portion of typical S_2 segment as seen on monitor screen, diameter 38.20 μm. *Bottom* Light intensity pattern across single raster line in above tubule. (From [3] with permission)

$\Delta \pi$ is the mOsm difference between the equilibration medium and the test medium as measured by vapor pressure technique.

To approximate J_{V_0} at time t = 0, we use only those tubule diameters and changes in relative tubule volume recorded and measured to be linear during the first few 1/60 s time intervals following osmotic challenge and change from steady state dimensions. The slope of that linear fit divided by the change in medium osmolality then gives the reflection coefficient of the test solute times the membrane hydraulic conductivity. Thus, if the solute has a reflection coefficient of one, as is the case for raffinose, the result is the membrane hydraulic conductivity, $L_P A$. Similarly, if two different solutes of equal measured osmolality are used in the same or different tubules, the ratio of the results is equal to the ratio of the reflection coefficients for the two different solutes employed. If one of the two solutes is raffinose, the result is a measure of the reflection coefficient of the second solute.

Results

Figure 2 shows the changes that occur in S_1, S_2, and S_3 proximal tubule segments after challenge with 240 mOsm hypotonic or 320 mOsm hypertonic raffinose medium. Note that the time scale is in units of 1/60 s and that only the first few time

Fig. 2. Typical responses of S_1, S_2, and S_3 segments during first several 1/60 s time increments after hypotonic or hypertonic challenge of approximately 40 mOsm. (From [2] with permission)

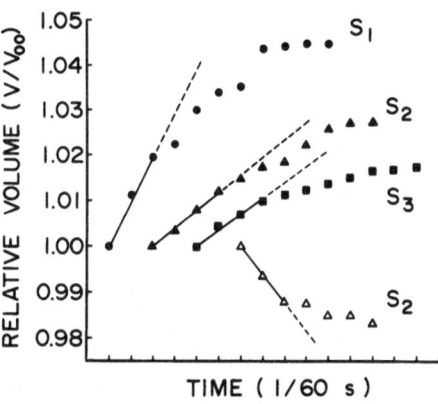

Fig. 3. Hydraulic conductivities of S_1, S_2, and S_3 segments given by the slopes of J_{V_0} vs magnitude of hypotonic challenge. (From [2] with permission)

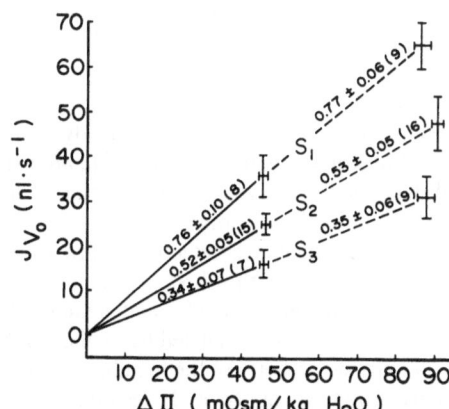

Fig. 4. Relationship in S_2 segments between J_{V_0} and magnitude of challenge produced by raffinose or NaCl. (From [3] with permission)

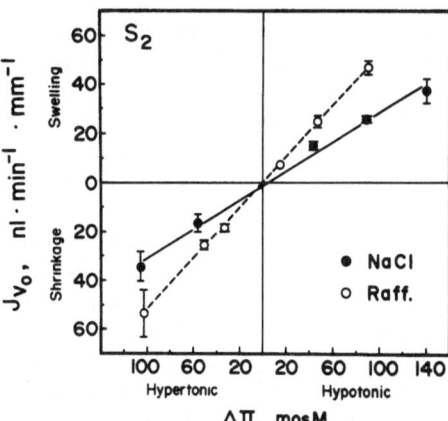

Table 1. Relative osmotic effectiveness of different solutes

n	A		B		σ_A
	Solute	$\sigma L_p A$/mm	Solute	$\sigma L_p A$/mm	σ_B
		nl·min⁻¹· min⁻¹·mOsm⁻¹		nl·min⁻¹· min⁻¹·mOsm⁻¹	
54	KCl	0.36 ±0.02	Raffinose	0.51 ±0.03	0.70 ±0.02
13	NaCl	0.27 ±0.02	KCl	0.36 ±0.03	0.76 ±0.06
6	KCl	0.28 ±0.02	KCl + BaCl$_2$	0.29 ±0.02	0.97 ±0.06
9	Na gluconate	0.33 ±0.03	Raffinose	0.40 ±0.03	0.84 ±0.06
10	K gluconate	0.37 ±0.05	Raffinose	0.39 ±0.06	0.97 ±0.07
8	Choline Cl	0.34 ±0.04	Raffinose	0.45 ±0.04	0.75 ±0.06

n, number of S_2 segments studied; σ, reflection coefficient of test solute; $L_p A$, basolateral membrane hydraulic conductivity per mm tubule length. All data mean ± SE

increments following a change from steady state volume have been considered. Note also the break in the volume vs time data after the first three or four data points and recall that calculations are based only on the slopes of the volume vs time data collected before that break point.

In Fig. 3 the hydraulic conductivities are given by the slopes of J_{v_0} vs magnitude of osmotic challenge for the three segment types. Clearly, hydraulic conductivity is greater in S_1 segments than in S_2, and greater in S_2 than in S_3. It is important to recognize, however, that the calculated hydraulic conductivities are in units of $L_p A$, where L_p is an intrinsic property of the membrane and A is the area of the membrane across which water movement occurs. If one divides by the known areas of basolateral membrane per millimeter tubule length [6], the result for all three segments is found to be about 300 μm·s⁻¹, not statistically different among the three segments, and approximately that calculated for mammalian red blood cell membrane [2].

The conclusion from these studies, therefore, is that proximal tubule basolateral cell membranes are quite leaky to water and that, in terms of cell volume regulation, membrane hydraulic conductivity is unlikely to be a limiting factor.

Figure 4 shows a comparison between the effects of raffinose in 59 S_2 segments and the effects of NaCl in 44 other S_2 segments. Since raffinose has a reflection coefficient of one, the ratio of these two effects is a measure of the NaCl reflection coefficient. The result from those data is a σNaCl of 0.56 ± 0.07. A very similar result was found in S_1 segments [3].

Because the experiments just described required a statistical comparison between separate groups of tubules, the procedure subsequently was changed to allow comparisons in individual tubules, each exposed to two hypertonic test solutions in random sequence and with intervening periods of equilibration in isotonic medium. To date, that new technique has been used to study the relative effects of KCl vs NaCl and of raffinose vs KCL, Na gluconate, K gluconate, or choline chloride [4]. The results are summarized in Table 1.

The first horizontal line of Table 1 shows that the osmotic efficiency of KCl is quite different from that of raffinose, $P < 0.001$. The ratio of the effects, and thus the reflection coefficient of KCl, is calculated there to be 0.73. In the next line it is seen that the efficiency of NaCl is less than that of KCl by a factor of about 0.76. In other words, although KCl is 0.7 times as efficient as raffinose, it still is 1.3 times more efficient than NaCl across the basolateral cell membrane. This is completely consistent with the earlier finding of a NaCl reflection coefficient of 0.56.

Regarding the other data in Table 1, note that the use of Na gluconate and choline Cl, in which the gluconate and choline can be assumed to be impermeant ions, results in calculated reflection coefficients statistically different both from unity and from the 0.56 value for NaCl. The result with K gluconate, however, is not different from that with raffinose.

Discussion

The findings in these studies lend themselves to discussion in two broad areas, one dealing with steady state osmotic balance in renal tubules and another dealing with the nature of the water and ion channels in the basolateral cell membrane. The starting point for both discussions is the recognition that while raffinose is a single species in solution, the other solutes used here are electrolytes that completely dissociate into their respective ions. Their observed effects, therefore, are the net effects of their component parts.

Consider first the proposition that the reflection coefficient for an electrolyte is the simple average of the reflection coefficients of its component ions. For example, $\sigma KCl = (\sigma K^+ + \sigma Cl^-)/2$, $\sigma NaCl = (\sigma Na^+ + \sigma Cl^-)/2$, etc. Now, if one considered only the σKCl and $\sigma NaCl$ results and the fact that chloride is common to both, it would be possible to establish broad ranges for the individual ion reflection coefficients. However, the more valuable information comes from the Na gluconate, K gluconate, and choline Cl studies in which we have the advantage of knowing that gluconate and choline have reflection coefficients of one. Thus, if σ Na gluconate = 0.84, σNa^+ must be approximately 0.68; if σK gluconate = 0.97, σK^+ must be approximately 0.94; and if σ choline Cl = 0.75, σCl^- must be approximately 0.50. Each of these values is, in fact, quite consistent with what would have been expected from the KCl and NaCl studies alone. That is, calculating from $\sigma Na^+ = 0.68$ and $\sigma Cl^- = 0.50$, $\sigma NaCl$ should have a value of about 0.59. That result is in good agreement with the 0.56 value actually observed. Furthermore, using $\sigma KCl = 0.73$ and $\sigma Cl^- = 0.50$, σK^+ should have a value of approximately 0.96, a value also in good agreement with that calculated from the K gluconate studies.

Returning now to the question of steady state osmotic balance, it is of interest to point out a seeming paradox in the maintenance of cell volume, namely, that under normal circumstances the cells of proximal renal tubule contain approximately 140 mM K^+, 10 mM Na^+, and 30 mM Cl^- (a total of 180 mM), while the bathing medium contains approximately 5 mM K^+, 150 mM Na^+, and 120 mM Cl^- (a total of 275 mM). Thus there is a 95 mM discrepancy which, if the reflection coefficients of the principal solutes were taken to be unity, would represent an osmolality difference of 95 mOsm/kg that presumably would have to be made up by other intracellular solutes. The nature of those solutes, however, is not readily apparent. On the other hand, if one multiplies the intra- and extracellular potassium, sodium, and chloride concentrations by the reflection coefficients from the present studies, the missing osmoles are reduced dramatically to about 13 mOsm. Furthermore, of those remaining, perhaps 5 mOsm might be accounted for by large impermeant solutes [7], and a variety of other solutes could easily contribute the rest. In any case, the point to be made is that any consideration of cell volume maintenance or adjustment, be it in the osmometric phase or the recovery phase, cannot disregard the reflection coefficients of the solutes involved.

The second broad area of discussion to which our results contribute is the nature of the water and ion channels in the basolateral membranes. Several comments can be made.

First, since the reflection coefficients for sodium and for chloride are found to be less than unity, those solutes and water must have common pathways through the cell membrane. Since solute movement thus must accompany water movement, the cell cannot be viewed as a perfect osmometer.

Second, it might be seen to be inconsistent that we find σNa^+ to be considerably less than σK^+ in spite of the well-known fact that the diffusional permeability of potassium exceeds that of sodium. That could be explained, however, if potassium mostly employs a highly permeable channel from which water is excluded, while sodium shares a pathway with water, as would all other solutes with reflection coefficients less than unity. Since potassium channels in this membrane are known to be blocked by barium [8], the present finding that the osmotic effect of KCl is not affected by $BaCl_2$ supports both the finding of a potassium reflection coefficient near unity and the suggestion that K^+ and water do not share a common pathway.

The last point of discussion has to do with the earlier assumption that the reflection coefficient of an electrolyte can be considered to be the average of the reflection coefficients of its dissociated ions. In spite of the fact that calculations based on that assumption yield internally consistent results and predict individual ion values quite appropriate for the maintenance of steady-state cell volume, it still should be asked how this can be reconciled with the fact that, for reasons of transmembrane charge conservation, electrolyte reflection coefficients would be weighted toward the least permeant ionic species with the highest reflection coefficients [9]. In other words, if gluconate and choline are indeed impermeant, how could the reflection coefficients of sodium gluconate and choline chloride have been anything other than unity?

To this we have no answer except to point out the very acute nature of the studies and the possibility that, at the initial instant of osmotic change, the membrane is just penetrated to various degrees by the several ionic species that still behave as hydrated particles in the bathing solution. Subsequently, as the particles proceed through the membrane and the transient state is diminished, there presumably would have to occur either a change in the effective reflection coefficient or a change in the steady state charge condition near the membrane. In the latter case, the reflection coefficient might even become a function of the ambient environmental conditions and the recent past history of the cell.

References

1. Dellesega M, Grantham JJ (1973) Regulation of renal tubule cell volume in hypotonic media. Am J Physiol 224:1288–1294

2. Welling LW, Welling DJ, Ochs TJ (1983) Video measurement of basolateral membrane hydraulic conductivity in the proximal tubule. Am J Physiol 245 (Renal Fluid Electrolyte Physiol 14):F123–F129
3. Welling LW, Welling DJ, Ochs TJ (1987) Video measurement of basolateral NaCl reflection coefficient in proximal tubule. Am J Physiol 253 (Renal Fluid Electrolyte Physiol 22):F290–F298
4. Welling LW, Welling DJ, Ochs TJ (1990) Relative osmotic effects of raffinose, KCl, and NaCl across basolateral cell membrane. Am J Physiol (Renal Fluid Electrolyte Physiol 28):F594–F597
5. Pedley TJ (1983) Calculation of unstirred layer thickness in membrane transport experiments: a survey. Q Rev Biophys 16:115–150
6. Welling LW, Welling DJ (1988) Relationship between structure and function in renal proximal tubule. J Electron Microsc Tech 9:171–185
7. Linshaw MA, Stapleton FB, Cuppage FE, Grantham JJ (1977) Effect of basement membrane and colloid osmotic pressure on renal tubule cell volume. Am J Physiol 233 (Renal Fluid Electrolyte Physiol 2):F325–F332
8. Welling PA, Linshaw MA, Sullivan LP (1985) Effect of barium on cell volume regulation in rabbit proximal straight tubules. Am J Physiol 249 (Renal Fluid Electrolyte Physiol 18):F20–F27
9. Kedem O, Leaf A (1966) The relation between salt and ionic transport coefficients. J Gen Physiol 49:655–662

Fluid Transport by Leaky Epithelia and Cell Volume Regulation

Kenneth R. Spring[1]

Summary. The mechanism and pathways of fluid absorption by leaky epithelia are subjects of considerable investigation and controversy. Theories and models of fluid transporting epithelia are briefly reviewed and related to fluid absorption across renal proximal tubules. The relevance of cell volume regulation to transepithelial fluid absorption is also discussed.

The Movement of Water Through Membranes and Tight Junctions

The means by which water may cross cell membranes have been recently reviewed in detail [1]. The movement of water may be treated theoretically in the same manner as the flow of any substance: water is driven by the difference in its electrochemical potential. Flow always occurs as a result of the driving forces which comprise the electrochemical gradient for a substance. In the case of water, the primary factors are the relative concentration of water across a barrier (i.e., the solute concentration difference) and the hydrostatic pressure difference. Electro-osmotically driven flow does not appear to be a significant factor in the movement of water across cell membranes [1–3].

Inasmuch as the flow of water is dependent on its gradient, the issue of the mechanism of transepithelial water flow may be reduced to two considerations: (1) Determination of the site and magnitude of the differences in water activity, and (2) Measurement of the water permeability of the relevant pathways across the epithelium. Most attempts to directly determine the magnitude of the water activity differences have not been successful because of difficulties in sampling the relevant

[1]Laboratory of Kidney and Electrolyte Metabolism, National Heart, Lung, and Blood Institute, Building 10, Room 6N307, Bethesda, MD 20892, USA

compartments and of precisely analyzing collected samples. It should be clear from the above considerations that there must be, within or adjacent to the epithelium, a region in which water activity differs from that of the bulk solutions. Determination of the site of this region of altered osmolality, as well as the magnitude of the osmotic pressure difference, has occupied the interest of transport physiologists for over 30 years.

Osmolality of the Transported Fluid

The earliest investigators were impressed by the lack of measurable difference in the composition of the bulk solutions bathing small intestine studied in vitro [4,5]. A number of studies in intestine [6] and renal proximal tubule [7] supported these earlier workers, showing that the calculated osmolality of the transported fluid agreed, within experimental error, with that expected for isosmotic transport. The subject of the osmolality of the transported fluid was investigated again in both gallbladder [8–10] and renal proximal tubule [11,12]. No measurable transepithelial differences in macroscopic osmolality were detected in these studies, supporting the conclusion that transepithelial osmotic pressure differences did not exist. Differences in solute reflection coefficients, and therefore the effective osmotic pressure generated by the bathing solutions, have been proposed as important factors in the generation of transepithelial driving forces for fluid movement across renal proximal tubule [13,14]. Although cryoscopic osmolality may not differ, the effective osmolality of solutions depends on the relative reflection coefficients of the solutes across the epithelial layer.

As studies of fluid absorption by mammalian proximal tubule have progressed, the issue of the composition of the transported fluid has received a great deal of attention [15]. Evidence has been obtained that the fluid filling the lumen of the proximal tubule may become slightly hypotonic as transport of solutes and water progresses [13,14,16]. Collection of the proximal tubular absorbate showed it to be significantly hypertonic to the lumenal perfusate, with much of the preferentially absorbed solute being glucose and other organic solutes [17,18]. In tissues such as the intestine, the underlying connective tissue (submucosa) precludes the type of fluid collection experiments done in perfused renal tubules and the composition of the transported fluid may be determined only indirectly. However, estimates of the osmolality of the subepithelial layer in small intestine support the conclusion that the osmolality of the interstitial fluid may be altered as a result of fluid absorption [19].

Models of Epithelial Fluid Transport

Although it was generally agreed that transepithelial water movement must be the result of osmosis, workers were perplexed by the fact that no transepithelial osmotic gradients could be detected. In most epithelia the transepithelial potential was also near zero [2,9,10,20], ruling out simple electro-osmosis as a mechanism for fluid transport. The most widely accepted solution to these problems was put forward by Diamond and Bossert [21] in their "standing gradient" model for fluid transport. This model was an outgrowth of an earlier three compartment model for epithelial fluid transport developed by Curran and MacIntosh [22]. Curran and MacIntosh developed a three compartment model which resulted in vectorial fluid transport consequent to solute injection into the middle compartment. The membrane between the middle compartment and the outer bath was assumed to be similar to a cell membrane, while the membrane facing the inner bath was assumed to be similar to a basement membrane. The outer membrane was an effective semipermeable barrier, while the inner membrane was ineffective as an osmotic barrier. Thus, as solute was injected into the middle compartment by active transport, water was osmotically drawn into this compartment from the outer bath. Water was not drawn into the middle compartment from the inner bath because of the lack of solute reflection by the inner membrane, i.e., because the inner membrane was not semipermeable, but was freely permeable to both solutes and water. As water entered the middle compartment the pressure within it rose and forced fluid out across the leaky inner membrane. The pressure caused predominant flow across the inner membrane because of its high hydraulic conductivity (water permeability) compared to that of the outer membrane.

An analysis of models for fluid-transporting epithelial was done by Weinstein and Stephenson [23,24]; they characterized all epithelial models as variants of the original scheme of Curran and MacIntosh. The essential conclusion is that transepithelial water flow arises because there is, within the epithelium, a region of higher osmolality than the bulk solutions. The exact location of the middle compartment of the Curran and MacIntosh scheme was not defined by those investigators, although the characteristics of the limiting membranes were strictly delineated.

Whitlock and Wheeler [25] suggested, on the basis of morphological studies of the rabbit gallbladder, that the middle compartment of the Curran and MacIntosh model was the lateral intercellular space separating epithelial cells. Tormey and Diamond [26] confirmed and extended the work of Whitlock and Wheeler and provided the morphological basis for the mathematical model developed by Diamond and Bossert [27]. It is worthwhile recalling why Diamond and Bossert rejected the simple three compartment scheme for osmotic flow as the mechanism of transepithelial fluid transport. They reviewed the literature values for epithelial hydraulic water permeability and concluded that the water permeability of the cell membranes was too low to enable water and solute to move out of the cell with equal speed. In other words, they concluded that salt actively transported out of the cell would rapidly diffuse away before exerting significant osmotic effect across the basolateral membrane. They therefore proposed a region of restricted solute diffusion within the epithelium where water and solute could equilibrate and achieve isotonicity. The lateral intercellular space was the postulated site of solute-solvent coupling. The space geometry and the location of the solute pumps figured prominently in this model. The spaces had to be sufficiently narrow and tortuous to restrict solute diffusion; the pumps had to be located near the blind, tight junctional end of the channel. Alterations of interspace geometry, such as widening or shortening of the space, resulted in the formation of hypertonic absorbate. Thus, a model was developed and widely accepted which assigned critical importance to the morphology of the epithelium.

What has followed in the last 20 years is a large number of morphological and theoretical studies concerned with the geometric alterations associated with variations in the rate of transepithelial fluid transport. It became evident that several of the key assumptions of the standing gradient model were incorrect. It was convincingly demonstrated that the tight junction was leaky to solutes [28,15] and that solute pumps were uniformly distributed [29,30], rather than clustered at the apical end of the channel as required by the standing gradient model. Model calculations showed that it was theoretically impossible to achieve true isotonic transport with the standing gradient [15] and that all acceptable models reduced to the three compartment system of Curran and MacIntosh [23,24,59]. Although serious questions about the standing gradient model for transepithelial fluid transport were raised by Hill [20], Diamond [2] had already noted that difficulties with the model were primarily associated with uncertainties about the values for the hydraulic water permeability of the basolateral cell membrane. Diamond [2] pointed out the need for direct determination of cell membrane water permeability, as well as the need for better estimates of epithelial water permeability, free of the errors due to solute polarization in the unstirred layers. Finally Weinstein and Stephenson [24] pointed out that there was no need for a standing gradient to achieve solute-solvent coupling when cell membrane water permeability was in the range of experimentally determined values for nonepithelial cell membranes.

Water Permeability of Epithelia

Epithelial hydraulic water permeability (L_p) has been measured in a number of preparations by the imposition of transepithelial osmotic pressure gradients. As previously discussed, unstirred layers adjacent to or within the tissue cause substantial underestimates of L_p [2,31–34]. The extent of the unstirred layer dependent error in L_p has been extensively discussed and it has been generally concluded that the L_p of most epithelial has been underestimated by an order of magnitude or more [1,2,34]. The exception to this conclusion is the renal tubule which, because of its small size, is essentially free of unstirred layer related errors [16,35]. Even in renal proximal tubule there is a relatively wide range (approximately ten-fold) of estimated L_p values [35]. Knowledge of the L_p of the epithelium is essential both to determination of the route of transepithelial fluid flow as well as to estimation of the magnitude of the osmotic forces required to achieve that flow [36]. Finally, estimates of epithelial reflection coefficient for individual ions or solutes are dependent on the epithelial L_p value [36].

The most reliable estimates of L_p in leaky, flat epithelia have come from work on rabbit gallbladder done by Van Os et al. [37] using rapid stirring and a fast response flow measurement apparatus developed by Wiedner [7]. These investigators determined L_p by imposition of either osmotic or hydrostatic pressures and determined the resultant volume flows by a capacitance method. Hydrostatic pressures can be used to measure L_p without concern about unstirred layer related effects. It should be noted that the imposition of hydrostatic pressure differences across the epithelium results in alterations of cell geometry which have consequences on the rate of fluid transport. Naftalin and Tripathi [38] used high speed optical measurements combined with the capacitance probe technique to simultaneously measure the volume flows across rabbit ileum and estimate the flows across the individual cell membranes. They used both osmotic and hydrostatic pressures to drive fluid across the tissue and examined the magnitude of unstirred layer effects as well as possible electro-osmosis. They concluded that apical unstirred layer related effects were negligibly small in their system and that electro-osmosis was demonstrable, as evidenced by streaming potentials. Although their measurements are probably the most accurate estimate of intestinal water permeability made to date, I find their arguments concerning electro-osmosis to be unconvincing and conclude, as others have done [3,20], that electro-osmosis does not result in a significant transepithelial flow of water. It is clear that unstirred layers and the unfavorable tissue geometry of flat epithelia prevent a complete assessment of the fluid flows across these tissues.

Direct determination of cell membrane water permeability of an epithelium was first reported by Persson and Spring [39]. They used quantitative light microscopy to measure rapid changes in cell volume subsequent to alteration of the osmolality of the apical or basolateral solution bathing the Necturus gallbladder. Other investigators [21,40–43] estimated basolateral cell membrane L_p from the rate of swelling of collapsed renal proximal tubules suddenly exposed to hypotonic bathing solution. The accuracy, speed, and validity of these studies were questioned [35], and subsequent investigations [43,44] led to somewhat higher values for basolateral membrane L_p. Apical membrane L_p was measured in renal proximal tubules by Gonzalez et al. [21]. The first direct determinations of apical and basolateral cell membrane L_p in cortical collecting tubules of rabbit have also been made [33]. The inherent difficulties in making L_p measurements in cells with the high surface area and small volume of mammalian cells have been reviewed [45].

The reported values of cell membrane L_p for all epithelia fall into a relatively narrow range after correction for surface amplification. Unfortunately the units used to define water permeability values are confusing and inconsistent [1,39], making it difficult to directly compare results from different laboratories. The most commonly used units for hydraulic water permeability, L_p, are cm/s-atm; while water permeability, Posm, is usually expressed in μm/s. (Posm=RTL_p/V_w, where R is the gas constant, T is temperature, V_w is the partial molar volume of water). Rather than expose the reader to a plethora of values, it is more instructive to recognize that all epithelial cell membranes studied have L_p or Posm values that differ by no more than an order of magnitude. Most epithelial cell membranes have Posm values of 40–50 μm/s; the only exception being the "poorly permeable" membranes such as the apical membrane of toad urinary bladder [46] or cortical collecting duct [33] in the absence of antidiuretic hormone. These membranes have Posm values in the 5–25 μm/s range [1,33]; Posm increases 6–10-fold upon addition of the hormone. The high apparent L_p of epithelia such as the renal proximal tubule comes from the great area amplification created by the microvilli and extensive infoldings [24]. Necturus gallbladder apical area is increased 8-fold by microvilli and basolateral area is increased 26-fold [47]. In all absorptive tissues investigated to date, basolateral membrane area exceeded apical area, with the result that the effective basolateral membrane L_p was much larger than that of the entire apical membrane, even though the L_ps of the unit membranes were similar [33,39].

The most significant aspect of the L_p of epithelial cell membranes is the realization that water permeability is sufficiently large that water moves "freely" across these barriers. Once both apical and basolateral membrane water permeabilities are known, the driving forces and routes of transepithelial water movement may also be estimated.

Route of Transepithelial Fluid Flow

Transcellular movement of water may not be the sole pathway for transepithelial flow, because the tight junction is known to be leaky to ions. There is no reason to believe that the junctions are not also permeable to water and that some fraction of transepithelial fluid flow is paracellular [36,48]. Most conclusions about the routes taken by water and solutes across epithelia have come from model calculations based on the geometry and structure of the tight junction and shunt pathway. Disputes about these parameters have led to a wide range of estimates of the relative flows across the cellular and shunt pathways. General agreement does exist about the relative areas of the cell and tight junction at the mucosal surface. In most epithelia, the area of the apical cell membrane is approximately 10^4 times that of the cross sectional area of the tight junction [48–50]. Significant rates of transepithelial flow of water and solutes across the tight junction occur when the area-adjusted permeability of that pathway approaches or exceeds that of the cellular pathway. The driving force for transepithelial volume flow is the osmotic pressure difference between the basolateral space and the apical bathing solution. If the same osmotic pressure exists across the tight junction and the entire cell, the relative flow through each path depends on the area-adjusted water permeability of each. As mentioned above, the basolateral membrane of epithelia is far more water permeable than the apical membrane, and interspace hypertonicity must therefore lead to volume flow across that membrane, with resultant increase in cell osmolality. The primary cellular barrier to osmotic pressure gradients is, then, the apical membrane. In Necturus gallbladder, the area-adjusted apical membrane Posm is 550 μm/s [48]; to achieve equal flows across junctional and cellular routes a junctional water permeability 10^4 times greater is required. The required junctional Posm, 5 m/s, is physically unreasonable, leading me to conclude that transjunctional flow of water is not a significant factor in fluid absorption. Other investigators have made similar calculations and reached the same conclusion [2,32,35,51]. However, the issue of the magnitude of the transjunctional volume flow remains controversial, with several reports favoring substantial paracellular water flux [25,36,43]. The route taken by water as it crosses the epithelium determines the epithelial solute reflection coefficients, as well as the magnitude of solvent drag effects. Until this issue is resolved interpretation of experimental results will be clouded.

Osmotic Driving Force Required for Transepithelial Flow

The osmotic driving force required to achieve the observed rate of fluid absorption may be calculated directly from the L_p of the epithelium. Such calculations for renal proximal tubule indicate that the osmotic pressure difference required is between 2 and 25 mosmol [19]. A similar calculation for Necturus gallbladder led to the conclusion that only 3.5 mosmol driving force was needed to achieve the observed rates of fluid absorption [39,48]. Such small differences in osmotic pressure are not readily detectable by conventional means [35,48,52], even when attempts are made to magnify the differences [19,53]. Assuming such osmotic pressure differences exist within the lateral intercellular spaces, it is instructive to consider the consequences of a hypertonic interspace.

Transcellular Osmosis

On the basis of the preceding discussion, it is possible to estimate the transmembrane driving forces required to obtain the observed rates of fluid absorption by transcellular osmotic flow for tissues in which cell membrane water permeabilities have been determined. Extensive work on the mechanism of fluid flow across Necturus gallbladder [39,48,54] has provided the necessary permeability and fluid flow rate information for calculations for that leaky tissue.

Knowledge of the cell membrane water permeabilities permits calculations to be made of the osmotic driving forces required to transport water across each membrane. The rate of fluid transport across Necturus gallbladder is about 1.6×10^{-6} cm/s [54]. If virtually all of this fluid enters the cells across the apical membrane, the osmotic pressure difference required to achieve this rate of fluid flow is about 1.6 mosmol/kg. The cell osmolality must be 1.6 mosmol higher than that of the apical solution to result in this flow. Vectorial water flow across epithelia must be the result of a gradient in water activity across the epithelial cell layer. The water activity in the fluid surrounding the basolateral membrane of the cell must be lower than that in the cell for water movement across that membrane. The calculated osmotic gradient across the basolateral membrane, based on its water permeability and a volume flow of 1.6×10^{-6} cm/s, is about 0.7 mosmol/kg. In other words, the osmolality of the interstitial fluid must be 0.7 mosmol/kg greater than that of the cell for water to move out of the cell at the required rate. Thus, the basolateral interstitial space must be about 2.3 mosmol/kg hypertonic to the apical bathing solution to result in normal rates of fluid transport [48]. The hyperosmolality of the interstitial fluid will result in an absorbate which is hyperosmotic to the bathing solutions by 1.5%. As mentioned above, such a small difference in osmolality would be very difficult to detect by present techniques. It is clear, however, that the cells become slightly anisotonic as a result of water entry across the apical membrane. Conversely, water would not enter the cells if there were no gradient in its activity.

Mechanism of Fluid Exit from the Basolateral Spaces

As Curran and MacIntosh [22] showed in their model of fluid transport, hydrostatic pressure constitutes the driving force for fluid exit from the middle compartment (lateral intercellular spaces and basolateral interstitium). The basement membrane and underlying connective tissue are highly permeable structures with virtually no solute reflection capabilities [55]. As a result of the low reflection coefficient of connective tissue, osmotic pressures cannot develop across these tissues. Fluid will only move across the submucosa by hydrostatic or oncotic forces. As fluid leaves the epithelial cells, driven by the osmotic pressure difference across the basolateral membrane, the lateral intercellular spaces fill and become dilated [26,56,57]. From the pressure volume curves of the spaces [56], it is possible to calculate the hydrostatic pressure within the spaces. For Necturus gallbladder this pressure difference amounts to 3 cm of water or less at normal rates of fluid transport. The hydraulic properties of the underlying basement membrane and connective tissue determine the magnitude of the pressure rise in the spaces. The pressure will increase until it is sufficient to drive the transported fluid across the submucosa. The magnitude of the restriction of fluid movement offered by the submucosal structures is an important factor in determination of the rate of transepithelial fluid flow [5,15,19,23,24,48].

Another mechanism could account for some of the fluid exit from the lateral inter-cellular spaces during transepithelial fluid transport. McGlaughlin and Mathias [3] proposed that water could be driven out of the lateral spaces by electro-osmotic flow parallel to the plane of the lateral cell membrane. This type of electro-osmosis had not been previously proposed for biological systems; it is dependent on close approx-imation of the lateral membranes of adjacent cells. If the lateral membranes of the epithelial cells are separated by a distance of 0.2 μm or less, the electric field created by the current through the Na-K pump could constitute a driving force for electro-osmotic movement of fluid out of the interspace. Mammalian renal proximal tubule cells may have the correct geometry for such electro-osmosis to occur, and McGlaughlin and Mathias [3] suggested several experiments to test their hypothesis in this epithelium. This mechanism will not account for significant fluid flows in epithelia in which the lateral spaces are widely separated during fluid transport, but it represents a possible class of water transport that has been overlooked as a biologi-cally relevant phenomenon.

Transjunctional Flows of Water and Ions

As discussed above, the tight junctions have been shown by many investigators to be leaky to solutes. It is unreasonable to assume that such an extracellular shunt pathway does not permit water to cross. The issue is not whether water will move across the junction, but the relative magnitude of the transjunctional fluid flux compared to the transcellular flow. Clearly, if one had accurate measurements of both epithelial and cell apical membrane L_p, the junctional contribution to transepithelial flow could be readily determined. Whittembury et al. [43] have attempted these measurements in renal proximal tubule and concluded that about one half of the transepithelial flow occurs across the tight junction. In other experiments Whittembury et al. [58] have attempted to demonstrate solvent drag of extracellular solutes across gallbladder. The demonstration of solvent drag is difficult, because the solutes employed diffuse across the junction into the interspace, while the fluid coming out of the cell across the lateral membranes is presumably free of these solutes. Thus the fluid within the spaces always has a lower concentration of the solute than does either bulk solution. Diffusion of solute from the apical bathing solution may then be mistaken for solvent drag [2,28].

In my opinion it is not possible to accurately estimate the magnitude of the trans-junctional flow of water at present. Weinstein [36] has recently calculated that the permeability and solute reflection properties of the rat renal proximal tubule cannot be reproduced by a mathematical model which does not permit substantial (50% or greater) transjunctional water flow. These calculations do not agree with my conclu-sion that transjunctional flow is negligible in leaky epithelial [48]. Resolution of this issue awaits future experimental results.

The conflict over the magnitude of the transcellular versus transjunctional water flow does not extend to the area of ion movements across these pathways. Boulpaep [59] first showed that the paracellular pathway, constituted by the tight junction and lateral intercellular spaces, was the primary route for transepithelial ionic currents. This conclusion has been supported by innumerable observations in many tissues, notably those of Frizzell and Schultz [60] in intestine. In most tissues the apical cell membrane permeability to ions is about 10^{-5}–$[10]^{-7}$ cm/s. Equal diffusional flows through the cellular and junctional paths would occur when the junctional permeability is in the range of $[10]^{-1}$–10^{-3} cm/s. Transjunctional ion flows would predominate when the junctional permeability exceeds that of the cell membrane. The calculated maximum diffusional permeability of the tight junction of Necturus gallbladder [48] is about 1.5 cm/s. Thus, junctional ion permeability could be about 10–500 times that of the cellular pathway without any physically unrealistic assumptions. The difference in the paths taken by water and salt in response to transepithelial gradients arises not because the junctions are selectively permeable to salt, but because the cell membrane restricts the flow of salt markedly compared to that of water.

Fluid Transport and the Regulation of Cellular Volume

The large volumes of fluid which move across epithelial cell membranes would result in significant dilution or concentration of the cytoplasm if fluid entry and exit were not balanced. As an example, the rates of fluid movement across renal proximal tubule cells are sufficiently great that the entire cellular volume is replaced every 20 seconds (or every 40 seconds if only half of the fluid absorption is transcellular as discussed above). If entry or exit rates change as a result of altered solute movements, cell volume should change dramatically. Substantial experimental evidence has been obtained which shows that stimulating solute entry, for example by the addition of a sugar or amino acid to the apical bathing solution, leads to significant cell swelling [61,62]. Similarly, interfering with solute exit results in cell swelling because solute entry continues [54,63–65]. In these cases cell swelling did not result in the rapid volume regulatory decrease usually observed when bathing solution osmolality is decreased. Necturus gallbladder is an example of an epithelium which shows cell volume regulatory behavior as well as transport related volume alterations.

When solute entry into Necturus cells is blocked by the removal of Na or Cl from the apical bathing solution [39,54,57], shrinkage of the cell occurs. The shrinkage results from the continued operation of the solute exit mechanism, primarily the Na,K-ATPase [54,64,65]. No sign of volume regulatory increase is observed, although the shrinkage is large (17%) compared to the osmotic stimulus (6%) required to activate volume regulatory increase. Blockage of solute exit, by the addition of ouabain, a specific inhibitor of the Na,K-ATPase results in cell swelling at a constant rate of 4% per minute [54,64]. This swelling has been shown to result from the continued entry of NaCl from the apical bath into the cell across the apical membrane. After 10–30 minutes, cell volume reaches a maximum of about 1.4 times that of control and a slow shrinkage begins that persists for many minutes or hours [64]. If at any time during the swelling phase resulting from ouabain addition an osmotic perturbation is imposed, volume regulatory behavior is activated [39,65,66]. It is apparent that changes in osmolality trigger a specialized response in Necturus gallbladder cells that differs from the response to perturbations in solute entry or exit. I have speculated in the past on the physiologic basis for volume regulation [48,65], and have concluded that volume regulation may be a misnomer. Volume is really not regulated, per se, the intracellular concentration of some key solute may be what is being regulated.

The kind of volume regulatory behavior exhibited by Necturus gallbladder epithelial cells raises questions about the relevance of volume regulation to transepithelial fluid transport. The response to a sudden perturbation of the osmolality of the bathing solution is a very rapid (60–90 seconds) readjustment of cell volume to control size, despite the continued presence of the anisotonic bath [65]. Such a perturbation may not be an appropriate stimulus for the study of the control of cell volume or composition, as discussed by Lohr and Grantham [61]. These investigators reported that the response of collapsed renal proximal tubules to a change in solution osmolality depended on the rate at which the osmolality change occurred. Changes of bath osmolality between 167 and 361 mosmol/kg did not cause a change in tubule volume if the rate of osmolality alteration did not exceed 1 mosmol/kg per min. The response to a sudden osmolality change may be due to changes in cell pH or calcium secondary to the change in cell osmolality [65]. In addition, the role of organic solutes in the maintenance of epithelial cell volume is not well understood.

At present the relationship between transepithelial fluid transport and cell volume regulation is not clearly defined. Inasmuch as fluid transport involves osmotic gradients across the cell membranes, it is possible to regard the regulatory responses to external osmolality changes as a manifestation of the osmoregulation required for balanced fluid entry and exit. The intracellular indicator(s) which trigger volume regulatory responses have not been identified in epithelia; their role, if any, in the regulation of transepithelial fluid transport is also unknown. Clearly, there is a great deal yet to be learned about fluid transport by epithelia.

References

1. Finkelstein A (1987) Water movement through lipid bilayers, pores, and plasma membranes. J. Wiley, New York
2. Diamond JM (1979) Osmotic water flow in leaky epithelia. J Membr Biol 51:195–216
3. McGlaughlin S, Mathias RT (1985) Electro-osmosis and the reabsorption of fluid in renal proximal tubules. J Gen Physiol 85:699–728
4. Goldschmidt S (1921) On the mechanism of absorption from the intestine. Physiol Rev 1:421–453
5. Reid W (1902) Intestinal absorption of solutes. J Physiol 28:241–256
6. Curran PF, Solomon AK (1957) Ion and water fluxes in the ileum of rats. J Gen Physiol 41:143–168
7. Wiedner G (1976) Method to detect volume flows in the nanoliter range. Rev Sci Intrum 47:775–776
8. Diamond JM (1962) The reabsorptive function of the gallbladder. J Physiol 161:442–473
9. Diamond JM (1964) Transport of salt and water in rabbit and guinea pig gallbladder. J Gen Physiol 48:1–14
10. Diamond JM (1964) The mechanism of isotonic water transport. J Gen Physiol 48:15–42
11. Andreoli TE, Schafer JA, Troutman SL (1978) Perfusion rate-dependence of transepithelial osmosis in isolated proximal convoluted tubules: Estimation of the hydraulic conductance. Kidney Int 14:263–269
16. Schafer JA (1984) Mechanisms coupling the absorption of solutes and water in the proximal nephron. Kidney Int 25:708–716

17. Barfuss DW, Schafer JA (1981) Collection and analysis of absorbate from proximal straight tubules. Am J Physiol 241 (Renal Physiology 10):F597–F604

18. Williams JC, Barfuss DW, Schafer JA (1986) Transport of solute in proximal tubules is modified by changes in medium osmolality. Am J Physiol 250 (Renal Fluid Electrolyte Physiol 19):F246–F255

19. Hallback D-A, Jodal M, Lundgren O (1980) Villous tissue osmolality, water and electrolyte transport in the cat small intestine at varying luminal osmolalities. Acta Physiol Scand 110:95–100

20. Hill A (1980) Salt-water coupling in leaky epithelia. J Membr Biol 55:117–182

21. Gonzalez E, Carpi-Medina P, Linares H, Whittembury G (1984) Osmotic water permeability of the apical membrane of proximal straight tubular (PST) cells. Pflugers Arch 402:337–339

22. Curran PF, MacIntosh JR (1962) A model system for biological water transport. Nature 193:347–348

23. Weinstein AM, Stephenson JL (1981) Coupled water transport in standing gradient models of the lateral intercellular space. Biophys J 35:167–191

24. Weinstein AM, Stephenson JL (1981) Models of coupled salt and water transport across leaky epithelia. J Membr Biol 60:1–20

25. Whitlock RT, Wheeler HO (1964) Coupled transport of solute and water across rabbit gallbladder epithelium. J Clin Invest 48:2249–2265

26. Tormey JM, Diamond JM (1967) The ultrastructural route of fluid transport in rabbit gallbladder. J Gen Physiol 50:2031–2060

27. Diamond JM, Bossert WH (1967) Standing-gradient osmotic flow. A mechanism for coupling of water and solute transport in epithelia. J Gen Physiol 50:2061–2083

28. Berry CA, Boulpaep (1975) Nonelectrolyte permeability of the paracellular pathway in Necturus proximal tubule. Am J Physiol 228:581–595

29. DiBona DR, Mills JW (1979) Distribution of Na pump sites in transporting epithelia. Fed Proc 38:134–143

30. Kyte J Immunoferritin determination of distribution of [Na+K] ATPase over plasma membranes of renal convoluted tubules. I. Proximal segment. J Cell Biol 68:287–303

31. Pedley TJ (1983) Calculation of unstirred layer thickness in membrane transport experiments, a survey. Q Rev Biophys 16:115–150

32. Schafer JA, Patlak CS, Andreoli TE (1974) Osmosis in cortical collecting tubules. J Gen Physiol 64:201–227

33. Strange KB, Spring KR (1987) Cell membrane water permeability of rabbit cortical collecting duct. J Membr Biol 96:27–43

34. Weinstein AM, Stephenson JL, Spring KR (1981) The coupled transport of water. In: Bonting SL, de Pont JJHHM (eds) New comprehensive biochemistry. Membrane transport, vol 2. Elsevier, Amsterdam, pp 311–351

35. Berry CA (1983) Water permeability and pathways in the proximal tubule. Am J Physiol 245 (Renal Fluid Electrolyte Physiology 14):F279–F294

36. Weinstein AM (1987) Convective paracellular solute flux. J Gen Physiol 89:501–518

37. Van Os CH, Wiedner G, Wright EM (1979) Volume flows across gallbladder epithelium induced by small hydrostatic and osmotic gradients. J Membr Biol 49:1–20

38. Naftalin RJ, Tripathi S (1985) Passive water flows driven across isolated rabbit ileum by osmotic, hydrostatic and electrical gradients. J Physiol 360:27–50

39. Persson B-E, Spring KR (1982) Gallbladder epithelial cell hydraulic water permeability and volume regulation. J Gen Physiol 79:481–505

40. Carpi-Medina P, Lindemann B, Gonzales E, Whittembury G (1984) The continuous measurement of tubular volume changes in response to step changes in contraluminal osmolality. Pflugers Arch 400:343–348

41. Gonzalez E, Carpi-Medina P, Whittembury G (1982) Cell osmotic water permeability in isolated rabbit proximal straight tubules. Am J Physiol 242 (Renal Electrolyte Fluid Physiol 11):F331–F330

42. Welling LW, Welling DJ, Ochs TJ (1983) Video measurement of basolateral membrane conductivity in the proximal tubule. Am J Physiol 245 (Renal Fluid Electrolyte Physiol 14):F123–F129

43. Whittembury G, Paz-Aliaga A, Biondi A, Carpi-Medina P, Gonzalez E, Linares H (1985) Pathways for volume flow and volume regulation in leaky epithelia. Pflugers Arch 405(Suppl 1):S17–S22

44. Verkman AS, Ives HE (1986) Water permeability and fluidity of renal basolateral membranes. Am J Physiol 250 (Renal Fluid Electrolyte Physiol 19):F633–F643

45. Strange KB, Spring KR (1986) Methods for imaging renal tubule cells. Kidney Int 30:P192–200

46. Kachadorian WA, Sariban-Sohraby S, Spring KR (1985) Regulation of water permeability in toad bladder at two barriers. Am J Physiol 248 (Renal Fluid Electrolyte Physiol 17):F260–F265

47. Suzuki K, Kottra G, Kampmann L, Fromter E (1982) Square wave pulse analysis of cellular and paracellular conductance pathways in Necturus gallbladder epithelium. Pflugers Arch 394:302–312

48. Spring KR (1983) Fluid transport by gallbladder epithelium. J Exp Biol 106:181–194

49. Bentzel CJ, Parsa G, Hare DK (1969) Osmotic flow across proximal tubule of Necturus: correlation of physiologic and anatomic studies. Am J Physiol 217:570–580

50. Blom H, Helander HF (1977) Quantitative electron microscopical studies on in vitro incubated rabbit gallbladder epithelium. J Membr Biol 37:45–61

51. Preisig PA, Berry CA (1985) Evidence for transcellular osmotic flow in rat proximal tubules. Am J Physiol 249 (Renal Fluid Electrolyte Physiol 18):F124–F131

52. Ikonomov O, Simon M, Fromter E (1985) Electrophysiological studies on lateral intercellular spaces of Necturus gallbladder epithelium. Pflugers Arch 403:301–307

53. Zeuthen T (1983) Ion activities in the lateral intercellular spaces of gallbladder epithelium transporting at low external osmolalities. J Membr Biol 76:113–122

54. Larson M, Spring KR (1983) Bumetanide inhibition of NaCl transport by Necturus gallbladder. J Membr Biol 74:123–129

55. Persson B-E, Spring KR (1984) Permeability properties of the subepithelial tissues of Necturus gallbladder. Biochim Biophys Acta 772:135–139

56. Spring KR, Hope A (1978) The size and shape of the lateral intercellular spaces in a living epithelium. Science 200:54–58

57. Spring KR, Hope A (1979) Fluid transport and the dimensions of cells and interspaces of living Necturus gallbladder. J Gen Physiol 73:287–305

58. Whittembury G, Verde-Martinez C, Linares H, Paz-Aliaga A (1980) Solvent drag of large solutes indicates paracellular water flow in leaky epithelia. Proc R Soc Lond [Biol] 211:63–81

59. Boulpaep EL (1967) Ion permeability of the peritubular and luminal membrane of the renal tubule cell. In: Kruck F (ed) Transport und Funktion Intracellularer Elektrolyte. Urban and Schwarzenberg, Munich, pp 98–107

60. Frizzell R, Schultz SG (1972) Ionic conductances of extracellular shunt pathway in rabbit ileum. Influence of shunt on transmural sodium transport and electrical potential differences. J Gen Physiol 59:318–348

61. Lohr JW, Grantham JJ (1986) Isovolumetric regulation of isolated S_2 proximal tubules in anisotonic media. J Clin Invest 78:1165–1172

62. Tune BM, Burg MB (1971) Glucose transport by proximal renal tubules. Am J Physiol 221:580–585

63. Guggino WB (1986) Functional heterogeneity in early distal tubule of Amphiuma kidney: evidence for two modes of Cl and K transport across the basolateral cell membrane. Am J Physiol 250 (Renal Fluid Electrolyte Physiol 19):F430–F440
64. Jensen PK, Fisher RS, Spring KR (1984) Feedback inhibition of NaCl entry in Necturus gallbladder epithelial cells. J Membr Biol 82:95–104
65. Spring KR, Ericson A-C (1982) Epithelial cell volume modulation and regulation. J Membr Biol 69:167–176
66. Larson M, Spring KR (1984) Volume regulation by Necturus gallbladder: basolateral KCl exit. J Membr Biol 81:219–233

Organic Compounds in Renal Volume Regulation

WALTER G. GUDER, MICHAEL SCHMOLKE[1], and FRANZ X. BECK[2]

SUMMARY. Four small organic molecules belonging to the chemical groups of trimethylamines (betaine and glycerophosphorylcholine) and polyols (sorbitol and inositol) have been identified as acting as organic osmolytes in the kidney. When measured along the corticopapillary axis, each substance exhibits a specific distribution pattern, indicating a specific localization and function. Studying their behavior under vasopressin treatment in diabetes insipidus rats and after insulin treatment in diabetes mellitus rats confirmed this conclusion: arginine vasopressin (AVP) led to a steady increase of sorbitol and glycerophosphorylcholine over 7 days with no effect on inositol levels. Insulin treatment of diabetic rats, on the other hand, decreased sorbitol with a concomitant increase in glycerophosphorylcholine, again without any effect on tubular inositol concentrations. From this and in vitro studies it can be concluded that both hormones act by indirect mechanisms, which alter interstitial osmolality. This in turn leads to a change in tubular osmolyte synthesis, uptake, and release rates. In addition, the concentration of the respective precursors, glucose and choline, influences the formation rates of sorbitol and betaine.

Introduction

Extracellular osmolality in mammalian kidney exhibits a corticopapillary gradient, which changes with renal concentrating and diluting functions depending on water load, vasopressin activity, and other osmoregulatory factors [1]. Whereas the osmolality of interstitium and intracellular space of renal cortex changes only in a narrow range, in parallel with plasma osmolality, papillary osmolality of these compartments can vary from near-isotonicity during diuresis to some thousand mosmol/kg H_2O

---

[1]Institute of Clinical Chemistry, Bogenhausen Hospital, D 8000 Munich 81, Federal Republic of Germany
[2]Physiologisches Institut der Universität, D 8000 Munich 81, Federal Republic of Germany

during water deprivation [2]. Such dramatic changes impose a severe osmotic stress on all medullary cells, which would lead to cell damage if it were not accompanied by adequate osmoregulatory mechanisms. In various medullary cells, several mechanisms have been found which lead to intracellular osmotic equilibration during changing extracellular osmolalities while keeping intracellular electrolyte concentrations rather constant [2], with or without cell volume regulation [3,4].

Recently, four small organic molecules have been found in high concentrations intracellularly in renal medullary cells, where they form corticopapillary concentration gradients in parallel to the osmotic gradients [5,6]. These substances were identified as the polyols sorbitol and inositol and the trimethylamines betaine and glycerophosphorylcholine. Besides carrying out their role as osmotic effectors, methylamines have been shown to counteract the destabilizing effect of urea on enzymes (non-perturbing solutes) [7].

After reliable methods were developed to quantify individual organic osmolytes we were able to document their intracellular concentrations in inner and outer medullary tubules [6,8]. When polyols and methylamines were measured in more defined kidney and nephron segments, it turned out that each substance exhibited an individual concentration pattern (Fig. 1). This result implies that each osmolyte may have different functions in different osmotic states and may be regulated by specific mechanisms. This hypothesis was further substantiated in two diuretic models, the Brattleboro (diabetes insipidus centralis) and the streptozotocin treated (diabetes mellitus) rat.

Materials and Methods

Brattleboro rats, kindly provided by D. Ganten, Heidelberg, were treated with AVP (100 ng/day per 100 g b.w.) for up to 14 days, via intraperitoneal osmotic mini-pumps [9]. Diabetes mellitus rats, (diabetes mellitus induced by a single i.v. injection of 100 mg/kg b.w. streptozotocin) were obtained in collaboration with E. Schleicher, Institute for diabetes research, Munich. These rats were treated for 8 days with insulin or for 6 days with insulin followed by 2 days omitting the hormone [10]. As a control group, untreated Sprague-Dawley rats were run in parallel. Kidneys were excised and cut into five sections along the corticopapillary axis (Fig. 1); the organic osmolytes were quantitated by high performance liquid chromatography (HPLC) [11] and by enzymatic methods [6] described previously.

Results

Distribution of Organic Osmolytes Along the Corticopapillary Axis

When analyzed by HPLC [12] and by enzymatic methods [6] each organic osmolyte exhibited an individual distribution pattern along the corticopapillary axis in normal rat kidney (Fig. 1). Sorbitol was found nearly exclusively in the inner medulla, forming a steep gradient from inner/outer medullary border to papillary tip. In sharp contrast, inositol increased at the corticomedullary border (Fig. 1) [5,6,9], but seemed to have no gradient along the entire medulla. Glycerophosphorylcholine concentra-

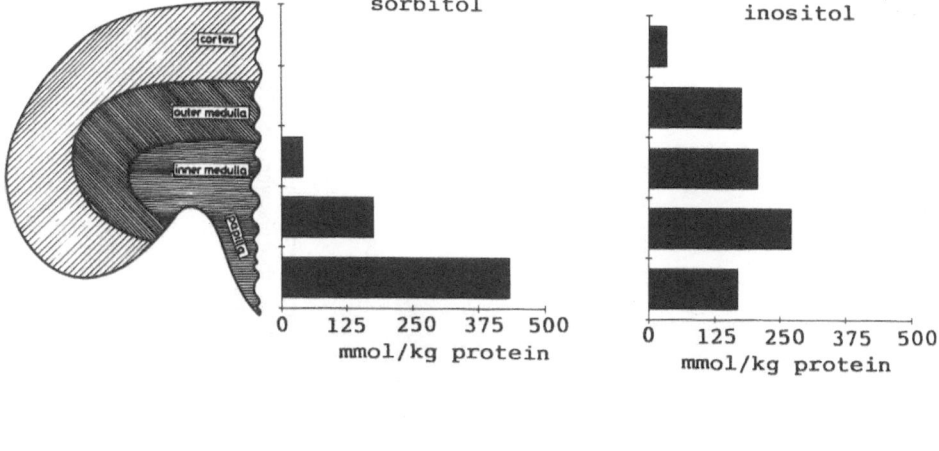

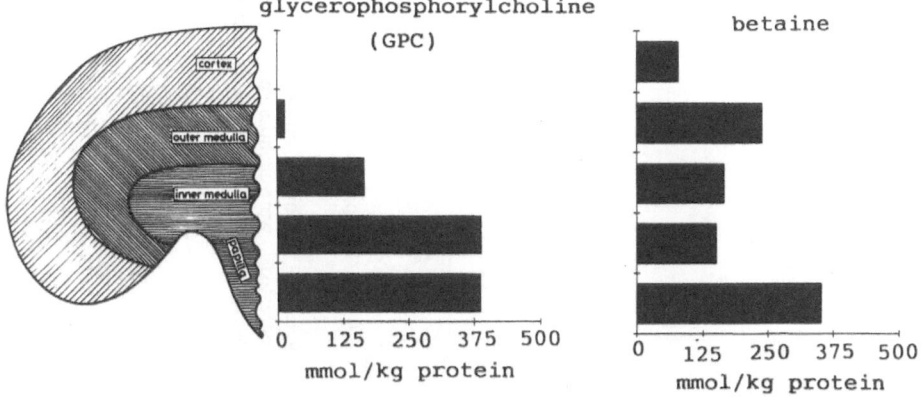

Fig. 1. Distribution of organic osmolytes in rat kidney. Sorbitol, inositol, glycerophosphorylcholine and betaine were quantitated in different sections of a normal rat kidney by the HPLC procedure described by Wolff et al. [11]. Results are given per tissue protein, measured by the biuret method in individual homogenates [6]

tion, on the other hand, increased from outer medullar to papilla, with negligible amounts in cortex. The betaine concentration increased in papillary tip, but in addition, it showed a unique gradient in the outer medulla decreasing to cortex. The latter finding has not been described before, whereas the other osmolyte patterns agree with those found in rabbit [12].

Changes in Diabetes Insipidus

Untreated Brattleboro rats were found to produce hypotonic urine (134 mosmol/kg, [9]). Under these conditions, sorbitol concentrations were reduced to 4–14% and glycerophosphorylcholine and betaine concentrations were reduced to 20–30%

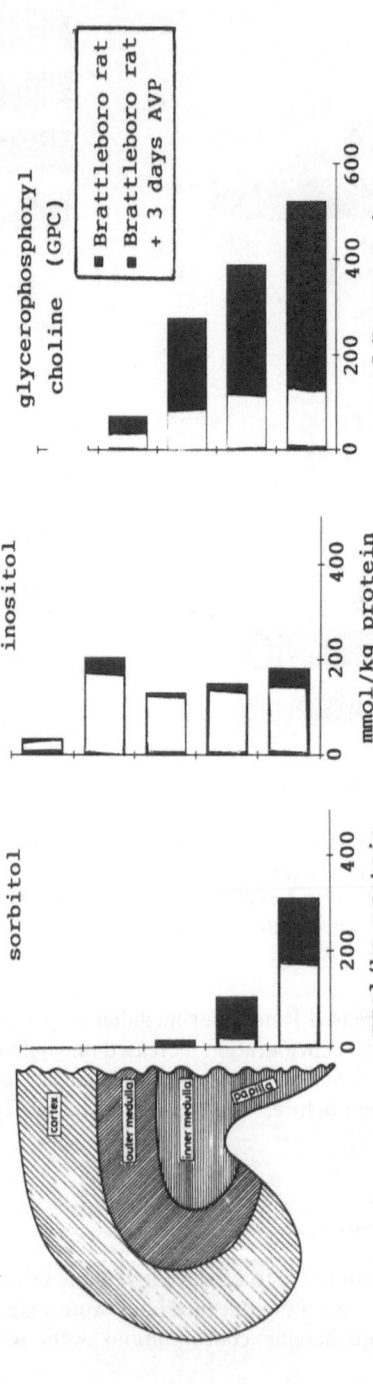

Fig. 2. Effect of arginine-vasopressin treatment on organic osmolyte concentrations in Brattleboro rat kidney sections. Brattleboro rats were treated with arginine vasopressin (*AVP*), 100 ng/100g bw per day, over 3 days, using osmotic mini-pumps; sorbitol, inositol, and glycerophosphorylcholine were quantitated by enzymatic methods as described elsewhere [9]. Results are means of four rats compared to those of three untreated Brattleboro rats

[9,13] of those found in control rats. In sharp contrast, inositol was little affected by diabetes insipidus, whereas furosemide, water and lithium diuresis decreased all four organic osmolytes [9,13,14,15,16].

Treatment with AVP led to normalization of organic osmolyte concentrations in 3 days (Fig. 2). Interestingly, urine osmolality increased before a significant effect of AVP on organic osmolyte content could be demonstrated. The conclusion that this finding indicates an indirect effect of AVP on organic osmolytes is confirmed by the lack of effect of this hormone on osmolyte content in isolated tubules (G Wirthensohn, unpublished work).

Osmolyte Content in Diabetes Mellitus

The sodium concentration of urine produced by insulin deficient diabetic rats was comparable to that in other diuretic states, but was of normal osmolality, due to high glucose concentration [10]. Therefore this model seemed to be suitable for the investigation of the possible role of sodium and glucose versus osmolality as possible triggers of organic osmolyte accumulation. In contrast to Brattleboro rats and furosemide diuresis, glycerophosphorylcholine was found to be only slightly decreased (Fig. 3) Inositol exhibited little change in diabetic animals. Sorbitol levels, on the other hand, increased 2–3-fold under these conditions, without significant changes in the distribution pattern (Fig. 3). Betaine was not measured in diabetic animals.

This glucose dependent increase in sorbitol, but not in inositol and glycerophosphorylcholine, was confirmed by in vitro experiments with inner medullary tubules: glucose increased sorbitol biosynthesis with a saturation above 10 mmol/l [6]. Distribution of newly synthesized sorbitol between cells and incubation medium was regulated by extracellular osmolality [6,8], pointing to a specific sorbitol export mechanism in papillary cells. In addition, diabetes mellitus was shown by Grunewald and Kinne [17] to increase the activity of the sorbitol forming enzyme, aldose reductase, known to be regulated at the gene level by extracellular osmolality in renal medullary cells [15].

Insulin treated diabetic rats showed a normalization of blood and urine glucose concentrations, urinary sodium, potassium, urea, and osmolality [10]. Accordingly, glycerophosphorylcholine increased slightly, inositol did not change, but sorbitol concentrations were reduced to levels between those of control and untreated diabetic rats. This decrease in cellular sorbitol was much less than expected from the normalization of glucose concentrations, indicating a time lag in adaptation of cellular osmolyte composition. Again the regional distribution pattern of organic osmolytes was not changed by insulin deficiency and insulin treatment.

Discussion

Why Four Different Organic Osmolytes?

The present findings and those of other investigators indicate that the four major substances found to be involved in renal medullary osmoregulation may have specific localization and specific regulation mechanisms, and may function under various physiological and pathophysiological conditions. This was confirmed by recent

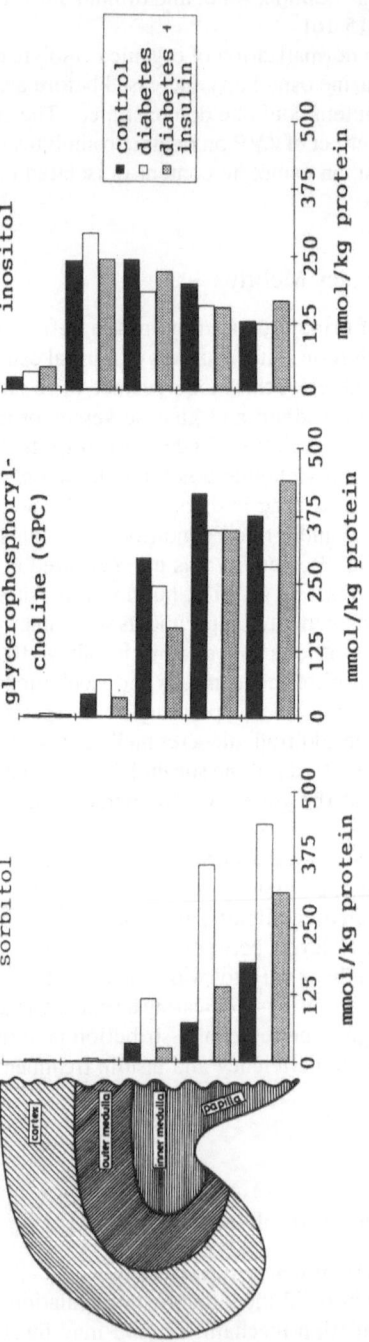

Fig. 3. Renal organic osmolytes in streptozotocin diabetic rats. Sorbitol, glycerophosphorylcholine, and inositol were measured by enzymatic methods in streptozotocin diabetic rats (100 mg/kg bw i.v.). *Black bars:* means of 3 untreated control rats run in the same series. *Open bars:* means of 9 diabetic animals, which were treated with insulin (2*5U per day) for 6 days after streptozotocin and analyzed on day 8, two days after insulin withdrawal. *Stippled bars:* means of 8 diabetic animals treated with insulin for 8 days

studies in microdissected nephron segments, showing a unique distribution of inositol in the segments of the thick ascending limb [18], whereas the enzymes for sorbitol synthesis [19] and sorbitol [18] were restricted to all tubular structures of the inner medulla. Choline oxidation to betaine, on the other hand, was shown to be highest in the S3 segment of the proximal tubule, but was also active in papillary tubules [20,21]. These findings point to a possible role of biosynthesis in regulating local osmolyte concentrations. On the other hand, cellular import and export mechanisms have been described as being involved in regulating tubular osmolyte concentrations [2].

Conclusions

From our present knowledge the following general conclusions may be drawn:

All four organic osmolytes described are present in papillary cells in concentrations which fill the osmotic gap between intracellular and extracellular salt concentration [2]. Moreover, betaine seems to play a specific role in cells at the corticomedullary border. Inositol forms high concentrations in loop cells of the thick ascending limb of Henle [20].

Betaine, glycerophosphorylcholine, and sorbitol are formed in tubular cells from their precursors choline [20,22] and glucose, [6,8,10] respectively; inositol and betaine, in addition, seem to be taken up by active transport from extracellular space [23]. All four osmolytes are highly concentrated in the cell, unless decreasing extracellular osmolality opens still undefined "gates" of cellular organic osmolyte export [6].

Besides their different locations along the nephron the presence of four different organic osmolytes in the renal papilla allows the kidney cell to adapt to various forms of changing osmolality in a flexible and specific way: Thus, vasopressin in vivo leads to an accumulation of all osmolytes [15], and water diuresis leads to rapid loss of all osmolytes [2] in the renal papilla, by changing interstitial osmolality. When sodium is replaced by glucose as extracellular osmolyte there is a specific increase in sorbitol [6,8,17].

Of all four organic osmolytes in the kidney, sorbitol is the best studied. The present study confirms that sorbitol is of special significance in diabetic states, where it seems to compensate for the high extracellular glucose concentrations [10,17,24]. Similar increases have been observed in diabetic eye lenses, nervous tissue, and blood cells [25]. The complications found in diabetes have partially been attributed to these changes. Consequently, aldose reductase inhibitors have been introduced to reduce tissue sorbitol levels. The present finding that, despite normoglycemia after two days of insulin treatment, sorbitol levels are still elevated, indicates slow adaptation of intracellular osmolality; this may help to explain osmoregulatory complications which appear during intensive treatment of hyperosmolar diabetic coma. On the other hand, aldose reductase inhibitors are expected to cause osmotic complications, if the missing sorbitol is not counterregulated by other osmolytes. The reciprocal changes in glycerophosphorylcholine and sorbitol concentrations in diabetic rats during treatment indicates that such mechanisms may exist in renal cells [10].

The lack of change in inositol concentration during AVP treatment in Brattleboro rats [9] and in diabetes mellitus [10] also contrasts with the behavior of the other polyols and suggests that the function of inositol in tubular osmoregulation differs from that of the other polyols.

In spite of our rapidly increasing knowledge of the mechanisms and sites of osmoregulation by organic osmolytes, major problems still remain to be investigated by future experiments: None of the transporters have been fully characterized, nor do we know the individual mediators that transfer the signal of changing extracellular osmolality to the intracellular sites. These unknown mediators seem to cause specific changes in the biosynthesis and transport of the individual osmolytes at the gene [15], protein [26], and membrane level [6,8,23]. Experiments in microorganisms, mammalian cell culture, and in vivo indicate that all kinds of mechanisms can be operative simultaneously, resulting in the specific osmolyte pattern observed in acute and chronic osmoregulation.

At present, little is known about the connection between cellular volume regulation and observed changes in organic osmolyte concentration. As extensively discussed in other contributions to these proceedings [2,4], cellular volume is expected to change upon rapid changes of intracellular osmolality. The rapidity and extent of volume regulatory changes may depend on the presence and velocity of changes in organic osmolyte concentrations. Thus, proximal tubule cells [27] and loop cells of the thick ascending limb of Henle [4] seem to be volume regulated, whereas in papillary collecting duct cells [2,3] this was not consistently observed.

Acknowledgment. The work reported herein was supported by the Deutsche Forschungsgemeinschaft (Gu 82/3-2 and Be 963/2-3).

References

1. Jamison RL, Kriz W (1982) Urinary concentrating mechanism. Oxford University Press, Oxford
2. Beck FX, Thurau K, Schmolke M, Guder WG (1991) Osmolytes and cell osmoregulation in the kidney. In: Proceedings of the XIth international congress of nephrology, July 15–20 1990. Tokyo, Japan
3. Law RO (1990) Adaptive volume responses of renal papillary cells exposed to hyperosmolal media. Renal Physiol Biochem 13:171–172
4. Hebert SC (1990) Rapid cell volume regulation. In: Proceedings of the XIth international congress of nephrology, July 15–20 1990. Tokyo, Japan
5. Bagnasco S, Balaban R, Fales H, Yang YM, Burg MB (1986) Predominant osmotically active organic solutes in rat and rabbit renal medullas. J Biol Chem 261:5872–5877
6. Wirthensohn G, Lefrank S, Schmolke M, Guder WG (1989) Regulation of organic osmolyte concentrations in tubules from rat renal inner medulla. Am J Physiol 256:F128–F135
7. Yancey P, Clark M, Hand S, Bowlus R, Somero G (1982) Living with water stress: evolution of osmolyte systems. Science 217:1214–1222
8. Schmolke M, Guder WG (1989) Metabolic regulation of organic osmolytes in tubules from rat renal inner and outer medulla. Renal Physiol Biochem 12:347–358
9. Schmolke M, Beck FX, Guder WG (1989) Effect of antidiuretic hormone on renal organic osmolytes in Brattleboro rats. Am J Physiol 257:F732–F737
10. Guder WG, Schleicher E, Schmolke M (to be published) Perturbation of renal polyols and glycerophosphorylcholine in streptozotocin diabetes and insulin treatment. Diabetologia
11. Wolff SD, Yancey PH, Stanton TS, Balaban RS (1989) A simple HPLC method for quantitating the major organic solutes of the renal medulla. Am J Physiol 256:F954–F956

12. Yancey PH, Burg MB (1989) Distribution of major organic osmolytes in rabbit kidneys in diuresis and antidiuresis. Am J Physiol 257:F602–F607
13. Blumenfeld J, Hebert S, Heilig C, Balschi J, Stromski M, Gullans S (1989) Organic osmolytes in inner medulla of the Brattleboro rat: effect of ADH and dehydration. Am J Physiol 256:F916–F922
14. Wirthensohn G, Lefrank S, Guder WG, Beck FX (1987) Studies of the role of glycerophosphorylcholine and sorbitol in renal osmoregulation. In: Kovacevic Z, Guder WG (eds) Molecular Nephrology: Biochemical aspects of kidney function. Walter de Gruyter, Berlin, pp 321–327
15. Cowley BD, Ferraris JD, Carper D, Burg MB (1990) In vivo osmoregulation of aldose reductase mRNA, protein, and sorbitol in renal medulla. Am J Physiol 258:F154–F161
16. Guder WG, Schmolke M, Lefrank S, Beck FX (1990) Specific changes of renal organic osmolyte pattern in different diuretic states (abstract). Renal Physiol Biochem 13:166–177
17. Grunewald W, Kinne RKH (1989) Sorbitol metabolism in inner medullary collecting duct cells of diabetic rats. Pflugers Arch 414:346–350
18. Schmolke M, Bornemann A, Guder WG (to be published) Polyol determination along the rat nephron. Biol Chem Hoppe Seyler
19. Sands JM, Terada Y, Bernard LM, Knepper MA (1989) Aldose reductase activities in microdissected rat renal tubule segments. Am J Physiol 256:F563–F569
20. Schmolke M, Bornemann A, Guder WG (to be published) Distribution and regulation of organic osmolytes along the nephron. In: Koide H, Endou H, Kurokawa H (eds) Cell Biology of Nephron Heterogeneity: Fine Structure and Functions. Karger Basel
21. Grossmann EB, Hebert SC (1989) Renal inner medullary choline dehydrogenase activity: characterization and modulation. Am J Physiol 256:F107–F112
22. Wirthensohn G, Guder WG (1982) Studies on renal choline metabolism and phosphatidylcholine synthesis. In: Morel F (ed) Biochemistry of kidney function. Elsevier, Amsterdam, pp 119–128
23. Nakanishi TR, Burg MB (1989) Osmoregulatory fluxes of myoinositol and betaine in renal cells. Am J Physiol 258:C964–C970
24. Burg MB (1988) Role of aldose reductase and sorbitol in maintaining the medullary intracellular milieu. Kidney Int 33:635–641
25. Burg MB, Kador PF (1988) Sorbitol, osmoregulation and the complications of diabetes: J Clin Invest 81:635–640
26. Bagnasco S, Uchida S, Balaban R, Kador P, Burg M (1987) Induction of aldose reductase and sorbitol in renal inner medullary cells by elevated extracellular NaCl. Proc Natl Acad Sci USA 84:1718–1720
27. Völkl H, Paulmichl M, Lang F (1988) Cell volume regulation in renal cortical cells. Renal Physiol Biochem 11:158–173

Volume Regulation in the Collecting Duct and Related Epithelia

KEVIN STRANGE[1]

SUMMARY. Under normal physiological conditions, cells of tight, Na^+-reabsorbing urinary epithelia, such as the collecting tubule, are exposed to both anisosmotic and isosmotic volume stress. A common but poorly understood response of these cells to volume perturbation is the activation of mechanisms that restore volume to its original resting value. The purpose of this article is to review briefly what is currently known about volume regulatory processes in the collecting tubule, amphibian and mammalian bladder, and frog skin. Specifically, the role of solute loss and accumulation pathways, transcellular cross-talk mechanisms, and volume sensor/transducer systems will be discussed. Key questions in need of future research will be emphasized.

Introduction

Under normal physiological conditions, cells of the renal collecting tubule are exposed to both anisosmotic and isosmotic volume stress. Anisosmotic volume changes are brought about by changes in extracellular osmolality, which fluctuates with the degree of diuresis or antidiuresis the animal is undergoing. In contrast, isosmotic volume perturbations occur when intracellular solute content changes. Variations in cell solute content take place during fluctuations in the activity of membrane transport processes.

In principle, it is teleologically desirable for cells to maintain a constant volume. Changes in cell volume can perturb flux through metabolic pathways, membrane transport processes, cellular signaling mechanisms, and the function of intracellular organelles. Excessive volume changes can result in cellular lysis. Many cell types, therefore, respond to volume perturbations by activating volume regulatory pathways. Cell volume regulation is brought about by the loss of, or accumulation of,

[1]The Children's Hospital, Division of Nephrology, Harvard Medical School, Boston, MA 02115, USA

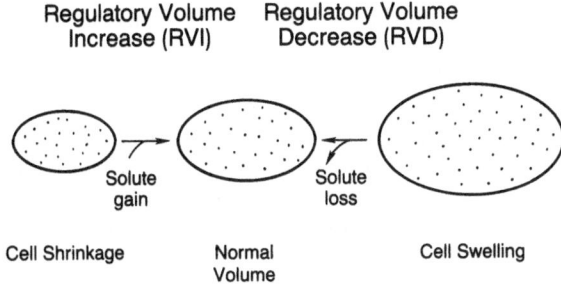

Fig. 1. Cells regulate their volume after swelling or shrinkage by the loss or gain of osmotically active solutes

inorganic ions and organic solutes, collectively referred to as osmolytes (Fig. 1). The purpose of this review is to discuss briefly the mechanisms and control of volume regulation in the renal collecting tubule and in three related epithelia, the amphibian bladder, the mammalian bladder, and frog skin. For additional discussions of cell volume regulation the reader should consult several articles published elsewhere in these proceedings (see List of Contents).

Volume Regulation Under Anisosmotic Conditions

One of the first studies of epithelial volume regulation was carried out by MacRobbie and Ussing in the frog skin [1]. These investigators demonstrated that dilution of the serosal bathing medium caused marked cell swelling, followed by a partial regulatory volume decrease (RVD) and significant loss of intracellular K^+. Ussing [2] demonstrated that RVD was inhibited by the Cl^- channel blocker, MK196, suggesting that parallel K^+ and Cl^- conductances mediate this process. Consistent with these observations are the recent microelectrode studies of Costa et al. [3], which suggest that cell swelling increases basolateral conductive K^+ permeability in this tissue.

MacRobbie and Ussing [1] also demonstrated that the frog skin was capable of undergoing regulatory volume increase (RVI). When volume-regulated skins were transferred from hypotonic to isosmotic medium, the cells shrank below their initial volume and then reswelled. Later studies by Ussing [4] demonstrated that this RVI process occurred only when Na^+, K^+, and Cl^- were present in the serosal bathing medium. In addition, the process was inhibited by furosemide and bumetanide, suggesting involvement of a basolateral Na/K/2Cl cotransport mechanism.

Optical studies carried out by Davis and Finn [5] have demonstrated that cells in the frog urinary bladder regulate their volume following exposure to serosal hypotonicity via a basolateral Ba^{2+}-sensitive K^+ channel. Interestingly, RVD is also blocked by luminal amiloride, which appears to decrease basolateral K^+ conductance via a transcellular cross-talk mechanism ([6]; discussed below). Studies by Lewis and coworkers [7–9] in both the toad and rabbit urinary bladders have indicated that cell shrinkage reduces basolateral K^+ conductance. Cell shrinkage also appears to inhibit the basolateral Cl^- conductance in rabbit bladder [8]. Downregulation of membrane ion permeability in these epithelia presumably reduces net cellular solute loss and aids in volume recovery. Donaldson and Lewis [9] have recently suggested that cell shrinkage in the rabbit bladder activates basolateral volume regulatory Na^+/H^+ and Cl^-/HCO_3^- exchangers.

Both principal and intercalated cells in the rabbit cortical collecting tubule (CCT) undergo nearly complete RVD following hypotonic cell swelling [10]. The mechanism by which this occurs, however, remains unknown. In this tissue RVD is not inhibited by bilateral addition of a variety of K^+ and Cl^- transport blockers (ouabain, bumetanide, Ba^{2+}, SITS, anthracene-9-carboxylic acid), bilateral HCO_3^- and CO_2 removal, bilateral elevation of K^+ concentration to 53 mM, or prolonged exposure of the tissue to K^+- or Cl^+-free media. These results suggest, very indirectly, that anisosmotic RVD may be mediated primarily by organic solute loss mechanisms such as occurs in medullary nephron segments and in cultured medullary cells [11].

The response of CCT cells to a volume decrease is variable. Principal cells show little or no capacity for RVI following 20–40 minutes of shrinkage [10,12]. In contrast, two populations of intercalated cell have been observed. One cell type shows no RVI capabilities, while the other undergoes a partial to complete volume recovery after shrinkage [10,12]. The mechanism of RVI and the relationship between volume regulation and the so-called type A and type B intercalated cell morphology is unknown.

Natke et al. [13] have reported that RVI can be activated in non-perfused rabbit CCT by exposure to low concentrations of butyrate. In perfused tubules, however, this organic acid has no effect on cell volume following hyperosmotic shrinkage (K. Strange, unpublished observations). It is interesting to speculate that the difference between the two preparations may be related to Na^+ transport. Sodium reabsorption in non-perfused tubules is blocked and, as such, it is likely that basolateral conductive pathways are downregulated (e.g., [6]; discussed below). Stimulation of solute influx pathways by butyrate (see [14]) may therefore allow net solute accumulation and RVI to occur.

Sun and Hebert [15] have examined volume regulation in the rat inner medullary collecting duct (IMCD). This nephron segment is normally exposed to variations in interstitial osmolality, which occur as part of the urinary concentrating mechanism. In the absence of antidiuretic hormone (ADH), the IMCD exhibits little or no RVI capabilities when exposed to a hypertonic medium. Peritubular addition of ADH or cAMP, however, stimulated a rapid RVI response following cell shrinkage. Volume regulation was inhibited by bilateral Na^+ or CO_2 and HCO_3^- removal and by peritubular addition of amiloride or DIDS, suggesting involvement of basolateral Na^+/H^+ and Cl^-/HCO_3^- exchangers. Luminal amiloride also inhibited RVI, suggesting that an apical cation channel or Na^+/H^+ exchanger may also mediate volume regulation.

The role of organic osmolyte transport and metabolism pathways in volume regulation has been examined in the intact renal medulla and in cultured renal medullary and Madin-Darby canine kidney (MDCK) cells (reviewed in [11]). Sands et al. [16] quantified aldose reductase activity in single, microdissected collecting tubule segments. The activity of this enzyme increased with depth into the medulla, suggesting that sorbitol is important for anisosmotic volume regulation in the medullary collecting duct. In suspensions of papillary tubules, Wirthensohn et al. [17] have observed high concentrations of inositol, sorbitol, and glycerophosphorylcholine. These organic compounds are transported out of the cell when extracellular osmolality is decreased, suggesting that they play an important role in RVD.

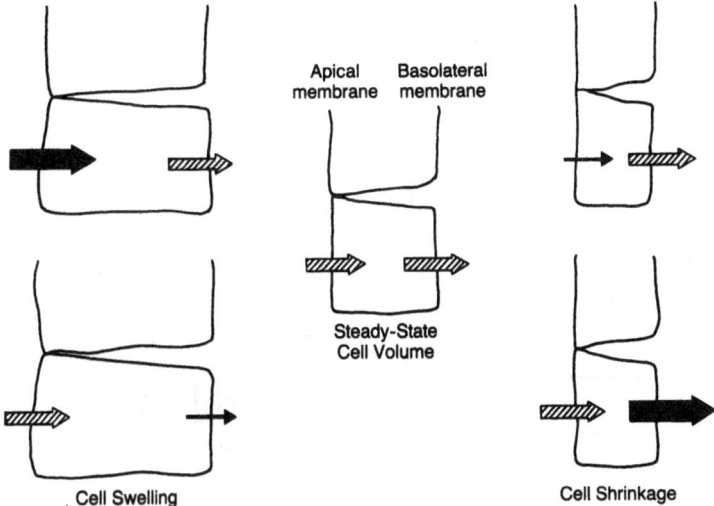

Fig. 2. Changes in the rates of apical and basolateral transport change epithelial cell volume. *Arrow size* reflects relative rate of solute influx or efflux (Modified from [30])

Volume Regulation Under Isosmotic Conditions

Under steady-state conditions, the rates of apical and basolateral membrane solute transport in epithelial cells are matched. These rates can, however, change independently of one another as the result of hormonal modulation of transport pathway activity and/or by variations in the concentration of transported solutes. This is particularly true in tight, Na^+-transporting, urinary epithelia. Tissues such as the collecting duct play a pivotal role in "fine tuning" whole animal salt and water balance. As such, transcellular transport rates can change rapidly and dramatically with changes in whole animal osmoregulatory demands. Figure 2 illustrates that independent changes in solute influx or efflux will alter intracellular solute content and cause cell swelling or shrinkage.

Regulation of epithelial cell volume during changes in transport is mediated by two distinct mechanisms. Transcellular cross-talk is a communication process that occurs between apical and basolateral cell membranes [18]. This communication allows epithelial cells to monitor rates of solute entry and exit and to adjust those rates so that they are matched. Return of epithelial cell volume to its original value following swelling or shrinkage is mediated by volume regulatory solute loss or accumulation pathways.

Transcellular Cross-Talk

The first observations of epithelial cross-talk were made by MacRobbie and Ussing in the frog skin [1]. These investigators noted that inhibition of basolateral Na^+ extrusion by ouabain caused an apparent reduction in apical Na^+, and basolateral K^+,

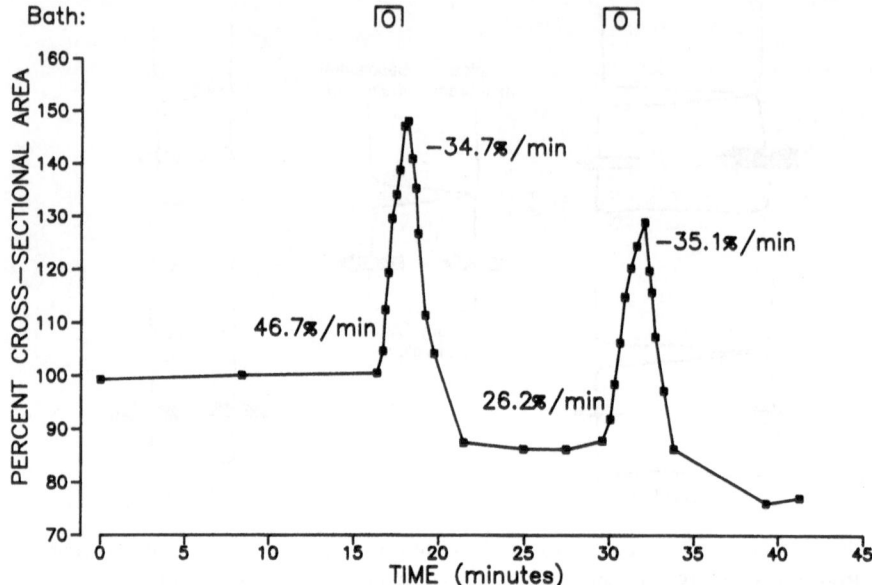

Fig. 3. Ouabain (O)-induced swelling in a principal cell of a CCT dissected from a mineralocorticoid-treated rabbit. The effects of ouabain on cell volume *per se* are readily reversible, but NaCl transport exhibits a long-term inhibition. Initial rates of cell swelling and shrinkage for the first and second periods of ouabain exposure and washout are shown. (See text and [20] for details)

permeability. Helman et al. [19] confirmed and extended these observations, using microelectrodes. Similar findings have also now been made in a variety of other Na^+ transporting epithelia [18].

In desoxycorticosterone acetate (DOCA)-treated rabbit CCT, ouabain causes principal cells to swell 50%–130% at rates of 25%–70%/min [20–21]. Cell swelling is due to net intracellular accumulation of NaCl and water during pump blockage. Sodium enters the cell primarily through an apical Na^+ channel. The mechanism and sidedness of Cl^- entry remains unclear at present.

As shown in Fig. 3, the effects of ouabain on principal cell volume are readily reversible. Removal of this inhibitor causes a rapid cell shrinkage as the pump is reactivated and NaCl is extruded from the cell. The effects of this compound on Na^+ reabsorption, measured as the rate of cell swelling, cannot be readily reversed, however. Brief, successive exposures to ouabain cause a rapid, concomitant reduction in the rate of Na^+ and/or Cl^- entry, while prolonged pump blockage results in a complete cessation of solute influx [20]. Reduction of apical solute entry during pump blockage prevents cell lysis and allows the cell to regulate its volume (discussed below).

Prolonged pump blockage also causes an apparent reduction of basolateral K^+ conductance in principal cells [21–22]. As discussed by Schultz [18], changes in basolateral K^+ permeability that occur with changes in Na^+ transport most likely reflect

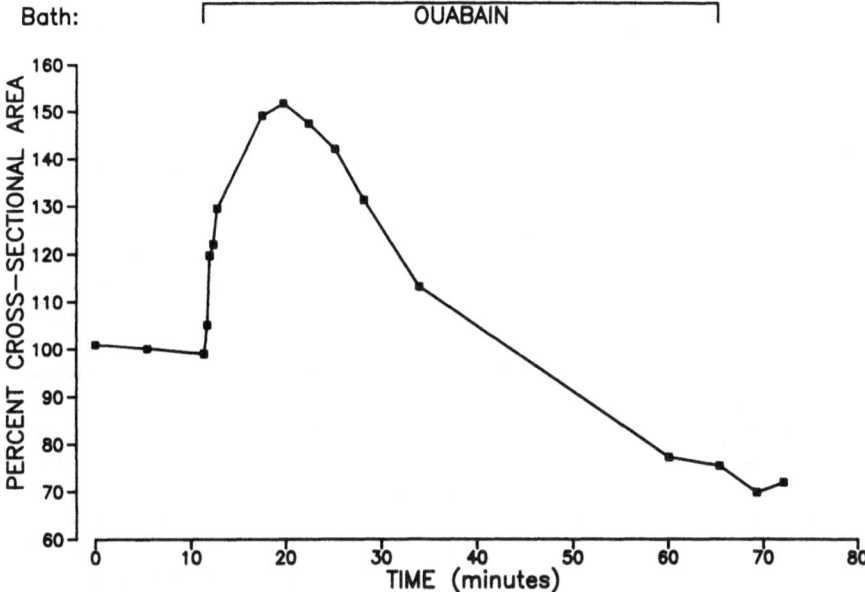

Fig. 4. Ouabain-induced swelling and RVD in a principal cell of a CCT dissected from a mineralocorticoid-treated rabbit

a close interaction between the Na^+/K^+ ATPase and K^+ channels. This pump-leak parallelism minimizes changes in cell K^+ when the activity of the Na^+ pump changes.

Primary changes in the rate of apical Na^+ entry also result in compensatory changes in rates of basolateral transport (see [18]). For example, in the amphibian urinary bladder, blockage of apical Na^+ channels with amiloride causes a rapid reduction in basolateral K^+ conductance [6].

Volume Regulatory Solute Loss and Accumulation

The mechanisms of isosmotic volume regulatory shrinkage or swelling are largely unknown. It is generally assumed that anisosmotic RVD and RVI pathways are the same as those activated following volume perturbations induced by changes in cell solute content. As discussed below, however, this may not be true in all cases.

The one tight epithelial cell type where isosmotic volume regulation has been examined in detail is the principal cell of the rabbit CCT. As discussed above, ouabain causes principal cells to swell rapidly. Attainment of the peak swelling volume is followed by volume regulatory shrinkage, which occurs at a rate of 4%-5%/min until a new volume 10%-15% below control is reached (Fig. 4). Bilateral addition of Ba^{2+} or tetraethylammonium (TEA)$^+$ inhibits [21] RVD 50%-60%. Bath addition of TEA$^+$ has no effect on RVD, but luminal perfusion with TEA$^+$ or quinidine inhibits the process by 50%-60%[21]. Since Ba^{2+}, TEA$^+$, and quinidine are blockers of K^+ channels, these results suggest that RVD is mediated in part by an apical K^+ conductance. Luminal K^+-induced cell swelling studies have indicated that the RVD channel is distinct from the resting apical K^+ conductance responsible for transepithelial K^+ secretion [21]. The RVD channel may be similar to the Ca^{2+}-activated high conductance channel described in patch clamp studies [23]. Ca^{2+}-sensitive, maxi K^+ channels mediate volume regulation in several cell types [24].

Volume regulatory K^+ loss must be accompanied by an equimolar loss of anion. The magnitude of the ouabain-induced volume increase requires that Cl^- accumulated in the cell be lost for RVD; no other intracellular anion is present in sufficient quantity to account for the magnitude of the observed volume regulatory shrinkage. Since K^+ efflux occurs via a conductive pathway, Cl^- loss should also occur by a channel mechanism. Recent studies from this laboratory have confirmed this prediction [22]. Reduction of peritubular Cl^- concentration transiently depolarizes the transepithelial potential by 35 mV and stimulates the rate of RVD 30-fold. Peritubular application of 0.5 mM DIDS inhibits RVD 74%. In contrast, luminal Cl^- reduction or application of DIDS has no effect on RVD.

Luminal K^+-induced swelling confirmed the presence of a Cl^- conductance in the basolateral membrane of volume-regulated principal cells [22]. The rate of K^+-swelling is unaffected by luminal Cl^- removal, but is inhibited 96%–99% by peritubular or bilateral replacement of Cl^- with isethionate. This unilateral inhibitory effect of Cl^- removal indicates clearly that the major pathway for KCl influx during luminal K^+-induced swelling is via K^+ and Cl^- channels located on opposing cell membranes.

K^+-swelling studies have demonstrated that the RVD Cl^- channel has a high selectivity for Cl^- over other anions [22]. Surprisingly, the channel has a very low NO_3^- permeability. Substitution of bath Cl^- for this anion inhibits the rate of K^+-swelling by 82%. The resting basolateral Cl^- channel also has a low NO_3^- permeability, suggesting, very indirectly, that it may be the predominant anion conductance responsible for RVD.

The volume regulatory response of principal cells to ouabain-induced swelling is likely to have a direct physiological correlate. Several endogenous substances have now been shown to inhibit the renal Na^+/K^+ ATPase, including prostaglandin E_2 (PGE_2), a potent natriuretic factor, and the vasoconstrictor substance, endothelin (reviewed in [21]). Rapidly accumulating evidence suggests that the hypothalamus produces a very high-affinity inhibitor of the Na^+/K^+ ATPase that functions in a manner similar to ouabain and may play a role in controlling renal salt and water excretion [25]. Doucet and Barlet [26] have suggested that the CCT may be a primary site of action of this so-called hypothalamic inhibitory factor (HIF).

An expected consequence of the action of endogenous pump blockers is cell swelling and volume regulation. In support of this prediction, Strange [21] has recently shown that micromolar concentrations of PGE_2 induce a pattern of swelling and RVD qualitatively identical to that seen with ouabain. Such results suggest strongly that the volume regulatory response to ouabain-induced swelling may occur with acute physiological downregulation of the Na^+ pump. Figure 5 illustrates a working model of isosmotic volume regulation in CCT principal cells.

It is interesting and important to note that anisosmotic and isosmotic volume regulation may not necessarily be carried out by the same transport pathways. As discussed above, hypotonic RVD in CCT principal cells does not appear to extensively involve passive KCl loss [10], whereas RVD following Na^+ pump blockage is clearly mediated by K^+ and Cl^- channels [21–22]. This suggests, indirectly, that the way in which cell volume is altered may influence the activity of volume regulatory path-

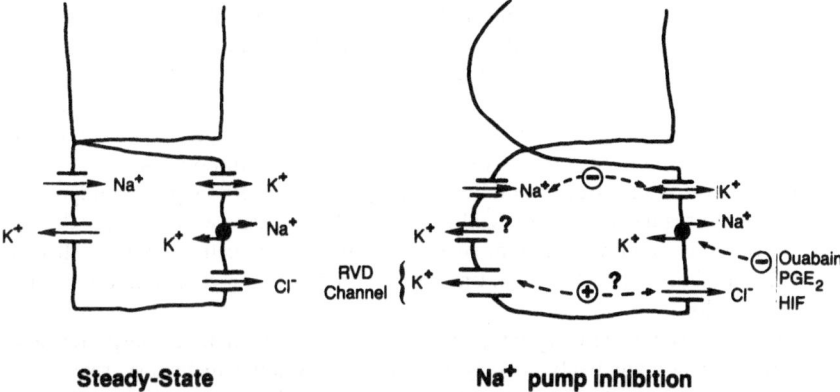

Steady-State   **Na⁺ pump Inhibition**

Fig. 5. Tentative cellular model of volume regulation in rabbit CCT principal cells following inhibition of the Na⁺ pump. HIF, hypothalamic inhibitory factor. (See text and [20–22] for details)

ways. Such a possibility is supported strongly by recent studies of Rome et al. [14,27]. These investigators quantified volume regulatory electrolyte loss and uptake in rabbit proximal tubules by electron microprobe analysis. Their results demonstrate clearly that the mechanisms utilized by proximal tubule cells for RVD or RVI are influenced by the rate at which cell volume is changed. For example, during gradual exposure to hyperosmotic solutions, 52% of the observed RVI was due to uptake of inorganic ions. The remainder of the RVI was mediated by some unknown organic solute(s). When proximal tubules were abruptly exposed to hyperosmotic solutions, however, only 21% of the observed RVI was due to inorganic ion accumulation [14]. Similar findings were made during exposure of proximal tubules to rapid or gradual reductions in extracellular osmolality [27].

Control of Volume Regulatory Pathways

Control of volume regulation requires the involvement of two distinct processes. First, the cell must have a means to sense a change in volume and/or intracellular composition. Second, the cell must be able to transduce the volume or compositional change into a regulatory response. Very little is known about these processes in either epithelial or symmetrical cells.

Intracellular Ca²⁺ has been implicated extensively in the control of cross-talk during fluctuations in transcellular Na⁺ transport [18]. Changes in cell Na⁺ concentration are "sensed" by the basolateral Na⁺/Ca²⁺ exchanger through changes in electrochemical driving forces. For example, increases in cell Na⁺ lead to a reduction in the inward driving force for Na⁺/Ca²⁺ exchange and lead to an elevation of cell Ca²⁺ concentration. Cell Ca²⁺, in turn, transduces the primary change in cell Na⁺ into a regulatory response by directly or indirectly inhibiting apical Na⁺ channels.

Elevation of cell Ca²⁺ may also activate Ca²⁺-sensitive, volume-regulatory solute loss mechanisms such as K⁺ channels. For example, anisosmotic RVD in frog bladder is blocked when serosal Ca^{2+} is removed [5]. In toad bladder, Wong et al. [28] have demonstrated that hypotonic swelling induces large increases in cell Ca^{2+} levels. Furthermore, removal of extracellular Ca^{2+} or buffering of intracellular Ca^{2+} changes inhibits RVD in this tissue (reviewed in [28]). Other cellular messengers, such as inositol phosphates, leukotrienes, G proteins, protein kinase activity, etc., are also likely to be involved in the control of volume regulatory pathways [24].

Stretch activated and stretch inhibited [24,29] ion channels may play an important role in volume regulation in some cell types. Mechanosensitive transport pathways apparently sense membrane stretch, such as that induced by cell swelling or shrinking. This membrane stretch is then transduced directly into a change in transmembrane solute flux.

For long-term volume stress, changes in the synthesis of membrane transporters and metabolic enzymes are likely to play an important volume regulatory role (e.g., [11,24]). In this case, the genome senses cell structural or compositional changes directly and then transduces those changes into altered gene expression. Genetic sensor-transducer systems are important in bacterial volume regulation (reviewed in [24]).

Conclusions

From the above discussion it is clear that an understanding of anisosmotic and isosmotic volume regulation in "tight," Na^+-transporting epithelia is still very much in its infancy. Future research must provide a detailed description of the transport and metabolic pathways and driving forces responsible for RVD and RVI. The possibility that cells possess multiple volume regulatory mechanisms that are activated under different conditions needs to be examined. Changes in cell solute content accompanying volume regulation must be quantified and volume sensors and intracellular signaling pathways need to be elucidated. The technical challenges involved in investigating these important areas are formidable. An integrated use of electrophysiological, optical, biochemical, and molecular biological approaches is required.

References

1. MacRobbie EAC, Ussing HH (1961) Osmotic behaviour of the epithelial cells of frog skin. Acta Physiol Scand 53:348–365
2. Ussing HH (1986) Epithelial cell volume regulation illustrated by experiments in frog skin. Renal Physiol 9:38–46
3. Costa PMF, Fernandes PL, Ferreira HG, Ferreira KTG, Giraldez F (1987) Effects of cell volume changes on membrane ionic permeabilities and sodium transport in frog skin (*Rana ridibunda*) J Physiol 393:1–17
4. Ussing HH (1985) Volume regulation and basolateral co-transport of sodium, potassium and chloride ions in frog skin epithelium. Pflugers Arch 405:S2–S7
5. Davis CW, Finn AL (1987) Interactions of sodium transport, cell volume, and calcium in frog urinary bladder. J Gen Physiol 89:687–702
6. Davis CW, Finn AL (1982) Sodium transport inhibition by amiloride reduces basolateral membrane potassium conductance in tight epithelia. Science 216:525–527
7. Lewis SA, Butt AG, Bowler MJ, Leader JP, MacKnight ADC (1985) Effects of anions on cellular volume and transepithelial Na^+ transport across toad urinary bladder. J Membr Biol 83:119–137

8. Donaldson PJ, Chen LK, Lewis SA (1989) Effects of serosal anion composition on the permeability properties of rabbit urinary bladder. Am J Physiol 256:F1125–F1134
9. Donaldson PJ, Lewis SA (1990) Effect of hyperosmotic challenge on basolateral membrane potential in rabbit urinary bladder. Am J Physiol 258:C248–C257
10. Strange K (1988) RVD in principal and intercalated cells of rabbit cortical collecting tubule. Am J Physiol 255:C612–C621
11. Wolff SD, Balaban RS (1990) Regulation of the predominant renal medullary organic solutes in vivo. Annu Rev Physiol 52:727–746
12. Strange K, Spring KR (1987) Cell membrane water permeability of rabbit cortical collecting duct. J Membr Biol 96:27–43
13. Natke E, Terranova R, DiScala VA (1989) Importance of butyrate in hypertonic volume regulation of cortical collecting tubule (CCT). Kidney Int 35:500
14. Rome L, Grantham J, Savin V, Lohr J, Lechene C (1989) Proximal tubule volume regulation in hyperosmotic media: intracellular K^+, Na^+, and Cl^-. Am J Physiol 257:C1093–C1100
15. Sun A, Hebert SC (1989) Rapid hypertonic cell volume regulation in the perfused inner medullary collecting duct. Kidney Int 36:831–842
16. Sands JM, Terada Y, Bernard LM, Knepper MA (1989) Aldose reductase activities in microdissected rat renal tubule segments. Am J Physiol 256:F563–F569
17. Wirthensohn G, Lefrank S, Schmolke M, Guder WG (1989) Regulation of organic osmolyte concentrations in tubules from rat renal inner medulla. Am J Physiol 256:F128–F135
18. Schultz SG (1981) Homocellular regulatory mechanisms in sodium-transporting epithelia: avoidance of extinction by "flush-through." Am J Physiol 241:F579–F590
19. Helman SI, Nagel W, Fisher RS (1979) Ouabain on active transepithelial Na transport in frog skin: studies with microelectrodes. J Gen Physiol 74:105–127
20. Strange K (1989) Ouabain-induced cell swelling in rabbit cortical collecting tubule: NaCl transport by principal cells. J Membr Biol 107:249–261
21. Strange K (1990) Volume regulation following Na^+ pump inhibition in CCT principal cells: apical K^+ loss. Am J Physiol 258:F732–F740
22. Strange K Volume regulatory Cl^- loss following Na^+ pump inhibition in CCT principal cells. Am J Physiol, in press
23. Frindt G, Palmer LG (1987) Ca-activated K channels in apical membrane of mammalian CCT, and their role in K secretion. Am J Physiol 252:F458–F467
24. Chamberlin ME, Strange K (1989) Anisosmotic cell volume regulation: a comparative view. Am J Physiol 257:C159–C173
25. Haber E, Haupert GT (1987) The search for a hypothalamic Na^+-K^+ ATPase inhibitor. Hypertension 9:315–324
26. Doucet A, Barlet C (1986) Evidence for differences in the sensitivity to ouabain of NaK-ATPase along the nephrons of rabbit kidney. J Biol Chem 261:993–995
27. Rome L, Lechene C, Grantham JJ (1990) Proximal tubule volume regulation in hypoosmotic media: intracellular K^+, Na^+, and Cl^-. J Am Soc Nephrol 1:211–218
28. Wong SME, DeBell MC, Chase HS (1990) Cell swelling increases intracellular free [Ca] in cultured toad bladder cells. Am J Physiol 258:F292–F296
29. Morris CE (1990) Mechanosensitive ion channels. J Membr Biol 113:93–107
30. Reuss L (1988) Cell volume regulation in nonrenal epithelia. Renal Physiol Biochem 3–5:187–201

Rapid Cell Volume Regulation by the Mouse Medullary Thick Ascending Limb of Henle

STEVEN C. HEBERT and ADAM M. SUN[1]

SUMMARY. In this paper, we summarize our current knowledge regarding cell volume regulation in mouse medullary thick ascending loop of Henle (MTAL) cells. It has become apparent that arginine vasopressin (ADH) plays a central role in this process (at least in certain species). During antidiuresis ADH increases the rate of NaCl absorption by the MTAL, thereby enhancing the single effect of countercurrent multiplication. In addition, ADH is required for MTAL cells to regulate their volume in the more hypertonic environment. ADH appears to activate normally quiescent basolateral $Na^+:H^+$ exchangers which mediate Na^+ uptake into MTAL cells during volume regulatory increase (VRI). This action of ADH may be mediated via an increase in cytosolic calcium. The trade off for this effect of ADH appears to be that the MTAL cells are no longer able to regulate their cell volume completely following reductions in interstitial osmolality. This is a direct result of an inverse relationship between the rates of salt absorption and volume regulatory decrease (VRD). This may not present a problem for the MTAL in vivo for two reasons. First, when interstitial osmolality is increased, NaCl absorption is reduced (see [1–3]). Second, when interstitial osmolality decreases during the transition from an antidiuretic to a water diuretic state the circulating level of ADH falls, and consequently, the rapid VRD response would be restored.

Introduction

Cell volume maintenance is one of the fundamental properties of renal epithelial cells. Over the last few years, much has been learned about how these cells maintain a constant, or nearly constant, cell volume under certain well-defined conditions. The medullary thick ascending limb of Henle (MTAL) has served as a valuable model

[1]Laboratory of Molecular Physiology and Biophysics, Renal Division, Department of Medicine, Brigham and Women's Hospital, Boston, MA 02115, USA

for the study of renal epithelial cell volume regulation. These studies have identified a new role for antidiuretic hormone (ADH, arginine vasopressin) in MTAL cells, that of activating normally quiescent, volume-responsive inorganic ion transporters.

Results and Discussion

Cell membranes are usually freely permeable to water, and thus, the distribution of water between cytosol and extracellular medium is in thermodynamic equilibrium. This is also true for "watertight" nephron segments such as the thick ascending limb of Henle (TAL). We have demonstrated in the isolated perfused MTAL that the apical cell membrane is the primary barrier that limits transcellular water movement and accounts for the very low hydraulic conductance of this nephron segment [4,5]. In contrast, the basolateral cell membrane of the MTAL is highly permeable to water, and differences in water activity between cell cytoplasm and the basolateral medium (interstitial fluid in vivo) provide the driving force for water movement into or out of these cells (i.e., changes cell volume).

Cell Volume Responses to Hypertonic Medium

Using quantitative morphological measurements of video images of cells obtained with differential interference contrast microscopy, we [4,6,7] have assessed the hypertonic Volume Regulatory Increase (VRI) responses of isolated perfused mouse CTAL and MTAL segments. The important observations are shown in Fig. 1. In the absence of ADH, MTAL cells behave as simple osmometers, showing no evidence of a rapid VRI response after cell shrinkage induced by a 50 mOsm increase in the osmolality of basolateral medium with mannitol (Fig. 1a). In contrast, following exposure of MTAL cells to physiological concentrations of ADH (25 µU/ml), a rapid VRI response is observed, with nearly complete recovery of cell volume in 2–5 minutes (Fig. 1b). The effect of vasopressin on the ability of mouse MTAL cells to express a VRI response is mimicked by the addition of dibutyryl cyclic AMP (Fig. 1c), and by direct activation of the catalytic subunit of adenylate cyclase with forskolin (Fig. 1d). These results indicate that the hypertonic VRI response of this medullary epithelial cell requires, at a minimum, an effect of ADH working through V_2 receptors. The increase in cell volume above baseline upon returning to the isotonic basolateral medium is consistent with net solute uptake into these cells during the VRI response. Since ADH has no effect on the negligible water permeability of the apical membrane [4], osmotic water uptake into these cells, which results from the increase in total cell osmoles, occurs exclusively across the basolateral membrane.

In contrast to the results in the MTAL, the mouse cortical thick ascending loop of Henle (CTAL) (Fig. 1e) shows no hypertonic VRI response even under conditions identical to those supporting VRI in the MTAL cells. The lack of a rapid hypertonic VRI response to a sudden increase in extracellular osmolality has also been observed in other renal cortical segments such as the proximal tubule [8] and cortical collecting duct. It should be noted, however, that Lohr and Grantham [9] have demonstrated that the rabbit proximal tubule is able to control cell volume when extracellular medium osmolality is increased slowly ($\cong 5$ mosom/min).

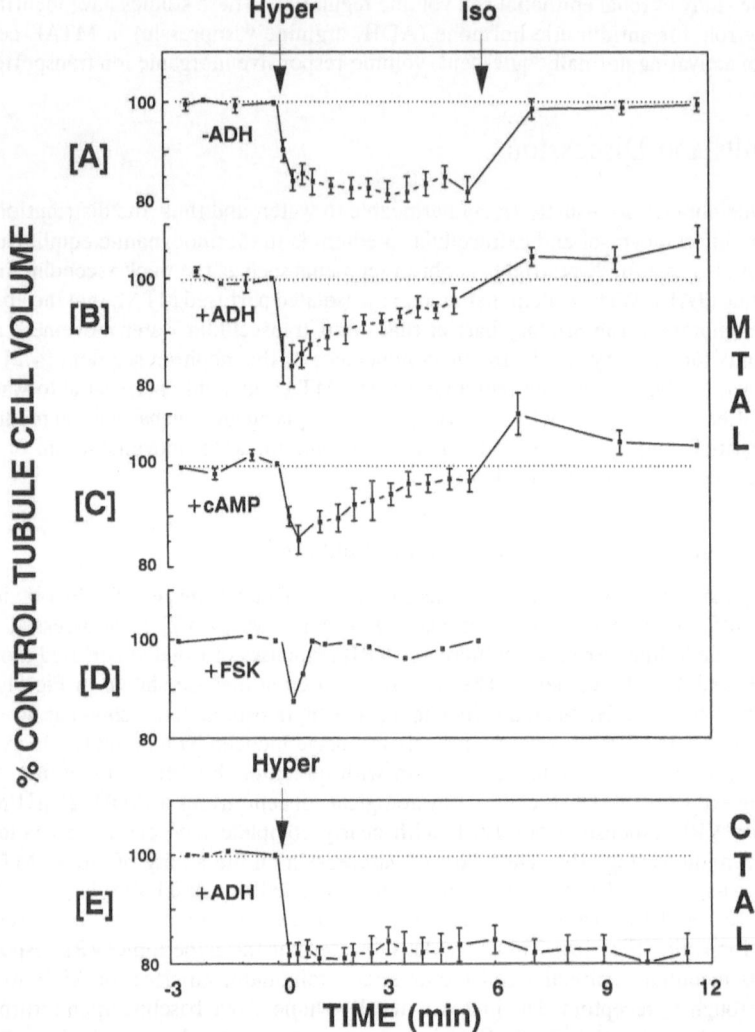

Fig. 1a-e. Hypertonic cell volume regulation in isolated perfused segments of mouse medullary (*MTAL*) or cortical (*CTAL*) thick ascending limbs of Henle. All studies were conducted at 37°C in HCO_3^-/CO_2-buffered media. At the *first arrow, hyper,* peritubular osmolality was increased from 290 to 340 mosm/Kg H_2O with mannitol. At the *second arrow, Iso,* peritubular medium was changed back to the isotonic solution. In the MTAL studies were performed: in the absence of arginine vasopressin (*ADH*), (a) or in the presence of peritubular ADH (25 µU/ml), (b), one mM dibutyryl cyclic AMP, (c), or one µM forskolin (*FSK*), (d). In the CTAL, (e), 25 µU/ml ADH was present in the peritubular medium. (Data from [4])

The requirement for ADH in expressing a VRI response is also seen when MTAL cells are shrunken upon re-exposure to an isotonic medium after a Volume Regulatory Decrease (VRD) response. The role of ADH in this post-VRD VRI response is shown in Fig. 2 [7]. This requirement for ADH is an unusual feature of volume regulation by MTAL cells since most renal (and nonrenal) cells show a VRI response with pre-exposure to hypotonic media in the absence of vasopressin, even if they don't express a hypertonic VRI response [10]. Finally, a more general role for ADH (via cyclic AMP) in the VRI responses of renal medullary-papillary cells has been suggested by the recent observation that ADH is also required for hypertonic VRI in rat inner medullary collecting duct cells [11].

Cell Volume Responses to Hypotonic Media

VRD responses have been assessed in isolated perfused mouse MTAL segments under the different states of salt absorption shown in Fig. 2 [7]. In the absence of ADH (Fig. 2a), cells first swell and then rapidly decrease their volume toward the control isotonic value when exposed to a 50 mOsm reduction in the bath osmolality. Upon returning to the isotonic medium cells shrink, consistent with cell solute loss during the VRD response. When salt absorption is increased with ADH (Fig. 2b), the VRD response is markedly reduced (compare Figs. 2a and 2b). This hormone-associated impairment of VRD is in sharp contrast to the ADH requirement for either post-VRD VRI (compare Figs. 2a and 2b) or hypertonic VRI (compare 1a and 1b). The blunting of the VRD response in ADH-activated MTAL segments is due to the hormone-mediated increase in NaCl absorption on the hypotonic-induced solute efflux mechanism(s) rather than to a direct inhibitory effect of hormone, via cyclic AMP, on the signal transduction pathway leading to activation of volume-responsive solute efflux [7]. The relevant observation, shown in Fig. 2c, is that the rate of VRD is increased four-fold when the ADH mediated increase in salt absorption is abolished with luminal furosemide.

When the rates of VRD are plotted for the varying rates of NaCl absorption for the three different transport conditions shown in Fig. 2a-2c, a highly significant inverse relationship is observed, i.e., increasing the rate of NaCl absorption decreases the rate of the VRD response [7]. This inverse relationship suggests that both an increase in cell solute traffic and a decrease in extracellular osmolality activate similar mechanisms to enhance salt exit. The recent observations that both ADH [12,13] and hypotonicity [14] activate Ba^{2+}-sensitive K^+ channels in apical membranes of the TAL provide strong support for the latter suggestion. A large conductance, maxi-K^+ channel appears to be activated by cell swelling and likely mediates K^+ loss during VRD.

Coupled Basolateral Na^+:H^+ and Cl^-:HCO_3^- Exchangers
and Apical Na^+:K^+:$2Cl^-$ Cotransporters Mediate VRI

Two types of electroneutral NaCl transport mechanisms have been proposed to mediate rapid hypertonic VRI responses. One process requires CO_2/HCO_3^- and involves parallel Na^+:H^+ and Cl^-:HCO_3^- exchangers; the other process is independent of CO_2/HCO_3^- and involves a loop diuretic-sensitive Na^+:K^+:$2Cl^-$ (or Na^+:Cl^-)

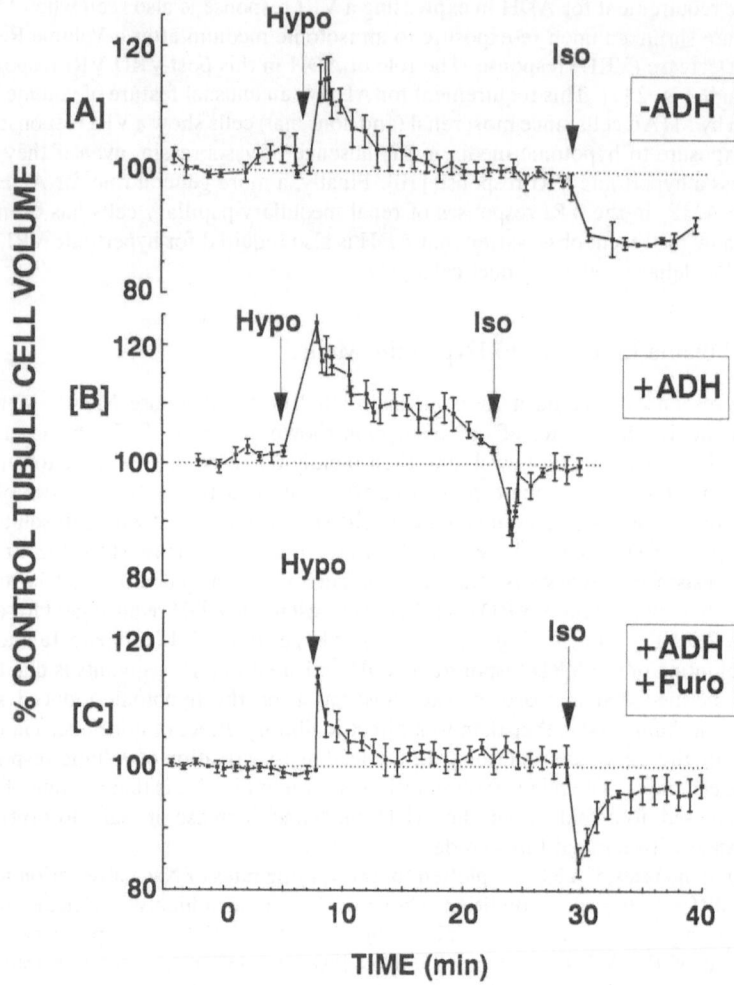

Fig. 2a-c. Hypotonic cell volume regulation in isolated perfused mouse medullary thick ascending loop of Henle (*MTAL*) segments. All studies were conducted at 37°C in HCO_3^-/CO_2-buffered media. At the *first arrow, hypo*, peritubular osmolality was decreased from 290 to 240 mosm/Kg H_2O by removal of 25 mM NaCl. At the *second arrow, Iso*, peritubular medium was changed back to the isotonic solution. Studies were performed: in the absence of arginine vasopressin (*ADH*), (**a**) or in the presence of peritubular ADH (10–25 μU/ml) (**b**), or in the presence of both ADH and 10^{-4} M luminal furosemide, (**c**). Cell volume changes following the return to isotonic basolateral media are referred to as post-volume regulatory decrease (*VRD*) VRI responses Furo, furosemide; VRI, volume regulatory increase. (Data from [7])

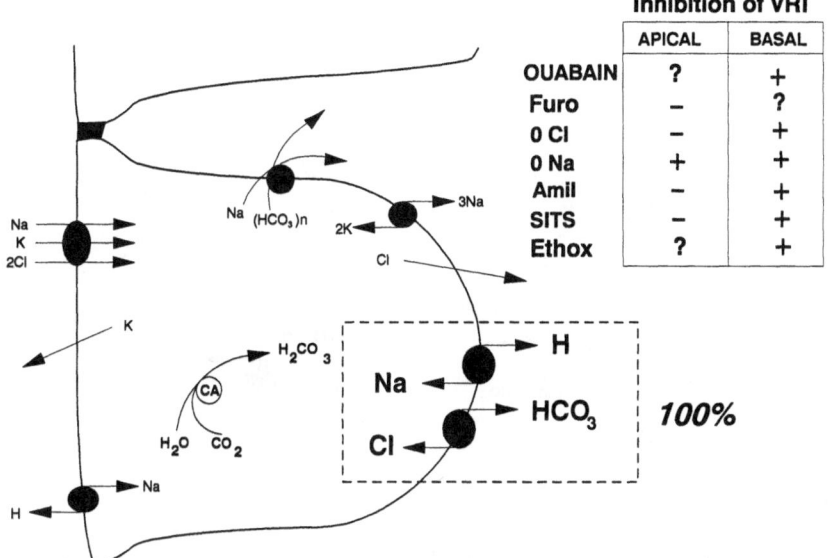

	Inhibition of VRI	
	APICAL	BASAL
OUABAIN	?	+
Furo	–	?
0 Cl	–	+
0 Na	+	+
Amil	–	+
SITS	–	+
Ethox	?	+

Fig. 3. Mechanism of ion uptake mediating the arginine vasopressin (*ADH*)-dependent hypertonic volume regulatory increase (*VRI*) response of the mouse medullary thick ascending loop of Henle (*MTAL*). All of the NaCl uptake mediating the VRI response appears to be mediated by basolateral $Na^+:H^+$ and $Cl^-:HCO_3^-$ exchangers. The *insert* lists the maneuvers utilized to deduce the VRI transport mechanism. Ouabain at 10^{-3} M, *Furo* is furosemide at 10^{-4} M, *Amil* is amiloride at 10^{-4} M, *SITS* is 4-acetamido-4'-isothiocyanostilbene-2,2'-disulfonic acid at 10^{-4} M, and *Ethox* is the carbonic anhydrase inhibitor, ethoxzolamide at 10^{-4} M. *CA* is carbonic anhydrase present in both the cytoplasm and along the basolateral membrane of mouse MTAL [30]

cotransporter [10,15–18]. Each of these transport mechanisms has been found to mediate NaCl uptake into mouse MTAL cells during the VRI response under certain conditions [4,6,7,19].

In both hypertonic and post-VRD VRI responses, NaCl uptake occurs via coupled $Na^+:H^+$ and $Cl^-:HCO_3^-$ exchangers located in basolateral membranes (Figs. 3 and 4). The relevant observations are (see insert in Fig. 3; [4,6,7]): (i) both the hypertonic and post-VRD VRI responses are abolished either by symmetrical Na^+ deletion from extracellular media or by basolateral, but not luminal, Cl^- removal; (ii) since either addition of ouabain to the basolateral solution or cooling the tissue to 15°C reduces or abolishes the hypertonic VRI response, NaCl uptake during VRI is an active (i.e., secondary active) process ultimately dependent on basolateral $Na^+:K^+$-ATPase; (iii) both types of VRI responses can also be abolished by basolateral, but not by luminal, amiloride, by the isohydric replacement of CO_2/HCO_3^- with HEPES, or by basolateral addition of 4-acetamido-4'-isothiocyanostilbene-2,2'-disulfonic acid (SITS); and (iv) inhibition of carbonic anhydrase (CA) activity with ethoxzolamide inhibits hypertonic VRI (CA appears to be required in order to maintain an adequate supply of H^+ and HCO_3^- to the basolateral exchangers).

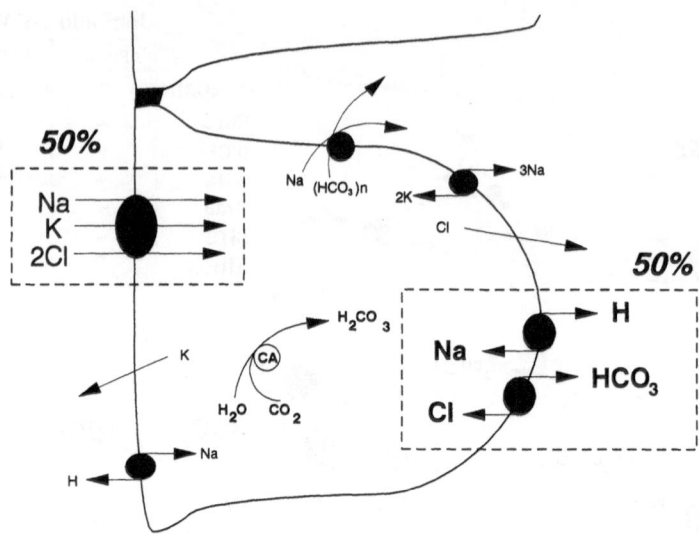

Fig. 4. Mechanism of ion uptake mediating the arginine vasopressin (*ADH*)-dependent post-volume regulatory decrease (*VRD*) VRI response of the mouse medullary thick ascending loop of Henle (*MTAL*). The apical Na^+:K^+:$2Cl^-$ cotransporter and the basolateral Na^+:H^+ and Cl^-:HCO_3^- exchangers each mediate about 50% of the net NaCl uptake during the VRI response. CA, carbonic anhydrase (see Fig. 3); VRI, volume regulatory increase

The contribution of the apical Na^+:K^+:$2Cl^-$ cotransporter to VRI depends explicitly on the method used to elicit the VRI response (see Table 1; Figs. 3 and 4). Inhibition of the apical Na^+:K^+:$2Cl^-$ cotransporter with furosemide (or the substitution of luminal Cl^- with isethionate) has no effect on the steady-state rate of VRI under hypertonic conditions (Fig. 3; [4,7]). On the other hand, the rate of post-VRD VRI is significantly reduced by this diuretic (Table 1; Figs. 2 and 4). The steady-state rate of post-VRD VRI is about three-fold higher than the rates of VRI under hypertonic conditions, with or without luminal furosemide, or the rate of post-VRD VRI in the presence of furosemide. Thus, the apical cotransporter provides a mechanism for enhancing ion uptake only during the post-VRD VRI response. In contrast, the contribution of the ADH-dependent, basolateral Na^+:H^+ and Cl^-:HCO_3^- exchangers to VRI does not appear to be altered by the method used to shrink MTAL cells.

ADH Activates Basolateral Na^+:H^+ Exchangers Mediating VRI

Our initial studies [4,6,7] suggested that the basolateral Na^+:H^+ and Cl^-:HCO_3^- exchangers involved in the VRI response of the mouse MTAL were either not functional, or not as active, during steady-state isotonic conditions. Using 2',7'-bis(carboxyethyl)-5(6)carboxyfluorescein (BCECF) to measure pH_i in isolated perfused MTAL tubules and in suspensions of MTAL segments from mouse kidney, we have demonstrated that a Na^+:H^+ exchanger is present on basolateral membranes in the absence of ADH; we have confirmed that this exchanger has a very acid pH_i set

Table 1. Role of the apical $Na^+:K^+:2Cl^-$ cotransporter in the VRI responses of the mouse MTAL

	ADH	FURO	Rate of VRI (nl/min per cm)
Hypertonic			
	+	–	0.105 ± 0.032
	+	+	0.167 ± 0.032
Post-VRD VRI			
	+	–	0.310 ± 0.050[a]
	+	+	0.138 ± 0.096

[a]indicates significantly different from the rate of post-VRD VRI in the presence of furosemide.
VRI, volume regulatory increase; VRD, volume regulatory decrease; MTAL, medullary thick ascending loop of Henle; ADH, arginine vasopressin; FURO, furosemide. (Data from [4,6,7])

point of $\cong 6.7$ so that it would be inactive at the resting pH_i ($\cong 7.23$ in the absence of CO_2/HCO_3^-) [19–22]. We also identified a $Na^+:H^+$ on apical membranes of the mouse MTAL. In contrast to the basolateral exchanger, this apical exchanger is active at the resting cell pH_i under isotonic conditions and in the absence of ADH ([19,20]; see Fig. 3) and functions importantly in pH regulation. The apical exchanger, however, appears to play no role in Na^+ uptake during VRI (luminal amiloride has no effect on the rate of cell volume recovery in either hypertonic VRI [6] or post-VRD VRI [7].

We have recently begun to assess the effects of ADH on both the apical and basolateral $Na^+:H^+$ exchangers in the isolated perfused mouse MTAL. The observation that VRI is supported by cyclic AMP (Fig. 1c) and forskolin (Fig. 1d) suggests that V_2 receptor-linked events may be involved in activation of the basolateral $Na^+:H^+$ exchanger by ADH. Interestingly, cyclic AMP, presumably working via activation of protein kinase A, inhibits $Na^+:H^+$ exchange activity in some cells [23–25], while this second messenger activates the exchanger in other cell types [26]. In fact, our recent preliminary studies in the mouse MTAL suggest that both effects of cyclic AMP may occur (see Table 2). The activity of the apical exchanger is reduced by ADH while the activity of the basolateral $Na^+:H^+$ exchanger is clearly enhanced by the hormone. We [21,22] have suggested that a hormone induced increase in cytosolic Ca^{2+} may be involved in the activation of the basolateral $Na^+:H^+$ exchanger by ADH. We found

Table 2. Effect of ADH on apical and basolateral $Na^+:H^+$ antiporters in mouse MTAL

	H^+ Efflux rate at $pH_i = 6.48$	
	(pmol/min per mm)	
ADH	Basolateral	Apical
–	3.40 ± 0.80	28.32 ± 1.81
+	8.41 ± 1.15[a]	14.61 ± 2.33[a]

[a]indicates $P < 0.05$ compared to the -ADH condition.
MTAL, medullary thick ascending loop of Henle; ADH, arginine vasopressin

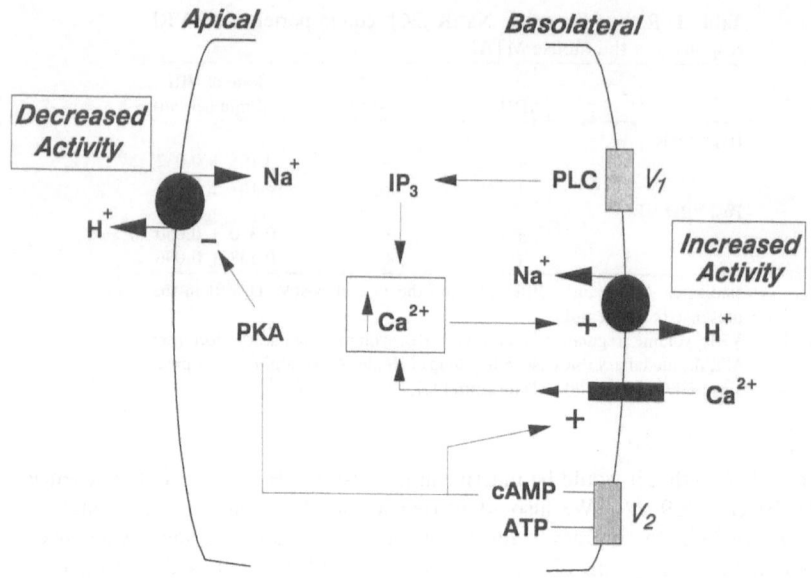

Fig. 5. Tentative model for the action of arginine vasopressin (*ADH*) on apical and basolateral Na$^+$:H$^+$ exchangers in the medullary thick ascending loop of Henle (*MTAL*)

that addition of one µM ionomycin to the basolateral solution in the absence of ADH markedly enhanced the activity of the basolateral Na$^+$:H$^+$ exchanger in isolated perfused mouse MTAL segments. A similar enhancement of Na$^+$:H$^+$ exchange activity by ionomycin-induced increases in cytosolic Ca^{2+} has previously been observed in lymphocytes by Grinstein and Cohen [27].

Although this effect of increased intracellular Ca^{2+} on exchanger activity might suggest that ADH-V$_1$ receptor-mediated events participate in the activation of the basolateral exchanger in the mouse MTAL, it is clear that cyclic AMP alone fully supports the VRI response. It is possible, however, that increased cytosolic Ca^{2+} may play a role in a further enhancement of the exchanger, mediated by cell shrinkage [27]. An alternative possibility is suggested by the recent preliminary studies of Hoffmann et al. [28] in the rabbit cortical collecting duct, which duct appears to possess both V$_1$ and V$_2$ receptors for ADH. These investigators found that a low concentration of ADH (100 µU/ml), working via V$_2$ receptor, increases the intracellular Ca^{2+} concentration of principal cells. This effect of hormone appears to be mediated virtually exclusively by an influx of Ca^{2+} from extracellular media, rather than by its release from intracellular Ca^{2+} stores.

A Tentative Model for the Action of ADH on Na$^+$:H$^+$ Exchangers

When taken together, our results suggested the tentative model for the action of ADH on apical and basolateral exchangers which is shown in Fig. 5. Activation of the basolateral exchanger is a two step process: an initial activation by ADH that prepares the cell for a second response induced by cell shrinkage. In the first step, ADH stimulates intracellular cyclic AMP production via activation of V_2 receptors. The increase in cyclic AMP, in turn, results in an enhanced activity of the basolateral $Na^+:H^+$ exchanger, possibly by induction of a Ca^{2+} influx, leading to an increase in cytosolic Ca^{2+} (how Ca^{2+} stimulates the exchanger is undetermined, but may also involve activation of a phosphorylation mechanism [27]). In the second step, cell shrinkage would further activate the exchanger, by as yet undetermined mechanisms. This latter activation step might lead to an additional alkaline shift in the pH_i dependence of the exchanger. Although it is possible that ADH-V_1 receptor-mediated events may play some role in augmenting the activation of the exchanger, we have not clearly identified this presence of the V_1 receptor on MTAL cells. Finally, the processes leading to activation of the basolateral $Cl^-:HCO_3^-$ exchanger involved in the VRI response of the mouse MTAL are completely unknown at present. However, it seems reasonable to speculate that ADH (via cyclic AMP) may also activate this exchanger by a process similar to that depicted in Fig. 5. As discussed above, the coupling of the $Na^+:H^+$ and $Cl^-:HCO_3^-$ exchangers appears to be critical to their function in volume regulation [29].

References

1. Hebert SC, Andreoli TE (1984) Control of NaCl transport in the thick ascending limb. Am J Physiol 246:F745–F75
2. Hebert SC, Culpepper RM, Andreoli TE (1981) NaCl transport in mouse medullary thick ascending limbs. III Modulation of the ADH effect by peritubular osmolality. Am J Physiol 241:F443–F45
3. Molony DA, Andreoli TE (1988) Diluting power of thick limbs of Henle: I. Peritubular hypertonicity blocks basolateral Cl channels. Am J Physiol 255:F1128–F1137
4. Hebert SC (1986) Hypertonic cell volume regulation in mouse thick limbs. I. ADH dependency and nephron heterogeneity. Am J Physiol 250:C907–C919
5. Hebert SC, Culpepper RM, Andreoli TE (1981) NaCl transport in mouse medullary thick ascending limbs. I Functional nephron heterogeneity and ADH-stimulated NaCl cotransport. Am J Physiol 241:F412–F431
6. Hebert SC (1986) Hypertonic cell volume regulation in mouse thick limbs. II. Na-H and Cl-HCO₃ exchange in basolateral membranes. Am J Physiol 250:C920–C931
7. Hebert SC, Sun A (1988) Hypotonic cell volume regulation in mouse medullary thick ascending limb: effects of ADH. Am J Physiol 255:F962–F969
8. Kirk KL, Schafer JA, DiBona DR (1987) Cell volume regulation in rabbit proximal straight tubule in vitro. Am J Physiol 252:F922–F932
9. Lohr J, Grantham JJ (1986) Isovolumetric regulation in anistonic media: A new approach to study compensated cell volume regulation in isolated proximal S2 segments. Kidney Int 29:419
10. Hoffmann EK, Simonsen LO (1989) Membrane mechanisms in volume and pH regulation in vertebrate cells. Physiol Rev 69:315–382
11. Sun A, Hebert SC (1989) Rapid hypertonic cell volume regulation in the perfused inner medullary collecting duct. Kidney Int 36:831–842
12. Hebert SC, Friedman PA, Andreoli TE (1984) Effects of antidiuretic hormone on cellular conductive pathways in mouse medullary thick ascending limbs of Henle: I. ADH increases transcellular conductive pathways. J Membr Biol 80:201–219
13. Reeves WB, McDonald GA, Mehta P, Andreoli TE (1989) Activation of K^+ channels in renal medullary vesicles by cAMP-dependent protein kinase. J Membr Biol 109:65–72

14. Taniguchi J, Guggino WB (1989) Membrane stretch: a physiological stimulator of Ca^{2+}-activated K^+ channels in thick ascending limb. Am J Physiol 257–26:F347–F352
15. Chamberlin ME, Strange K (1989) Anisotonic cell volume regulation: a comparative view. Am J Physiol 257(26):C159–C173
16. Hebert SC (1987) Volume regulation in renal epithelial cells. Semin Nephrol 7:48–60
17. Eveloff JL, Warnock DG (1987) Activation of ion transport systems during cell volume regulation. Am J Physiol 252:F1–F10
18. Blumenfeld JD, Grossman EB, Sun AM, Hebert SC (1989) Sodium-coupled ion cotransport and volume regulatory increase response. Kidney Int 36:434–440
19. Kikeri D, Azar S, Sun A, Zeidel ML, Hebert SC (1990) $Na^+:H^+$ antiporter and $Na^+(HCO_3^-)_n$ symporter regulate intracellular pH in mouse medullary thick limbs. Am J Physiol 258:F445–F456
20. Kikeri D, Sun A, Zeidel ML, Hebert SC (1989) Cell membranes impermeable to NH 3. Nature 339:478–480
21. Hebert SC, Sun A, Kikeri D (1990) Interrelationships among cell volume, pH and salt transport in thick ascending limb (TAL) and inner medullary collecting duct (IMCD) cells from mammalian kidney: Effects of vasopressin (abstract). Renal Physiol Biochem 13:168–169
22. Sun A, Hebert SC (1990) Antidiuretic hormone (ADH) and cytosolic Ca^{2+} regulate the basolateral (BI) $Na^+:H^+$ antiporter involved in the rapid volume regulatory increase (VRI) response of mouse medullary thick limbs (MTAL) (abstract). Clin Res 38:313A
23. Grinstein S, Rothstein A (1986) Mechanism of regulation of the Na^+/H^+ exchanger. J Membr Biol 90:1–12
24. Ussing HH (1960) Active and passive transport of the alkali metal ions. In: Ussing HH, Kruhoffer P, Thaysen JH, Thorn NA (eds) The alkali metal ions in biology. Springer, Berlin, pp 45–143
25. Weinman EJ, Shenolikar S, Kahn AM (1987) cAMP-associated inhibition of Na^+-H^+ exchanger in rabbit brush-border membranes. Am J Physiol 252:F19–F25
26. Borgese F, Garcia-Romeu F, Motias R (1987) Control of cell volume and ion transport by β-adrenergic catecholamines in erythrocytes of rainbow trout, Salmo gairdneri. J Physiol (Lond) 382:123–144
27. Grinstein S, Cohen S (1987) Cytoplasmic $[Ca^{2+}]$ and intracellular pH in lymphocytes. Role of membrane potential and volume-activated Na^+/H^+ exchange. J Gen Physiol 89:185–213
28. Hoffmann EK, Simonsen LO (1989) Membrane mechanisms in volume and pH regulation in vertebrate cells. Physiol Rev 69:315–382
29. Mason MJ, Smith JD, Garcia-Soto JD-J, Grinstein S (1989) Internal pH-sensitive site couples Cl^--HCO_3^- exchange to $Na^+:H^+$ antiport in lymphocytes. Am J Physiol 256-25: C428–C433
30. Dobyan DC, Magill LS, Friedman PA, Hebert SC, Bulger RE (1982) Carbonic anhydrase histochemistry in rabbit and mouse kidneys. Anat Rec 204:185–197

Mechanisms of Renal Cell Injury of Acute Renal Failure

Chair: Haskel E. Eliahou (Israel)
Robert W. Schrier (USA)

Evidence of Renal Cell Injury in Acute Renal Failure

H.E. Eliahou, C. Falconi, and L. Shulman[1]

The basis of the early irreversible stage of acute tubular necrosis (ATN), i.e., of established acute renal failure (ARF), is the cell injury and dysfunction which seem to be responsible for the lack of glomerular filtration. The loss of glomerular filtration occurs despite the fact that the initially raised plasma renin activity and the diminished renal blood flow (RBF) have returned to normal levels. Even at the onset of established acute renal failure in man, the RBF does not decrease to levels below 45% of normal [1], a rate which should allow some glomerular filtration. Thus, earlier conclusions that vasoconstriction is the factor responsible for the cessation of glomerular filtration seem inadequate to explain the phenomenon of renal failure following traumatic or hypovolemic shock.

It is well-known from experimental animal models of ARF that GFR remains negligible despite the return of renal blood flow to normal levels within 24 to 72 h after the injury. Renal failure persists in mercuric chloride-induced ARF, even though renal blood flow returns to normal by 24 h, after reaching 20% in the first 3–6 h after injection (Biber et al. [2]).

Similar findings of normal RBF after 1 or 2 days of mercuric chloride injection were described by Churchill et al. and Sherwood et al. [3,4]; findings after 3 days were described by Baehler et al. [5]. Renal blood flow was normal within 24 h in the glycerol model [6] and in the nor-epinephrine model [7] of ARF. Additional support for the dissociation between return to normal RBF and return to normal GFR has come from Blantz [8] who reported decreased glomerular permeability in the absence of detectable structural abnormalities in uranyl nitrate-induced ARF.

There is a similar dissociation between the RBF and GFR in man. For instance, Reubi [1] also showed adequate RBF in the presence of suppressed GFR in man in ARF after shock. Nevertheless, with the discovery of the extremely potent vasoconstrictor endothelin, and with the improvement in glomerular function obtained by the anti-endothelin antibodies in short term ischemic ARF, the question of continu-

---

[1]Department of Nephrology, Chaim Sheba Medical Center, S2621, Tel-Hashomer, Israel

ous sustained vasoconstriction has, once again, become important in understanding the pathogenesis of the renal failure in ARF.

Recently, Kon et al. [9] showed that continuous infusion of endothelin in a first-order branch of the left main renal artery was sufficient to induce ARF in Munich Wistar rats [9]. It was found by micropuncture that SNGFR was decreased by 35% in the glomeruli exposed to endothelin. Glomerular plasma flow was also reduced. This hypofiltration/hypoperfusion was associated with an increase in the afferent and efferent arteriolar resistance. The study of the effect of anti-endothelial antibodies on kidney function 48 hours after 25 min of renal artery clamping is even more interesting. The infusion of anti-endothelin antibody into one of the branches of the main renal artery ameliorated the characteristic post-ischemic vasoconstriction and significantly improved SNGFR. These findings tend to show that sustained vasoconstriction is important in the pathogenesis of ARF which results from 25 minutes of complete ischemia. However, the effect of deviation from the currently accepted 50–60 min period of ischemia required to produce ARF in the rat is not clear. The question is whether the anti-endothelin antibody would have acted to the same extent had the renal artery occlusion lasted 60 rather than 25 min, with the resultant, more definite, cell injury.

Conger et al. [10] produced ARF in uninephrectomized Sprague Dawley rats by the infusion of nor-epinephrine 0.6µg/kg per min for 90 min, using a micropipette directly into the renal artery. Seven days after this injury, the response to changes in renal perfusion pressure and renal nerve stimulation was measured.

Their investigation showed that, following nor-epinephrine induced ARF (NE-ARF), there was a marked sensitivity of the renal vessels to reductions in renal perfusion pressure (RPP) and to renal nerve stimulation. This was shown by a marked decrease in RBF with a decrease in RPP or renal nerve stimulation. Conger and colleagues were able to reverse this hypersensitivity with the calcium channel blockers verapamil or diltiazem. This seems to indicate that this hypersensitivity is dependent on intracellular calcium concentration. The use of endothelium-derived relaxing factor (EDRF) dependent agents, such as acetyl choline or bradykinin, was not successful in reversing this hypersensitivity. This would favor the possibility that endothelial injury results in a decrease in EDRF release, which allows sustained vasoconstriction. The authors claim that in such a condition, even subclinical reductions in blood pressure in the ARF patient could cause a great deal of vasoconstriction, which may result in ATN. Since this hypersensitivity is reversed by calcium channel blockers, it seems to be modulated by perturbations in cell calcium. Thus, endothelial cell injury resulting in the decreased release of EDRF, and therefore in vasoconstriction, may be the cause of the lack of filtration at the glomerulus. This vasoconstriction resulting from the high endothelin and the decreased release of EDRF is, in itself, a consequence of endothelial cell injury and dysfunction.

Calcium entry blockers were found to reverse the initial stages of ARF. In the renal artery clamping model in the rat, we found that orally administered verapamil was able to alleviate the functional damage of the involved kidney [11].

Verapamil also significantly improved renal function and was accompanied by less histologic damage in a rat model in which ARF was induced by cyclosporin treatment combined with mild renal ischemia of only 20 min. The authors concluded that trans-cellular calcium ion transport disturbances seemed to be important in the pathogenesis of ischemic as well as nephrotoxic ARF [12].

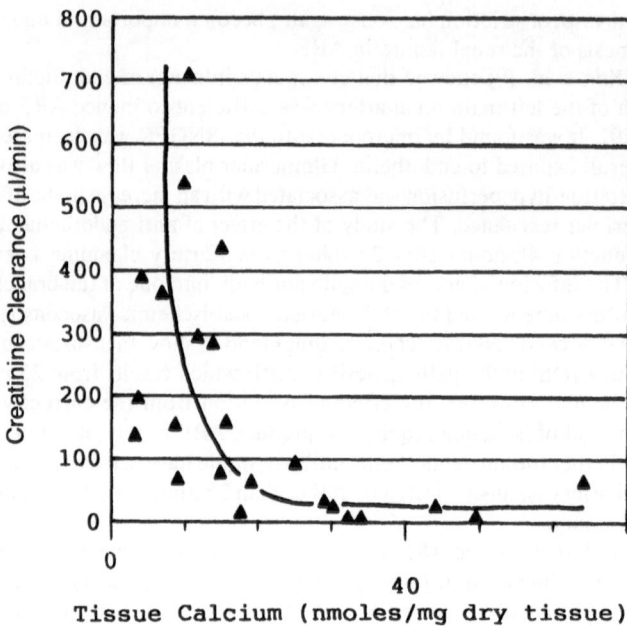

Fig. 1. Verapamil and mifedipine in rat ARF correlation of tissue Calcium and Ccr. Ccr, creatinine clearance; ARF, acute renal failure.

In our studies in rats, in which ARF was induced by uninephrectomy and contralateral clamping of the renal artery for one h, the tissue calcium content of the renal cortex correlated very well with creatinine clearance on the day following the operative procedure (Fig. 1).

Epithelial cell polarity is lost in ischemia [13]. The ARF produced in Sprague Dawley rats by 50 min clamping of the renal pedicle resulted in a loss of Na-K-ATPase polarity in the proximal tubular cells. This was demonstrated cytochemically and biochemically by the redistribution of Na-K-ATPase to apical membranes, where it should not be found. Furthermore, the relative percentage of sphingomyelin content at the apical membrane of the proximal tubular cell was considerably decreased allowing a decreased sphingomyelin/phosphatidyl choline ratio. This ratio is important in the determination of membrane fluidity [14] and therefore of transmembrane transport. The postulate is that one needs a re-establishment of lipid and protein polarity for the normalization of tubular cell function. An additional finding affecting another cell compartment was the significant decrease in the activity of sphingomyelinase in gentamicin-induced ARF in rats (50mg/kg per d for 4 days or 4 mg/kg per d for 8 days). This enzyme is responsible for the intra-lysosomal breakdown of sphingomyelin [15].

More evidence which demonstrates cell dysfunction in ARF is the finding, by microprobe analysis, of a marked increase in proximal tubule intracellular sodium and chloride concentrations. This seems to indicate that there is a marked disturbance in the sodium potassium pump [16].

What is the evidence for an effect of cell dysfunction on glomerular filtration? It has been claimed that when elevated arteriolar resistance in post-ischemic ARF is lowered by saline volume expansion, the rate of glomerular ultrafiltrate formation remains very depressed [17]. Thus, there is an intrinsic loss of normal ultrafiltration capacity at the glomerular capillary wall. This decrease in permeability is still undefined. A similar finding occurs in the tubule, where it has been shown that recovery from ARF coincided with the restoration of tubular impermeability to inulin [18].

Treatment of Wistar rats with either 4 or 40 mg gentamicin/kg per day for 10 days resulted in a marked decrease in the glomerular capillary ultrafiltration coefficient, Kf, in both gentamicin treatment groups. The ultrastructural changes in the proximal tubules (focal loss of brush border, myeloid bodies and cell vacuoles) were typical of gentamicin toxicity. Nevertheless, it seems surprising that there were no apparent ultrastructural differences between the control and experimental groups in the 3 different component layers of the glomerular capillary wall, i.e., the endothelium, GBM, and epithelial cell layer, despite the significant decrease in Kf [19].

Ultrastructural studies in the clamp model of ischemic ARF show that cell swelling, even in the glomeruli, is a predominant feature of this model. This feature occurred, together with a normal RBF measured with the Xenon-washout technique, 6 and 24 h after reflow [20]. In norepinephrine-induced acute renal failure in dogs, scanning electron microscopy revealed a marked abnormality in the epithelial structure of the glomerulus [17]. These studies indicate that ultrastructural changes may be an important aspect of the cell dysfunction which contributes considerably to lack of filtration.

In ischemic ARF the renal tissue calcium content is increased, as is the cytosolic Ca^{2+}. Calcium channel blockers improved experimental ischemic ARF. Observations on mitochondrial respiration, as assessed by state 4 and state 3 oxidative phosphorylation and by uncoupled respiration, show that the detrimental effects of ischemia on these various states of mitochondrial respiration are prevented by calcium channel blockers.

During ischemia, renal beta-ATP, as assessed by 31P-NMR in the renal cortex, fell rapidly to about 10% of control levels. During reflow and recovery, the tissue ATP returned slowly to near normal, but in rats given ATP-$MgCl_2$, the return of ATP levels to normal was accelerated [21].

Creatinine kinase determinations in freeze clamped kidney cortex in rats showed normal values in both control and experimental (60 min clamping of renal pedicle) kidneys, 24 h following the episode of ischemia (Shulman LM, Eliahou HE, unpublished work, 1990). This, together with the finding that cortex ATP returned to near normal within 24 h following the ischemia, seems to indicate that the energy system was functioning during this period, yet the glomerulus was not able to filter normally.

In 1974 Cox et al. [17] described nor-epinephrine-induced acute renal failure (NE-ARF) in a dog, induced by the intrarenal infusion of NE 0.75µg/kg per min for 2 h. In this model, the RBF decreased considerably (from 190ml/min to 116ml/min), 48 h after the NE infusion. The administration of 10% of body weight Ringer's solution resulted in a marked redistribution of flow to inner cortical nephrons in both control and experimental kidneys, with a marked increase in total RBF. In the experimental kidney, the increase was from 116 to 235 ml/min. Over 99% of the 15 µM spheres were extracted in one pass through the experimental kidney. However, despite the marked increase in RBF, there was essentially no urine flow.

Micropuncture showed that the surface tubules were collapsed with no evidence of tubular obstruction or leakage of filtrate. Scanning electron microscopy revealed a marked abnormality in the epithelial structure of the glomerulus. The authors suggest a decrease in the capillary permeability in this model of ARF. In this paper, the NE was infused for 2 h and therefore the damage was very severe, and probably of the irreversible type.

An interesting, somewhat similar, finding in the glomeruli was described by Kobayashi et al. [22]. They induced ARF, with uranyl acetate (2mg/Kg body weight IV), in rabbits. Five days later, scanning electron microscopy revealed a loss of epithelial foot processes and fattening and spreading of podocyte cell bodies. These changes were most pronounced in the maintenance stage of the ARF. In many areas the glomerular capillaries were covered by a continuous sheet of podocyte cytoplasm and the fine structure of the foot processes was not found. There was a decrease in the density of fenestrae in some areas. The authors found no correlation between the morphological findings and serum creatinine levels. Following ischemia, the mitochondria were severely affected. Immediately following 60 min of ischemia, the cells were seen to be swollen, but not necrotic, and the tubules were filled with eosinophilic debris. Six h after recovery from ARF, partial necrosis of tubular walls with some cell swelling was seen in the cytoplasm. At 12 h, severe necrosis of tubules was already seen. Electron microscopy showed large clear intracristal spaces, with swollen and distended microvilli and rounded swollen mitochondria [23].

In summary, there is much evidence to indicate that there is cellular injury and dysfunction in ARF. Such disturbances have been studied mainly in the tubule, apparently because the glomerulus does not lend itself to the study of the individual type of cell. Direct studies on the permeability at the glomerulus are needed to clarify the lack of filtration during ARF. Our present studies are being directed towards defining new molecules and biological response systems which can serve as markers of cell dysfunction in acute renal failure.

References

1. Reubi FC, Vorburger C (1976) Renal hemodynamics in acute renal failure after shock in man. Kidney Int 10:S137–S143
2. Biber TUL, Mylle M, Baines AD, Gottsschalk CW (1968) A study by micropuncture and microdissection of acute renal damage in rats. Am J Med 44:664–705
3. Churchill S, Zarlengo MD, Carvalho GF, Gottlieb MN, Oken D (1977) Normal renal cortical blood flow in experimental acute renal failure. Kidney Int 11:246–255
4. Sherwood T, Lavender JP, Russell SB (1974) Mercury induced renal vascular shutdown: Observations in experimental acute renal failure. Eur J Clin Invest 4:1–8
5. Baehler RW, Kotchen TA, Burke JA, Galla H, Bhathena D (1977) Considerations in the pathophysiology of mercuric chloride induced acute renal failure. J Lab Clin Med 90: 330–340
6. Kurtz TW, Maletz RM, Hsu CH (1976) Renal cortical blood flow in glycerol induced acute renal failure. Circ Res 38:30–35
7. Conger GD, Robinette JB, Guggenheim SJ (1981) Effect of acetyl choline on the early phase of reversible nor-epinephrine induced acute renal failure. Kidney Int 19:399–409
8. Blantz RC (1975) The mechanism of acute renal failure after uranyl nitrate. J Clin Invest 55:621–635

9. Kon V, Yoshioka T, Fogo A, Ichikawa I (1989) Glomerular actions of endothelin in vivo. J Clin Invest 83:1762-1767

10. Conger JD, Robinette JB, Schrier RW (1988) Smooth muscle calcium and endothelium-derived relaxing factor in the abnormal vascular responses of acute renal failure. J Clin Invest 82:532-537

11. Goldfarb D, Iaina A, Serban I, Gavendo S, Kapuler S, Eliahou HE (1983) Beneficial effect of verapamil in ischemic acute renal failure in rats. Proc Soc Exp Biol Med 172:389-392

12. Iaina A, Herzog D, Cohen D, Gavendo S, Kapular S, Schiby G, Eliahou HE (1986) Calcium entry blockade with verapamil in cyclosporin A plus ischemia induced acute renal failure in rats. Clin Nephrol 25(Suppl 1):S168-S170

13. Spiegel DM, Wilson PD, Molitoris BA (1989) Epithelial polarity following ischemia: A requirement for normal cell function. Am J Physiol 256 (Renal Fluid Electrolyte Physiol 25):F430-F436

14. Pottel H, VanDer Meer W, Herreman W (1983) Correlation between the order parameter and the steady state fluorescence anisotropy of 1,6 diphenyl-1,3,5 hexatriene and an evaluation of membrane fluidity. Biochim Biophys Acta 730:181-186

15. Morin JP, Viotte G, Vandewalle A, Van Hoof F, Tulkens P, Fillastre JP (1980) Gentamicin-induced nephrotoxicity: A cell biology approach. Kidney Int 18:583-590

16. Mason J, Beck F, Dorge A, Rick R, Thurau K (1981) Intracellular electrolyte composition following ischemia. Kidney Int 20:61-70

17. Cox JW, Baehler RW, Sharma H, O'Dorisio T, Osgood RW, Stein JH, Ferris TF (1974) Studies on the mechanism of oliguria in a model of unilateral acute renal failure. J Clin Invest 53:1546-1558

18. Finn WF, Chevalier RL (1979) Recovery from postischemic acute renal failure in the rat. Kidney Int 16:113-123

19. Baylis C, Rennke HR, Brenner BM (1977) Mechanisms of the defect in glomerular ultrafiltration associated with gentamicin administration. Kidney Int 12:344-353

20. Frega NS, DiBona DR, Guestler B, Leaf A (1976) Ischemic renal injury. Kidney Int 10:S17-S25

21. Siegel NJ, Avison MJ, Reilly HF, Alger JR, Shulman RG (1983) Enhanced recovery of renal ATP with postischemic infusion of ATP-MgCl$_2$ determined by 31P-NMR. Am J Physiol 245:F530-F534

22. Kobayashi S, Nagase M, Honda N, Hishida A (1984) Glomerular alterations in uranyl acetate acute renal failure in rabbits. Kidney Int 26:808-815

23. Glaumann B, Glaumann H, Trump BF (1977) Studies of cellular recovery from injury. Virchows Arch [Cell Pathol] 25:281-308

Pathogenetic Role of Calcium in Renal Cell Injury

ROBERT W. SCHRIER, JOHN D. CONGER, and THOMAS J. BURKE[1]

Introduction

In 1981 at the VIIIth International Congress of Nephrology in Athens, Greece, and subsequently at the Tel Aviv Satellite Symposium on Acute Renal Failure (ARF) in Israel, the first studies pointing to a pathogenetic role of Ca^{2+} in renal ischemic injury were reported by our group [1–3]. In those initial experiments it was shown that infusion of a calcium channel blocker (CCB) or mannitol prevented or greatly attenuated the severity of the functional defect in experimental, norepinephrine- (NE) induced ARF in dogs. Moreover, mitochondrial function assessed by mitochondrial Ca^{2+} content, respiration, and efflux rates was normal at 24 h after these treatments. Subsequent investigations in our laboratories have not only provided insight into the mechanism of Ca^{2+}-related tubular epithelial cell injury, but have also suggested that smooth muscle cell Ca^{2+} may contribute to the abnormal vascular reactivity that follows renal ischemia [4].

This report will first review evidence that CCBs, assumedly by attenuating increases in cell Ca^{2+}, are protective in the ischemic ARF. Next, experiments will be described that focus on the pivotal role of disordered Ca^{2+} metabolism in tubular epithelial cell ischemia and, finally, the potential mechanistic role of Ca^{2+} in the functional aberrations of the renal vasculature following transient interruption of renal blood flow (RBF) will be examined.

Effects of CCB in Ischemic ARF

In one of our early studies, verapamil or nifedipine was infused into the renal artery of dogs prior to the infusion into the renal artery of a dose of NE that resulted in total renal ischemia [5]. Dogs infused with these CCB did not develop ARF, as assessed

[1]Department of Medicine, University of Colorado School of Medicine, Denver, CO 80262, USA

by inulin clearance (C_{In}). Although we could find no evidence for an attentuation of the severe renal ischemia induced during the NE infusion, it was possible that the failure of ARF to develop was simply due to a small, continued level of RBF, undetected by flow meter methodology. However, improved C_{In} was also observed in dogs in which CCB were infused after, rather than before, NE. Since publication of our report, others have demonstrated protection against ischemic ARF in both rat and dog models when CCBs are infused while a totally occlusive clamp is in place on the renal artery. Such maneuvers should not be associated with a lessening of the ischemia during clamping induced by this mechanical obstruction to RBF.

The functional improvement we noted occurred as early as one hour after NE infusion was terminated and persisted at 24 h. In addition, the morphologic appearance of the kidney by light and electron microscopy was dramatically improved. The results of these experiments demonstrating an impressive protective effect of CCB in ischemic ARF suggested an important role of Ca^{2+} in cell injury. The pathogenesis of Ca^{2+}-mediated cell injury may relate to the dissipation of the very large gradient for Ca^{2+} ions between extracellular and intracellular fluid, since maintenance of this gradient requires expenditures of energy and, thus, O_2 dependent adenosine triphosphate (ATP) synthesis. In ischemia or anoxia where O_2 levels are very low or absent, the mechanisms for the control of cytosolic-free Ca^{2+} ($[Ca^{2+}]_i$), such as Na^+/Ca^{2+} exchange, CaATPase, and mitochondrial buffering, fail, with the result that $[Ca^{2+}]_i$ increases and, in parallel, cell injury ensues.

Ca^{2+} in Tubular Epithelial Cell Ischemic Injury

Studies from our laboratories [6,7] and from those of other investigators [8] have demonstrated the critical contribution of tubular injury and obstruction to the acute deterioration in renal function following ischemia. Tubular obstruction from cellular debris and, to a varible extent, tubular fluid backleak as a result of disrupted tubular wall integrity are central factors in the reduction in glomerular filtration. Thus, an examination of Ca^{2+} kinetics in tubules or tubular epithelial cells was a logical first step in determining the mechanism of protection conveyed by CCB.

However, neither the mechanism of ischemic injury to tubules nor the site(s) at which CCB convey protection are precisely identified during in vivo studies. For example, it is difficult to argue against the suggestion that some of the improvement in glomerular filtration rate (GFR) or reduction in blood urea nitrogen (BUN) occurs as a direct result of the effects of improved renal hemodynamics which are induced by intrarenal or systemic CCB to cause improvement in O_2 and substrate delivery to the previously ischemic renal epithelial tissue. For this reason, we have turned to several in vitro models of tubular ischemic injury. Each model has, of course, its limitations and pitfalls, but use of the models in combination with the results of whole animal studies provides important data which help explain both the pathogenesis and prevention of ischemic injury.

One example of the in vitro model is that of the isolated perfused kidney (IPK) in which the vasculature is already maximally dilated (or nearly so) such that improved C_{In} is unlikely to be due solely to improved RBF. We have found that both low dose (2.5 and 5.0 μM) verapamil and high dose (100 μM) verapamil improved C_{In} after 40 min of warm ischemia in the rat IPK, and ATP regeneration was enhanced. Cold

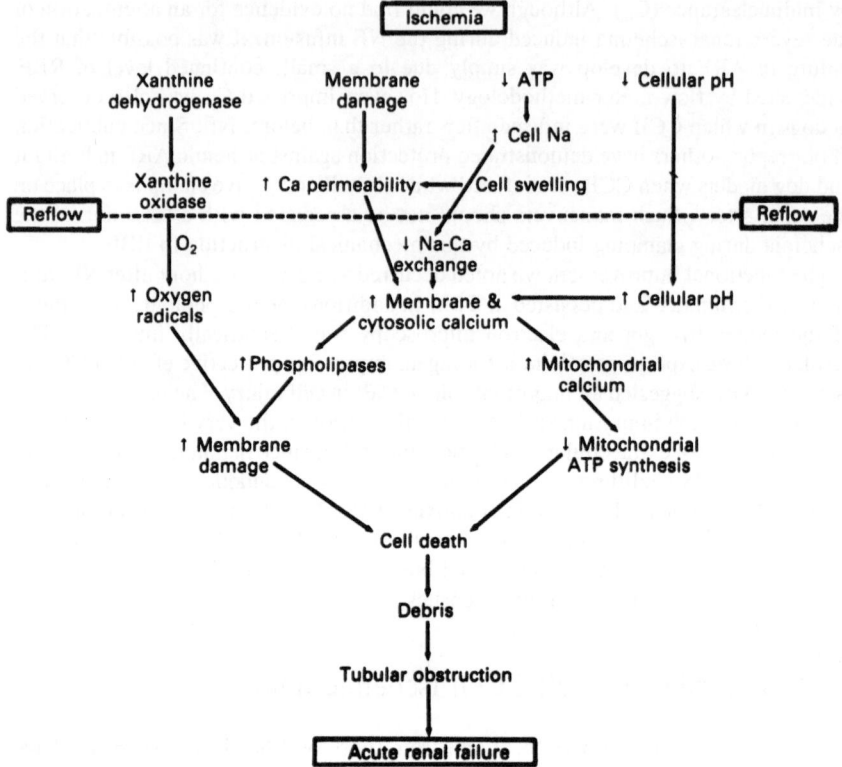

Fig. 1. Mechanisms of renal epithelial cell injury during ischemia and reflow. (From [20] with permission)

ischemia, a model of organ harvesting and storage prior to transplantation, also leads to renal injury and this can be attenuated, as assessed by better tubular Na$^+$ reabsorption (T_{Na}) when verapamil is added to the initial flush solution [9].

Together, the in vivo and in vitro demonstration of less renal tubular injury following ischemia when CCB are added led us to the hypothesis that ischemia is associated with an increased [Ca^{2+}]$_i$ burden, which may play a role in inducing epithelial (tubular) cell injury, thereby providing the source of tubular debris that causes nephron obstruction, as shown in Fig. 1. It is also likely that, at various times during reperfusion, the influx of Ca^{2+} into the mitochondria of tubular epithelial cells occurs at high but different rates, due in part to differences in the state of mitochondrial energization.

Mitochondrial respiration is impaired during ischemia (prior to reflow), subsequently improves during the first 3 h of reflow, and thereafter begins to deteriorate. The lowest values for basal respiration (S_4), adenosine diphosphate-stimulated (S_3), and uncoupled respiration are usually seen prior to reflow and after 24 h of reflow. Associated with reflow, mitochondrial Ca^{2+} content increases, reaching its highest level at 24 h post-ischemia [10].

To determine if the increase in renal mitochondrial Ca^{2+} noted at 24 h of reflow was simply a result of cell death, we measured the Ca^{2+} content of mitochondria harvested from renal cortical tissue of rat kidneys immediately after ischemia (prior to reflow) and after 1, 3, 6, 12, 18, and 24 h of reflow [11]. These data reveal that during the first 3 h of reflow, mitochondrial Ca^{2+} content increases only slightly, but that between 3 and 24 h, a progressive, significant, and further rise in mitochondrial Ca^{2+} content occurs. The 3 h time point appears to be a critical turning point, because during reflow, mitochondrial respiration steadily improves for the first 3 h and then becomes progressively impaired thereafter.

To determine if the mitochondria harvested from ischemic kidneys had been damaged in some way other than simply by the exposure to Ca^{2+} in vivo, we isolated normal rat kidney mitochondria in an isolation buffer that contained increasing concentrations of Ca^{2+}, much as might occur when calcified renal tissue is disrupted during the isolation of mitchondria. These mitchondria, exposed to a normal cytosolic-like fluid containing progressively higher Ca^{2+} concentrations, exhibited progressively more severe inhibition of mitchondrial respiration, even when all isolation and centrifugation steps were conducted at 4°C [11].

Since Ca^{2+} translocation across the mitchondrial inner membrane can be blocked by ruthenium red, we reexamined the interrelationship between mitchondrial Ca^{2+} overload and mitchondrial respiration during reperfusion when ruthenium red was present during isolation [11]. The magnitude of the rise in Ca^{2+} and the depression in respiration were reduced somewhat by this maneuver but the temporal changes were similar to those observed without ruthenium red. We conclude that tissue and mitchondrial Ca^{2+} overload occur after complete ischemia in vivo, primarily during reflow.

The uniqueness of mitchondrial injury was demonstrated by isolation of endoplasmic reticulum (ER) from ischemic kidneys [12]. This membrane preparation exhibited normal Ca^{2+} transport characteristics, unlike the decrement in mitchondrial respiration, 24 h after ischemia, for 50 or even 90 min duration. Thus, ischemic injury to renal cortical tissue, primarily epithelial tissue, may be manifested mainly by Ca^{2+}-mediated damage to mitochondria. The associated impairment in S_3 respiration limits the ability of the cells to reestablish normal structure and function. Provision of exogenous ATP to ER in vivo, 24 h after reflow, shows that this organelle's function of transporting Ca^{2+} is essentially intact. It is likely, however, that the reduction in S_3 respiration and the decreased mitchondrial ATP synthesis may impair Ca^{2+} uptake by the ER in vivo.

Ca^{2+} Handling by Injured Renal Tissue

As noted above, tissue and mitchondrial Ca^{2+} accumulation occur with reperfusion and, without ATP to extrude Ca^{2+}, could reflect the effect simply, of normal rates of Ca^{2+} uptake. Since it is possible that Ca^{2+} uptake rate from extracellular fluid (ECF) to tubules is increased following a period of O_2 deprivation, we have measured $^{45}Ca^{2+}$ uptake rates in isolated rat proximal tubules (RPT) [13]. Our data show that $^{45}Ca^{2+}$ uptake rate is increased in vitro during reoxygenation at a PH of 7.4 and that reduction in ECF pH to 6.9 normalizes $^{45}Ca^{2+}$ uptake. We have also shown that cellular death can be attenuated in primary cultures of rabbit tubule segments by removal of

Ca^{2+} from the media during the first 2 h of reoxygenation after anoxia; all tubule segments including S_1, S_2, and S_3 segments of the proximal tubule, as well as the cortical collecting duct and the medullary ascending limb were protected [14].

ATP and Cell Injury

As noted above, we have observed a decrease in mitchondrial respiration beginning about 3 h after reflow following ischemia. ATP is synthesized under normal conditions by substrates metabolized by mitchondria. In several glycolytic reactions, consumption of ATP is necessary and when ATP availability is reduced, as it is shortly after an ischemic insult, glycolytic processes, and thus mitchondrial respiration, are at risk.

We have attempted to increase ATP synthesis by addition of fructose 1,6-diphosphate to the perfusate in an isolated perfused kidney subjected to 40 min of warm ischemia. Both C_{In} and T_{Na} were markedly increased. Nuclear magnetic resonance spectroscopy of these kidneys showed that ATP concentrations had indeed improved quite substantially.

Together, data obtained in the experiments described above led to a tentative hypothesis as to how Ca^{2+} derangements occurring during ischemia and during reflow contribute to epithelial cell injury and manifest themselves as ARF (Fig. 1).

Mechanisms and Magnitude of Increased Ca^{2+} Uptake in O_2 Deprivation

We have begun to examine the cause(s) of incresed Ca^{2+} uptake which leads to time dependent, tissue Ca^{2+} overload during hypoxia. After determining that there was indeed a "window" of severe hypoxia (pO_2 range 40–60 mmHg) during which rat proximal tubule (RPT) Ca^{2+} content increased, as had been previously demonstrated by two groups in the rabbit proximal tubule, $^{45}Ca^{2+}$ uptake was measured in RPT during total anoxia ($pO_2 = 0$ mmHg). These results demonstrated that $^{45}Ca^{2+}$ uptake was indeed increased during anoxia, but only during the first 10 min; by 20 min of anoxia $^{45}Ca^{2+}$ uptake had returned to control levels. Verapamil reduced $^{45}Ca^{2+}$ uptake to near normal levels during the first 10 min of either anoxia or hypoxia, suggesting that at least one of the influx pathways for Ca^{2+} was via a potential operated channel (POC). Because one similarity between hypoxic or anoxic epithelial tissue and excitable tissues, which normally respond to CCB, is an altered transmembrane K^+ gradient, we have questioned whether K^+ loss from ischemic tissues and chronic membrane depolarization induced by O_2 deprivation may be related to the 1) opening of potential operated Ca^{2+} channels and to the 2) efficacy of CCB in preventing epithelial injury during O_2 deprivation.

The approach we have taken is to expose normoxic RPT to various drugs or incubation conditions which have the capacity to alter the transmembrane K^+ gradient (and therefore the membrane potential). We have used 3 and 30 μM valinomycine, 10 μM ouabain, 30 μM amphotericin, and 40 mM extracellular KCl. The Krebs Henseleit buffer (KHB) was modified by reducing NaCl, in order to keep extracellular osmol-

Fig. 2. $^{45}Ca^{2+}$ uptake, in freshly isolated rat proximal tubules incubated under normoxic conditions, is increased when the transcellular K^+ gradient is reduced. Studies were performed at 10 (*top panel*) and 20 min (*bottom panel*) after exposure to the experimental conditions. Val, valinomycin; Ampho, amphotericin; Ouab, ouabain; KCl, 40 mM extracellular potassium chloride

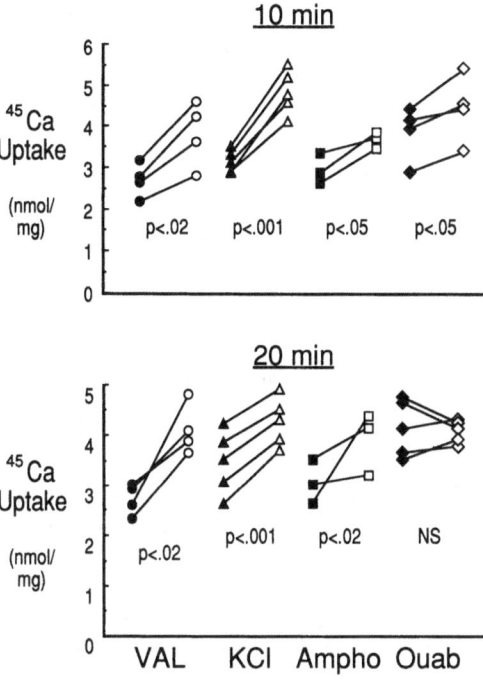

ality constant when KCl was increased from 4 to 40 mM and in other studies the independent effects of reducing NaCl by 40 mM and replacing it with choline chloride were also tested. The results of these studies demonstrate that each of the four different maneuvers increases $^{45}Ca^{2+}$ uptake rate (Fig. 2). This increase can be blocked by verapamil. Blockade of $^{45}Ca^{2+}$ uptake in depolarized, hypoxic tissue is not unique to verapamil because flunarizine, a non-specific CCB, also prevents $^{45}Ca^{2+}$ uptake and lessens lactate dehydrogenase (LDH) release.

Our final question concerned the mechanism for the abrupt cessation of Ca^{2+} uptake by anoxic RPT after an initial early increased rate. Takano and colleagues had suggested that the hypoxic rabbit proximal tubule accumulates Ca^{2+} in a time-dependent manner because the mitchondria remain partially energized, providing a site for sequestration of Ca^{2+} and therefore for sustained high Ca^{2+} uptake rates [15]. In anoxic tissue there would be no partially energized mitchondria, so that Ca^{2+} sequestration would not occur and any early increase in $^{45}Ca^{2+}$ uptake would simply increase the concentration of free Ca^{2+} in the cytosol. If this reasoning is correct then free Ca^{2+} ($[Ca^{2+}]_i$) measured by Fura2 should be similar in control and in hypoxic tissue but increased in anoxic tissue. Figure 3 demonstrates that this indeed is the case, since in anoxic RPT, $[Ca^{2+}]_i$ is 2- to 3-fold higher after 10 min of anoxia compared to normoxic RPT and there is virtually no difference in $[Ca^{2+}]_i$ between hypoxic and normal RPT. Furthermore, if hypoxic but not anoxic RPT accumulate Ca^{2+} in their mitochondria, then administration of FCCP, which collapses the mitochondrial membrane potential, should lead to release of Ca^{2+} from mitochondria of hypoxic RPT and to a much higher

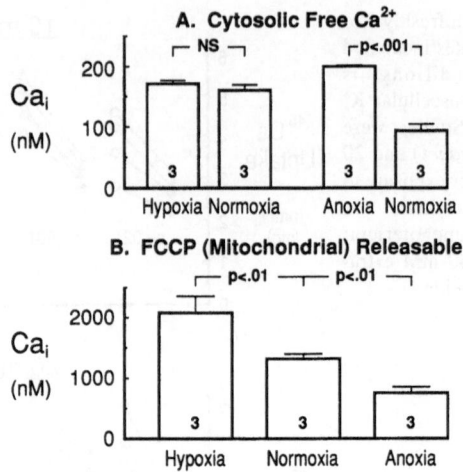

Fig. 3. Fura2 measurements of cytosolic free calcium ($[Ca^{2+}]_i$) in freshly isolated rat proximal tubules (*RPT*) under conditions of O_2 deprivation

Ca^{2+} signal (using Fura2) than in normoxic tissue, which in turn, should be higher than in anoxic tissue. Figure 3 also demonstrates that this is exactly what occurs.

Ca^{2+} in Vascular Ischemic Injury

While there has been considerable focus on post-ischemic tubular injury and the pathogenetic role of Ca^{2+}, there is a growing body of evidence indicating that renal ischemia results in specific abnormalities of the renal vasculature as well. There is also evidence that disordered smooth muscle cell Ca^{2+} metabolism may be a factor in the aberrations of vasoreactivity.

Following ischemic ARF induction, there are two recognized functional defects of the arterial system of the kidney: persistent focal pre-glomerular vasoconstriction and a loss of normal RBF autoregulation [7,16]. The former defect results in decreased driving forces for glomerular filtration and, in conjunction with tubular obstruction and tubular fluid backleak, is a significant pathogenetic mechanism in ischemic ARF. Persistent vasoconstriction is a focal rather than a diffuse process, as indicated by the heterogeneity of glomerular capillary pressure and glomerular plasma flow measurements by micropuncture and the near restoration of total kidney blood flow in established ARF [7]. Recently, we examined basal tone in afferent arterioles (AA) isolated from kidneys of rats that had undergone ARF induction with NE one week previously and had RBF and GFR that were 80% and 30% of control values, respectively. Mean lumen diameter of AA from ARF kidneys was less than that of sham-ARF control kidney over a physiologic pressure range (Fig. 4). These data indicate that there was an intrinsically greater arteriolar tone in AA from ARF kidneys. (It should be noted, however, that while there was a statistically lesser lumen diameter at physiologic pressures, there were occasional AA with diameters

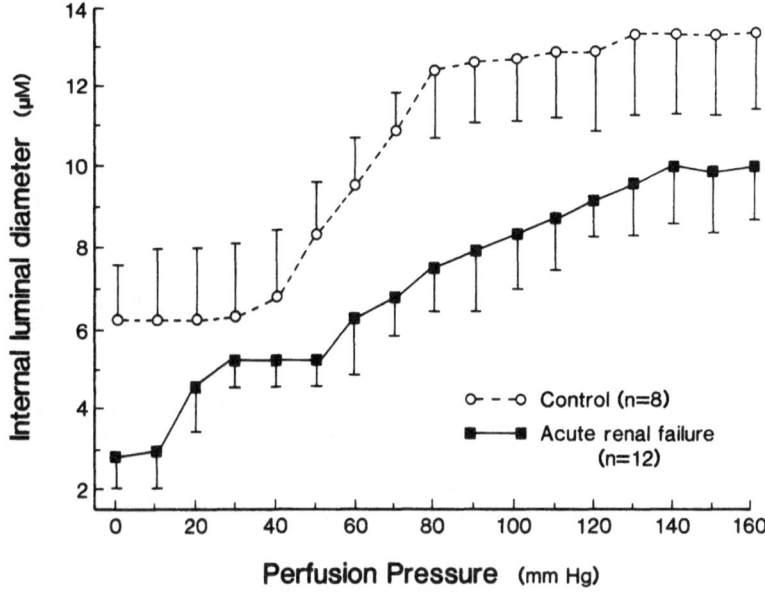

Fig. 4. Pressure-related changes in lumen diameter of afferent arterioles isolated from control and post-ischemic ARF rat kidneys. Over a physiologic range (60–100 mmHg) lumen diameter was less in the afferent arterioles from ARF kidneys ($P < .02$)

similar to sham-ARF controls, consistent with the heterogeneity of the vascular abnormality.) To assess the basis for differences in tone between AA from ARF and control kidneys, we examined smooth muscle $[Ca^{2+}]_i$ in these vessels at 80 mmHg pressure before and after the addition of the vasoconstrictor agonist angiotensin II by dual excitation fluorescence ratio imaging using Fura2. As can be seen from Fig. 5, the basal $[Ca^{2+}]_i$ was more than 2-fold higher in ARF vessels (equivalent to 200 vs 70 nM). There was an abrupt increase in $[Ca^{2+}]_i$ in response to angiotensin II in the control AA, but no detectable response in the AA from ARF kidneys. While one interpretation of these data is provided by the recent study of Kon et al. [17] indicating that persistent post-ischemic vasoconstriction is due to the paracrine action of endothelin, another explanation is possible. As in tubular epithelial cells, increases in smooth muscle Ca^{2+} may be a consequence of ischemia, per se, secondary to a loss of transmembrane potential difference. Although indirect evidence, the lack of receptor activation by angiotensin II in AA from ARF kidney suggests a loss of receptors from smooth muscle cells. If there was a similar loss of receptors to endothelin, then the latter explanation for increased $[Ca^{2+}]_i$ would be more tenable. In any case, the increase in post-ischemic smooth muscle cell Ca^{2+} is consistent with the demonstrated increase in basal tone in the majority of AA examined from ARF kidneys.

The second defect in post-ischemic vascular reactivity, loss of RBF autoregulation, is actually a paradoxical vasoconstriction to a reduction in renal perfusion pressure, when examined in the NE-induced ARF rat model [18]. The aberrant vasoconstriction in the autoregulatory pressure range, over which vasodilation is the normal

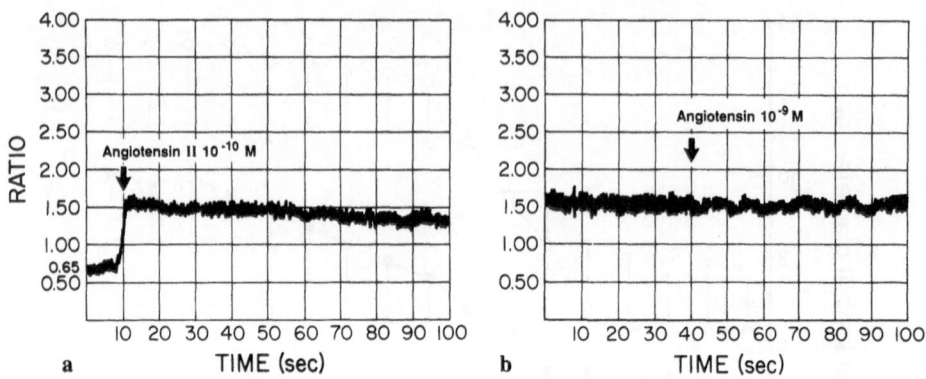

Fig. 5a-b. Real time cytosolic free calcium $[Ca^{2+}]_i$ transients in smooth muscle cells of afferent arterioles from normal (**a**) and post-ischemic ARF rats (**b**) in basal state and after addition of angiotensin II as determined by dual excitation fluorescence ratio imaging using Fura2. Note that basal state $[Ca^{2+}]_i$ was higher in afferent arterioles from ARF kidneys, but did not respond to angiotensin II despite the higher concentration used in comparison with AA from normal kidneys

response, is intimately related to a renovascular hypersensitivity to autonomic nerve activity. There is an increased vasoconstriction to renal nerve stimulation and a complete attenuation of the paradoxical vasoconstriction to renal perfusion pressure reduction if the kidney is denervated [18]. Interestingly, while renal denervation

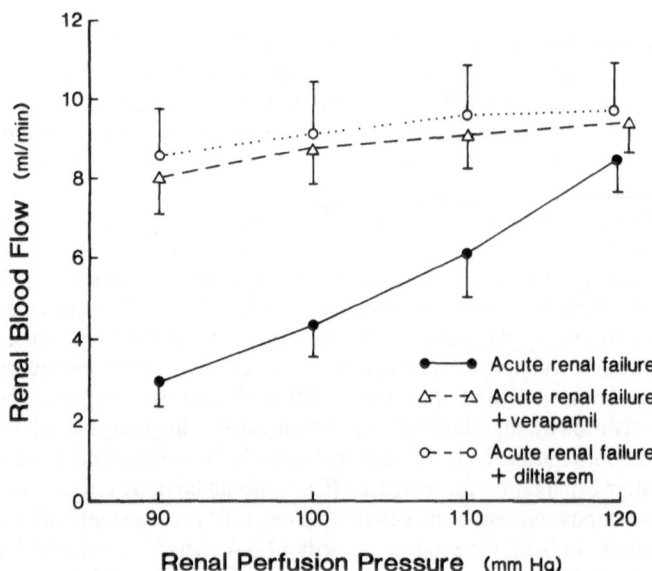

Fig. 6. Renal blood flow (*RBF*) response to reduction in renal perfusion pressure over the physiologic autoregulatory range in post-ischemic acute renal failure (*ARF*) kidneys without and with 90 min intrarenal infusion of calcium channel blockers

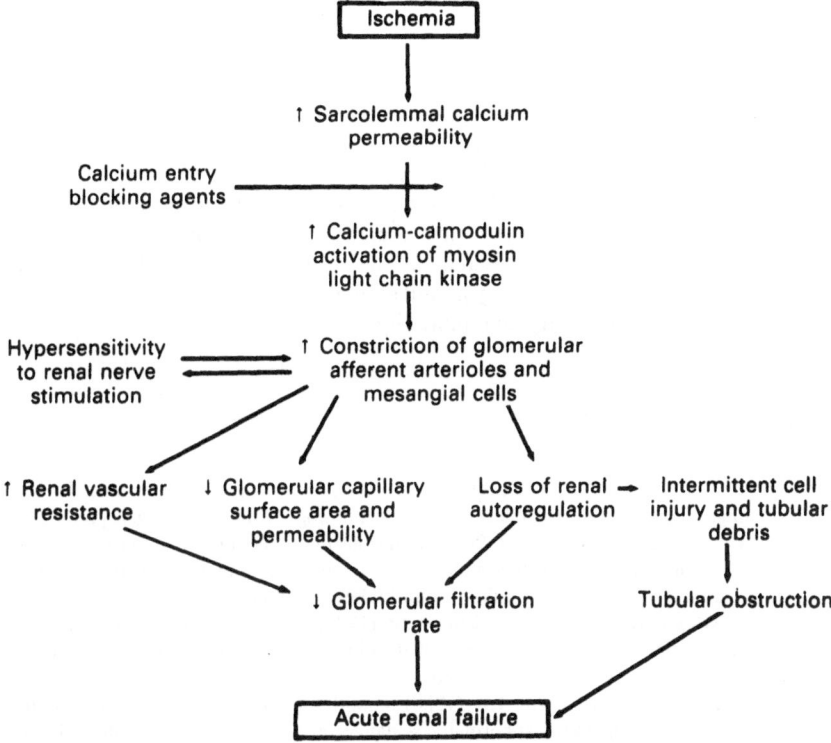

Fig. 7. Vascular and tubular contribution to ischemic acute renal failure (*ARF*). (From [20] with permission)

blocks the paradoxical vasoconstriction to renal perfusion pressure reduction, normal autoregulatory vasodilation is not restored. The abnormal vasoreactive response to renal perfusion pressure reduction following ischemic renal injury is complex and, likely, involves more than one mechanism, including an augmented release of neurotransmitter to autonomic nerve activity [19]. However, it is possible that abnormal smooth muscle cell Ca^{2+} also plays a role in this disordered autoregulatory response. We have found that 90 min, but not 30 min, intraarterial infusion of the CCB verapamil and diltiazem will completely block the renovascular hypersensitivity to renal nerve stimulation and renal perfusion pressure reduction [4]. In addition, the normal autoregulatory vasodilation is restored, as shown in Fig. 6. It is postulated that prolonged CCB infusion reduces smooth muscle cell Ca^{2+} (assuming continued Ca^{2+} extrusion and blocked Ca^{2+} entry) restoring a more nearly normal response to adrenergic neurotransmitters and appropriate vasodilation to renal perfusion pressure reduction. The inference derived from this postulate is that increased arteriolar $[Ca^{2+}]_i$, as demonstrated by Fura2 fluorescence of isolated AA, contributes both to exaggerated vasoconstriction to stimuli such as renal nerve stimulation, and to the failure to dilate appropriately to renal perfusion pressure reduction in the autoregulatory range (Fig. 7).

Conclusion

Our understanding of the pathogenesis and prevention of ARF has progressive dramatically over the last 20 years, from observations of whole animals in the 1970s to cells and organelles in the 1980s. Much of this information was recently synthesized in an editorial [20]. Nevertheless, even with present therapeutic approaches, the mortality in ARF is 35%–75% and thus there continues to be a dire need for interventional strategies. With the demonstration of altered Ca^{2+} kinetics in both vascular and epithelial tissue in ARF, further research into the mechanisms by which Ca^{2+} is mishandled by ischemic renal tissues may permit clinicians, in the near future, to reverse or eliminate this extraordinarily high mortality rate.

References

1. Schrier RW, Burke RJ, Conger JD, Arnold PE (1981) New aspects of acute renal failure. Proceedings of the 8th International Congress Nephrology, Athens. S Karger, pp 63–69
2. Schrier RW, Arnold PE, Burke TJ (1982) Alterations in mitchondrial respiration and calcium movements in norepinephrine-induced acute renal failure: modification by mannitol. In: Eliahou HE (ed) Acute renal failure. John Libbey, London, pp 21–22
3. Burke TJ, Arnold PE, Grossfeld PD, Schrier RW (1982) Effect of calcium membrane inhibition on norepinephrine-induced acute renal failure. In: Eliahou HE (ed) Acute renal failure. John Libbey, London, pp 239–240
4. Conger JD, Robinette JB, Schrier RW (1988) Smooth muscle calcium and endothelium-deprived relaxing factor in the abnormal vascular responses of acute renal failure. J Clin Invest 82:532–537
5. Burke TJ, Arnold PE, Gordon JA, Bulger RE, Dobyan DC, Schrier RW (1984) Protective effect of intrarenal calcium membrane blockers before or after renal ischemia. J Clin Invest 74:1830–1841
6. Burke TJ, Cronin RE, Duchin KL, Peterson LN, Schrier RW (1980) Ischemia and tubule obstruction during acute renal failure in dogs: Role of mannitol in protection. Am J Physiol 238:F305–F314
7. Conger JD, Robinette JB, Kelleher SP (1984) Nephron heterogeneity in ischemic acute renal failure. Kidney Int 26:422–429
8. Tannen GA, Sophasan S (1976) Kidney pressures after temporary renal artery occlusion in the rat. Am J Physiol 230:1173–1179
9. Shapiro JI, Cheung C, Itabashi A, Chan L, Schrier RW (1985) The effect of verapamil on renal function after warm and cold ischemia in the isolated perfused rat kidney. Transplantation 40:596–600
10. Wilson DR, Arnold PE, Burke TJ, Schrier RW (1984) Mitochondrial calcium accumulation and mitchondrial respiration in ischemic acute renal failure in the rat. Kidney Int 25:591–526
11. Arnold PE, Lumlertgul D, Burke TJ, Schrier RW (1985) In vitro versus in vivo mitchondrial calcium loading in ischemic acute renal failure. Am J Physiol 248:F845–F850
12. Schieppati A, Wilson PD, Burke TJ, Schrier RW (1985) Effect of renal ischemia on cortical microsomal calcium transport. Am J Physiol 249:C476–C483
13. Burnier M, Van Putten VJ, Schieppati A, Schrier RW (1988) Effect of extracellular acidosis on $^{45}Ca^{2+}$ uptake in isolated hypoxic proximal tubules. Am J Physiol 254:C839–C846
14. Wilson PD, Schrier RW (1986) Nephron segment and calcium as determinants of anoxic cell death in primary renal cell cultures. Kidney Int 29:1172–1179

15. Takano T, Soltolf SP, Murdaugh S, Mandel LJ (1985) Intracellular respiratory dysfunction and cell injury in short-term anoxia of rabbit renal proximal tubules. J Clin Invest 76:2377-2384
16. Conger JD (1983) The role of blood flow autoregulation in pathophysiology of acute renal failure. Circ Shock 11:235-244
17. Kon V, Yoshioka T, Fogo A, Ichikawa I (1989) Glomerular actions of endothelin in vivo. J Clin Invest 83:1762-1767
18. Kelleher SP, Robinette JB, Conger JD (1984) Sympathetic nervous system in the loss of autoregulation in acute renal failure. Am J Physiol 15:F379-F386
19. Robinette JB, Conger JD (1990) The roles of angiotensin II and thromboxanes in the hypersensitivity to renal nerve stimulation in acute renal failure. J Clin Invest 86:1532-1539
20. Schrier RW, Arnold PE, Van Putten VJ, Burke TJ (1987) Cellular calcium in ischemic acute renal failure: Role of calcium entry blockers. Kidney Int 32:313-321

Cyclosporine Nephrotoxicity in the 1990s

Kim Solez[1] and Lorraine C. Racusen[2]

SUMMARY. As we approach the 18th year since the discovery of cyclosporine's immunosuppressive properties, the drug has now "come of age." Despite the advent of newer agents such as FK506, 15-deoxyspergualin, and rapamycin, cyclosporine is such a highly successful therapeutic agent that it is likely to remain in use for many years. Therefore, cyclosporine nephrotoxicity, the major side effect of the drug, will continue to be an important problem. Renal vasoconstriction appears to be the primary mechanism of toxicity, and thromboxane is likely to be the principal mediator of this effect. Thromboxane receptor blockade or inhibition of thromboxane synthesis may be a clinically effective means of lessening cyclosporine nephrotoxicity.

Introduction

It has now been 18 years since the discovery of the immunosuppressive properties of cyclosporine A by Borel et al., 12 years since the first clinical trials in kidney transplantation and graft-versus-host disease, 10 years since the total synthesis of the molecule, and 7 years since its approval and release for use as an immunosuppressive agent in the U.S. [1] Cyclosporine has moved from the status of a new drug to that of an established pharmaceutical agent which has had a major impact on medical practice.

Cyclosporine represents not only a major therapeutic and pharmacologic advance but also a major phenomenon in the medical literature. As depicted in Fig. 1, the number of articles per year devoted to cyclosporine, dubbed "the drug of the 1980s," has steadily risen from 3 in 1976 to nearly 1600 in 1988. The decline since 1988 has been more or less compensated for by a burgeoning literature on newer powerful and potentially clinically useful immunosuppressive agents, such as FK506, 15-deoxy-

---

[1]Department of Pathology, 5B4.02 Mackenzie Health Sciences Centre, University of Alberta, Edmonton, Alberta, T6G 2R7 Canada. Recipient of a Sandoz Travel Fellowship
[2]Department of Pathology, Johns Hopkins Hospital, Baltimore, Maryland 21205, USA

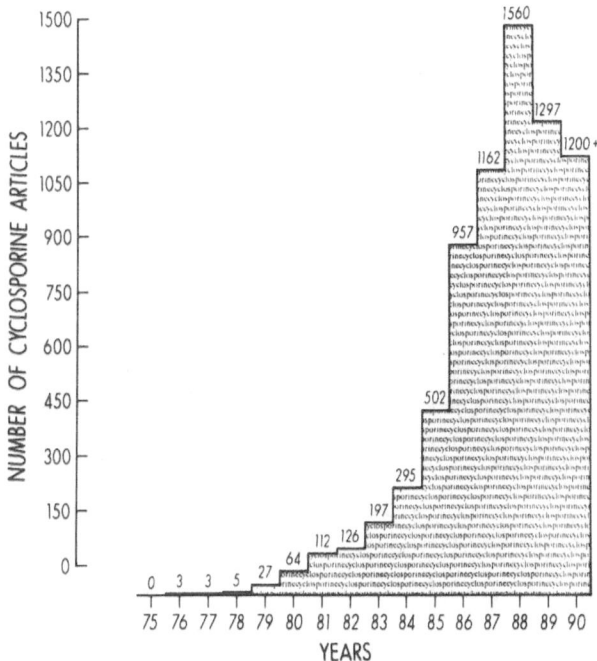

Fig. 1. Number of cyclosporine articles published per year, 1975-1990

spergualin, and rapamycin [2–14]. The best characterized of these three new agents, FK506, appears to have a mechanism of action similar to that of cyclosporine [15–20]. It has some potential for nephrotoxicity [21], but apparently lacks direct endothelial toxicity [22,23].

Much of the immense literature on cyclosporine deals with its nephrotoxicity, reflecting the fact that the renal toxicity of the drug, which manifests itself clinically in over half the patients who receive it, is the major side effect limiting its use [24] (Table 1). The 8000 articles on cyclosporine published between 1976 and 1990 could logically be expected to generate confusion. It is important in the nephrotoxicity area to try to provide some clarity and consensus out of the morass of conflicting studies. Clinical cyclosporine nephrotoxicity can be divided into six forms [24]:

1) Acute reversible renal functional impairment
2) Delayed renal allograft function
3) Acute vasculopathy (thrombotic microangiopathy)
4) Chronic nephropathy with interstitial fibrosis
5) Functional toxicity
6) Tubular toxicity

It is now clear that, clinically, the most important of these forms are 1, 4, and 5, and that these three clinical syndromes represent a spectrum of functional and morphologic abnormalities brought about in the kidney by cyclosporine-induced

Table 1. Reported adverse effects of cyclosporine-A in 3518 renal transplant recipients[a]

Adverse effect	Percentage
Renal dysfunction	54.3
Hypertension	42.4
Infections	
Bacterial	15.4
Viral	14.8
Fungal	3.3
Hypertrichosis	32.5
Tremor	22.1
Hepatic dysfunction	18.2
Gum hyperplasia	16.2
Nausea, vomiting	9.0
Paresthesia	5.2
Hyperuricemia	4.1
Gl ulcer hemorrhage	3.2
Convulsions	1.8
Hyperkalemia	1.7
Malignancy (including 0.4% lymphoma)	1.3
Joint/muscle pain	1.1
Anemia	1.1

[a](Modified from [31])

vasoconstriction. Possible suggested mechanisms for this vasoconstriction have included:

1) A direct vasoconstrictive effect
2) Endothelin mediated vasoconstriction
3) Enhancement of local production of angiotensin in renal vessels
4) Decreased atrial natriuretic peptide
5) Increased production of thromboxane
6) Activation of the sympathetic nervous system

The renal vasoconstriction induced by cyclosporine is clearly not secondary to tubular injury, since it can be observed in the hydronephrotic rat model in which most tubular structures have been obliterated [25]. Enhanced thromboxane release is likely to be the most important mechanism of cyclosporine-induced renal vasoconstriction. Several studies document amelioration of cyclosporine nephrotoxicity after thromboxane receptor blockade or modulation of thromboxane metabolism in experimental animals [26–28]. Inhibition of thromboxane synthetase has recently been shown to improve renal allograft function in patients taking cyclosporine [29]. It is of interest that thromboxane synthetase inhibition has also been shown to be beneficial in another condition in which renal vasoconstriction plays an important role, acute renal failure accompanying systemic sepsis [30].

Concluding Remarks

Cyclosporine is such a successful drug that it is likely to remain in use for many years despite the discovery of other potent immunosuppressive agents. Elucidation of the mechanisms of cyclosporine-induced renal vasoconstriction will enable the development of better strategies to avoid this important side effect of the drug.

References

1. Borel JF (1982) The history of Cyclosporin A and its significance. In: White DJG (ed) Cyclosporin A. Elsevier Biochemical, Amsterdam, pp 5–17
2. Kino T, Hatanaka H, Miyata S, Inamura N, Nishiyama M, Yajima T, Goto T, Okuhara M, Kohsaka M, Aoki H, Ochiai T (1987) FK-506, a novel immunosuppressant isolated from *A Streptomyces*. II: Immunosuppressive effect of FK-506 *in vitro*. J Antibiot (Tokyo) 40(9):1256–1265
3. Goto T, Kino T, Hatanaka M, Nishiyama M, Okuhara M, Kohsaka M, Aoki H, Imanaka H (1987) Discovery of FK-506, a novel immunosuppressant isolated from *Streptomyces Tsukubaensis*. Transplant Proc 19(5):4–8
4. Starzl TE, Todo S, Fung J, Demetris AJ, Venkataramman R, Jain A (1989) FK 506 for liver, kidney and pancreas transplantation. Lancet II:1000–1004
5. Ochiai T, Sakamoto K, Gunji Y, Hamaguchi K, Isegawa N, Suzuki T, Shimada H, Hayashi H, Yasumoto A, Asano T, Isono K (1989) Effects of combination treatment with FK506 and cyclosporine on survival time and vascular changes in renal-allograft-recipient dogs. Transplantation 48:193–197
6. Hoffman AL, Makowka L, Banner B, Cai X, Cramer DV, Pascualone A, Todo S, Starzl TE (1990) The use of FK-506 for small intestine allotransplantation. Transplantation 49:483–490
7. Inagaki K, Fukuda Y, Sumimoto K, Matsuno K, Ito H, Takahashi M, Dohi K (1989) Effect of FK506 and 15-deoxyspergualin in rat orthotopic liver transplantation. Transplant Proc 21:1069–1071
8. Ishibashi M, Jiang S, Kokado Y, Takahara S, Sonoda T (1989) Immunopharmacologic effects of immunosuppressive agents explored by a new effector monocyte generation assay. Transplant Proc 21:1854–1858
9. Nakajima K, Sakamoto K, Ochiai T, Asano T, Isono K (1989) Effects of 15-deoxyspergualin and FK506 on the histology and survival of hamster-to-rat cardiac xenotransplantation. Transplant Proc 21:546–548
10. Ochiai T, Nakajima K, Sakamoto K, Nagata M, Gunji Y, Asano T, Isono K, Sakamaki T, Hamaguchi K (1989) Comparative studies on the immunosuppressive activity of FK506, 15-deoxyspergualin, and cyclosporine. Transplant Proc 21:829–832
11. Dumont FJ, Staruch MJ, Koprak SL, Melino MR, Sigal NH (1990) Distinct mechanisms of suppression of murine T cell activation by the related macrolides FK-506 and rapamycin. J Immunol 144:251–258
12. Dumont FJ, Melino MR, Staruch MJ, Koprak SL, Fischer PA, Sigal NH (1990) The immunosuppressive macrolides FK-506 and rapamycin act as reciprocal antagonists in murine T cells. J Immunol 144:1418–1424
13. Calne RY, Collier DStJ, Lim S, Pollared SG, Samaan A, White DJG (1989) Rapamycin for immunosuppressants in organ allografting. Lancet II:227
14. Thomson AW, Woo J (1989) Immunosuppressive properties of FK-506 and rapamycin. Lancet II:443–444
15. Harding MW, Galat A, Uehling DE, Schreiber SL (1989) A receptor for the immunosuppressant FK506 is a *cis-trans* peptidyl-prolyl isomerase. Nature 341:758–760
16. Siekierka JJ, Hung SHY, Poe M, Lin CS, Sigal NH A cytosolic binding protein for the immunosuppressant FK506 has peptidyl-prolyl isomerase activity but is distinct from cyclophilin. Nature 341:755–757
17. Freedman RB (1989) Convergence of drug action. Nature 341:692

18. Tocci MJ, Matkovich DA, Collier, Kwok P, Dumont F, Lin S, Degudicibus S, Siekierka JJ, Chin J, Hutchinson NI (1989) The immunosuppressive FK506 selectively inhibits expression of early T cell activation genes. J Immunol 143:718–726

19. Siekierka JJ, Staruch MJ, Hung SHY, Sigal NH (1989) FK-506, a potent novel immunosuppressive agent, binds to a cytosolic protein which is distinct from the cyclosporin A-binding protein, cyclophilin. J Immunol 143:1580–1583

20. Suzuki N, Sakane T, Tsunematsu T (1990) Effects of a novel immunosuppressive agent, FK506, on human B cell activation. Clin Exp Immunol 79:240–245

21. Stephen M, Woo J, Hasan NU, Whiting PH, Thomson AW (1989) Immunosuppressive activity, lymphocyte subset analysis, and acute toxicity of FK-506 in the rat. Transplantation 47:60–65

22. McCauley J, Bronsther O, Fung J, Todo S, Starzl TE (1989) Treatment of cyclosporin-induced haemolytic uraemic syndrome with FK506. Lancet II:1516

23. Brown Z, Neild GH (1990) FK-506 and haemolytic uraemic syndrome. Lancet I:412

24. Racusen LC, Solez K (1988) Cyclosporine nephrotoxicity. Int Rev Exp Pathol 30:107–157

25. Zimmerhackl LB, Fretschner M, Steinhausen M (1990) Cyclosporin reduces renal blood flow through vasoconstriction of arcuate arteries in the hydronephrotic rat model. Klin Wochenschr 68:166–174

26. Rossini M, Belloni A, Remuzzi G, Perico N (1990) Thromboxane receptor blockade attenuates the toxic effect of cyclosporine in experimental renal transplantation. Circulation 81:61–68

27. Spruney RF, Mayros SD, Collins D, Ruiz P, Klotman PE, Coffman T (1989) Thromboxane receptor blockade improves cyclosporine nephrotoxicity in rats. Prostaglandins 39:135–146

28. Teraoka S, Takahashi K, Tanabe K, Yamaguchi Y, Kawai T, Tojinbara T, Nakajima I, Nakagawa Y, Fujikawa H, Hayashi T, Oba S, Tagisama T, Honda H, Fuchinoue S, Toma H, Agishi T, Ota K (1989) Improvement in renal blood flow and kidney function by modulation of prostaglandin metabolism in cyclosporine-treated animals. Transplant Proc 21:937–940

29. Coffman TM, Smith SR, Creech EA, Schaffer AV, Martin LL, Rakhit A, Douglas FL, Klotman PE (1990) The thromboxane (TX) synthetase inhibitor CGS 13080 improves renal allograft function in patients taking cyclosporine (CYA). Kidney Int 37:604

30. Cumming AD, McDonald JW, Lindsay RM, Solez K, Linton AL (1989) The protective effect of thromboxane synthetase inhibition on renal function in systemic sepsis. Am J Kidney Dis 13:114–119

31. Krupp P, Gülich A, Timonen P (1986) Side effects and safety of Sandimmune in long-term treatment of renal transplant patients. Transplant Proc 18:991–992

Heterogeneity of Nephron Energy Metabolism: Implications for Response to Hypoxic Insult

HITOSHI ENDOU and KYU YONG JUNG[1]

SUMMARY. The mammalian kidney is known to consume ATP at high rates for various transporting processes. In order to evaluate energy metabolism and response to hypoxic insult along the nephron, we measured ATP content in each of the microdissected nephron segments from three animal species under various conditions using the luciferin/luciferase technique.

When proximal tubules from rats or mice were incubated at 37°C for 15 min without substrate, ATP content decreased rapidly in the following order; terminal (S_3) > middle (S_2) > early (S_1) segments, in rabbits, however, the order was reversed. This ATP decrease was restored with a sole preferred substrate at 2mM. ATP production from glucose was minimal in S_1 from three species, but was substantial in S_3. Glutamine or pyruvate was a preferred substrate in the proximal tubule. In lower nephron segments, although ATP was not reduced after 15 min incubation without substrate, a monovalent cationic ionophore, monensin, (10 μg/ml) decreased ATP, and this decrease was restored by 2mM glucose or pyruvate as preferred substrates.

In order to identify the portion within the proximal tubule most sensitive to hypoxic insult, each of three proximal segments was incubated with antimycin A, and ATP content was determined. In rats, antimycin A, at 5×10^{-7}M, decreased ATP content dramatically in S_3, moderately in S_2 and slightly in S_1, even in the presence of a preferred substrate.

These results suggest that energy metabolism differs from segment to segment, and that, in response to hypoxic insult, S_3 is the most fragile segment in rats.

Introduction

For active transporting systems, ATP is the major high-energy compound. To generate this energy source, the kidney metabolizes various substrates [1–3]. For each

---

[1]Department of Pharmacology, Faculty of Medicine, University of Tokyo, 113 Tokyo, Japan

defined nephron segment, however, with the exception of our recent reports [4,5], no clear-cut information is available about major substrates used for ATP synthesis along the nephron. We, therefore, report here that renal energy metabolism and its functions possess intranephron heterogeneity.

In addition, the kidney is very vulnerable to changes in metabolism and function caused by anoxia or by various chemicals such as drugs and hazardous xenobiotics. Since, in the field of renal toxicology, the relationship between ATP synthesis and consumption, as affected by exogenous materials in each nephron segment, has not yet been demonstrated, we also report here the effect of antimycin A, instead of anoxia, on cellular ATP within the rat proximal tubule.

Materials and Methods

Tissue preparation and tubule microdissection techniques used in this study have been previously described [6,7]. Incubation of microdissected nephron segments for ATP turnover determination and ATP assay were carried out as reported elsewhere [4,5]. Monensin and antimycin A were dissolved in ethanol, and the final concentration of vehicle was 0.2%. In preliminary experiments, this concentration of vehicle did not interfere with ATP biosynthesis.

Bovine serum albumin (BSA), collagenase (type 1, 240 U/mg), monensin, antimycin A, β-hydroxybutyrate, and DL-lactate were purchased from Sigma Chemical (St. Louis, Mo). Monitoring reagent for ATP was purchased from LKB-Wallac. All other compounds and reagents were of the highest grade available.

Values were expressed as means $\pm$ SE. Analysis of variance for multiple group comparisons and the Student's t test for unpaired data were used to determine statistical significance.

Results

Effect of Incubation Time on Cellular ATP Content in Individual Nephron Segments

When isolated nephron segments from kidneys of three animal species were incubated without any substrates, cellular ATP content was reduced dramatically in the proximal tubule, but not so conspicuously in the lower nephron segments (Table 1). In mice, the glomerulus also showed a decrease of ATP similar to that in the proximal tubule, where the straight portion (S_2 and S_3) showed a larger decrease than S_1. In rats, the most fragile segment was S_3, followed by S_2. In contrast, in rabbits, S_1 was the most sensitive suggesting a clear species difference in metabolic properties within the proximal tubule.

Substrate Specificities in the Maintenance of ATP Content in the Glomerulus and Proximal Tubule

When rat proximal tubules were incubated at 37°C for 15 min without exogenous substrate, cellular ATP content decreased significantly (Fig. 1). When glucose was

Table 1. Effect of incubation time on cellular ATP content in isolated nephron segments from three animal species

Species incubation	Mouse		Rat		Rabbit	
	0	30 min	0	[a]20 or 30 min	0	25 min
Glm	6.3±0.5	1.9±0.3	12.1±1.2	ND	14.3±1.9	11.1±1.5
S_1	12.2±1.2	2.2±0.4	17.4±2.2	[a]4.8±2.3	24.2±2.1	6.9±1.0
S_2	24.8±1.7	1.7±0.3	20.9±3.7	[a]4.9±1.4	29.8±2.8	12.4±3.0
S_3	25.2±2.8	2.7±0.3	20.0±1.7	[a]2.4±0.6	25.7±1.4	21.2±0.8
MAL	17.3±1.8	15.9±1.2	17.5±0.4	14.9±0.4	18.6±2.9	ND
CAL	12.8±1.2	10.3±1.3	9.9±0.4	ND	10.2±0.8	ND
DT	23.0±2.8	14.7±2.4	13.1±0.7	13.6±0.8	27.3±1.8	ND
CCT	20.8±2.8	15.2±1.5	13.9±0.7	ND	23.5±2.5	ND
MCT	14.0±1.2	10.0±1.3	17.6±1.1	16.0±0.6	29.2±2.2	ND

[a]S_1, S_2, and S_3 of rat were incubated for 20 min and MAL, DT, and OMCT were incubated for 30 min. Values ($\times 10^{-13}$ mol/glm or mm tubule) are means ± SE of 4–7 experiments. ND, not done; Glm, glomerulus; S_1 to S_3, first to third segments of the proximal tubule; MAL and CAL, medullary and cortical thick ascending limbs of Henle's loop; DT, distal tubule; CCT and MCT, cortical and outer medullary collecting tubules

added to the incubation medium as an exogenous substrate, ATP production by the proximal tubule cells was minimal (Fig. 1), whereas glutamine or pyruvate caused cellular ATP contents higher than those of other substrates used in this study. Figure 1 also shows that cellular ATP produced by lactic acid and β-hydroxybutyric acid was relatively high in the proximal tubule. In the glomerulus, however, no remarkable difference in ATP production was observed among these substrates. The order of preferred substrates for cellular ATP maintenance in the proximal tubule was pyruvate = glutamine > lactic acid > β-hydroxybutyric acid > glucose.

Substrate Specificities for Maintaining ATP in the Distally Located Nephron Segments

As shown in Table 1, a simple incubation of the distally located nephron segments does not change ATP content. Therefore, it is difficult to identify their preferred substrates by the same protocol as that used for the glomerulus or the proximal tubule. It should be possible to demonstrate that increasing the rate of active sodium transport by addition of a cationic ionophore, monensin, decreases cellular ATP content. Although the data are not shown, concentrations of monensin higher than 10μg/ml decreased ATP content significantly in the medullary thick ascending limb of Henle's loop (MAL), the distal tubule (DT), and the medullary collecting tubule (MCT).

In the presence of 10μg/ml monensin, cellular ATP content in distally located nephron segments decreased significantly without substrate (Fig. 2). When the ionophore was added to the incubation medium, the differences in each substrate's ability to maintain the ATP level also became clear in the distally located nephron segments. The pattern of substrate specificity in these segments (Fig. 2) was different from that in the proximal tubule (Fig. 1). The order of preferred substrates for cellular ATP maintenance in distally located nephron segments was glucose = pyruvate = lactate > β-hydroxybutyric acid > glutamine.

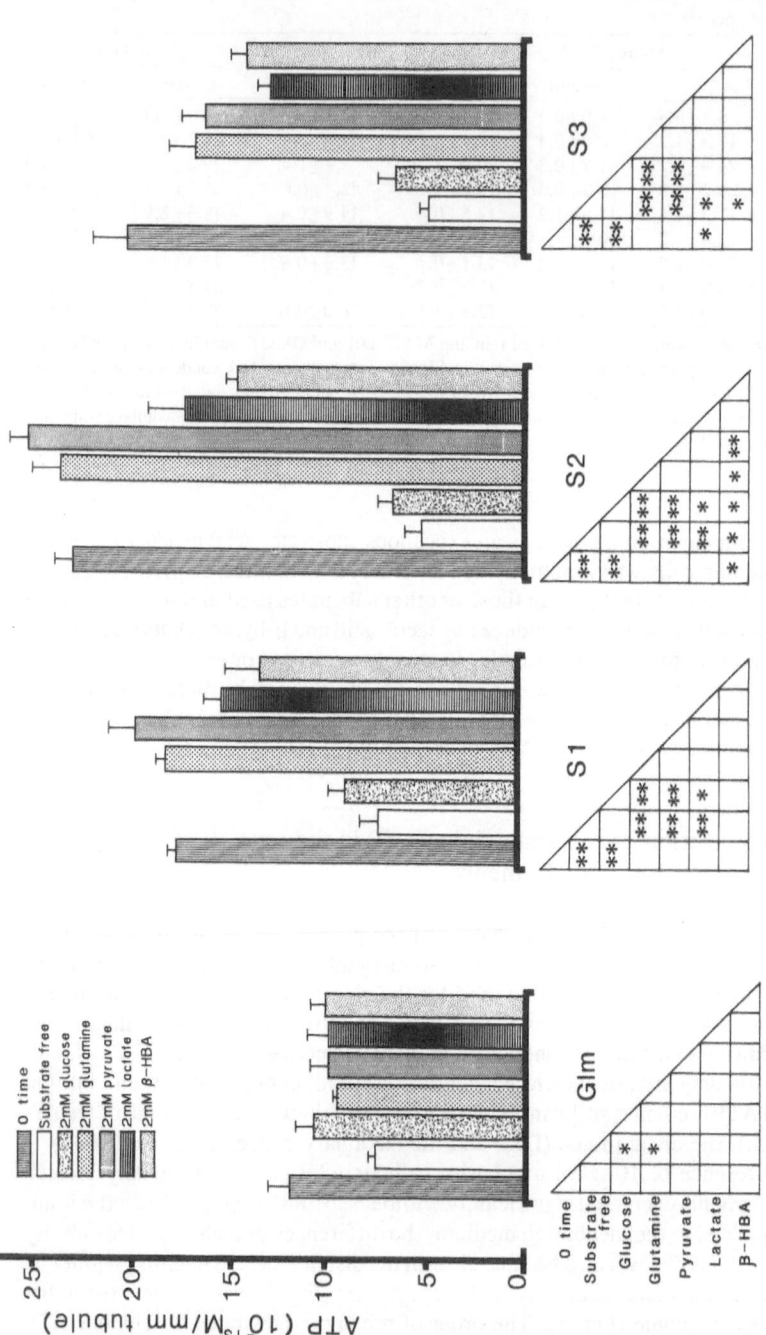

Fig. 1. Specificity of substrate utilization in maintaining cellular ATP content in the glomerulus and the proximal tubule. Immediately after microdissection, cellular ATP contents of the isolated glomerulus and proximal tubule were determined by microchemiluminescence (0 time). After 15 min of incubation at 37°C in Hanks' medium (oxygen saturated, pH 7.40) with each substrate (2 mM) cellular ATP was measured. β-HBA, β-hydroxybutyric acid. Statistical analysis was carried out by ANOVA ($*P < 0.05$, $**P < 0.01$). Values are means ± SE ($n = 5$) [5]

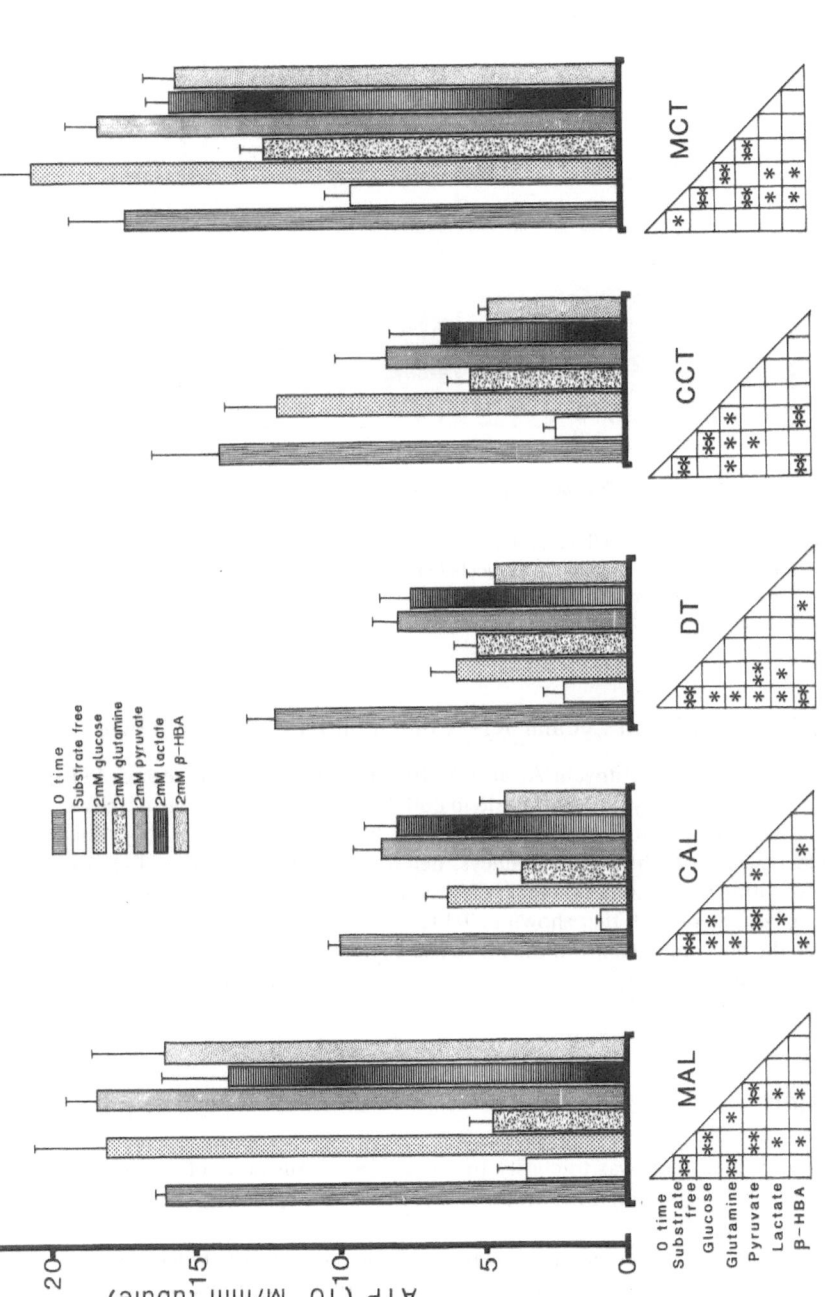

Fig. 2. Substrate specificity in the maintenance of cellular ATP content in distally located nephron segments. Assay protocol was the same as that described in Fig. 1, except that the incubation medium (pH 7.40) contained 10 μg/ml monensin to delete ATP by stimulating Na⁺, K⁺-ATPase activity. MAL and CAL, medullary and cortical thick ascending limbs of Henle's loop; DT, distal tubule; CCT and MCT, cortical and medullary collecting tubules; β-HBA, β-hydroxybutyric acid Asterisks denote significant differences among various substrates by ANOVA (*$P < 0.05$, **$P < 0.01$). Values are means ± SE ($n = 5$) [5]

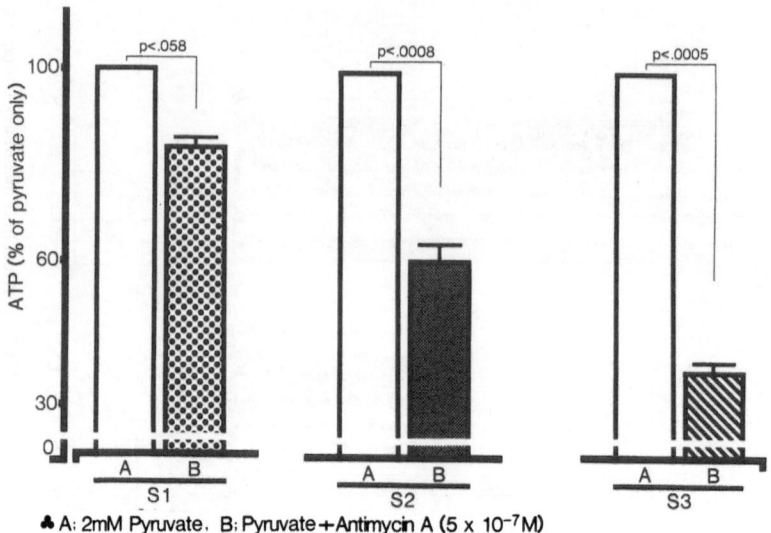

♣ A: 2mM Pyruvate. B: Pyruvate + Antimycin A (5 x 10⁻⁷M)

Fig. 3. Effect of antimycin A on cellular ATP content in rat proximal tubule. Each nephron segment isolated from male SD rat kidneys was incubated in the presence of 2mM pyruvate, with or without 5×10^{-7}M antimycin A, at 37°C for 15 min, and ATP content was assayed by the luciferin/luciferase method

Effect of Antimycin A on Cellular ATP Content in Rat Proximal Tubule

As illustrated in Fig. 3, antimycin A, at 5×10^{-7}M, significantly decreased ATP which had been restored by 2mM pyruvate in both S_2 and S_3; however, the decrease was insignificant in S_1. The decreased amount in S_3 was higher than that in S_2. This finding clearly suggests that, in rat kidneys, heterogeneity in response to hypoxic insult exists within the proximal tubule, where S_3 is most fragile. This result, shown in Fig. 3, is consistent with that shown in Table 1.

Although the data are not shown, the MAL and CAL (the cortical thick ascending limb of Henle's loop) of mouse kidneys are more sensitive to antimycin A than the CCT or MCT [4].

Discussion

The purpose of this study was to clarify the specificity of substrate utilization for ATP production along the single nephron and to identify the nephron segment(s) sensitive to hypoxic insult.

Since ATP is the most efficient high-energy compound used by the kidney to support its various functions, it is worthwhile to study nephron heterogeneity of ATP consumption and production. Levels of ATP in microdissected nephron segments have previously been reported [8]; however, information concerning the efficiency of ATP extraction from nephron segments was not provided. We found that the conventional ATP extracting agents, such as Extralight and Triton X-100, did not adequately extract ATP from the segments tested. Although there was no direct proof that TCA extraction used in this study was complete, the estimated ATP concentration, on the basis of the value obtained by TCA extraction, was calculated to be 3–6mM, using the available morphometry [9], values that are in accord with the physiological concentrations previously reported in in vivo freeze-clamp studies [10,11].

It became evident in this study that each nephron segment has its own distinct ability to utilize specific substrates. Studies on enzyme distribution in different nephron segments have also revealed distinct patterns, suggestive of specific substrate metabolism [12]. In glucose metabolism particularly, hexokinase, phosphofructokinase, pyruvate kinase, and pyruvate dehydrogenase are key enzymes [13]. Hexokinase activity was low in the proximal tubules, especially in S_1, but was slightly increased in S_3 [14]. Our results in Fig. 1 indicate that S_3, but not S_1 or S_2, could metabolize glucose to produce ATP. As predicted by hexokinase distribution [14], all distally located nephron segments tested readily utilized glucose to maintain cellular ATP.

We observed that a relatively low concentration of substrate ($10^{-4}M$) was sufficient to maintain cellular ATP in almost all segments (data not shown). Considering the physiological concentrations of these substrates, glomeruli and tubules would normally be surrounded by sufficient metabolic fuels in vivo. Endogenous substrates may also play a role in energy metabolism. The amount of glycogen stored in the kidney has been reported to be small [15], but Bastin et al. [10] showed that thick ascending limb and papilla had a tenfold larger glycogen content than did the proximal tubule. In our study, the decrease of ATP content after 30-min incubation without substrate (Table 1) was greater in proximal tubules than in distally located segments. Moreover, this conserved ATP content in MAL or CAL decreased remarkably when the MAL or CAL were incubated with antimycin A [4]. These observations suggest that the distally located nephron segments may contain more endogenous substrate(s) than do the proximal tubules, and that they might be more resistant to hypoxia. Indeed, S_3 is most vulnerable to ischemia [16], and this might be related to the observation that ATP content in proximal tubules, especially in S_3, decreased faster than that in distally located segments. In addition, we have recently found that the superoxide generating enzyme, xanthine oxidase, was densely distributed in the proximal tubule [17]. This factor may also be directly related to the vulnerability of that tubule.

In order to gain better understanding of unsolved species differences the remarkable difference between rats and rabbits, within the three portions of the proximal tubule, in ATP decrease after incubation without substrate (Table 1), should be further investigated.

Acknowledgments. This work was supported by grants from the Japanese Ministry of Education, Science, and Culture (Nos. 01480136 and 01870111), and by the Japanese Ministry of Health and Welfare, Hoansya and Shimabara Science Promotion Foundation.

References

1. Weidemann MJ, Krebs HA (1969) The fuel of respiration of rat kidney cortex. Biochem J 112:149–166

2. Pitts RF, Macleod MB (1975) Metabolism of blood glucose by the intact functioning kidney of the dog. Kidney Int 7:130–136
3. Wirthensohn G, Guder WG (1986) Renal substrate metabolism. Physiol Rev 66:469–497
4. Uchida S, Endou H (1988) Substrate specificity to maintain cellular ATP along the mouse nephron. Am J Physiol 255:F977–F983
5. Jung KY, Uchida S, Endou H (1989) Nephrotoxicity assessment by measuring cellular ATP content. Toxicol Appl Pharmacol 100:369–382
6. Morel F, Chabardes D, Imbert M (1976) Functional segmentation of the rabbit distal tubule by microdetermination of hormone-dependent adenylate cyclase activity. Kidney Int 9:264–277
7. Nonoguchi H, Uchida S, Shiigai T, Endou H (1985) Effect of chronic metabolic acidosis on ammonia production from L-glutamine in microdissected rat nephron segments. Pflügers Arch 403:229–235
8. Kiebzak GM, Yusufi ANK, Kusano E, Braun-Warness J, Dousa TP (1985) ATP and cAMP system in the in vitro response of microdissected cortical tubules in PTH. Am J Physiol 248:F152–F159
9. Pfaller W, Guder WG, Gstraunthaler G, Kotanko P, Jehart I, Purschel S (1984) Compartmentation of ATP within renal proximal tubular cells. Biochim Biophys Acta 805:152–157
10. Bastin J, Canbon N, Thompson M, Lowry OH (1987) Changes in energy reserves in different segments of nephron during brief ischemia. Kidney Int 31:1239–1247
11. Guder WG, Wagner S, Wirthensohn G (1986) Metabolic fuels along the nephron: pathways and intracellular mechanisms of interaction. Kidney Int 29:41–45
12. Guder WG, Ross B (1984) Enzyme distribution along the nephron. Kidney Int 26:101–110
13. Ross BD, Espinal J, Silva P (1986) Glucose metabolism in tubular function. Kidney Int 29:54–67
14. Vandewalle A, Wirthensohn G, Heidrich HG, Guder WG (1981) Distribution of hexokinase and phosphoenolpyruvatecarboxykinase along the rabbit nephron. Am J Physiol 240:F492–F500
15. Needleman P, Passonneau JV, Lowry OH (1968) Distribution of glucose and related metabolites in the kidney. Am J Physiol 215:655–659
16. Venkatachalam MA, Bernard DB, Donohoe JF, Levinsky NG (1978) Ischemic damage and repair in the rat proximal tubule; difference among S1, S2, and S3 segments. Kidney Int 14:31–49
17. Endou H, Yamada T, Takahashi T, Tamura K, Ito S (1987) Intranephron distribution and properties of xanthine oxidase, superoxide dismutase, and guanase activities in control and nephrotic rats. In: Kovacevic Z, Guder WG (eds) Molecular nephrology. Walter de Gruyter, Berlin, pp 347–352

Ischemia-Induced Loss of Epithelial Polarity

BRUCE A. MOLITORIS[1]

SUMMARY. Proximal tubular cells play a major role in the reabsorption of ions, water and solutes from the glomerular filtrate. This process is accomplished, in large part, by the cells having a polarized surface membrane with structurally, biochemically, and physiologically distinct apical and basolateral membranes separated by cellular junctional complexes. Establishment and maintenance of these unique membrane domains is essential for the normal functioning of proximal tubular cells. Ischemia results in the duration-dependent loss of apical and basolateral surface membrane lipid and protein polarity. This loss of surface membrane polarity is associated with disruption of the microfilament network and opening of cellular tight junctions. Surface membrane lipids and proteins are then free to diffuse laterally within the bilayer into the alternate membrane domain. Functionally, ischemia-induced loss of epithelial polarity is responsible for reduced sodium and glucose reabsorption and for the enhanced susceptibility of proximal tubular cells to aminoglycoside-induced nephrotoxicity. With recovery, proximal tubular cells undergo remodeling of the surface membrane, such that the unique apical and basolateral membrane domains are reestablished, allowing normal cellular function to return.

Introduction

Renal proximal tubular epithelial cells function to provide and regulate the unidirectional movement of ions, water, and macromolecules between the glomerular filtrate and the blood. This is accomplished, in large part, by having a surface membrane polarized into apical and basolateral components which are structurally, biochemically, and physiologically distinct membrane domains that contain different ion channels, transport proteins, enzymes, and lipids [1,2]. The establishment and maintenance of these unique surface membrane domains is dependent upon the polarized

---

[1]Denver VA Medical Center, Denver, CO 80220, USA

delivery of newly synthesized surface membrane components, cytoskeletal surface membrane interactions, and cell-cell junctional complexes which serve as a barrier between apical and basolateral domains [1,2]. The purpose of this review is to highlight the polar nature of proximal tubule cells, describe how ischemia disrupts the ability of proximal tubule cells to maintain polarity, and to discuss the cellular mechanisms involved and the functional consequences of loss of surface membrane polarity in proximal tubular cells.

Proximal Tubular Cells as a Polarized Epithelium

Renal proximal tubular cells possess highly polarized apical and basolateral membrane domains (Table 1). The apical membrane faces the urinary lumen (external compartment) and is composed of membrane proteins with specialized properties related to the reabsorption of water, electrolytes, and macromolecules. The basolateral membrane domain faces the internal milieu (blood compartment) and has a complement of intrinsic and extrincis membrane proteins which are involved in the maintenance of the normal physiologic state of the cell and also in signal recognition and transduction [1]. Extensive differences also exist between apical and basolateral membrane lipids, which are responsible for large physicochemical differences between the two different membrane domains [3–5]. Differences in membrane lipids also influence the function of numerous membrane proteins and the binding of certain macromolecules [6].

The functional necessity of the polarized distribution of surface membrane components into apical and basolateral domains is well illustrated by considering the

Table 1. Asymmetery of the surface of membrane of proximal tubular cells

Characteristics	Apical membrane	Basolateral membrane
Proteins		
Enzymes	Leucine aminopeptidase	Adenylate cyclase
	Maltase	
	GPI-linked proteins (alkaline phosphatase)	
Receptors		Insulin
		Parathyroid hormone
		Epidermal growth factor
ATPases	H^+-ATPase	Na^+-K^+-ATPase
	Mg^{2+}-ATPase	Ca^{2+}-ATPase
Carriers	Na^+-dependent cotransporters	Cl^-/HCO_3 exchanger
	Na^+-H^+ antiporter	Na^+-independent glucose carrier
Lipids		
Cholesterol/		
phospholipid	High	Low
Sphinogomyelin	High	Low
Phosphatidylcholine	Low	High
Phosphatidylinositol	Low	High
Physical properties		
Electrical resistance	High	Low
Membrane fluidity	Low	High

GPI, glycosyl-phosphatidylinositol

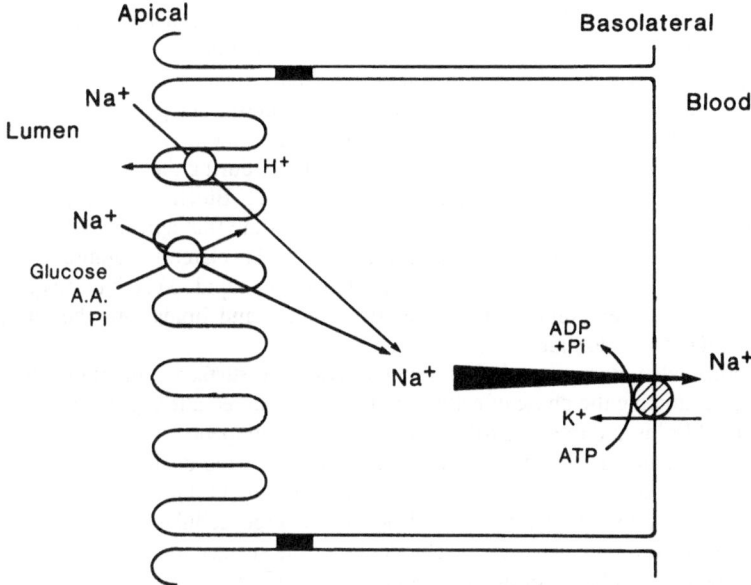

Fig. 1. Polarized proximal tubular cell. Sodium enters across the apical membrane down its electrochemical gradient providing the driving force for hydrogen ion secretion and the cellular uptake of glucose, amino acids, and phosphate, via co-transport processes. Sodium is then pumped up its electro-chemical gradient by NaK-ATPase, which is specifically localized to the basolateral membrane. This is an energy requiring process which also results in the inward movement of potassium

basolateral localization of NaK-ATPase (Fig. 1). NaK-ATPase is synthesized in the endoplasmic reticulum, transported to the Cis aspect of the golgi complex, buds off the Trans aspect of the golgi complex and is delivered in a polarized fashion to the basolateral membrane [7]. Upon arrival it associates with the actin cytoskeleton via a direct linkage of the alpha subunit to an ankryn-fodrin complex [2,8]. In this location the enzyme functions to bring about the ATP-dependent outward movement of sodium up its electro-chemical gradient, and the inward movement of potassium. This action, in conjunction with specialized apical membrane sodium-dependent carriers, results in the efficient reabsorption of sodium from the glomerular filtrate (Fig. 1).

Ischemia Alters Surface Membrane Protein and Lipid Polarity

That ischemia resulted in the loss of surface membrane protein and lipid polarity was suggested by our initial study, in which we were only able to isolate apical membrane fractions, following ischemia, that were markedly enriched for NaK-ATPase (our basolateral membrane marker) [9]. This redistribution of basolaterally associated NaK-ATPase into the apical membrane occurred rapidly during ischemia, with significant differences being documented following 10 minutes of ischemia [10,11].

Subsequent biochemical, histochemical, and immunocytochemical studies have now clearly demonstrated that ischemia induced a time-dependent loss of surface membrane lipid and protein polarity. Marked decreases in apical sphingomyelin and cholesterol content and increases in apical phosphatidylcholine and phosphatidylinositol content occurred within 5 minutes of generalized ischemia induced by renal pedicle clamping [10]. These lipid alterations occurred rapidly during the first 15 minutes of ischemia, and at a much slower rate thereafter [10,11]. Biochemical and immunocytochemical studies have also been used to demonstrate that apical lipids and proteins (leucine aminopeptidase) redistribute into the basolateral membrane during ischemic injury [11]. In summary, ischemia induced the rapid redistribution of apical and basolateral membrane domain specific proteins and lipids into the alternate surface membrane domain.

We have also documented that repolarization of surface membrane polarity occurred following the phase of cellular injury. The marked alterations in apical and basolateral lipids and the redistribution of leucine aminopeptidase and NaK-ATPase into the alternate surface membrane domain was corrected during reperfusion following reversible ischemic injury [11,12]. Since proximal tubule cells recover from ischemic injury by cellular repair and do not undergo cellular division [12], the changes observed represent actual remodeling of the surface membrane domains of recovering cells and are not due to cellular proliferation.

Functional Significance of Ischemia-Induced Loss of Epithelial Polarity

While loss of surface membrane polarity could lead to numerous alterations in the cell's ability to conduct its normal functions, my laboratory has concentrated on two specific areas known to be fundamentally important in proximal tubular function. The first area involved transcellular transport (reabsorption). Since ischemia led to the duration-dependent redistribution of NaK-ATPase into the apical membrane we reasoned that the redistributed enzyme could be functional and therefore able to carry out the transport of intracellular sodium to the nephron lumen (Fig. 2). This would lead to reduced effective Na^+ reabsorption and would also uncouple ATP and sodium reabsorption, resulting in inefficient utilization of an already limiting source of cellular energy (Fig. 2). Two approaches were used to test this hypothesis. Our first approach involved the use of in vivo micropuncture techniques to measure sodium reabsorption under control situations and then following 15 minutes of ischemia and two hours of reperfusion in the same nephron segment. Following two hours of reperfusion, cellular ATP, cellular morphology, and apical sodium permeability had all normalized. However, there was a marked reduction in both the reabsorption of sodium (37.4% vs 23.0%, $P < 0.01$) and water (48.6% vs 36.9%, $P < 0.01$) in these paired tubule studies [13]. In an additional in vivo study, following 50 minutes of ischemia, normalization of the transcellular transport sodium and lithium, a specific marker of proximal tubular reabsorption, was dependent upon the reestablishment of surface membrane NaK-ATPase polarity in proximal tubular cells. Normalization of glucose transport across proximal tubular cells following ischemic injury was also found to be dependent upon the reestablishment of surface

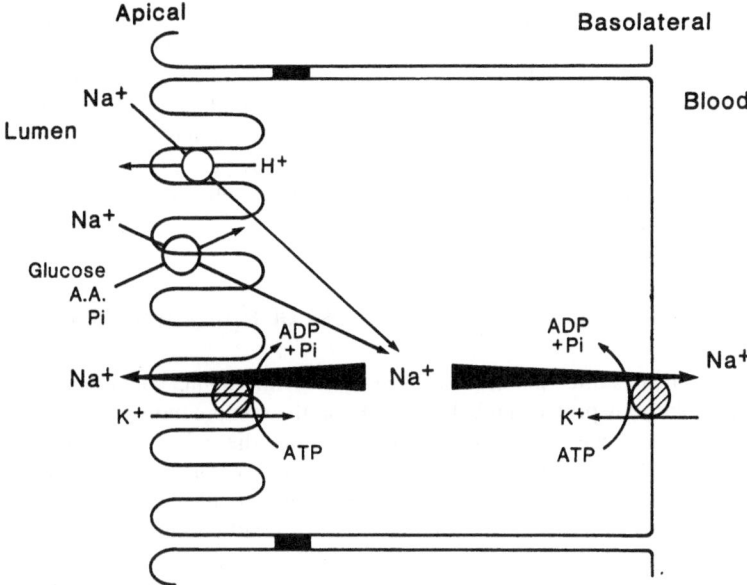

Fig. 2. Non-polarized renal proximal tubular cell following ischemic injury. Following ischemic injury NaK-ATPase is found in both the basolateral and the apical membrane domains. In the apical membrane NaK-ATPase maintains its functional activity and is, therefore, capable of competing for intracellular sodium ions. This markedly diminishes the efficiency of sodium transport and results in a high urinary excretion of sodium following ischemic injury. By pumping sodium back out of the lumen a futile cycle is also set up which uncouples ATP utilization and sodium transport

membrane apical lipid polarity [12]. In brush border membrane vesicle studies, alteration in the ability of the apical membrane to transport glucose was directly related to a decease in membrane fluidity and to the sphingomyelin/phosphatidylcholine ratio. These data suggest that the rapid ischemia-induced alteration in these lipids was responsible for reduced reabsorption of glucose following ischemic injury [14]. Furthermore, glucose transport increased to control levels concurrently with the reestablishment of the apical sphingomyelin/phosphatidylcholine ratio [12]. Taken together, these data indicate that the reabsorption of ions, water, and solutes by proximal tubular cells is dependent upon the establishment and maintenance of domain-specific lipid and protein polarity in apical and basolateral membranes. Furthermore, following ischemic injury, proximal tubular cells are unable to function properly until surface membrane polarity has been reestablished.

Recent evidence from our laboratory also indicates that alterations in the phospholipid content of the apical membrane may be of critical importance in determining the nephrotoxicity of aminoglycoside antibiotics. Aminoglycoside antibiotics are known to bind to phosphatidylinositol phospholipids with increased affinity [15] and are internalized via the endocytic process. Ischemia is known to rapidly increase the apical content of phosphatidylinositol [9–11]. We have now shown that mild, functionally insignificant, ischemia occurring prior to aminoglycoside administration, markedly enhanced the nephrotoxicity of gentamicin [16]. Additional preliminary evidence indicated that, following ischemic injury, gentamicin binding to the apical membrane increased markedly [17]. These data, when taken together, suggest the ischemia-induced increase in apical phosphatidylinositol content is directly responsible for enhanced gentamicin binding. This, in turn, may play a role in the ischemia-induced enhancement of aminoglycoside nephrotoxicity observed by our laboratory and others [16,18].

Mechanism of Ischemia-Induced Loss of Epithelial Polarity

Figure 3 indicates three potential avenues by which ischemia could induce loss of epithelial polarity in proximal tubular cells. First, the random (non-polar) delivery of newly synthesized membrane components to either the apical or the basolateral membrane could be responsible. This, however, seems unlikely because both the synthesis and intracellular translocation of these membrane components is ATP-dependent and during ischemia cellular ATP drops rapidly to non-detectable levels [13]. Second, abnormal migration and fusion of previously existent endocytic and

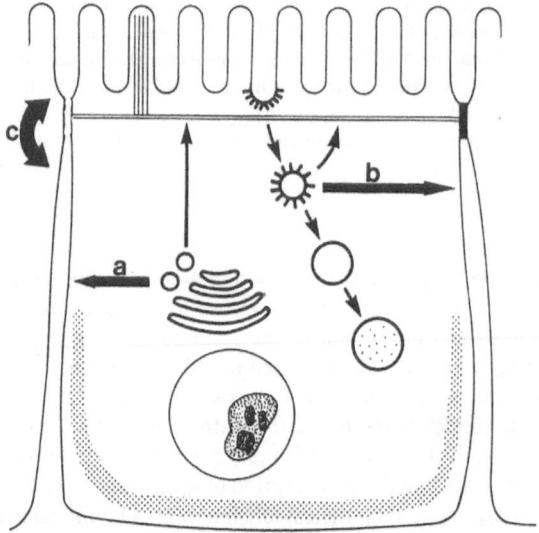

Fig. 3. Potential mechanisms for loss of epithelial polarity during ischemic injury. The first potential mechanism (a) involves the abnormal (random) translocation of newly synthesized membrane components from the trans golgi to the incorrect surface membrane domain. The second mechanism (b) involves the abnormal (random) intracellular movement of endocytic and exocytic vesicles and fusion with the alternate surface membrane domain. The final potential mechanism, resulting in loss of epithelial polarity (c) involves the opening of cellular tight junctions which then allows for the lateral diffusion of surface membrane lipids and proteins within the plane of the bilayer into the alternate surface membrane domain

exocytic vesicles to the alternate membrane domain could also lead to the loss of epithelial surface membrane polarity. Studies from our laboratory, published in preliminary form, indicate that this mechanism was also not involved in the loss of epithelial polarity [19]. We have, however, accumulated data which indicated that disruption of the tight junction is involved in the loss of surface membrane polarity during ischemic injury. In proximal tubular cells tight junctions between cells consist of one or two discontinuous strands. Proximal tubular cells are classified as "leaky" epithelia, as the electrical resistance across a monolayer of these cells is low. Since disruption of tight junctions by several mechanisms (calcium, chelation, monoclonal antibodies) results in loss of epithelial polarity, we investigated the effect of ischemia on tight junction functional integrity. In vivo microperfusion of early loops of proximal tubules with ruthenium red in glutaraldehyde was used to gain selective access to and outline the apical surface membrane and tight junctions. Ischemia resulted in a time-dependent stepwise increase in the number of tight junctions penetrated by ruthenium red, from less than 10% in control situations to 29%, 50%, and 62% after 5, 15, and 30 minutes of ischemia, respectively [10]. This was associated with the rapid duration-dependent redistribution of basolateral membrane domain specific lipids and NaK-ATPase into the apical membrane domain. We, therefore, believe that ischemia leads to rapid deterioration in the cells' ability to maintain the tight junction. Following the disassociation of the tight junction cellular barrier, apical and basolateral lipids and proteins are free to diffuse laterally within the plane of the bilayer and redistribute into the alternate membrane domain. That lipids moved more rapidly into the alternate membrane domain is consistent with their increased lateral mobility, as compared to proteins [20].

Since the tight junction is under the direct control of the microfilament cytoskeleton [21], we next undertook studies to determine the effect of ischemia on the proximal tubular cell microfilament network. Ischemia was associated with the rapid duration-dependent disruption of the apical microfilament network, with loss of the polarized distribution of microfilaments from the apical aspect of the cell into the entire cell cytoplasm. Disruption of the apical microfilament network was noticeable following only five minutes of ischemia and was present in all cells following 15 minutes of ischemia. To determine the functional significance of selective microfilament disruption, a microfilament selective dose of cytochalasin D (10 μM) was utilized in an isolated perfused kidney system. Structurally, cytochalasin D resulted in extensive disruption of the apical surface, with blebbing, vacuolization, fusion, and patchy loss of microvilli. Cytochalasin D also brought about a decrease in the reabsorption of sodium, from 97.1% $\pm$ 0.7% to 64.3% $\pm$ 7%, which occurred in a linear fashion throughout the duration of cytochalasin D exposure [22]. In control kidneys the reabsorption of Na$^+$ remained unchanged throughout the duration of the perfusion. Lithium reabsorption also decreased linearly and there was a high degree of correlation in individual kidneys between sodium and lithium reabsorption, indicating that the defect in Na$^+$ reabsorption induced by cytochalasin-mediated microfilament disruption was localized to proximal tubular cells. These data indicate that the selective disruption of microfilaments results in proximal tubular structural and functional alterations similar to those seen during ischemia. The data, therefore, imply that microfilament disruption may play an important role in the pathophysiology of ischemic injury.

In summary, ischemia leads to the duration-dependent loss of surface membrane polarity in proximal tubular cells. This appears to occur via loss of the cells' ability to maintain the actin cytoskeleton, and via the opening of cellular tight junctions. Following ischemic injury, proximal tubular cells function as non-polar cells until cellular remodeling occurs, allowing for the return of unique apical and basolateral membrane domains which can then function together in a coordinated fashion to bring out the vectorial transport ions, water, and macromolecules transcellularly. Further understanding of ischemia-induced loss of surface membrane polarity and cytoskeletal alterations will greatly enhance the understanding of the pathophysiology of ischemic injury and cellular recovery.

References

1. Molitoris BA, Nelson WJ (1990) Alterations in the establishment and maintenance of epithelial cell polarity as a basis for disease processes. J Clin Invest 85:3–9
2. Rodriquez-Boulan E, Nelson WJ (1989) Morphogenesis of the polarized epithelial cell phenotype. Science 245:718–725
3. Molitoris BA, Simon FR (1985) Renal cortical brush-border and basolateral membranes: cholesterol and phospholipid composition and relative turnover. J Membr Biol 3:207–215
4. Carmel G, Rodriquez F, Carriere S, LeGrimellec C (1985) Composition and physical properties of lipids from plasma membranes of dog kidney. Biochim Biophys Acta 818:149–157
5. Molitoris BA, Hoilien C (1987) Static and dynamic components of renal cortical brush border and basolateral membrane fluidity: role of cholesterol. J Membr Biol 99:165–172
6. Molitoris BA (1987) Membrane fluidity: measurement and relationship to solute transport. Semin Nephrol 7:61–67
7. Caplan MJ, Anderson HC, Palade GE, Jamieson JD (1986) Intracellular sorting and polarized cell surface delivery of Na⁺, K⁺-ATPase, an endogenous component of MDCK cell basolateral plasma membranes. Cell 46:623–631
8. Nelson WJ, Hammerton RW (1989) A membrane-cytoskeletal complex containing Na⁺, K⁺-ATPase ankyrin, and fodrin in Madin-Darby canine kidney (MDCK) cells. Implications for the biogenesis of epithelial cell polarity. J Cell Biol 108:893–902
9. Molitoris BA, Wilson PD, Schrier RW, Simon FR (1985) Ischemia induces partial loss of surface membrane polarity and accumulation of putative calcium ionophores. J Clin Invest 76:2097–2105
10. Molitoris BA, Dahl RH, Falk SA (1989) Ischemia-induced loss of epithelial polarity. Role of the tight junction. J Clin Invest 84:1334–1339
11. Molitoris BA, Hoilien CA, Dahl RH, Ahnen DJ, Wilson PD, Kim J (1988) Characterization of ischemia-induced loss of epithelial polarity. J Membr Biol 106:233–242
12. Spiegel DM, Wilson PD, Molitoris BA (1989) Epithelial polarity following ischemia: a requirement for normal cell function. Am J Physiol (Renal Fluid Electrolyte Physiol) 256:F430–F436
13. Molitoris BA, Chan LK, Shapiro JI, Conger JD, Falk SA (1989) Loss of epithelial polarity: A novel hypothesis for reduced proximal tubule Na⁺ transport following ischemic injury. J Membr Biol 107:119–127
14. Molitoris BA, Kinne R (1987) Ischemia reduces surface membrane dysfunction. Mechanism of altered Na⁺-dependent glucose transport. J Clin Invest 80:647–654
15. Hume HD (1988) Aminoglycoside nephrotoxicity. Kidney Int 33:900–911
16. Spiegel DM, Shanley PF, Molitoris BA (to be published) Mild ischemia predisposes the S₃ segment to gentamicin toxicity. Kidney Int
17. Molitoris BA, Geerdes A, Meyer C (1990) Ischemia enhanced gentamicin toxicity: Role of increased apical phosphatidylinositol. Clin Res 38:141A

18. Zager RA (1988) Gentamicin nephrotoxicity in the setting of acute renal hypoperfusion. Am J Physiol 254:F574–F581
19. Molitoris BA, Falk S, Dahl R (1989) Mechanism of ischemia-induced loss of epithelial polarity. Clin Res 37:497A
20. Salas PJI, Vega-Salas E, Hochman J, Rogriquez-Boulan E, Edidin M (1988) Selective anchoring in the specific plasma membrane domain. A role in epithelial cell polarity. J Cell Biol 107:2363–2376
21. Madara JL (1989) Loosening tight junctions. Lessons from the intestine. J Clin Invest 83:1089–1094
22. Kellerman PS, Clark PAF, Hoilien CA, Linas SL, Molitoris BA (to be published) Role of microfilament in maintenance of proximal tubule structural and functional integrity. Am J Physiol

Acquired Resistance to Rechallenge Injury to Acute Renal Failure

Akira Hishida, Hideo Yamada, Taisuke Isozaki, and Nishio Honda[1]

Summary. A smaller dose of uranyl acetate (0.8–0.9 mg/kg) lessened the severity of acute renal failure (ARF) following a rechallenge with a larger dose of the agent (2 mg/kg). This resistance to the rechallenge was not attributed largely to renal hemodynamic alterations, suppressed glomerular contractile response to vasoactive substances, smaller amount of uranium bound to regenerated tubular cells, and altered active oxygen scavenging enzyme and Na-K-ATPase activities in regenerated tubular cells.

Introduction

A number of studies have demonstrated that prior nephrotoxic acute renal failure (ARF) affords resistance to a rechallenge with the same or a different agent [1,2,3,4,5], though this is not a universal finding [5]. The mechanisms for acquired resistance to ARF are poorly understood, but possible mechanisms include renal hemodynamic alterations, suppressed glomerular response to vasoactive substances, altered glomerular capillary ultrafiltration coefficient (K_f), and the resistance of regenerated tubular epithelium to a rechallenge with renal failure insult [5]. In this paper, we summarize our data regarding the mechanisms for acquiring resistance to ARF.

Acquired Resistance to Uranyl Acetate(UA)-Induced ARF

Studies were performed on uranium-induced ARF rabbits. In this model, major determinants of ARF seem to be a decrease in glomerular filtration rate (GFR) due to reduced K_f, back-leakage of the filtrate across damaged tubular epithelia and, probably, tubular obstruction due to casts.

---

[1]The First Department of Medicine, Hamamatsu University School of Medicine, 3600 Handa-cho, Hamamatsu, 431–31 Japan

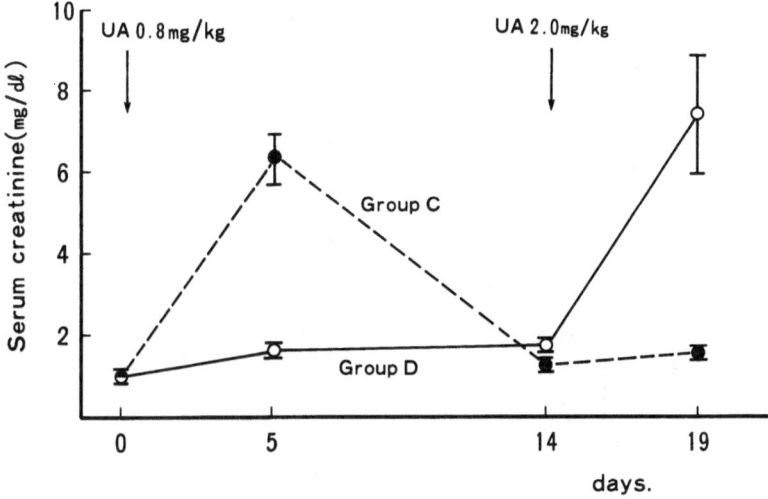

Fig. 1. Effects of a rechallenge with uranyl acetate (*UA*) on serum creatinine. *Group C*, rabbits which developed azotemia by UA (0.8 mg/kg) injection; *Group D*, rabbits which did not develop azotemia by UA (0.8 mg/kg) injection

In experiments, rabbits were classified into 4 groups: group A, normal controls; group B, in which a single dose of 2 mg/kg of UA was injected i.v.; groups C and D, in which a smaller dose of UA (0.8–0.9 mg/kg) was administered 14 days before a rechallenge with UA (2 mg/kg). In half of the rabbits examined (group C), 0.8–0.9 mg/kg of UA induced a decrease in GFR but in the remainder (group D), it did not induce a decrease. In groups B and D 2 mg/kg of UA induced a decrease in creatinine or inulin clearance and an increase in plasma creatinine, though these changes were much less in group D. In contrast, the animals recovering from ARF (group C) did not develop renal failure after the second UA injection [3] (Fig. 1). This resistance to ARF disappeared 4 weeks after the initial injection of UA [6].

Mechanisms for Resistance to a Rechallenge with UA

Vascular Factors

Renal blood flow (RBF) and intracortical blood flow distribution were estimated in all groups 5 days after the vehicle or UA (2mg/kg) injection. There was no significant difference in RBF or intracortical flow distribution between groups, except for redistribution of the regional flow toward the deep cortex in group B [3]. The data suggest that altered renal hemodynamics makes a minor contribution to resistance to ARF. Recent studies suggest that a decrease in K_f accounts for UA-induced reduction in GFR [7,8], and that this reduction in K_f is mediated by increased renin-angiotensin activity [8]. In our experiments, the plasma renin activity increased in both ARF-resistant (group C) and -less resistant (group D) rabbits following the rechallenge, as in animals subjected to a single UA injection. There was no significant difference in the plasma renin activity between groups [9].

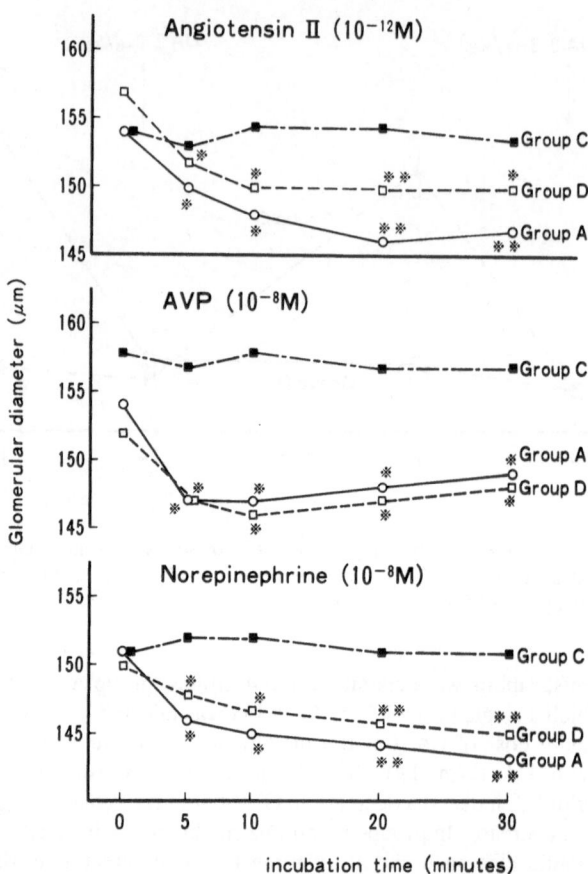

Fig. 2. Changes of glomerular diameter induced by angiotensin II, arginine vasopressin (*AVP*), and norepinephrine in rabbits. *Group A*, normal controls; *Group C*, ARF-resistant rabbits; *Group D*, ARF-less resistant rabbits

Unfortunately, K_f has not yet been estimated in ARF-resistant animals. Morphologic studies with scanning electron microscopy, including our study in UA-induced ARF, disclosed changes in the glomerular ultrastructure in various models of ARF [10,11,12,13]; this was characterized by a flattening and spreading of podocyte cell bodies associated with loss of epithelial foot processes, and reduction in the density of endothelial fenestrae, and suggested a causative role of these alterations in the diminution of K_f and thereby GFR [10,11,12]. To evaluate these glomerular changes semiquantitatively, we measured the percent fraction of the glomerular capillary surface covered only by processes narrower than 1 μm in width, percent fraction of the interpedicular space on the glomerular epithelial surface, and the density and diameter of the endothelial fenestrae in groups B, C, and D, 5 days after the UA (2 mg/kg) injection. No significant difference between groups, in changes of these parameters, was found [14].

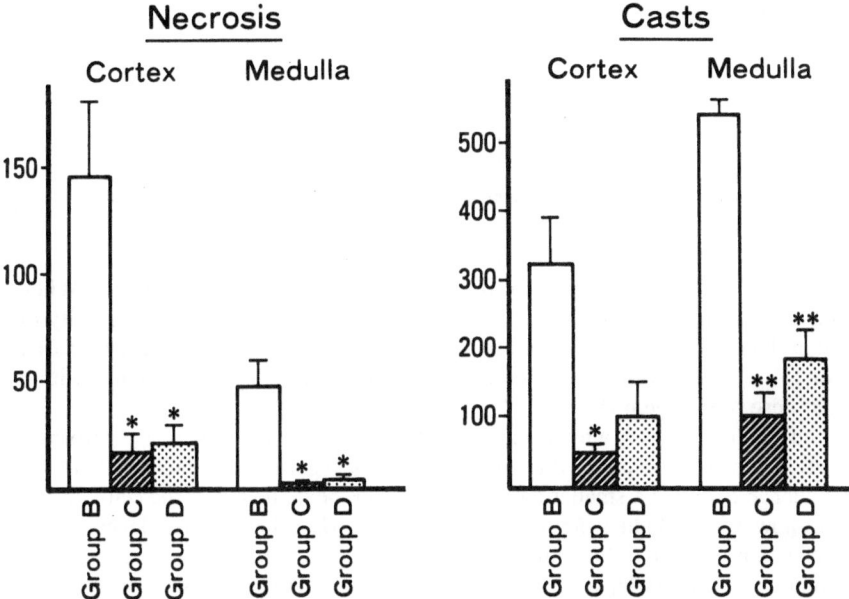

Fig. 3. The number of necrotic renal tubules (*necrosis*) and intratubular casts (*casts*) on day 5 after injection of uranyl acetate (2mg/kg). The number was counted in 50 fields at 400 magnification with a light microscope. *Group B*, UA (2mg/kg) single injection; *Groups C* and *D*, rechallenge with UA (2mg/kg) 14 days after 0.8mg/kg of UA injection; Group C developed azotemia and Group D did not. *$P < 0.05$ and **$P < 0.01$ compared with Group B

Wilkes et al. [15] demonstrated that the glomerular contractile response to angiotensin II(AII) was totally inhibited in rats recovering from glycerol-induced ARF; they suggested that loss of glomerular response to angiotensin contributed, at least in part, to the resistance to a subsequent renal failure challenge. We examined the glomerular response to AII, norepinephrine (NE), and arginine vasopressin (AVP) in controls (group A), ARF-resistant (group C), and ARF-less resistant (group D) rabbits, 14 days after the vehicle or the first UA injection. Angiotensin II, NE, and AVP significantly reduced the diameter of glomeruli derived from normal controls and ARF-less resistant animals. In contrast, these vasoactive substances did not provoke glomerular contraction in ARF-resistant rabbits [10] (Fig. 2). The suppressed glomerular response to the vasoactive substances was still observed 4 weeks after the initial UA injection, a time at which resistance to ARF disappeared. It is unlikely, therefore, that resistance to ARF is largely due to suppressed glomerular contractile response to vasoactive substances.

Tubular Factors

Previous studies suggested that tubular obstruction by casts [16] and back-leakage of the filtrate across damaged epithelia [7] also contributed to developing and maintaining UA-induced ARF. Following rechallenge with UA, intratubular cast formation and tubular necrosis lessened, in ARF-resistant (group C) than in ARF-less resis-

Table 1. Effects of uranyl acetate (*UA*) (0.9mg/kg) injection on kidney tissue enzyme activities

	n	SOD (U/mg)	GSH-Px (nmol/mg per min)	Catalase (U/mg)
Control	6	16.8 ± 0.6	330 ± 18	228 ± 22
UA 14 days	9	14.6 ± 0.5 P < 0.02	351 ± 33 NS	220 ± 26 NS

SOD, superoxide dismutase; GSH-Px, glutathione peroxidase; NS, not significant

tant (group D) rabbits, though the difference was not statistically significant. When compared to group B subjected to a single UA injection, however, the severity of tubular damage was significantly less in groups C and D. This finding suggests that prior UA administration attenuates tubular damage caused by a rechallenge with a larger dose of the agent (Fig. 3).

A question arises as to why regenerated tubular cells are resistant to a nephrotoxic agent. There is a possibility that the resistance of regenerated tubular cells to the rechallenge is due to a smaller amount of uranium being bound to the cells. In our study, however, the kidney previously challenged by UA achieved tissue levels of uranium similar to those of the untreated kidney subjected to the second UA injection.

Some investigators have suggested that the peroxidative process contributes to heavy metal-mediated tubular damage [17,18]. An alternative possibility may be, therefore, that active oxygen scavenging enzymes might have been activated by the first UA injection, and thereby protect against the peroxidative action enhanced by the second UA injection. We measured the superoxide dismutase, glutathion-peroxidase, and catalase activities in the kidney tissue before, and 14 days after, the initial UA injection. There was no significant increase in the enzyme activities in the kidney tissues in previously UA-treated rabbits (Table 1).

Uranium and mercury have been found to inhibit Na-K-ATPase activity [19,20]. Kirschbaum and Oken [21] demonstrated that Mg-ATPase activity in the brush border membrane increases to 310% of the control value 10 days following $HgCl_2$-induced ARF. There is a possibility, therefore, that regenerated tubular cells are rich in Na-K-ATPase and resistant to the inhibition of Na-K-ATPase by uranium. In our experiment, however, no significant difference was found between normal controls and rabbits subjected to prior UA injection in Na-K-ATPase activity in tissue homogenates of whole kidney (control 30.8±6.9 vs. 14 days after UA 26.6±5.9 μmol Pi/mg prot per hr).

Acknowledgment. This work was supported by a research grant for Cardiovascular Diseases from the Ministry of Health and Welfare in Japan.

References

1. MacNider W deB (1929) The functional and pathological response of the kidney in dogs subjected to a second subcutaneous injection of uranium nitrate. J Exp Med 49:411–431
2. Elliott WC, Houghton DC, Gilbert DN, Baines-Hunter J, Bennett WM (1982) Gentamicin nephrotoxicity. II. Definition of conditions necessary to induce acquired insensitivity. J Lab Clin Med 100:513–525

3. Honda N, Sudo M (1982) Resistance to uranyl acetate-induced acute renal failure in rabbits: renal function and morphology. In: Eliahou HE (ed) Acute renal failure. John Libbey, London, pp 105–107

4. Yonemura K (1986) Acquired resistance to acute renal failure in ischemic and uranium-induced renal failure of rabbits. Nippon Jinzo Gakkai Shi 28:1221–1227

5. Honda N, Hishida A, Ikuma K, Yonemura K (1987) Acquired resistance to acute renal failure. Kidney Int 31:1233–1238

6. Ikuma K, Honda N, Yonemura K, Ohishi K, Hishida A, Nagase M (1988) Glomerular refractoriness to contractile stimuli in rabbits recovering from ischemic acute renal failure. Nephron 48:306–309

7. Blantz RC (1975) The mechanism of acute renal failure after uranyl nitrate. J Clin Invest 55:621–635

8. Blantz RC, Pelayo JC, Gushwa LC, Myers RR, Evan AP (1985) Functional basis for the glomerular alterations in uranyl nitrate acute renal failure. Kidney Int 28:733–743

9. Ikuma K, Honda N, Hishida A, Nagase M (1986) Loss of glomerular responses to vasoconstrictor agents in rabbits recovering from ARF. Kidney Int 30:836–841

10. Avasthi PS, Evan AP, Hay D (1980) Glomerular endothelial cells in uranyl nitrate-induced acute renal failure in rats. J Clin Invest 65:121–127

11. Avasthi PS, Evan AP, Huser JW, Luft FC (1981) Effect of gentamicin on glomerular ultrastructure. J Lab Clin Med 98:444–454

12. Solez K, Racusen LC, Whelton A (1981) Glomerular epithelial cell changes in early postischemic acute renal failure in rabbits and man. Am J Pathol 103:163–173

13. Kobayashi S, Nagase M, Honda N, Hishida A (1984) Glomerular alterations in uranyl acetate-induced acute renal failure in rabbits. Kidney Int 26:808–815

14. Kobayashi S, Yonemura K, Ikuma K, Hishida A, Nagase M, Honda N (1985) Glomerular alterations in acute renal failure-resistant rabbits (abstract). Nippon Jinzo Gakkai Shi 27:700

15. Wilkes BM, Caldicott WJH, Schulman G, Hollenberg NK (1981) Loss of the glomerular contractile response to angiotensin in rats following myohemoglobinuric acute renal failure. Circ Res 49:1190–1195

16. Hishida A, Yonemura K, Ohishi K, Yamada M, Honda N (1988) The effect of saline loading on uranium-induced acute renal failure in rats. Kidney Int 33:942–946

17. Gstraunthaler G, Pfaller W, Kotanko P (1983) Glutathione depletion and in vitro lipid peroxidation in mercury or maleate induced acute renal failure. Biochem Pharmacol 32:2969–2972

18. Shukla GS, Hussain T, Srivastava RS, Chandra SV (1989) Glutathione peroxidase and catalase in liver, kidney, testis and brain regions of rats following cadmium exposure and subsequent withdrawal. Ind Health 27:59–69

19. Nechay BR, Thompson JD, Saunders JP (1980) Inhibition by uranyl nitrate of adenosine triphosphatases derived from animal and human tissues. Toxicol Appl Pharmacol 53:410–419

20. Kramer HJ, Gonick HC, LU E (1986) In vitro inhibition of Na-K-ATPase by trace metals: relation to renal and cardiovascular damage. Nephron 44:329–336

21. Kirschbaum BB, Oken DE (1979) The effect of mercuric chloride on renal brush border membrane. Exp Mol Pathol 31:101–112

Cellular and Integrative Regulation of Renal Circulation

Chair: Hans R. Ulfendahl (Sweden)
Kenjiro Yamamoto (Japan)

Hormonal Control of Medullary Blood Flow

LOTHAR BERND ZIMMERHACKL[1]

SUMMARY. The medullary microcirculation is part of the countercurrent exchange system which is necessary for the regulation of salt and water homeostasis. To maintain mass balance, solute and fluid reabsorbed by tubular transport mechanisms are removed directly from the medullary tissue by the vasa recta. This role of the medullary microcirculation during the physiological changes of diuresis and water diuresis, regulated by the antidiuretic hormone, is firmly established.

Technical constraints still influence the investigation of medullary vascular regulation. New animal models — in-vitro perfusion of juxtamedullary nephrons and the split hydronephrotic rat kidney — stimulate the study of medullary blood flow regulation.

Besides its part in nephro-vascular coupling, the microvascular-tubular unit supports the tissue with energy. Oxygen delivery may be hampered by low medullary hematocrit. With regard to the high energy demand of active transport of solute in the thick ascending limb of Henle, the medullary blood flow has an important role under pathophysiological conditions of toxicity or ischemia.

The hormonal regulation of medullary blood flow differs from the regulation of cortical blood flow. Under physiological conditions, medullary blood flow is influenced by the renin-angiotensin system. Inhibition of angiotensin by converting enzyme antagonists significantly increase medullary blood flow. Infusion of angiotensin II decreases medullary blood flow. This action can be reversed by the activation of prostaglandins.

Cyclosporine reduces medullary blood flow after short term ischemia. This may reflect local activation of endothelin release.

---

[1]Department of Pediatrics, Albert-Ludwigs-University, Mathildenstr. 1, D-7800 Freiburg, Federal Republic of Germany

Introduction

Under physiologic conditions, the medullary microcirculation has three major tasks: (1) it plays an important role in nephro-vascular coupling; (2) it supports tissue energy supply and, (3) it participates passively in solute reabsorption from interacting tubules [1,2].

Under pathophysiologic conditions, in particular after renal ischemia, medullary congestion, with damage to the outer stripe of the medulla, is evident [3,4].

Medullary blood supply is distinct from renal cortical blood supply and may have different tasks [1,2,5]. The influence of vasoactive hormones under physiological and pathophysiological conditions may thus be important for the outcome of any renal disturbance.

New Animal Models for Studying Medullary Blood Flow

Technical constraints still hamper the investigation of medullary vascular regulation. New animal models – in-vitro perfusion of juxtamedullary nephrons [6,7] and the split hydronephrotic rat kidney [8] – stimulate the study of medullary blood flow regulation. These two new animal models may be important in the investigation of medullary blood flow in vitro and in vivo. In vitro perfusion of the excised medulla has been put forward by Casellas and co-workers [6,7]. With this animal model the influence of hormones, without the interaction of other systemically activated hormones, can be studied. With the hydronephrotic kidney model it is possible to investigate the influence of hormones on juxtamedullary glomerulus and the presumed vasa recta structures directly, without the interaction of tubular parameters. This model has no tubular structures remaining. According to Steinhausen et al. [7], sex difference may play an as yet neglected role in medullary flow regulation. In his preparation, female animals demonstrate medullary autoregulation, whereas male animals do not! This is in contrast to earlier observations in a different rat model [9]. However, both models allow the study of acute changes only. Long-term effects still cannot be studied with present techniques.

Fluid Reabsorption and Medullary Blood Flow: Effects of Furosemide and Adenosine

According to the mathematical concept of countercurrent exchange, medullary tonicity is inversely correlated to medullary blood flow [1,2,5]. During physiological changes in diuresis, total renal blood flow is unchanged. Medullary blood flow is diminished during diuresis, due to a direct vasoactive effect of vasopressin through its V_1-receptor [10]. The vasa recta are able to remove water from the medulla [5]. Under furosemide-induced diuresis (10 mg/kg/per h) vasa recta fluid flow was increased [11,12]. Red cell flux, an indicator of blood supply, was slightly elevated as well (Fig. 1; [11,12]). This situation of passive removal of fluid was already demonstrated in 1971 by Jamison and coworkers [13]. In several experimental protocols, the "passive" role of the medullary microcirculation as the route of fluid removal

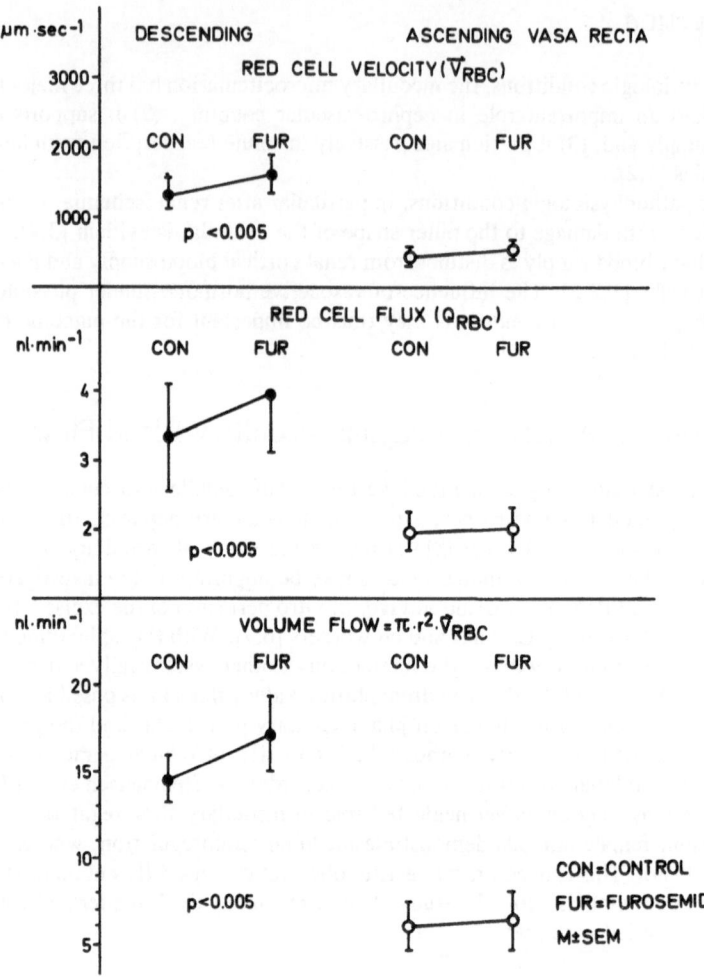

Fig. 1. Effect of furosemide on medullary erythrocyte velocity, red cell flux, and volume flow in rats, using videomicroscopy with fluorescent red cells and fluorescent plasma. After furosemide infusion significant increase occurred in volume flow, red cell velocity, and red cell flux. CON, control period; FUR, furosemide period (10 mg/kg i.v.); RBC, red blood cell

from the medulla, necessary for the maintenance of mass balance, could be confirmed [1,2].

Under experimental conditions, the "medullary washout" hypothesis was demonstrated by Thurau and collaborators in the dog [14]. Several studies in rats are in conflict with this thesis [1,2,15]. In a recent study by Miyamoto et al. [16] the influence of intrarenal adenosine on medullary blood flow was studied. Adenosine caused a dramatic natriuresis and diuresis with an infusion of as little as 2µg/min. In contrast, vasa

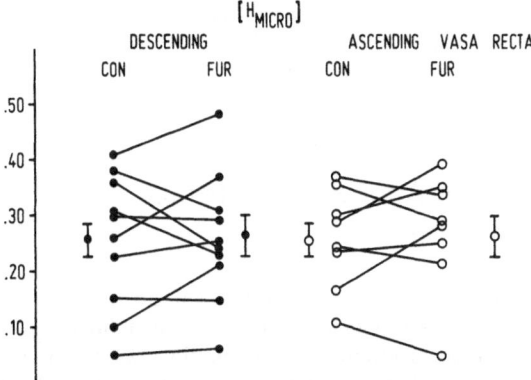

Fig. 2. Dynamic hematocrit in vasa recta in ascending and descending vessels of the rat. Hematocrit was calculated from flux of fluorescent red cells and volume flow was derived from diameter and red cell velocity (without correction for Fahräus effect). CON, control period; FUR, furosemide period

recta blood flow was increased at much higher infusion rates only. Although this study does not disprove the notion that medullary washout exists, it does not support it.

Medullary Congestion?

During pathophysiological situations, hormonal influence on medullary blood flow may be crucial in the maintenance of solute balance. Following the hypothesis of Epstein et al. [4] and Mason et al. [3], electrolyte transport of the thick ascending loop of Henle may be influenced by energy support from the vasa recta. Medullary hematocrit [1] is lower than cortical hematocrit (Fig. 2). In ischemic acute renal failure in particular, medullary congestion plays an important role. Recently Hellberg et al. [17] reported that neutrophils are involved in intravascular erythrocyte aggregation, particularly in the outer medulla. This finding supports the concept of a vulnerable region in the outer medulla, which is particularly prone to damage under conditions of high tubular transport activity and low medullary blood flow [3,4].

Influence of Angiotensin II

Under physiological conditions, medullary blood flow is influenced by the renin-angiotensin system. Exogenous infusion of angiotensin II in pharmacological concentrations reduces cortical and medullary blood flow by afferent and efferent arteriolar vasoconstriction [18]. Inhibition of angiotensin-mediated action by the angiotensin converting enzyme (ACE) antagonists captopril or enalapril significantly increases medullary blood flow without influence on water excretion [19–21]. Even under normal conditions blood flow is increased after saralasin or ACE-inhibition. Infusion of angiotensin II decreases medullary blood flow [18]. The effect of angiotensin on salt regulation is still not fully understood. In particular, understanding of the interaction between angiotensin, vasopressin, and prostaglandins [21] is incomplete. This is a situation of important clinical relevance, since the application of prostaglandin antagonists under conditions of hypovolemia (activation of angiotensin and vasopressin) can cause acute renal failure with medullary damage.[2]

Hormonal Influence After Renal Ischemia: Effects of Cyclosporin A

After short-term renal ischemia, medullary blood flow is maintained, or even enhanced. Using direct microscopic techniques, several authors were able to demonstrate early reflow with normal to increased blood flow [22,23], after 45–60 minutes of renal ischemia. However, ischemic endothelia may be prone to damage by nephrotoxic agents [24,25]. Acute infusion of Cyclosporine A (20 mg/kg i.v.) reduces cortical blood flow at the level of the arcuate arteries in the split hydronephrotic kidney model [26]. The same infusion rate in the intact kidney of the rat had no effect on medullary blood flow [27]. After ischemia, however, medullary blood flow was considerably reduced [27]. In addition, ischemia and cyclosporine can cause medullary tubular damage in humans as well [28]. Whether this is a direct action of cyclosporine or an indirect effect of local endothelin, as shown by Kon et al. [29] is under investigation.

Acknowledgment. This work was supported by the German Research Foundation.

References

1. Zimmerhackl B, Robertson CR, Jamison RL (1985) The microcirculation of the renal medulla. Circ Res 57:657–667
2. Chou S-Y, Porush JG, Faubert PF (1990) Renal medullary circulation: Hormonal control. Kidney Int 37:1–13
3. Brezis M, Seymour R, Silva P, Epstein FH (1984) Renal ischemia: a new perspective. Kidney Int 26:375–383
4. Mason J, Welsch J, Torhorst (1987) The contribution of vascular obstruction to the functional defect that follows renal ischemia. Kidney Int 31:65–71
5. Jamison RL, Kriz W (1982) Urinary concentrating mechanisms: structure and function. Oxford University Press, Oxford
6. Casellas D, Moore LC (1990) Autoregulation and tubuloglomerular feedback in juxtamedullary glomerular arterioles. Am J Physiol 258:F660–F669
7. Casellas D, Carmines PK, Navar LG (1985) Microvascular reactivity of in vitro blood perfused juxtamedullary nephrons from rats. Kidney Int 28:752–759
8. Steinhausen M, Ballantyne D, Fretschner M, Parekh N (1990) Sex differences in autoregulation of juxtamedullary glomerular blood flow in hydronephrotic rats. Am J Physiol 258:F863–F869

---

[2]This is, for example, the situation in preterm infants with open ductus arteriosus. These patients receive indomethacin for duct closure. Under hypovolemic and antidiuretic conditions these patients are prone to acute renal failure, which can be prevented by inducing water diuresis before the application of the prostaglandin antagonist.

9. Cohen HJ, Kayser B, Marsh DJ (1983) Autoregulation in vasa recta of the rat kidney. Am J Physiol 245:F32–F40

10. Zimmerhackl B, Jamison RL, Robertson CR (1985) Effect of arginine vasopressin on renal medullary blood flow. J Clin Invest 76:770–778

11. Zimmerhackl B, Dussel R, Steinhausen M (1986) Nieren Hochdruckkrankheiten 15:371

12. Spitalewitz S, Chou PF, Faubert PF, Porush JG (1982) Effects of diuretics on inner medullary hemodynamics in the dog. Circ Res 51:703–710

13. Jamison RL, Buerkert F, Lacy F (1971) A micropuncture study of collecting tubule function in rats with hereditary diabetes insipidus. J Clin Invest 50:2444–2452

14. Thurau K (1964) Renal hemodynamics. Am J Med 36:698–719

15. Sjöquist M, Görannson A, Hansell P, Ulfendahl HR (1985) Regulation of filtration rate and blood flow in juxtamedullary nephrons of the rat kidney. Acta Physiol Scand 123:4A

16. Miyamoto M, Yagil Y, Larson T, Robertson CR, Jamison RL (1988) Effect of intrarenal adenosine on renal function and medullary blood flow in the rat. Am J Physiol 255:F1230–F1234

17. Hellberg POA, Källskog ÖT, Öjteg G, Wolgast M (to be published) Peritubular permeability and intravascular RBC aggregation after ischemia: effects of neutrophils.

18. Zimmerhackl B, Parekh N, Kücherer H, Steinhausen M (1985) Influence of systemically applied angiotensin II on the microcirculation of glomerular capillaries in the rat. Kidney Int 27:17–24

19. Hansell P, Sjöquist M, Ulfendahl HR (1988) Effect of a converting-enzyme inhibitor on vasa recta blood flow in the rat kidney. Am J Physiol 254:F492–F499

20. Roman RJ, Kaldunski ML, Scicli AG, Carretero OA (1988) Influence of kinins and angiotensin II on the regulation of papillary blood flow. Am J Physiol 255:F690–F698

21. Cupples WA, Sakai T, Marsh DJ (1988) Angiotensin II and prostaglandins in control of vasa recta blood flow. Am J Physiol 254:F417–F424

22. Böttcher W, Steinhausen M (1976) Microcirculation of the renal papilla of rats under control conditions and after temporary ischemia. Kidney Int 10:S74–S80

23. Yagil Y, Miyamoto M, Jamison RL (1989) Inner medullary blood flow in postischemic acute renal failure in the rat. Am J Physiol 256:F456–F461

24. Brenner BM, Troy JL, Ballermann BJ (1989) Endothelium-dependent vascular responses. J Clin Invest 84:1373–1378

25. Devarakan P, Kaskel FJ, Arbeit LA, Moore LC (1989) Cyclosporine nephrotoxicity: blood volume, sodium conservation, and renal hemodynamics. Am J Physiol 256:F71–F78

26. Zimmerhackl LB, Fretschner M, Steinhausen M (1990) Cyclosporin reduces renal blood flow through vasoconstriction of arcuate arteries in the hydronephrotic rat model. Klin Wochenschr 68:166–174

27. Yagil Y (1990) Acute effect of cyclosporin on inner medullary blood flow in normal and postischemic rat kidney. Am J Physiol 258:F1139–F1144

28. Steidel K, Brandis M, Leititis JU, Kramer M, Zimmerhackl LB (1990) Cyclosporin causes hyperuricemia in renal transplants, not in children treated for nephrotic syndrome. Renal Failure 12:193–198

29. Kon V, Sugiura M, Inagami T, Harvie BR, Ichikawa I, Hoover RL (1990) Role of endothelin in cyclosporin-induced glomerular dysfunction. Kidney Int 37:1487–1491

On the Intrinsic Control of Capillary Permeability

M. Wolgast, Ö. Källskog, K. Nygren, and G. Öjteg[1]

SUMMARY. The permeability of the renal capillary membranes is suggested to be controlled not only by external forces, but also by the prevailing Starling pressures, in the sense that a large net driving force is followed by a large hydraulic resistance, and vice versa. This means that, in spite of variations of the net driving force, the fluid transfer may remain fairly constant—in other words an *autoregulation* of the membrane permeability is suggested. The need for such a mechanism would seem obvious, i.e., since otherwise even small changes in glomerular filtration and/or peritubular capillary uptake might lead to drastic changes in the urinary output. The hypothesis has its basis in a new model, in which it is supposed that a *flexible* gel/fiber-matrix, rather than a rigid porous membrane, constitutes the membrane. The size, shape, and permeability characteristics of such a membrane will be the result of the balance between, on the one hand, the above mentioned physical forces and, on the other, the mechanics of the gel/fiber structure. Here, the tension of the fibers acts to restrict expansion, whereas membrane-fixed negative charges, via the resulting electroosmotic pressure and balancing hydrostatic pressure, act to resist compression. Regarding the intra-membranous net driving force, the hydrostatic pressure gradient valid in the Starling model will be replaced by an electroosmotic net driving force, i.e., where the magnitude and direction of the force is governed by the electric field. A gel/fiber-matrix membrane can furthermore be predicted to possess a self-rinsing ability, a feature typical of, e.g., the glomerular capillary membrane. Regarding external control of the membrane permeability, all factors which affect the isoelectric point of the structure carrying the charges can be predicted to govern the membrane characteristics.

[1]Department of Physiology and Medical Biophysics, University of Uppsala, S-75123 Uppsala, Sweden.

Introduction

The present paper aims to analyze whether the permeability of renal capillary membranes is governed not only by "external factors" (humoral factors, the action of contractile elements etc.), but also by physical factors such as the transmembranous Starling forces. More specifically, it is suggested that a high net driving force will induce a high hydraulic resistance, whereas a low net driving force will be concomitant with a reduced resistance such that the fluid transfer may remain largely unaltered – in other words, an autoregulation of the hydraulic permeability of the membrane is suggested.

The need for such a mechanism would seem obvious. Thus, if the permeability of the two renal capillary membranes would remain constant, even a minute increase in, e.g., the hydrostatic pressure would lead to a very large difference between fluid filtration and reabsorption and hence to a large urinary output.

The basis for the above hypothesis is a new model, in which it is suggested that flexible gel/fiber matrix, rather than a rigid porous membrane, constitutes the capillary membrane. From an anatomical point of view, this suggestion would not seem particularly provocative. Morphologists [1–6] have since long denied the existence of a rigid membrane penetrated by discrete cylindrical pores, but have claimed that capillary membranes are composed of highly specialized structural elements with a network of collagenous fibrils and, immobilized in this network, medium-sized polysaccharides known as glycosaminoglycans.

From a biophysical point of view, however, the assumption of a gel/fiber-matrix membrane does not merely imply a change of wording, but indeed a change of concept. The key point refers to the fact that, in the absence of rigid elements, other means of preserving membrane integrity have to be considered. Furthermore, since at least "dilute" gels do not allow for the development of hydrostatic pressure gradients, "new" forces accounting for the fluid transfer have to be considered. The ability of charged gel/fiber-matrix membranes to rinse themselves from entrapped proteins, a feature typical of biological membranes, will also be examined.

Model

Figure 1 depicts a capillary membrane with a network for fibers attached to each other by interconnecting filaments. If this membrane is exposed to a hydraulic pressure gradient, the pressure on the right hand side of each fiber will be higher than that on the left hand side. The fibers will then move in the left hand direction until eventually they will be packed one next to the other, with the formation of a very dense and tight capillary membrane. It is also evident that, on the plasma side, the plasma proteins will drag water out of the fiber-matrix, which again results in the formation of densely packed fibers.

In Fig. 2, this complete collapse of the membrane has been prevented by replacing the interconnecting fibers with strings able to resist both expansion and compression. Still, however, the fiber density will be dependent on the hydraulic pressure gradient, such that a low net driving force is followed by a low hydraulic resistance,

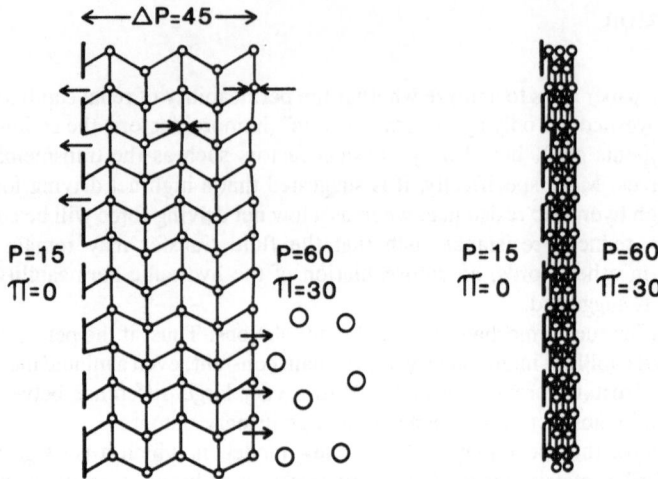

Fig. 1. Fiber-matrix of the glomerular capillary membrane. Since the pressure on the right hand side of the individual fibers is higher than that on the left hand side, the fibers will move in the right hand direction until they become packed, one next to the other, with the formation of a very dense tight matrix. At the plasma side of the membrane, the plasma proteins will drag water out of the membrane, which again results in a dense packing of the matrix fibers

whereas a high net driving force is followed by a high hydraulic resistance. As a result, fluid transfer may remain largely unaltered.

In order to test the expected dependency between net driving force and hydraulic resistance, the data on 1) the glomerular and 2) the peritubular capillary membranes, obtained in our previous investigation [7], were applied. The experimental condi-

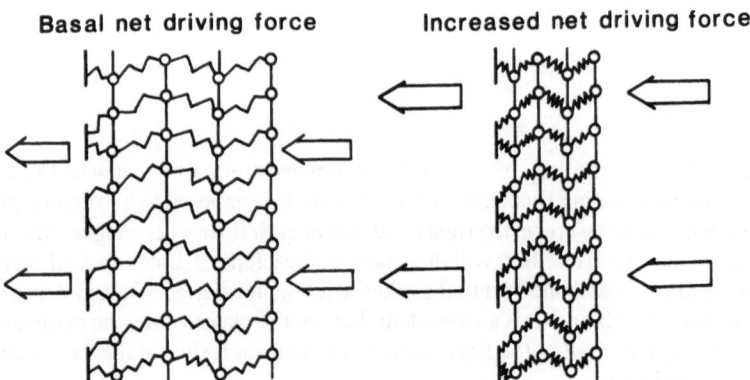

Fig. 2. The same fiber matrix as in Fig. 1, but where the interconnecting filaments are assumed to possess a "string-like" action, i.e., an action which prevents the complete collapse seen in Fig. 1. A higher net driving force (*right panel*) will nevertheless lead to an increased hydraulic resistance such that the fluid flow may be largely unaltered

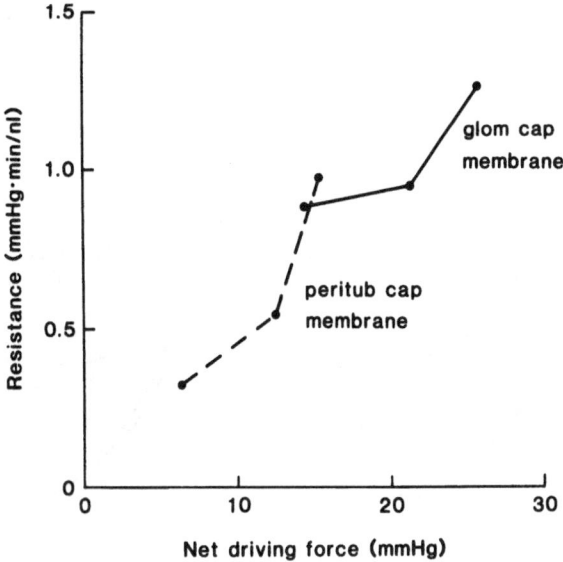

Fig. 3. Relation between the net driving force and hydraulic resistance in the glomerular and peritubular capillary membranes

tions were: a) control antidiuresis, b) 4% saline expansion, and c) 10% saline expansion. As shown from the two points in the middle of Fig. 3, the control net driving force and also the hydraulic resistance of the glomerular and peritubular capillary membrane would seem to be about the same. After saline expansion, however, the net driving force across the glomerular capillary membrane will increase, whereas in the peritubular capillaries, the same dilution leads to a reduction of the driving force. In both cases, however, a rise in the net driving force will be accompanied by an increased hydraulic resistance. The biological data thus supports the expected dependency between net driving force and hydraulic resistance.

Nature of the Elastic Forces

As regards the mechanical characteristics of a fiber matrix, it is easy to imagine that the collagenous fibers act to resist expansion of the gel/fiber-matrix. In contrast, however, they are probably less effective in restricting compression, i.e., unless the matrix is very dense.

A chemical osmotic force would also seem less likely, simply because the *molar concentration* of the structural elements is very small.

A third possibility arises from charged groups fixed to the matrix filaments [7–11]. Altough such charges, in themselves, do not induce an osmotic force, they will attract mobile ions of opposite charge, and it is these ions that induce the osmotic force. The consequent fluid entry and rise in the intramembranous hydrostatic pressure now enables the membrane to resist compression. Indeed, the charges will have a true

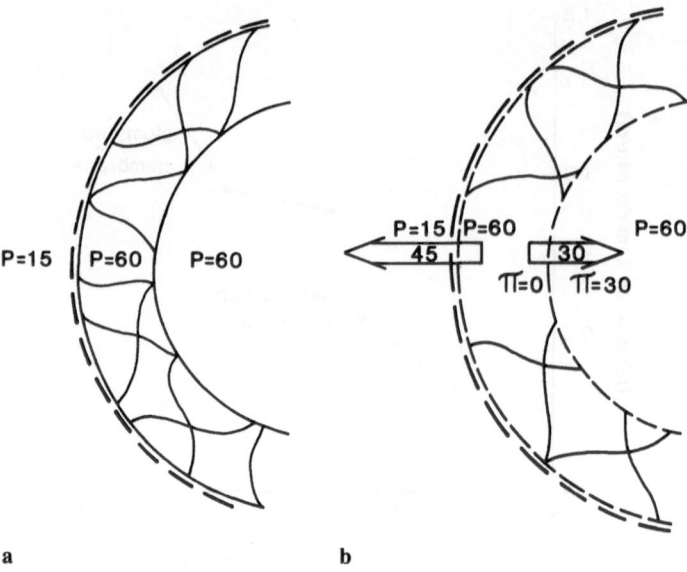

a   b

Fig. 4a,b. Structure of the glomerular capillary membrane consisting of a "loose" gel/fiber-matrix enclosed into two sheets; in **a** the two sheets are assumed to be watertight, in **b** they are permeable. In both cases the basement membrane offers mechanical support. Note that, since a gel (like water) is able to transmit pressures, the intra-membranous hydrostatic pressure must equal the glomerular capillary hydrostatic pressure of 60 mm Hg

"string-like" action in the sense that compression leads to a rise in the fixed charge density and hence to an increased electro-osmotic pressure, and vice versa.

It should be pointed out that the electro-osmotic pressure is independent of the sign of the charges. However, in most biological structures negatively charged groups seem to predominante.

Where the concentration of membrane-fixed charges is concerned, there are two alternatives, which both allow for the preservation of membrane integrity. In the first and simplest case, the charge density is so high that the resulting electoosmotic pressure and the balancing intramembranous hydrostatic pressure outrange the pressures in the free fluid phases surrounding the membrane. Since such an "overstretched" membrane thereby will be unaffected by the Starling forces in its surroundings, it will in fact behave as a rigid porous membrane.

In the second, and more probable, alternative the hydrostatic and osmotic pressures of the membrane are in balance with those in its surrounding free fluid phases. In the evaluation of this alternative, we may first assume (Fig. 4a) that the gel/fiber-matrix is enclosed between two flexible and *watertight* sheets, the sheet to the left faces the interstitium (or Bowman's space) and that to the right faces the capillary plasma. In order to prevent rupture of the structure, the membrane is supported by a relatively rigid (though still tensile) basement membrane (the heavy interrupted line in Fig. 4).

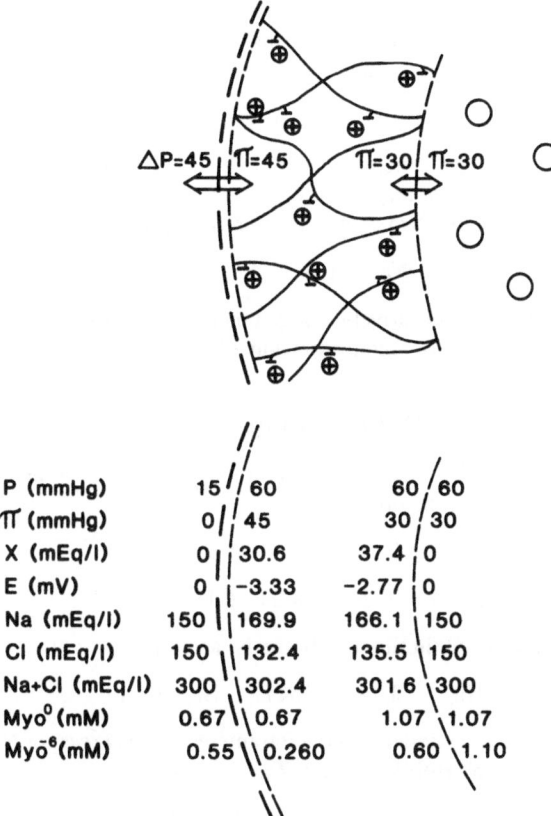

Fig. 5. Gel/fiber-matrix of the glomerular capillary membrane, where the electroosmotic force offered by positive mobile ions attracted to negative membrane-fixed charges enables fluid equilibria at the two interphases of the membrane

Since the membrane gel, like water, transmits hydrostatic pressures, exposure to a capillary hydrostatic pressure of 60 mm Hg (i.e., as in the glomerular capillaries) results in an intramembranous hydrostatic pressure of the same 60 mm Hg. However, since the two sheets enclosing the gel/fiber-matrix are watertight there will be no exchange of fluid. The integrity of the capillary membrane will thus be maintained.

Water-tightness is, however, not an obligatory prerequisite. We may also assume a fluid equilibrium across the two interphases. In this case, we have to balance a pressure difference of 45 mm Hg on the Bowman's space (interstitial) side and, on the plasma side, the glomerular plasma colloid osmotic pressure of 30 mm Hg (Fig. 4b).

This is accomplished (Fig. 5, upper panel) by introducing membrane-fixed negative charges such that the electroosmotic pressure becomes 45 mm Hg and 30 mm Hg, at the two sides of the membrane, respectively.

In order to calculate the fixed charge density producing the desired electroosmotic pressure, the distribution of the small mobile ions has first to be considered. Here,

Donnan equilibrium predicts that the concentrations of the mobile positive and negative ions (here denoted as Na and Cl) in the inside (index i) and outside (index o) solution are related to the electric potential, E, as:

$$E = z_{Na} \cdot F/RT \cdot \ln(Na_i/Na_o) = z_{Cl} \cdot F/RT \cdot \ln(Cl_i/Cl_o) \quad (1a)$$

where z_{Na} and z_{Cl} are the valences of Na and Cl, F is Faradays constant, R the gas constant, and T the absolute temperature.

The equality between the two expressions on the right hand side means that:

$$Na_i/Na_o = (Cl_i/Cl_o)^{-1} = Cl_o/Cl_i \quad (1b)$$

Utilizing the fact that in a negatively charged membrane with a charge density of X mEq/l, the intra-membranous concentration of chloride, $Cl_i = (Na_i - X)$, we obtain:

$$Na_i/Na_o = Cl_o/(Na_i - X) \quad (2)$$

Since Na_o and Cl_o in the outside solution are known, the intra-membranous concentrations of the ions can be obtained:

$$Na_i = X/2 + [(X/2)^2 + Na_o \cdot Cl_o]^{1/2} \quad (3a)$$

$$Cl_i = -X/2 + [(X/2)^2 + Na_o \cdot Cl_o]^{1/2} \quad (3b)$$

The sum of Na and Cl within the membrane is, accordingly:

$$Na_i + Cl_i = 2 \cdot [(X/2)^2 + Na_o \cdot Cl_o]^{1/2} \quad (4)$$

The osmotic force, Π, generated by the intramembranous *excess* of Na and Cl, can now be obtained by van't Hoff's law, $\pi = RT \cdot \Delta C$, as:

$$\begin{aligned} \pi &= RT \cdot [(Na_i + Cl_i - (Na_o + Cl_o)] \\ &= RT \cdot \{2 \, [(X/2)^2 + Na_o \cdot Cl_o]^{1/2} - (Na_o + Cl_o)\} \end{aligned} \quad (5)$$

Evidently, the electroosmotic force is dependent on both the fixed charge density, X, and the ionic strength (Na_o and Cl_o). If Na_o and Cl_o approach zero, the electroosmotic force will approach $RT \cdot X$, i.e., it is directly proportional to the fixed charge density. For higher ionic strengths the electroosmotic presssure shows a progressive decrease; the figures at physiological ionic strength, where $Na_o = Cl_o = 150$ mEq/l, are shown in Fig. 6.

Utilizing this figure, we may obtain the fixed charge densities, X, for the sought electroosmotic pressures of 45 mm Hg and 30 mm Hg, respectively, valid for the glomerular capillary membrane discussed in Fig. 4. These figures, the electric potentials, the distributions of Na and Cl and sums, (Na+Cl), are given in the lower panel of Fig. 5. As expected from a negatively charged membrane, the intramembranous concentration of Na is higher than that of Cl.

Valididification of the Hypothesis

As shown in Fig. 5, a low concentration of negative ions not only applies to Cl, but also to a negatively charged polyion such as Myoglobin:

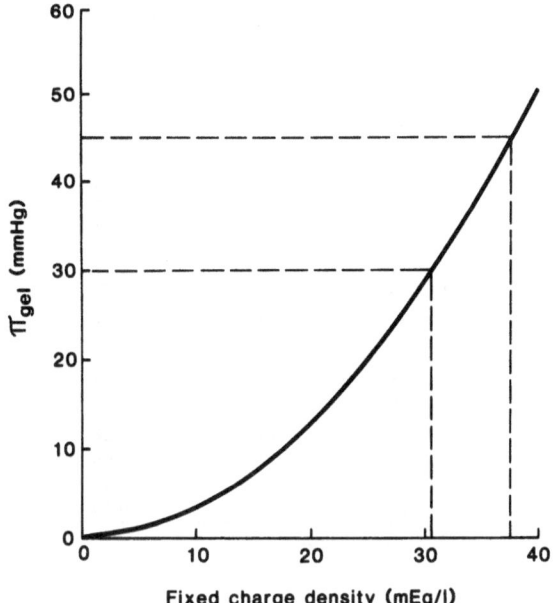

Fig. 6. Relation between fixed charge density and electroosmotic pressure at a physiological ionic strength

$$E = z_{Cl} \, F/RT \cdot \ln(Cl_i/Cl_o) = z_{Myo} \, F/RT \cdot \ln(Myo_i/Myo_o) \qquad (6)$$

The transport, M, of myoglobin across the membrane is governed by Nernst's equation:

$$M = -A_p D' \, dC(x)/dx + V \, (1-\sigma) \, C(x) - A_p D' \, C(x) \cdot dE(x)/dx \qquad (7)$$

where A_p is the pore area, D' the coefficient for restricted diffusion, V the hydraulic fluid flow (in the glomerulus the glomerular filtration rate), σ the reflection coefficient and $dE(x)/dx$ the electric field.

Assuming a constant electric field, i.e., $dE(x)/dx = \Delta E/\Delta x$, integration between $x=0$ (plasma side) and $x=\Delta x$ (Bowman's space side) gives:

$$M = [V \, (1-\sigma) - D'Ap/\Delta x \, (\Delta EzF/RT)] \cdot [C(\Delta x) - C(0) \exp K]/[1-\exp K],$$

where $K = [V \, (1-\sigma) - D'Ap/\Delta x \, (\Delta EzF/RT)]/[D'Ap/\Delta x]$

Details of analyses of pertinent parameters have been given elsewhere [11]. In brief, the terms $A_p/\Delta x$, D' and σ are obtained (Table 1) from the transport of a series of neutral probes: inulin, myoglobin, horse radish peroxidase (HRP), and lactate dehydrogenase (LDH). Knowing the electric potential difference, ΔE (Fig. 5, lower panel), the transport, and hence also the interstitial (Bowman's space) concentration, of their negatively charged counterparts could be predicted. The latter figures, for both the glomerular and peritubular capillary membranes are shown in Table 1. As is evident from this table, the experimental data support the hypothesis.

Table 1. Experimental and predicted concentration of a series of neutral and charged molecular probes in Bowman's space (*upper panel*) and renal interstitium (*lower panel*). The concentration in systemic plasma is put at 1.0

Probe (plasma concentration)	Size	Valency	Experimental concentration	Predicted concentration
Bowman's space				
Inulin (1.01)	11 Å	0	0.94	0.94
Myoglobin (1.07)	17.5 Å	0	0.67	0.67
HRP (1.20)	32 Å	0	0.07	0.06
Myoglobin (1.10)	17.5 Å	−6	0.51	0.55
Myoglobin (1.05)	17.5 Å	+2	0.74	0.70
HRP (1.20)	32 Å	−14	0.01	0.01
Renal interstitial field				
HRP (1.13)	32 Å	0	0.32	0.32
LDH (1.13)	46 Å	0	0.12	0.12
HRP (1.13)	32 Å	−14	0.28	0.29
LDH (1.13)	46 Å	−19	0.08	0.07
LDH (1.13)	46 Å	+2	0.13	0.13
Myoglobin (1.13)	17.5 Å	−6	0.66	0.66

HRP, horseradish peroxidase; LDH, lactate dehydrogenase

Net Driving Force for Fluid Transfer

On inspecting the numbers in the lower panel of Fig. 5 one can see that gel osmotic pressures of 45 mm Hg and 30 mm Hg at the two sides of the membrane, respectively, are shown. The resulting net driving force will then be 15 mm Hg, i.e., the same as that calculated conventionally from the Starling forces in glomerular plasma and Bowman's space.

This force derives from the difference in osmolality on the two sides of the membrane; on the Bowman's space side (Na+Cl) = 302.4 mOsm/kg and at the plasma side (Na + Cl) = 301.6 mOsm/kg, i.e., a difference of 0.8 mOsm/kg. Utilizing van't Hoff's relation, $\pi = RT\Delta C$, the osmotic pressure difference would be the same − 15 mm Hg.

Such a calculation assumes, however, that the membrane is impermeable to the particles in question. Considering the small size of Na and Cl, this assumption most certainly is not valid. Instead, the required "impermeability" results from the electric potential difference (0.56 mV), which prevents a *net transport* of both Na and Cl. To be more precise, the momentum and hence the presssure generated by Na and Cl in the two directions will be the same. The only source of a difference in momentum or pressure is then that resulting from the difference in the water activity, i.e., from the difference of 0.8 mOsm/kg. Since this force is dependent on electric field, it should be denoted an electroosmotic force.

A second, and perhaps more adequate, mode of expressing the electroosmotic force π_{EI}, is as:

$$\pi_{EI} = -[Na(x) - Cl(x)] \cdot F \cdot dE(x)/dx = -X(x) \cdot F \cdot dE(x)/dx \qquad (8)$$

The advantage of this formulation is inherent in the fact that it more clearly demonstrates that the osmotic force is dependent on the magnitude and direction of the electric field. As regards the pressure in the direction perpendicular to the electric field, it remains the same (60 mm Hg, see Fig. 5) in all parts of the membrane. The membrane is thereby able to withstand the same pressure – 60 mm Hg – in glomerular capillary plasma.

So far, the analysis is based on the assumption of an equilibrium, i.e., no net transport of fluid, including its ions. This would, however, lead to the false conclusion that, since the intramembranous concentration of Na is higher than that of Cl, the bulk flow transport, $\dot{M} = \dot{V} (1-\sigma) C(x)$, for Na would exceed that of Cl, i.e., the prerequisite of electroneutrality would not be fulfilled. For this reason we have to adjust the electric potential difference, such that the transport of negative and positive ions becomes the same. However, since the adjustment needed is only of the order of 1%, this consideration does not alter the figures for the ion distribution outlined in Fig. 5.

Pore Structure of the Gel/Fiber Matrix

Figure 7a aims to illustrate the structure in a fenestra of the glomerular capillary membrane. It is assumed that the fibers (probably synthesized by the endothelial cells) carry specific binding sites able to form the regular network depicted in the figure. In order to prevent collapse of the meshes in the network, the fibers are also assumed to carry negatively charged groups, which, via the attraction of positive mobile ions, cause an inward transport of fluid and expansion of the meshes. This process will proceed until the "dilution" of the charges has resulted in an electroosmotic pressure equal to the colloid osmotic pressure of glomerular plasma (30 mm Hg).

At a given plasma colloid osmotic pressure, the size of the meshes is thus governed by the number of charges on each fiber. Many charges would thus lead to large meshes, and vice versa, i.e., providing that the fibers are tensile. Obviously, the density of the fiber network in the plasma-Bowman's space direction may also contribute to the resultant fixed charge density.

At the Bowman's space side of the membrane the electroosmotic pressure has to be somewhat higher (45 mm Hg). This might be accomplished either by 1) a larger number of charges on each fiber, or 2) by a slight narrowing of the meshes, or 3) by a compression of the matrix at this side of the membrane.

Rinsing of Entrapped Proteins from the Membrane

In Fig. 7b, a protein molecule has been trapped into one of the meshes of the membrane (the single mesh depicted above the fenestra). The space available for the positive mobile ions needed to neutralize the fixed negative charges is thereby reduced. Consequently, the *concentration* of the mobile ions, and hence the osmotic force, will increase. Fluid will then enter into the space between the protein molecule and the fibers, widen the mesh, which thence will allow the entrapped protein to move in the downstream direction until it will be expelled into the Bowman's space. A charged gel/fiber-matrix can thus be predicted to possess a self rinsing ability, an essential feature of membranes such as, e.g., the glomerular capillary membrane.

a

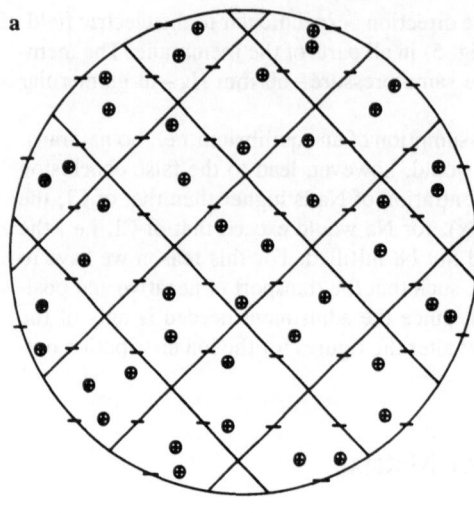

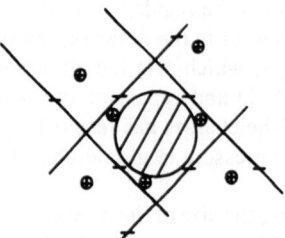

Fig. 7. a Capillary fenestra, where positive mobile ions attracted to membrane-fixed negative charges have induced an inward fluid flow and hence expansion of the meshes to the form depicted in the figure. **b** In this figure a relatively large protein molecule has been trapped into one of the meshes in the gel/fiber-matrix (the single mesh depicted above the fenestra). Since the space available for the positive mobile ions (needed to neutralize the membrane-fixed negative charges) is thereby reduced, the local concentration (not the number) of the mobile positive ions will be increased. The consequent fluid entry will then widen the mesh such that the protein molecule is free to move in the downstream direction

b

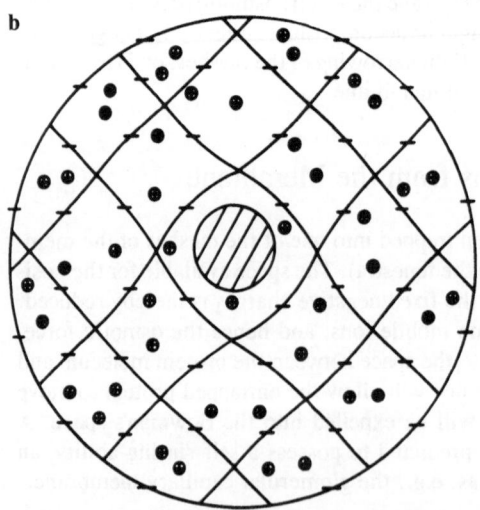

Discussion

The prediced dependency of the hydraulic resistance on the driving forces for fluid transfer will in fact constitute an "edema preventing mechanism." It will thereby add to the more classical mechanism, in which capillary fluid loss is prevented by a compensatory increase in the hydrostatic, and decrease in the colloid osmotic, pressure of the interstitial fluid.

In the kidney, the constancy of the glomerular filtration rate would be a result not only of autoregulation of the renal blood flow, but also of the mechanism discussed here. Where the peritubular capillaries are concerned, the above mentioned mechanism would seem even more essential. Thus, considering that, in man, the transcapillary fluid flow is about 150 l/day, a depression of the hydrostatic pressure in the two capillary beds of as little as 1.5 mm Hg (in both the capillary beds equal to 10% of the normal net driving force) would thus result in a urinary loss as excessive as 30 l/day!! Evidently, the delicate task of controlling extracellular volume cannot be attributed to such "unreliable" forces as the capillary Starling forces. If, on the other hand, the permeability of the peritubular capillary membrane adjusts itself such that, in all instances, the capillaries reabsorb all of the tubular reabsorbate, renal fluid handling will be regulated by the tubular epithelial cells, seemingly a more suitable target for systems aimed to control extracellular volume.

It should be noted, however, that although this reasoning speaks against a strict coupling between the capillary Starling forces and tubular reabsorption, it does not rule out the possibility of some sort of "peritubular control" of, e.g., proximal tubular fluid reabsorption. A further conclusion is that factors altering the fixed charge density might be powerful regulators of capillary permeability. A decline in the isoelectric point of the fibers carrying the charges, for instance, would thus increase the fixed charge density and hence increase capillary permeability.

References

1. Kritz W, Kaissling B (1985) Structural organization of the mammalian kidney. In: Seldin DW, Giebisch G (eds) The kidney: physiology and pathophysiology. Raven, New York, pp 265–306
2. Maul GG (1971) Structure and formation of pores in fenestrated capillaries. J Ultrastruct Res 36:768–782
3. Maunsbach AB, Olsen TS, Christensen EI (1980) Functional ultrastructure of the kidney. Academic, New York
4. Milici AJ, Lérnhault N, Palade GE (1985) Surface density of diaphragmed fenestrae and transendothelial channels in different murine capillary beds. Circ Res 56:709–717
5. Simioneski M, Simionescu N (1984) Ultrastructure of the microvascular wall: functional correlations. In: The Cardiovascular System. Microcirculation. American Physiology Society, Bethesda, pp 41–101 (Handbook of Physiology, sect 2, vol 4)
6. Levick JR, Smaje LH (1987) An analysis of the permeability of a fenestra. Microvasc Res 33:233–256
7. Larsson M, Nygren K, Sjöquist M, Wolgast M (1983) Functional characteristics of the peritubular capillary membrane in the rat kidney. Acta Physiol Scand 117:251–261
8. Deen WM, Satvat B, Jamieson JM (1980) Theoretical model for glomerular filtration of charged solutes. Am J Physiol 238:F126–F139

9. Deen WM, Bridges CR (1982) Molecular charge of horse radish peroxidase. Am J Physiol 242:F750–F762
10. Ötjeg G, Nygren K, Wolgast M (1987) Permeability of renal capillaries. II. Transport of neutral and charged protein molecular probes. Acta Physiol Scand 129:287–294
11. Öjteg G, Wolgast M (1988) Permeability of renal capillaries. III. Theoretical analysis of hydraulic conductivity, pore structure and electric properties. Acta Physiol Scand 133:459–468
12. Wolgast M, Öjteg G (1988) Electrophysiology of renal capillary membranes: gel concept applied and the Starling model challenged. Am J Physiol 254:F364–F373

Regulation of Renal Vascular Resistance: Studies Using Pharmacological Probes

Yasuharu Aki, Toshiaki Tamaki, Hideyasu Kiyomoto, Hiroshi Iwao, and Youichi Abe[1]

Introduction

The kidney has two resistance vessels, the afferent and the efferent arterioles, located in the pre- and post-glomerulus. Different reactions of each arteriole to endogenous and exogenous vasoactive agents regulate renal blood flow (RBF) and glomerular filtration rate (GFR). Functional and anatomical heterogeneity among nephrons has also been well recognized. Therefore, it might be expected that differences exist among nephrons in the relative tonus of afferent and efferent arterioles. However, there is no literature concerning these differences.

To understand the regulatory mechanisms of renal hemodynamics, we must have good pharmacological tools which act selectively either on the afferent arteriole or the efferent arteriole. For this purpose we have examined the effects of various renal vasodilators on renal hemodynamics and determined the intrarenal vascular action sites of these agents. Then, using these pharmacological tools, we clarified the vasodilatory characteristics of the afferent and efferent arterioles. In addition, the differences in the relative tonus of the afferent and efferent arterioles between the superficial and juxtamedullary nephron were also determined.

In the present study, we used glucagon, adenosine, dipyridamole, ATP, acetylcholine, forskolin and dibutyryl cyclic AMP as pharmacological tools. Adenosine has been noted to be one of the endogenous regulators of renal hemodynamics [1–3]. Osswald and colleagues [1] reported that adenosine is a mediator in the tubuloglomerular feedback mechanism. According to their hypothesis, increased GFR enhances sodium reabsorption and elevates renal oxygen consumption and energy utilization, thereby increasing ATP hydrolysis and adenosine production. Increased adenosine levels in renal tissue would then preferentially constrict the afferent arterioles, helping to return the GFR toward the control level. However, it has

[1]Department of Pharmacology, Kagawa Medical School, 1750-1 Ikenobe, Miki-cho, Kita-gun, Kagawa, 761-07 Japan

been reported that adenosine has both renal vasoconstrictive action, via the inhibition of adenylate cyclase and renal vasodilatory action, via the activation of adenylate cyclase [4,5]. In addition, the renal vasoconstrictive action of adenosine was found to be transient when it was infused into the renal artery [6,7]. Therefore, in this study we have focused on the renal vasodilatory action and have examined whether the vasodilation induced by adenosine might be induced via the activation of adenylate cyclase.

The vascular action sites of these agents were determined by an analysis of the renal arterial pressure (RAP)–RBF relationship. RBF remains relatively constant over a wide range of RAPs through adjustments in the resistance of the preglomular afferent arteriole [8–12]. Also, it is generally accepted that the resistance of the preglomerular vessels attains a minimum value at the RAP near the lower limit of the autoregulatory pressure range [11]. If a vasodilator such as adenosine impairs autoregulatory efficiency within an autoregulatory pressure range and has no potency to increase RBF at the lower limit of the autoregulatory pressure range, it should mainly dilate the afferent arterioles. In contrast, if a vasodilator maintains autoregulatory efficiency despite a higher RBF level, it should mainly dilate the efferent arterioles. Based on the above idea, RAP–RBF relationships were obtained during the infusion of adenosine, ATP and glucagon.

The vasodilatory capabilities of the superficial and the juxtamedullary nephrons were determined by flow measurements in the superficial and deep cortex zone, using the radioactive microsphere method. Based on the differences in the zonal flow responses to various agents, the relative tonus of the afferent and the efferent arterioles in each nephron was estimated.

Methods

Preparations

Experiments were performed on mongrel dogs of both sexes, weighing 12–19 kg, which were maintained on a standard sodium diet. Animals were anesthetized with sodium pentobarbital (30 mg/kg, i.v.), which was followed by a maintenance dose if necessary. A tracheotomy was performed, and the right brachial artery and vein were catheterized for the measurement of systemic blood pressure, sampling of arterial blood, and the infusion of saline and inulin. Another catheter was inserted into the left ventricle via the right carotid artery in order to inject the microspheres. The left kidney was exposed through a retroperitoneal flank incision. The kidney was denervated by a division of all visible periarterial nerve fibers and a sharp dissection of the tissue connected to the renal hilum cephalad to the renal artery. RAP was measured via a catheter inserted into the right femoral artery and advanced into the abdominal aorta just below the bifurcation of the left renal artery. An adjustable aortic clamp was placed on the aorta between the bifurcation of the right and left renal arteries. RAP was varied by means of that clamp. RBF was measured by an electromagnetic flowmeter (MPV-1200, Nihonkohden, Japan). RBF and RAP were continuously monitored and recorded on a polygraph (model No. 361, NEC San-ei, Japan). A curved 23-gauge needle was inserted into the left renal artery for the infusion of saline and drug solutions. The needle was maintained patent by a continuous infusion of saline at a rate of 0.19 ml/min. After the completion of surgery, an intravenous infusion of saline was initiated at the rate of 2 ml/min. For the measurement of GFR, a priming dose of inulin (100 mg/kg) was given intravenously, followed by a continuous infusion of inulin at a rate of 100 mg/kg per hr to maintain a constant plasma level. GFR was obtained by the renal clearance of inulin; inulin was determined by the method of Walser et al [13].

Protocols

The experiments were divided into the following groups: A; Effects of adenosine (20 µg/kg per min, n = 12), ATP (40 µg/kg per min, n = 5), glucagon (0.5 µg/kg per min, n = 10), and acetylcholine (ACh, 4 µg/kg per min, n = 8) on RAP–RBF relationships, B; Effects of glucagon, adenosine, and ACh on the intrarenal distribution of blood flow, C; Effects of dipyridamole (10 µg/kg per min) on RBF and GFR with and without a low dose of adenosine (1 µg/kg per min, n = 5), D; Effects of forskolin (0.2 µg/kg per min, n = 6), dibutyryl cyclic AMP (0.3 mg/kg per min, n = 7) and a calcium channel blocker (nitrendipine, 0.5 µg/kg per min, n = 7), and forskolin (0.2 µg/kg per min, n = 7) on RBF and GFR. In group A, the RAP–RBF relationships were obtained during the infusion of each agent and also for control. RAP was sequentially altered in the 5 steps indicated in Fig. 1, i.e., normal pressure, 100, 75, 60 and 45 mmHg. Each pressure level was maintained for several minutes to allow for a complete autoregulatory response.

Analytical Procedures

The distribution of cortical blood flow was determined using the radioactive microsphere technique [14–16]. A suspension of microspheres labeled with different gamma emitters (85-Sr or 141-Ce), 15 µm in diameter and containing 0.5 mg of bead mass, was inserted into the left ventricle at control and 20 min after the start of the adenosine, glucagon, or ACh infusion. Then the kidney was excised and the renal cortex was cut, parallel to the surface, into four zones of equal thickness. These four cortex zones were analyzed for individual isotope counts, and the flow rate of each zone was calculated.

Data are presented as means ± SEM. The Student's t-test for paired comparisons was used for statistical analysis. Probability values of less than 0.05 were accepted as being statistically significant differences.

Results and Discussion

Intrarenal Vascular Sites of Action of Glucagon, Adenosine and ATP

The effects of glucagon, adenosine and ATP on RBF, GFR, and filtration fraction are shown in Table 1. The dose of each agent used was the respective submaximum dose on the basis of its renal vasodilatory action. In intrarenal infusion of adenosine caused a biphasic response in RBF. Following the initiation of the infusion, RBF decreased transiently and then increased to about 40% above the control level within 5 min, as reported previously [6,17]. This high level of RBF continued thereafter

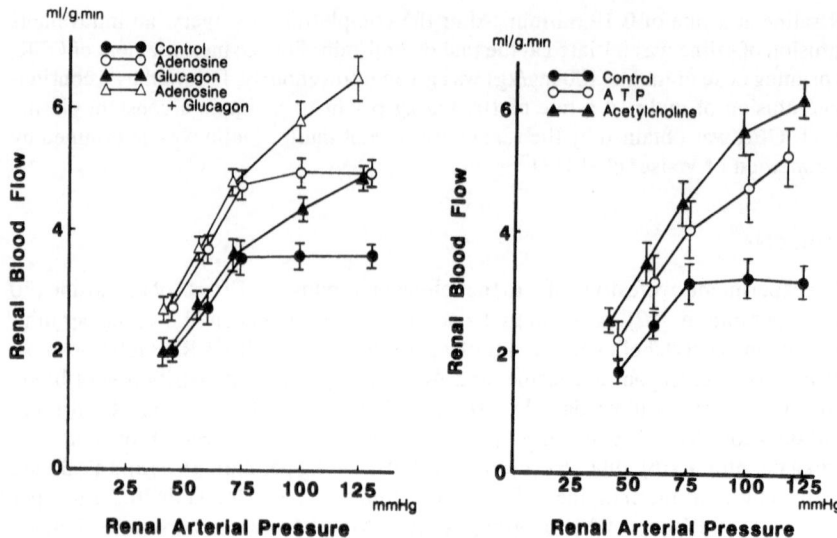

Fig. 1. The *left hand panel* shows the effects of adenosine alone, glucagon alone, and adenosine plus glucagon on the relationship between renal arterial pressure (RAP) and renal blood flow (RBF). Adenosine increased RBF at RAPs below, as well as within, the autoregulatory pressure range. In contrast, glucagon increased RBF at RAPs within the autoregulatory range. The superimposition of glucagon to adenosine infusion resulted in a further vasodilation which occurred at RAPs within the autoregulatory pressure range. The *right hand panel* shows the effects of ATP and acetylcholine (ACh) on the relationship between RAP and RBF. Both ATP and ACh increased RBF at RAPs below, as well as within, the autoregulatory pressure range and significantly impaired the autoregulation of RBF

during the infusion, but GFR was reduced significantly. As a result, the filtration fraction decreased significantly. Glucagon, which activates the adenylate cyclase [18,19], also increased RBF without the initial reduction seen during adenosine infusion. This renal vasodilation induced by glucagon was similar in magnitude to that produced by adenosine, however GFR increased significantly.

Fig. 1 compares the respective effects of adenosine, glucagon, and adenosine plus glucagon on RAP–RFB relationships. Although both adenosine and glucagon elicited vasodilation, the effects on the overall relationships were quite different. Adenosine increased RBF at RAPs below, as well as within, the autoregulatory pressure range. Although the autoregulatory capability was not perceptibly impaired by adenosine, the autoregulatory plateau was shifted upward. The responses obtained by the infusion of adenosine were consistent with the responses previously reported [6]. During the infusion of glucagon, RBF decreased in proportion to the reduction of RAP. At RAPs lower than the autoregulatory range, there were no significant differences between RBF in the absence of or in the presence of glucagon. That is, the vasodilation induced by glucagon was restricted to the RAPs within the autoregulatory pressure range. Glucagon completely abolished the autoregulation of RBF.

It is generally considered that autoregulation-induced resistance changes occur predominantly at the afferent arteriole and that the resistance of an afferent arteriole

Table 1. Effects of various vasodilators on renal hemodynamics in dogs

	Renal blood flow ml/g.min	Glomerular filtration rate ml/g.min	Filtration fraction
Control	3.67±0.18	0.75±0.03	0.32±0.02
glucagon (0.5 µg/kg/min)	5.08±0.23*	0.98±0.04*	0.32±0.02
Control	3.60±0.15	0.74±0.05	0.34±0.02
adenosine (20 µg/kg/min)	5.07±0.15*	0.55±0.04*	0.18±0.01*
adenosine + glucagon	6.63±0.33*⁺	0.73±0.02⁺	0.22±0.03⁺
Control	3.03±0.36	0.72±0.06	0.38±0.03
ATP (40 µg/kg/min)	5.03±0.44*	0.66±0.07	0.20±0.03*
Control	3.36±0.18	0.74±0.04	0.36±0.04
acetylcholine (4 µg/kg/min)	6.41±0.33*	0.74±0.04	0.20±0.02*
Control	3.40±0.20	0.72±0.05	0.35±0.05
forskolin (0.2 µg/kg/min)	4.15±0.30*	0.86±0.06*	0.34±0.05
Control	3.15±0.13	0.64±0.06	0.33±0.02
dibutyryl cyclic AMP (0.3 mg/kg/min)	5.10±0.38*	0.89±0.09*	0.30±0.03
Control	3.29±0.21	0.72±0.04	0.32±0.02
nitrendipine (0.5 µg/kg/min)	4.80±0.31*	0.96±0.04*	0.31±0.02

All values are means±S.E. * indicates significant difference from control ($P<0.05$); + indicates significant difference from adenosine alone ($P<0.05$)

attains a minimum value at the lower limit of the autoregulatory pressure range. Therefore, the observation that glucagon selectively interferes with the autoregulatory component suggests that glucagon dilates the afferent arteriole primarily. In contrast to the action of glucagon, adenosine increased RBF even at the RAP of 75 mmHg, having a minimum value of the afferent arteriolar resistance. This observation indicates that adenosine may dilate the postglomerular efferent arterioles preferentially. The RAP–RBF relationships obtained during the infusions of ACh, which dilates both afferent and efferent arterioles [10,20], and ATP are shown in the right hand panel of Fig. 1. During infusion of ATP or ACh RBF decreased in proportion to the reduction of RAP. But, unlike the effect of glucagon, during infusion of ACh or ATP RBF was significantly higher than the control at each pressure level. Thus, both ACh and ATP induced significant vasodilation characterized by a leftward shift in the RAP–RBF relationship. Thus, these findings show that both ATP and ACh dilate both arterioles. The superimposition of glucagon onto adenosine induced further vasodilation at RAPs within the autoregulatory pressure range. However, at RAPs lower than 75 mmHg there was no difference in RBF between the infusion of adenosine alone and the infusion of adenosine plus glucagon (Fig. 1). The superimposition of glucagon onto adenosine dilated the renal blood vessels such that there was a marked attenuation of the autoregulatory efficiency. Also, there were no significant differences between the RAP–RBF relationship obtained during the infusion of ACh and adenosine plus glucagon. These findings indicate the differences in the action sites of glucagon and adenosine, and support our conclusion.

Osswald et al. [21] reported that adenosine preferentially constricts the afferent arterioles in the superficial nephron of the canine kidney. It is well known that adenosine causes both vasoconstriction and dilation of renal blood vessels unlike that in other organ vascular beds [6,7,22]. The vasoconstriction may appear immediately after the start of infusion whereas the vasodilation appears gradually. Transient

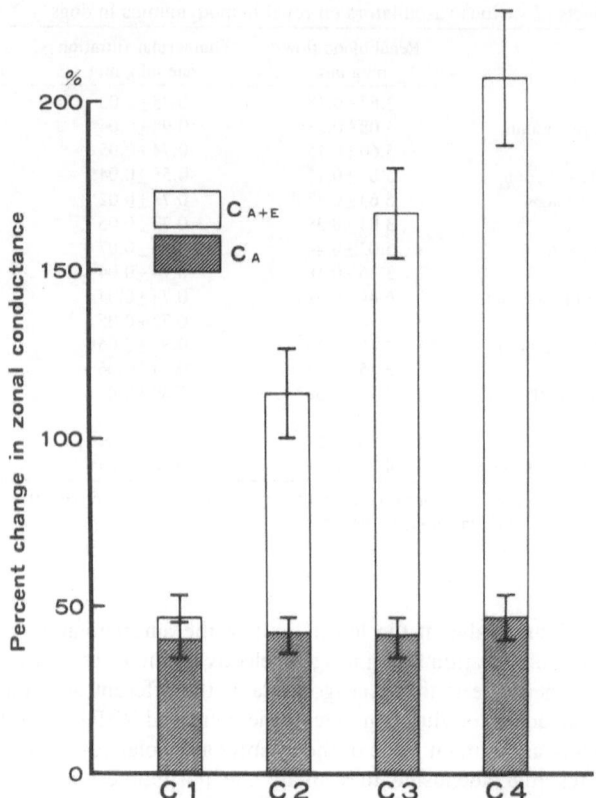

Fig. 2. Vasodilatory capabilities of the afferent and efferent arterioles in the renal cortex zone. The vasodilatory capability of the afferent arteriole (▨) was uniform among zones. That of the efferent arteriole (▢) was not uniform and was characterized by a progressively proportional increase from the superficial to the deep cortex

reduction of RBF may be observed by the summation of both actions of adenosine. So, it could be considered that an abrupt change in adenosine concentration may induce transient vasoconstriction, but the gradual increase of adenosine concentration may not cause such transient vasoconstriction. To test the above hypothesis, the effect of dipyridamole, which inhibits the cellular uptake of adenosine [23] and the degradation of adenosine [24] on RBF, was examined. The intrarenal infusion of dipyridamole alone at a rate of 1 μg/kg per min did not affect RBF, but dipyridamole at a rate of 10 μg/kg per min increased RBF significantly, from 3.32 ± 0.15 to 3.75 ± 0.26 ml/g per min ($P < 0.05$). The superimposition of dipyridamole at a rate of 1 μg/kg per min on adenosine infusion (0.05 μg/kg per min), which did not affect RBF, significantly increased RBF from 3.25 ± 0.20 to 3.81 ± 0.30 ml/g per min without any transient reduction of RBF ($P < 0.05$). Thus, the moderate and gradual changes in adenosine concentration may not induce net vasoconstriction on a whole kidney basis. At present, the speed of changes of adenosine concentration in the renal tissue under various conditions is unknown. Nevertheless, it can be considered that the possible physiological action of adenosine may be preferential dilation of the efferent arterioles.

Differences Among Nephrons in the Vasodilatory Capacities and the Relative Tonus of the Afferent and Efferent Arterioles

In the previous section, the intrarenal action sites of adenosine and glucagon were determined. Glucagon preferentially dilates the afferent arteriole, while adenosine dilates the efferent arteriole. We examined the effects of both of these agents, and ACh, on the intrarenal distribution of blood flow. At basal condition, the flow rate of each cortex zone differed significantly from that of the other three. The inner zones were characterized by the lower perfusion rates. The response to glucagon (0.5 μg/kg per min) was characterized by an almost uniform increase in the flow rates in all four cortex zones. On the other hand, although adenosine induced a significant increase in flow rates in all zones, the zonal response pattern was not uniform. The response pattern was characterized by a progressively proportional increase in flow from the superficial to the deep cortex. Thus, glucagon, which dilates the afferent arterioles, increased the zonal flow rates by the same degree. Adenosine, which dilates the efferent arterioles, increased the inner cortical flow more than the outer cortical flow. These results indicate that the vasodilatory capability of the afferent arteriole is uniform among nephrons, whereas the vasodilatory capability of the efferent arteriole is not uniform and is highest in the juxtaglomerular nephron (Fig. 2). ACh, as well as adenosine, increased the deep cortical flow more than the superficial flow, but the flow response to ACh in each zone was higher than that to adenosine. Renal vasodilation induced by ACh reached a maximum at a dose of 4 μg/kg per min because other vasodilators such as bradykinin and prostaglandin E2 could not dilate the renal blood vessels more than ACh [15,25]. In addition, as shown in Table 1 and in Fig. 1, adenosine plus glucagon achieved almost the same degree of dilation as that achieved by ACh. Thus, it seems that glucagon and adenosine selectively dilate the afferent arteriole and the efferent arteriole, respectively, to the maximum extent.

Vasodilatory Mechanisms of Adenosine

Forskolin, which activates adenylate cyclase in various tissues, increased RBF and GFR concomitantly. Conversely, adenosine, which shows bi-directional action to adenylate cyclase, increased RBF and decreased GFR. If the efferent arteriolar dilation induced by adenosine is exerted exclusively by the activation of adenylate cyclase, it is unlikely that there are significant differences between GFR responses, even though adenosine dilates renal blood vessels in the same magnitude as forskolin. Thus, it is possible that the vasodilatory action of adenosine may not be induced via the activation of adenylate cyclase. The intrarenal infusion of dibutyryl cyclic AMP caused significant increases of both RBF and GFR, which were similar to those seen during the glucagon infusion.

We have previously reported that forskolin stimulated cyclic AMP production in the isolated canine afferent arteriole [26]. However, at present we do not have any data concerning the cyclic AMP production ability of the efferent arteriole. However, it seems likely that the efferent arteriole is also able to produce cyclic AMP. The present findings, that both forskolin and dibutryl cyclic AMP produced the same renal hemodynamic actions, suggest that differences between the intracellular signal-transduction systems of the afferent arteriole and the efferent arteriole may exist.

Conclusions

The present study clearly shows that glucagon and adenosine preferentially dilate the afferent arteriole and the efferent arteriole, respectively. Both agents can be considered to be useful pharmacological tools for clarifying the regulatory mechanisms of renal hemodynamics. The action of adenosine has demonstrated the importance of adenosine as a physiological controller of renal hemodynamics. The increase of adenosine production indicates the negative balance of oxygen supply. Adenosine reduced oxygen consumption in the kidney via the reduced GFR and increased the oxygen supply via the increased RBF. Thus, we suggest that adenosine plays an important role in linking the control of RBF and GFR with changes in renal metabolism. In addition, renal vasodilation by adenosine might not be mediated via the activation of adenylate cyclase. Both forskolin and dibutyryl cyclic AMP produced the same renal hemodynamic actions. These results substantiate the differences between the intracellular signal-transduction systems of the afferent arteriole and the efferent arteriole.

References

1. Osswald H, Hermes H, Nabakowski G (1982) Role of adenosine in signal transmission of tubuloglomerular feedback. Kidney Int 22: S136–S142
2. Osswald H, Nabakowski G, Hermes H (1980) Adenosine as a possible mediator of metabolic control of glomerular filtration rate. Int J Biochem 12: 263–267
3. Spielman WS, Thompson IC (1982) A proposed role for adenosine in the regulation of renal hemodynamics and renin release. Am J Physiol 242: F423–435
4. Van Calker D, Miller M, Hamprecht B (1978) Adenosine inhibits the accumulation of cyclic AMP in cultured brain cells. Nature 276: 839–841
5. Londos C, Cooper DMF, Wolff J (1980) Subclasses of external adenosine receptors. Proc Natl Acad Sci USA 77: 2551–2554
6. Premen AJ, Hall EJ, Mizelle LH, Cornell EJ (1985) Maintenance of renal autoregulation during infusion of aminophylline or adenosine. Am J Physiol 248 (Renal Fluid Electrolyte Physiol 17): F366–F373
7. Ueda J, Abe Y, Okahara T, Yamamoto K (1974) Adenine nucleotides and renal function: Special reference with intrarenal distribution of blood flow. Osaka City Med J 20: 33–50
8. Schmid HE, Garrett CR, Spencer PM (1964) Intrinsic hemodynamic adjustments to reduced renal pressure gradients. Circ Res 15(Suppl): 170–177
9. Selkurt EE, Hall WP, Spencer PM (1949) Influence of graded arterial pressure decrement of renal clearance of creatinine, p-aminohippurate and sodium. Am J Physiol 159: 359–378
10. Abe Y, Dixon F, McNay JL (1970) Dissociation between autoregulation of renal blood flow and glomerular filtration rate. Am J Physiol 219: 986–993
11. Navar LG (1970) Minimal preglomerular resistance and calculation of normal glomerular pressure. Am J Physiol 219: 1658–1664

12. Robertson CR, Deen MW, Troy LJ, Brenner MB (1972) Dynamics of glomerular ultra-filtration in the rat: III. Hemodynamics and autoregulation. Am J Physiol 223:1191–1200
13. Walser M, Davidson GD, Orloff J (1955) The renal clearance of alkali-stable inulin. J Clin Invest 34: 1520–1523
14. McNay JL, Abe Y (1970) Pressure dependent heterogeneity of renal cortical blood flow in dogs. Circ Res 27: 571–587
15. Abe Y, Okahara T, Kishimoto T, Yamamoto K, Ueda J (1973) Relationship between intrarenal distribution of blood flow and renin secretion. Am J Physiol 225: 319–323
16. Abe Y, Kishimoto T, Yamamoto K, Ueda J (1973) Intrarenal distribution of blood flow during ureteral and venous pressure elevation. Am J Physiol 224: 746–751
17. Ueda J (1972) Adenine nucleotides and renal function: Special reference with intrarenal distribution of blood flow (abstract). Jpn J Pharmacol 22: 5
18. Broadns AE, Kaminsky NI, Northcutt RC, Hardman JC, Sutherland EW, Liddle GW (1970) Effects of glucagon on adenosine 3', 5'-monophosphate and guanosine 3', 5'-monophosphate in human plasma and urine. J Clin Invest 49: 2237–2244
19. Mulvehill JB, Hui YS, Barnes LD, Palumbo PJ, Dousa TP (1976) Glucagon sensitive adenylcyclase in human renal medulla. J Clin Endocrinol Metab 42: 380–386
20. Abe Y (1971) Intrarenal blood flow distribution and autoregulation of blood flow and glomerular filtration rate. Jpn Circ J 35: 1163–1173
21. Osswald H, Spielman SW, Knox GF (1978) Mechanism of adenosine mediated decreases in glomerular filtration rate in dogs. Circ Res 43: 465–469
22. Murray RD, Churchill CP (1985) Concentration dependency of the renal vascular and renin secretory responses to adenosine receptor agonists. J Pharmacol Exp Ther 232: 189–193
23. Klabunde RE, Althouse DG (1981) Adenosine metabolism in dog whole blood: effects of dipyridamole. Life Sci 28: 2631–2641
24. Bunag RD, Douglas CR, Imai S, Berne RM (1964) Influence of a pyrimido-pyrimidine derivative on determination of adenosine by blood. Circ Res 15: 83–88
25. Imanishi M, Abe Y, Okahara T, Yukimura T, Yamamoto K (1980) Effects of prostaglandin I2, and E2 on renal hemodynamics and function and renin release. Jpn Circ J 44: 875–882
26. Tamaki T, Hura CE, Kunau RT (1989) Dopamine stimulates cAMP production in canine afferent arterioles via DA1 receptors. Am J Physiol 256: H626–H629

Role of Intracellular Calcium in the Regulation of Renal Hemodynamics

L. Gabriel Navar[1], Pamela K. Carmines[1], Kenneth D. Mitchell[1], and P. Darwin Bell[2]

SUMMARY. Intracellular calcium contributes to renal hemodynamic regulatory mechanisms in multiple ways. Calcium channel blockers elicit a selective vasodilation of preglomerular arterioles leading to increases in renal blood flow (RBF), glomerular filtration rate (GFR), and glomerular pressure, with marked attenuation of autoregulatory capability. The effects of these agents seem to be restricted to the component of renal vascular resistance responsible for autoregulation and contrast with other agents which vasodilate the kidney at arterial pressures below, as well as within, the autoregulatory range. This component of renal vascular resistance that is not influenced by calcium entry blockade can be altered by angiotensin converting enzyme inhibition. Studies at the microvascular level have demonstrated that the effects of angiotensin II on afferent arterioles are dependent upon calcium entry whereas the vasoconstrictor actions on efferent arterioles are not influenced by calcium channel blockade. The macula densa cells responsible for mediating tubular glomerular feedback (TGF) appears to utilize a different type of intracellular calcium mechanism for transmission of feedback signals. Increases in the intralumenal solute concentration at the macula densa elicit feedback signals to constrict the afferent arterioles and reduce glomerular pressure. These effects can be artificially induced by the intralumenal addition of calcium ionophores; however, intralumenal addition of calcium channel blockers or variation in intralumenal calcium concentration do not interfere with signal transmission. In contrast, agents that interfere with intracellular calcium mobilization can block TGF responses. Thus, intracellular mobilization of cytosolic calcium within the macula densa cells leads to transmission of TGF signals to the vascular cells. At the afferent arteriolar effector site, transmembrane calcium flux appears to serve as the dominant mechanism for regulating intracellular calcium, since TGF-mediated vasoconstrictor responses are abolished by calcium channel blockade. The efferent arterioles may be

[1]Department of Physiology, Tulane University School of Medicine, 1430 Tulane Ave., New Orleans, LA 70112, USA
[2]Department of Physiology, Nephrology Research and Training Center, University of Alabama at Birmingham, Birmingham, AL 35294, USA

less responsive to TGF signals because of their relative insensitivity to agents that alter transmembrane calcium flux.

Introduction

Although it is well recognized that activation of cytosolic calcium is a pivotal step in many intracellular processes, including vascular smooth muscle contraction, the mechanisms by which increases in cytosolic calcium can be achieved are varied [1–3]. Cytosolic calcium can be activated either by increasing calcium influx from the extracellular compartment through several mechanisms or by increased mobilization of intracellular calcium from sequestered sites. In many systems there is a complex coupling between intracellular mobilization mechanisms and calcium influx mechanisms [1–4]. For this presentation emphasis will be placed on the role of intracellular calcium in two specific aspects related to renal hemodynamic regulatory mechanisms. Initially, attention will be focused on the role of calcium entry mechanisms in regulating afferent arteriolar resistance in response to changes in perfusion pressure and in response to certain vasoactive peptides, such as angiotensin II. In the second part of this paper, consideration will be given to the role of intracellular calcium in the mediation of tubular glomerular feedback (TGF) signals from the macula densa cells to the afferent arterioles.

Vascular Control Mechanisms

The fact that transmembrane calcium flux is very important in mediating vascular contraction [2–4] should not be taken as evidence that fluctuations in the ionized calcium levels in the extracellular fluid environment within the physiologic range cause major effects. Indeed, because of the exquisite power which very small changes of cytosolic calcium have to cause major alterations in cellular function, the cell membrane has developed a high degree of impermeability to calcium ions. Calcium ions generally leak in very slowly from the extracellular fluid compartment and can be removed by a number of powerful transport mechanisms that return calcium to the extracellular fluid or compartmentalize it within the cell in an inactive form. Thus, although calcium concentration in the extracellular fluid is in the millimolar range, the intracellular concentration of free calcium is less than one micromolar [1–4]. In spite of this extremely large calcium gradient between the extracellular and the intracellular environments, the influx is considered to be rather limited and to be controlled primarily by mechanisms which activate calcium influx through specific calcium channels. Accordingly, previous studies have demonstrated that changes in plasma calcium concentration within the physiologic range elicit only subtle changes in renal vascular resistance and have rather negligible effects on renal autoregulatory capability [5].

Pharmacological agents which can directly alter transmembrane calcium influx have been shown to have powerful renal hemodynamic effects [6]. Systemic or intrarenal arterial infusion of calcium channel blockers increases RBF and GFR and causes a marked attenuation of the ability of the vasculature to respond to changes in arterial pressure with appropriate autoregulatory resistance adjustments [7,8].

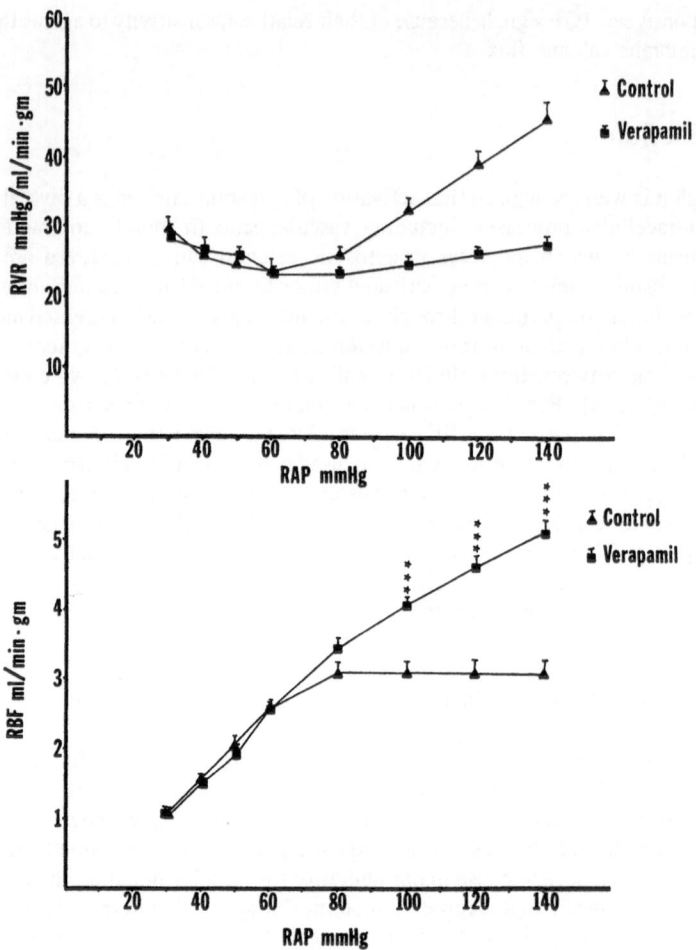

Fig. 1. Effects of verapamil on renal autoregulatory behavior. Data show the relationship between renal arterial pressure (*RAP*) and renal blood flow (*lower panel*) and between RAP and renal vascular resistance (*RVR*) (*upper panel*). (Data from [7])

Examples of such responses are shown in Fig. 1, which demonstrates the shift from a normal autoregulatory pattern to a near passive RBF response to decreases in renal arterial pressure which occurs during the intraarterial infusion of verapamil. Importantly, the verapamil-induced increase in RBF was restricted primarily to the range of arterial pressures associated with autoregulation. At these higher renal arterial pressures, the loss of autoregulatory capability resulted in the magnitude of the renal vasodilation being highly dependent on the level of renal arterial pressure. However, at arterial pressures below the autoregulatory range, there was little or no difference between RBF during control conditions and during calcium channel blockade. Coincident with the loss of RBF autoregulation, calcium channel blockers also attenuated

GFR autoregulation [7]. When these responses are assessed as changes in renal vascular resistance during reductions in arterial pressure, it can be observed that calcium channel blockers decrease renal vascular resistance only down to the minimal level achieved at the reduced levels of arterial pressure. Thus, calcium channel blockers appear to be unique in their ability to vasodilate the kidney. In contrast to other types of vasodilators, such as acetylcholine, which can vasodilate at renal arterial pressures below as well as within the autoregulatory range [9], or angiotensin converting enzyme (ACE) inhibitors, which increase RBF at all pressures but do not alter renal autoregulatory behavior [7,10], the calcium channel blockers seem to uniquely influence the autoregulatory portion of the curve with little or no effect on other components. Interestingly, pharmacological agents that interfere with intracellular mobilization of calcium are not as effective in blocking autoregulatory mediated changes in vascular resistance [11]. These observations suggest that one unique property of the renal vascular resistance segment responsible for autoregulation is its sensitivity to stimuli which alter transmembrane calcium flux.

In further studies it was demonstrated that infusion of an angiotensin converting enzyme inhibitor during calcium channel blockade caused additional dilation of the renal vascular bed [7]. The effect could be reversed by angiotensin II even though it was apparent that overall angiotensin II sensitivity was markedly reduced by calcium channel blockade. Thus, there is also an angiotensin sensitive vascular resistance component that is not susceptible to calcium channel blockers.

The whole kidney data suggest that calcium channel blockers predominately dilate the preglomerular resistance vessels responsible for mediating autoregulatory adjustments in renal vascular resistance. More recent micropuncture experiments using the peritubular capillary infusion technique have provided direct confirmation of this conclusion [12]. Peritubular capillary infusion is a particularly useful technique, because it allows infusion of high concentrations of hormones or pharmacological agents into the blood flow of a single large peritubular capillary welling point on the surface of the kidney. The infused agents diffuse out of the peritubular capillary network and infiltrate the surrounding interstitial spaces and can thus expose the adjoining microvasculature to high concentrations of vasoactive agents without affecting systemic arterial pressure. With this technique, the effects of maximally effective doses of calcium channel blockers on the superficial nephron vascular function can be assessed without the hypotensive effects elicited by intravenous or intraarterial infusion of these agents. One purpose of our study was to evaluate the effects of calcium entry blockers on glomerular pressure and glomerular pressure autoregulation, as assessed by proximal tubule stop flow pressure (SFP) measurements. As shown in Fig. 2, verapamil caused substantial increases in SFP and also increased the slope of the relationship between renal arterial pressure and SFP. Thus, even though the control SFP responses reflect only the residual autoregulatory capability occurring in the absence of the contribution of TGF influences from the nephron with interrupted distal flow [13], calcium entry blockade caused a further preglomerular dilation and a near passive relationship between arterial pressure and glomerular pressure.

Another important objective of this study was to evaluate the sensitivity of the effector component of the TGF mechanism to calcium channel blockers [12]. As shown in Fig. 3, SFP feedback responses were nearly abolished during peritubular capillary infusion with verapamil or nifedipine. These results provide further support for the

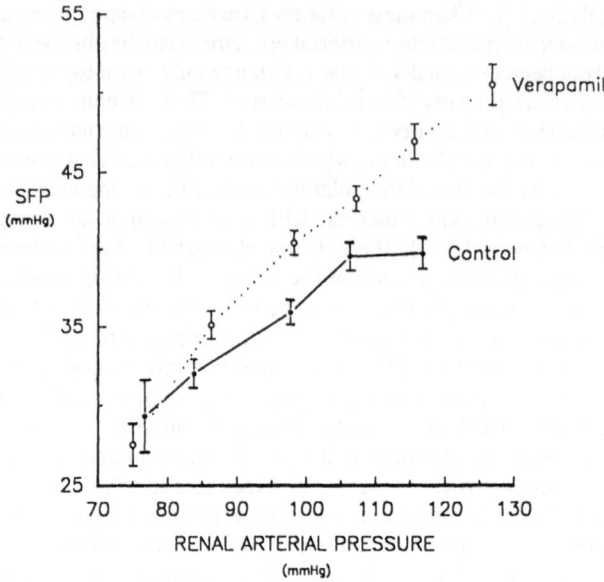

Fig. 2. Relationships between RAP and stop flow pressure (*SFP*) obtained during control conditions and during peritubular infusion of verapamil. (Data from [12])

contention that the preglomerular contractile elements responsible for autoregulatory capability, as well as for TGF responsiveness, can essentially be rendered passive by calcium entry blockers and suggest that transmembrane calcium flux through voltage-dependent channels serves as a common effector mechanism for both feedback-mediated and autoregulation-induced adjustments in preglomerular resistance.

Because of the evidence suggesting that complex intrarenal vascular control mechanisms are only partially dependent on transmembrane calcium movement through voltage-dependent channels, videomicroscopic measurements of vascular dimensions were performed on in vitro blood perfused juxtamedullary nephrons [14]. The effects of calcium channel blockers on control arteriolar diameters and on the vascular responsiveness to angiotensin II were evaluated. In particular, attention was focused on differences between afferent and efferent arterioles. The in vitro blood perfused juxtamedullary nephron technique is unique in that it provides accessibility to the preglomerular and postglomerular microvasculature, allowing videometric evaluation under well controlled in vitro conditions [14]. Kidney donors are heparinized and the right kidney is perfused through a double-barreled cannula with an oxygenated Tyrode's solution containing albumin. During continued perfusion, the kidney is removed and sectioned longitudinally to expose the pelvic cavity, leaving the papilla intact. Since the papilla normally overlies the tissue of interest, it is reflected back and the pelvic mucosa, adipose, and connective tissues which normally cover the inside cortical surface are removed and the veins are cut open. This procedure exposes the tubules and superficial microvasculature of juxtamedullary nephrons. The terminal portions of the vasculature giving rise to arterioles

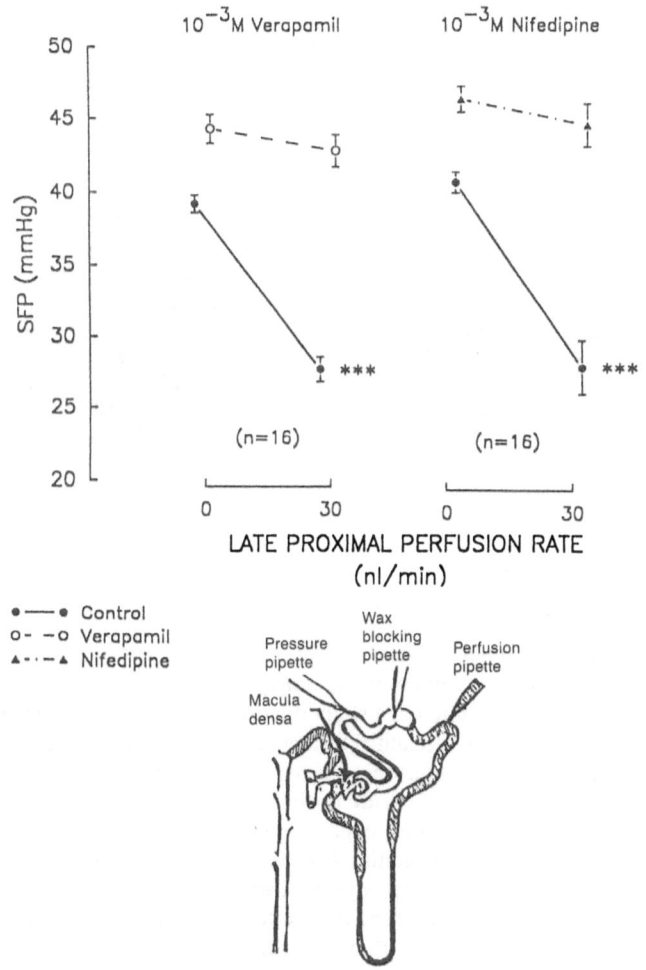

Fig. 3. Effects of calcium channel blockers on tubuloglomerular feedback responses. For these experiments, the normal TGF-mediated decrease in stop flow pressure (*SFP*) was assessed by increasing orthograde perfusion rate to 30 nl/min. After recovery, peritubular capillary infusion with either verapamil or nifedipine was started. After maximal response in SFP was achieved, the tubular perfusion rate was again increased to 30 nl/min. TGF-mediated vasoconstriction was nearly abolished during treatment with these agents. (Data from [12])

associated with these "superficial" juxtamedullary nephrons are isolated with tight ligatures [15]. It is important to emphasize that, although the technique for exposing these structures is extensive, the actual nephron segments and arterioles are not dissected and anatomical tubular-vascular relationships are not interrupted [15].

Videometric techniques were used to evaluate the afferent and efferent arteriolar responses to calcium channel blockade in this unique experimental setting. As shown in Fig. 4, these experiments provide direct confirmation of previous results showing

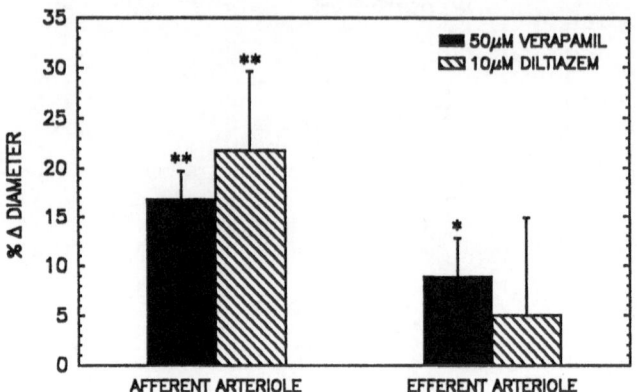

Fig. 4. Effects of calcium channel blockers on the afferent and efferent arteriolar diameters. Arteriolar inside diameters were measured utilizing videometric microscopy techniques. Control diameters averaged 23.0 ± 1.6 and 21.2 ± 2.2 μm for afferent and efferent arterioles, respectively. Verapamil and diltiazem were administered topically via the superfusing bathing solution. *, $P < 0.05$ vs control diameter; **, $P < 0.01$ vs control (Data from [14])

the ability of calcium channel blockers to dilate the afferent arterioles with maximal dilation of 17%–22% being observed. Interestingly, there was a mixed response of the efferent arteriole. Verapamil elicited a slight dilation of the efferent arterioles (9%), whereas diltiazem did not significantly influence efferent arteriolar caliber. Thus, these studies demonstrate further that calcium channel blockers predominantly dilate the afferent arterioles and provide further support to the interpretation based on whole kidney and micropuncture experiments. Other recent data have demonstrated that the calcium channel agonist, BAY K8644, constricts the preglomerular arterioles more than efferent arterioles [16]. Also, KCl-induced depolarization is a more effective constrictor of afferent than efferent arterioles [17]. In a recent micropuncture study, it was shown that manganese, which is capable of blocking transmembrane calcium flux through voltage gated as well as other entry pathways, exerted selective preglomerular vasodilation [18]. Collectively, these data support the premise that there is a fundamental difference between the intracellular calcium activation mechanisms in afferent and efferent arterioles, with voltage gated calcium channels being of predominant importance in afferent arterioles and intracellular mobilization mechanisms playing a greater role in efferent arterioles.

The influence of calcium channel blockers on the arteriolar responsiveness to angiotensin II was particularly intriguing. As shown in Fig. 5, both verapamil and diltiazem abolished the afferent arteriolar constrictor effect of angiotensin II at concentrations up to 10 nanomolar. In contrast to this effect, the responses of the efferent vessels were virtually unaffected by these calcium entry blockers. These results indicate that angiotensin II elicits its vasoconstrictor actions on afferent and efferent arterioles through different mechanisms of calcium entry, mobilization, or activation. At the afferent arterioles, essentially all of the contractile response can be explained on the basis of an increased transmembrane calcium influx. In contrast, the finding that angiotensin sensitivity persists in the presence of calcium channel block-

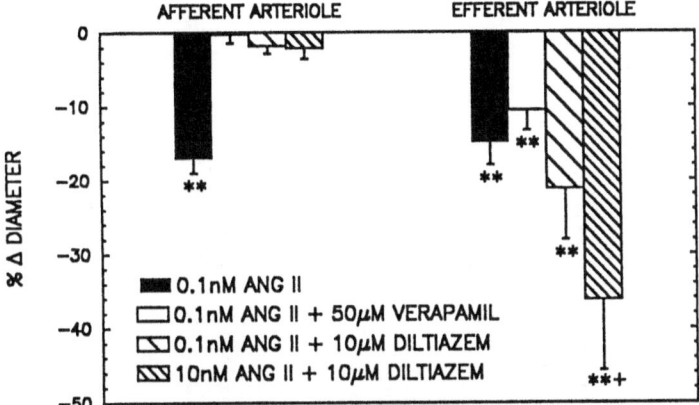

Fig. 5. Effects of calcium channel blockers on angiotensin-induced vasoconstriction of afferent and efferent arterioles. Arteriolar diameters were measured as described for Fig. 4. Responses to topical application of angiotensin II (ANG II) were assessed before and during exposure to either diltiazem or verapamil. **, P <0.01 vs control diameter; +, P <0.05 vs response to 0.1 nm ANG II plus 10 μm diltiazem. (Data from [14])

ade in efferent arterioles suggests a more complicated mechanism operating through receptor operated channels not sensitive to these blockers, or involving calcium mobilization from intracellular storage sites, as has been demonstrated for cultured vascular smooth muscle cells of aortic origin [19]. These results may have important implications that will help us to understand how, in certain pathophysiological states, the preglomerular vessels become unresponsive to angiotensin II. Such a selective loss of preglomerular sensitivity could have detrimental consequences due to altered glomerular pressure in conditions where the renin-angiotensin system is activated and only the efferent arterioles have retained their sensitivity to the elevated angiotensin II levels. Furthermore, such a setting may explain how the administration of ACE inhibitors could lead to the paradoxical reductions in glomerular function not infrequently observed in some patients [20]. These intriguing differential mechanisms of intracellular calcium activation of the afferent and efferent arterioles in response to angiotensin II emphasize the importance of studies on discrete segments of the renal microvasculature.

Macula Densa Intracellular Calcium Activating Mechanism

As already mentioned, the TGF mechanism serves as a communication link from the macula densa cells of the ascending limb of the loop of Henle to the afferent arterioles. Although signalling mechanisms remain uncertain, the effector responses at the level of the afferent arteriole appear to be dependent on voltage-dependent calcium entry mechanisms [12]. In contrast, the macula densa cells which are responsible for mediating TGF signals to the afferent arterioles appear to utilize a completely different intracellular calcium activating mechanism for the transmission of feedback

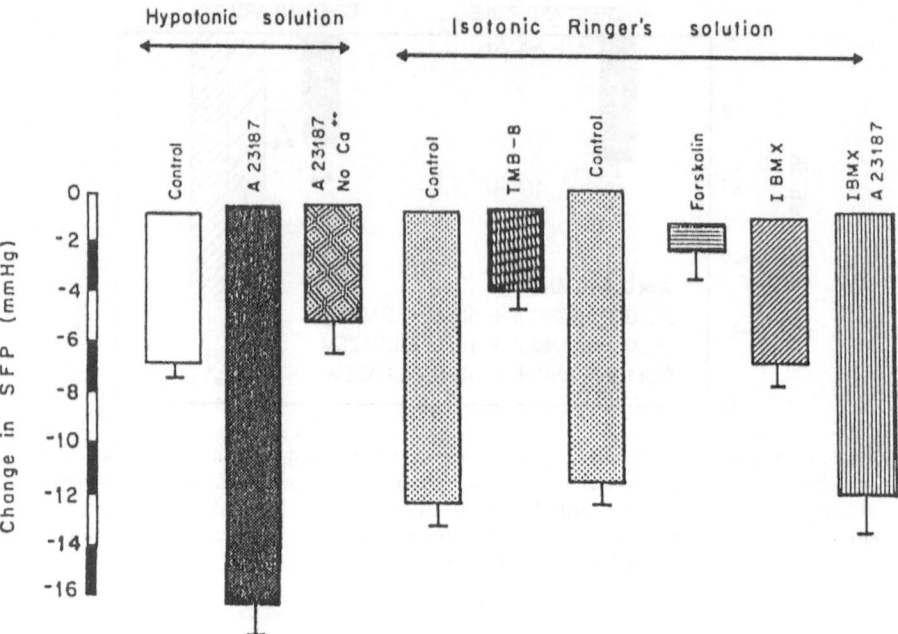

Fig. 6. Summary of the TGF responses during retrograde intralumenal perfusion with various agents that alter cytosolic calcium or cAMP. SFP, stop flow pressure. (Results taken from data in [23–25])

signals. Under normal conditions, tubular fluid osmolality at the level of the macula densa is in the range of 100 mOsm, but varies directly with flow [21]. The flow-dependent changes in solute concentration are sensed by the macula densa cells which initiate a sequence of events leading to the mediation of vasoactive signals to the afferent arteriole. Several studies have indicated that a critical intracellular event requisite for the transmission of these signals from the macula densa cells is activation of intracellular calcium [21,22].

Because of the frequent role of cytosolic calcium as a regulator of various cellular processes in other systems, we were prompted to consider how it may be involved in the mediation of TGF responses. This possibility was initially addressed by evaluating the consequences of increases in cytosolic calcium concentrations. TGF responses were assessed by the retrograde microperfusion technique, which involves perfusion of the macula densa segment with solutions of different solute concentrations. Previous studies have demonstrated that the magnitude of the TGF-mediated decrease in SFP depends on the total solute concentration of the perfusion solution, with maximum responses achieved with solutions of 120 mOsm/Kg [21]. A calcium ionophore (A23187) was utilized to artificially induce an increase in lumenal calcium permeability. As shown in Fig. 6, addition of the calcium ionophore to the perfusion solution (5–500 μM) elicited a marked augmentation of the TGF response during perfusion with a hypotonic solution (60 mOsm/Kg) which normally does not elicit substantive TGF-mediated decreases in SFP [23]. This effect of the calcium iono-phore appeared to be due to calcium entry, as indicated by further studies in which calcium was eliminated from the tubular fluid perfusion solution. These results indi-cated that A23187 artificially increased macula densa cytosolic calcium concentra-tion by allowing an entry of calcium from the tubular fluid into the cells. However, in further experiments in which the calcium ionophore was not used it was clear that changes in lumenal fluid calcium concentration normally had no significant effects. For example, total elimination of calcium from the perfusion solution or the addition of a calcium chelator to the perfusion solution did not inhibit normal TGF responses. Furthermore, the addition of verapamil in high concentrations to the perfusion solu-tion did not interfere with the ability of increases in tubular fluid osmolality to induce feedback-mediated vasoconstriction [24].

These results support the hypothesis that an increase in intracellular calcium is a critical step in the mediation of TGF signals, but that under normal conditions, trans-membrane calcium flux is probably not responsible for this increase in intracellular calcium. Additional experiments were conducted to evaluate the potential role of intracellular calcium mobilizing mechanisms in this phenomenon. TMB-8 (8-(N,N-diethylamino)-octyl-3,4,5-trimethoxybenzoate), an agent which binds to intracellu-lar calcium and prevents the release of calcium from calcium sequestering sites, was utilized in this study. During perfusion with solutions containing TMB-8 in concen-trations up to 500 micromolar, a normal feedback response was observed initially; however, the response slowly waned and was markedly attenuated after 3–5 minutes. Thus, it appeared that TMB-8 entered the macula densa cells and formed a stable complex with the intracellular calcium, thus preventing its release. Furthermore, it appeared that this inhibition of calcium release was a critical step necessary for nor-mal mediation of feedback responses. In order to determine if the effects of TMB-8 were specifically related to alterations of intracellular calcium, we combined the cal-cium ionophore with the TMB-8. Under those conditions, the A23187 completely reversed the effects of TMB-8 and a maximal feedback response was restored [24]. These results provide further evidence that the effects of TMB-8 were not non-specific, and support the concept that activation of the TGF signaling pathway nor-mally includes an intracellular calcium mobilizing event. It should also be noted that these effects were probably due to direct alterations in macula densa cell function, since it has been shown that systemic infusion of TMB-8 does not elicit renal vasodi-lator effects or interfere with renal autoregulatory behavior [11].

A number of other experiments have been conducted to probe the potential interac-tions between intracellular calcium mobilization and other signal transduction sys-tems. Experiments using calmodulin inhibitors revealed little or no role for a calcium calmodulin-interaction in the mediation of feedback signals [25]. This is another important difference between the role of intracellular calcium in the macula densa signal mediating system compared to its role in vascular smooth muscle. Interest-ingly, calmodulin antagonists significantly prolonged the recovery response follow-ing cessation of perfusion, suggesting that one potential role of calmodulin in the TGF mechanism could be to promote calcium resequestration after termination of the stimulus.

Further experiments were conducted to evaluate the potential role of cAMP as a mediator of TGF signals. Various studies have previously suggested that cAMP might be involved, because treatment with agents capable of increasing cell cAMP levels led

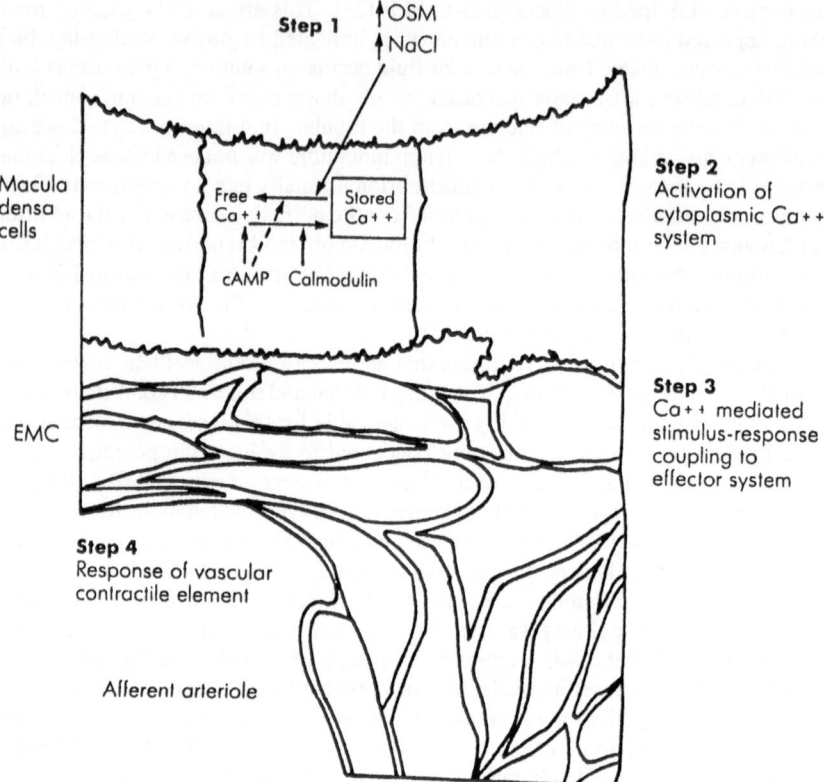

Fig. 7. Schematic presentation of macula densa signalling mechanism and the interaction of signal transduction mechanisms which regulate cytosolic calcium

to attenuation of TGF responses [26]. The inclusion of IBMX, a methylxanthine capable of increasing cAMP because of its action as a phosphodiesterose inhibitor, in the perfusion solution markedly attenuated the magnitude of the feedback response. This attenuation appeared to be primarily related to an increase in cell cAMP levels, because the increase in cellular cAMP levels elicited by treatment with dibutyryl cAMP in the presence of small concentrations of IBMX resulted in a similar attenuation of TGF vasoconstrictor responses [27]. Further experiments with forskolin, an activator of the catalytic subunit of adenylate cyclase, also caused a marked attenuation of the TGF response. Interestingly, the effects which increased cell cAMP had in attenuating TGF responses were completely abolished when we added A23187 to the perfusion solution [27]. Thus, the increase in intracellular calcium caused by the calcium ionophore reversed the inhibitory effects elicited by elevations in cAMP. These results suggest that the increases in cAMP are probably interacting with a cytosolic calcium system and may be causing TGF inhibition by reducing macula densa cytosolic calcium and preventing appropriate activation during intralumenal perfusion (Fig. 7). This conclusion, based on the results of micropuncture experiments, has received further support from recent studies on isolated perfused thick ascending limbs in which the cytosolic calcium level in the macula densa cells has been measured directly using fluorescence microscopy [28]. In response to increases in intratubular sodium chloride concentration, there was an increase in cytosolic calcium in the macula densa cells as assessed by changes in fura-2 fluorescence intensity.

Thus, one can conclude that the macula densa cells are capable of responding to increases in tubular fluid solute concentration by eliciting an increase in cell calcium that is primarily due to mobilization of calcium from intracellular sites. At present it is not clear how the increase in cell calcium may mediate feedback signals. It is possible that an increase in cytosolic calcium leads to the formation of a vasoactive agent which is secreted from the macula densa cells into the extraglomerular mesangial area and vascular cleft of the glomerulus. In turn, this agent may directly cause increase in calcium entry into afferent arteriolar smooth muscle cells by activating voltage-dependent calcium channels. It is likely that the relative insensitivity of the efferent arteriole to TGF signals is due to its lack of responsiveness to agents which influence voltage gated calcium channels and its ability to maintain vascular responsiveness to angiotensin II, even during exposure to calcium channel blockers. In terms of the TGF signal transmission pathway, some of the critical steps which remain uncertain relate to the membrane and transport events at macula densa cells which are actually responsible for detection of changes in lumenal fluid solute concentration and the ever elusive substance which is released by the macula densa cell and serves as the communication link with the smooth muscle cells of the afferent arteriole.

Acknowledgments. We would like to acknowledge the technical assistance of Anthony K. Cook and Lynn Debose and assistance from Agnes C. Buffone in preparing the manuscript. This work was supported by the National Institute of Health Grants HL18426, HL26371, and DK39202. P.K. Carmines and P.D. Bell are Established Investigators of the American Heart Association.

References

1. Exton JH (1985) Role of calcium and phosphoinositides in the action of certain hormones and neurotransmitters. J Clin Invest 75:1753–1757
2. Williamson JR, Monck JR (1989) Hormone effects on cellular calcium fluxes. Annu Rev Physiol 51:107–129
3. Cauvin C, Loutzenhiser R, Van Breemen C (1983) Mechanisms of calcium antagonist-induced vasodilation. Annu Rev Pharmacol Toxicol 23:373–396
4. Loutzenhiser R, Leyten P, Saida K, Van Breemen C (1985) Calcium compartments and mobilization during contraction of smooth muscle. In: Graver AK, Daniel EE (eds) Calcium and contractility. Humona, pp 61–92
5. Chomdej B, Bell PD, Navar LG (1977) Renal hemodynamic and autoregulatory responses to acute hypercalcemia. Am J Physiol (Renal Fluid Electrolyte Physiol 6) 232:F490–F496
6. Loutzenhiser R, Epstein M (1985) Effects of calcium channel antagonists on renal hemodynamics. Am J Physiol 249:F619–F629
7. Navar LG, Champion WJ, Thomas CE (1986) Effects of calcium channel blockade on renal vascular resistance responses to changes in perfusion pressure and angiotensin-converting enzyme inhibition in dogs. Circ Res 58:874–881

8. Ono H, Kokubun H, Hashimoto K (1974) Abolition by calcium antagonists of the autoregulation of renal blood flow. Naunyn Schmiedebergs Arch Pharmacol 285:201–207

9. Baer PG, Navar LG (1973) Renal vasodilation and uncoupling of blood flow and filtration rate autoregulation. Kidney Int 4:12–21

10. Rosivall L, Youngblood P, Navar LG (1986) Renal autoregulatory efficiency during angiotensin-converting enzyme inhibition in dogs on a low sodium diet. Renal Physiol 9:18–28

11. Ogawa N, Ono H (1988) Effect of 8-(N,N-diethylamino)octyl-3,4,5-trimethoxybenzoate (TMB-8), an inhibitor of intracellular Ca^{2+} release, on autoregulation of renal blood flow in the dog. Naunyn Schmiedebergs Arch Pharmacol 338:293–296

12. Mitchell KD, Navar LG (1990) Tubuloglomerular feedback responses during peritubular infusions of calcium channel blockers. Am J Physiol (Renal Fluid Electrolyte Physiol 27)258:F537–F544

13. Navar LG, Chomdej B, Bell PD (1975) Absence of estimated glomerular capillary pressure autoregulation during interrupted distal delivery. Am J Physiol 229:1596–1603

14. Carmines PK, Navar LG (1989) Disparate effects of Ca channel blockade on afferent and efferent arteriolar responses to ANG II. Am J Physiol (Renal Fluid Electrolyte Physiol 25)256:F1015–F1020

15. Casellas D, Navar LG (1984) In vitro perfusion of juxtamedullary nephrons in rats. Am J Physiol (Renal Fluid Electrolyte Physiol 15)246:F349–F358

16. Steinhausen M, Baehr M (1989) Vasomotion and vasoconstriction induced by a Ca^{2+}-antagonist in the split hydronephrotic kidney. Prog Appl Microcirc 14:25–39·

17. Loutzenhiser R, Hayashi K, Epstein M (1989) Divergent effects of KCl-induced depolarization on afferent and efferent arterioles. Am J Physiol 257:F561–F564

18. Lafferty HM, Gunning M, Brady HR, Brenner BM, Anderson S (1990) Renal hemodynamic and natriuretic effects of manganese and interactions with atrial natriuretic peptide. Am J Physiol (Renal Fluid Electrolyte Physiol 27)258:F998–F1004

19. Smith JB (1986) Angiotensin-receptor signaling in cultured vascular smooth muscle cells. Am J Physiol (Renal Fluid Electrolyte Physiol 19)250:F759–F769

20. Curtis JJ, Luke RG, Welchel JD, Diethelm AG, Jones P, Dustan HP (1983) Angiotensin converting enzyme inhibition in renal transplant patients with hypertension. N Engl J Med 308:377–381

21. Bell PD, Navar LG (1982) Macula densa feedback control of glomerular filtration: Role of cytosolic calcium. Miner Electrolyte Metab 8:61–77

22. Bell PD, Franco M, Navar LG (1987) Calcium as a mediator of tubuloglomerular feedback. Annu Rev Physiol 49:275–293

23. Bell PD, Navar LG (1982) Cytoplasmic calcium in the mediation of macula densa tubuloglomerular feedback responses. Science 215:670–673

24. Bell PD, Reddington M (1983) Intracellular calcium in the transmission of tubuloglomerular feedback signals. Am J Physiol 245:F295–F302

25. Bell PD (1986) Tubuloglomerular feedback responses in the rat during calmodulin inhibition. Am J Physiol 250:F715–F719

26. Schnermann J, Osswald H, Hermle M (1977) Inhibitory effect of methylxanthines on feedback control of glomerular filtration in the rat kidney. Pflugers Arch 369:39–48

27. Bell PD (1985) Cyclic AMP-calcium interaction in the transmission of tubuloglomerular feedback signals. Kidney Int 28:728–732

28. Bell PD, Franco-Guevara M, Abrahamson DR, Lapointe JY, Cardinal J (1988) Cellular mechanism for tubuloglomerular feedback signalling. In: Persson AEG, Boberg U (eds) The juxtaglomerular apparatus. Elsevier, Amsterdam, pp 63–77

The Role of Angiotensin in the Control of Renal Vascular Resistance

László Rosivall[1]

Introduction

Not only does the kidney play an essential role in regulating the renin-angiotensin system by secreting renin in response to a variety of stimuli, but it also serves as an important target tissue for angiotensin II. The renal action of angiotensin II to conserve sodium and maintain appropriate extracellular fluid volume under the condition of volume and/or salt deprivation is evoked by the direct hemodynamic and also by the tubular effects of angiotensin II, and by the consequent indirect alterations in renal peritubular Starling forces. The details of these complex effects of angiotensin on kidney function have been widely studied for a long time, raising many different issues and utilizing many different approaches. Consequently, in the literature so much—in many cases conflicting—information has been gathered that the realistic aim of this review shouldn't be more than to select some topics and focus on issues that seem to be promising for future experimental and clinical research.

Effects of Angiotensin on Renal Hemodynamics

With the interesting exception of the large arteries of the kidney, the renal vasculature is highly sensitive to angiotensin II, although some heterogeneity of response has been noted within the renal vascular beds [1-6].

Angiotensin II elicits a dose-dependent decrease in renal blood flow and similar but more variable effects on glomerular filtration rate [2-4,7]. Also, infusions of moder-

[1]Department of Pathophysiology, Semmelweis University Medical School, Budapest P.O. Box 370, H-1445, Hungary

ate amounts of angiotensin do not prevent normal autoregulatory adjustment in vascular resistance following reductions in arterial pressure [8,9].

In micropuncture experiments it has been observed that angiotensin II infusions reduce single nephron glomerular filtration rate (SNGFR) and glomerular plasma flow, the latter reduction being proportionally greater [10,11]. Afferent and efferent arteriolar resistance increased and the glomerular filtration coefficient (K_f) was decreased [10–12]. These studies suggest that the changes in afferent arteriolar resistance are greater than could be attributed specifically to the autoregulatory mechanism. Uncertainty exists, however, as to whether angiotensin II normally has a direct vasoconstrictor effect on preglomerular vessels under physiological conditions. While in most of the cases it was found that either the infusion of angiotensin or the administration of converting enzyme inhibitor altered both pre-and post-glomerular resistances in anesthetized dog [3,11,13], it has been also demonstrated that angiotensin II infusions, in pharmacological concentrations, affected preglomerular resistance only when other autoregulatory mechanisms (tubuloglomerular feedback activating and myogenic mechanism) were intact, thereby negating direct constrictor effects of angiotensin II on preglomerular vessels [14]. Even the latter investigators, however, have reported that in the presence of high intrarenal levels of adenosine or under blockade of renal prostaglandin synthesis, angiotensin II appears to have a direct vasoconstrictor effect on the preglomerular vessels [15]. Also, protective effects of vascular prostaglandins, mainly on the afferent arteriole, against the vasoconstriction due to the circulating angiotensin II was recently suggested by others [16].

In another study, the pressure in the interlobular arteries was measured in anesthetized rats by micropuncture through conicotomy and the relative interlobular arterial resistance was calculated by utilizing the pressures and renal blood flow values [17]. It was demonstrated that angiotensin II infusion had a direct vasoconstrictor effect even in the interlobular arteriole as a preglomerular response, but the constriction of interlobular arteries elicited by intravenous angiotensin II reflected more autoregulatory response and less direct effect.

In normotensive rats there is a pressure drop along the interlobular arteries, resulting in different hemodynamic conditions in the outer and inner cortical nephrons [18]. The superficial afferent arterioles are almost maximally dilated, whereas the juxtamedullary ones are significantly constricted under the condition of normo-hydration [19]. Recently it was shown that inhibition of angiotensin converting enzyme in these deep nephrons markedly changed SNGFR [20], medullary plasma flow [21], and intratubular free-flow pressure [4], indicating that angiotensin II plays a role in the regulation of juxtamedullary vascular resistance. This conclusion is also supported by the recent demonstration of significant increase in red cell flux in the vasa recta in the exposed papilla during converting enzyme inhibition [22]. Earlier studies from the same laboratories have shown that captopril increased SNGFR to a lesser extent than it increased the inner medullary blood flow [4,20,21]. Thus the overall data suggest that both afferent and efferent arteriolar resistances are under the influence of angiotensin II in the juxtamedullary nephrons.

These data indicate that angiotensin II can serve to regulate both pre- and post-glomerular resistances. It is possible, however, that under some steady state conditions the influence of angiotensin on the preglomerular vessels is counteracted, either partially or completely, by other intrarenal humoral systems.

Direct Assessment of the Effects of Angiotensin II on Renal Segmental Vascular Diameter

The inaccessibility of renal vessels in vivo under normal experimental conditions has hindered assessment of the specific segmental vascular effects of angiotensin II. This holds true particularly for the intrarenal vasculature located in the juxtamedullary area. During the past few years this issue has benefitted from the development of a variety of in vivo or in vitro techniques which allow visualization of the vessels and direct approach to renal microcirculation [5].

Utilizing the technique of transplantation of renal tissue into hamster cheek pouch it was demonstrated that afferent and efferent arterioles responded to angiotensin II and that these responses were augmented in hypertension [23]. The effects appeared to be slightly greater on the efferent arteriole. Edwards [24], however, was able to document constriction of efferent, but not afferent arterioles during exposure of isolated microvessels to angiotensin II. More recently, in similarly isolated vessel segments, it was also demonstrated that the efferent arteriole was more sensitive than the afferent arteriole to angiotensin II, whereas the sensitivity of both arterioles to norepinephrine was similar [25].

In contrast to this, an extensive study using the split hydronephrotic kidney preparation demonstrated that 1] acute intravenous administration of angiotensin II produced a significant constriction of pre- and postglomerular vessels, 2] the constriction of the preglomerular vessels in response to acute angiotensin II infusion was greater than the postglomerular constriction, 3] the constriction of preglomerular vessels primarily resulted from a direct angiotensin II constrictor action mediated by angiotensin II receptors, and to much lesser extent, from a myogenic response due to elevation of blood pressure [6]. It is of interest that, in this preparation, these workers observed attenuated vascular responses to angiotensin II, following long-term exposure, similar to those which were earlier demonstrated in dog [7]. In these experiments several segments of the renal vasculature were studied by precise identification of proximal and distal parts of a. arcuata, vas afferens and vas efferens. The diameter of a. interlobularis was measured at the distal site, near the branching point of the terminal afferent arteriole. Approximate changes in vessel diameter at controlled blood pressure were as follows: a. arcuata, -15%, -20%; a. interlobularis, -25%; vas afferens, -18%, -20%; vas efferens, -16%, -8%. It is worth noting that the diameter of certain preglomerular vessels progressively increased following angiotensin II infusion, probably reflecting the action of vasodilator substances released by the peptide.

To gain further insight, both micropuncture and videometric technique have been used to elucidate the influence of angiotensin II on various segments of the in vitro blood perfused juxtamedullary nephrons. It was demonstrated that intravascular bolus injection of angiotensin II (12.5–20 ng) increased total vascular resistance, as revealed by a rise in perfusion pressure, and induced dose-dependent and reversible decreases in glomerular capillary pressure [26]. Such a change is indicative of predominantly preglomerular vasoconstriction which could not be attributed to an autoregulatory response. In subsequent studies on the same preparation, topical application of angiotensin II induced significant reductions in diameter of arcuate and interlobular arteries, as well as of afferent and efferent arterioles [27,28,9].

Table 1. Percent changes in vessel diameter during angiotensin II treatments

AII treatment	BP controlled	A. arcuata Early	A. arcuata Late	A. interlobularis	Afferent arteriole Early	Afferent arteriole Mid	Afferent arteriole Late	Efferent arteriole Early	Efferent arteriole Mid	Efferent arteriole Late	Doses	Ref. no	Preparation
Systemic	−	−17	−20	−30	−17		−11	−12		−7	50mg/min per kg	[6]	Hydronephrotic split kidney
	−	−18	−26	−35	−29		−22	−13		−3	100mg/min per kg		
	±	−13	−20	−25	−19		−20	−17		−7	100mg/min per kg		
Topical		−4	−5	−5	−2		−9	−9		−5	10^{-9}M	[6]	Hydronephrotic split kidney
		−28	−22	−39	−35		−36	−33		−9	10^{-7}M		
						−5			−9		10^{-13}M	[23]	Tissue transplant (cheek pouch)
						−24			−31		10^{-12}M		
				±0		±0			−10		10^{-12}M	[24]	Isolated vessel
				±0		±0			−60		10^{-8}M		
						±0			−5		10^{-12}M	[25]	Isolated vessel
						−20			−60		10^{-10}M		
						−80			−95		10^{-8}M		
				−18		−20	−14		−17		10^{-12}–10^{-9}M	[27]	Isolated nephron
						−17			−15		10^{-10}M	[28]	Isolated nephron

Taken together, these observations indicate that both circulating and extravascularly administered angiotensin II can, in most cases, induce major resistance effects at both preglomerular and efferent arteriolar sites (Table 1). The angiotensin-induced changes in the caliber of a. arcuata and a. interlobularis probably represent a relatively small overall effect on preglomerular resistance, due to the big size of these vessel segments and their minor contribution to the normal pressure drop along the renal vasculature. Nevertheless, it seems clear that angiotensin II is capable of influencing the renal microcirculation at all vascular levels. The reason why the isolated renal afferent arteriole is less responsive to angiotensin II than the efferent arteriole [24,25], which observation makes this preparation clearly distinct from others, is not obvious. This observation of efferent, but of no, or significantly fewer, preglomerular effects of angiotensin II was made under conditions of stop flow in the arteriole, when there were no tubular elements and there was no blood etc. It is important to emphasize that even under these conditions, angiotensin is able to constrict preglomerular arterioles, proving the presence of angiotensin receptors in this segment, but there is a decreased sensitivity [25]. This finding, however, may also indicate that angiotensin II-induced effects on pre- and postglomerular vessel segments operate through complex and/or disparate mechanisms [28,29].

Effects of Locally Formed Angiotensin II on Renal Hemodynamics

The significance of this issue depends on two basic problems: (1) Is there enough intrarenal angiotensin formation to substantially alter renal function? and (2) Is there any difference between the effects of angiotensin II formed intrarenally, versus delivered systemically, on renal hemodynamics?

Previous studies have demonstrated that a substantial amount of angiotensin II is formed within the kidney and that this formation shows a significant correlation with renin secretion [30]. In this study it was not possible to determine the source of angiotensin I (endogenously generated vs systemically delivered) utilized by the kidney to generate angiotensin II. It was suggested earlier, however, that 90% of angiotensin I is a result of an extravascular local production [31]. This is supported by recently published data, obtained in hypertensive patients, showing that there is a rapid metabolism of angiotensin in the kidney, while there is no difference between the arterial and venous angiotensin I concentrations [32]. It was calculated that less than 20%–30% of the de novo-produced angiotensin I could be accounted for by circulating renin, indicating that most of the intrarenally formed angiotensin II comes from locally produced angiotensin I. Whatever the source of angiotensin I in the kidney, it is important that at least 20% of the angiotensin I is converted to angiotensin II in a single passage through the kidney [33]. This conversion probably occurs not only intravascularly, but also extravascularly [34] and is induced not only by the angiotensin converting enzyme, but also by other enzymes [29,34,35]. Because the angiotensin I concentration in the blood may well be several-fold higher (10–15x) than the angiotensin II concentration, as was demonstrated in dog and in human [33,36], it is probable that most of the angiotensin effects on kidney function are due to the effect of intrarenally formed angiotensin II.

It cannot yet be determined what percentage of the angiotensin I formed in the kidney originates from circulating or from intrarenally produced angiotensinogen. Recent studies show that in the kidney angiotensinogen mRNA expression is altered by sodium intake and by various pathophysiological conditions such as hypertension and cardiac failure [37,38]. The change in angiotensinogen mRNA is not necessarily parallel with renal renin gene expression [39]. These findings support the theory that intrinsic renin-angiotensin may play a substantial role in the regulation of renal function under experimental and clinical conditions.

There are many—partly overlooked—examples of data in the literature that are indicative of differences in effects on renal hemodynamics induced by circulating or by locally formed angiotensin II. Intrarenally converted angiotensin II produced somewhat different intrarenal blood flow distribution than did circulating angiotensin II [40]. Topical administration of angiotensin II in the hydronephrotic kidney preparation produced concentration-dependent reductions in the diameter of all preglomerular vessels; results just like those achieved with intravenous infusion of angiotensin II. The constrictor response of afferent arteriole to local angiotensin II, however, was not followed by a dilation during the control period, as was the case with i.v. infusion [6].

In a recent series of experiments, where angiotensin I and angiotensin II infusion were studied concurrently, it was recognized that even equiconstrictor doses of these peptides might produce slightly different effects on renal hemodynamics, i.e., GFR was more consistently decreased during angiotensin I infusions [3]. According to the above-mentioned effects of topically administered angiotensin II, it is possible that locally formed angiotensin II causes less release of protective vasodilators than does the circulating peptide. These data also indicate that intrarenal conversion of circulating angiotensin I occurs at vascular sites early enough to allow the locally formed angiotensin to decrease glomerular function. Micropuncture data show that this augmented intrarenal conversion of circulating angiotensin I reduces GFR as a consequence of decreases in glomerular filtration coefficient as well as in glomerular plasma flow, the latter being due to concomitant increases in preglomerular and efferent arteriolar resistances in superficial nephrons [11]. The existence of the difference between the effects of circulating and locally formed angiotensin II is also supported by the observation that in the sodium restricted dog, intravenous angiotensin II infusion alone, even in doses sufficient to restore renal blood flow (RBF) to control during captopril treatment when both the circulating and local formation of angiotensin II is blocked, failed to restore the increase in GFR [41].

In a micropuncture study, angiotensin I or II was infused into peritubular capillary; the objective was to determine whether angiotensin I infusion could lead to sufficient de novo generation of angiotensin II, in the peritubular or interstitial environment, to elicit effects on glomerular function. It was found that angiotensin II formed beyond the glomerular circulation could reduce SNGFR and enhance proximal tubular reabsorption [42]. Presumably, angiotensin generated from interstitially formed angiotensin I due to the enhanced renin release into the interstitium would act in a similar manner.

In a subsequent study, peritubular infusion of both angiotensin I and II, in doses which did not effect base-line glomerular capillary pressure, increased the sensitivity of the tubuloglomerular feedback mechanism [43]. Angiotensin I or angiotensin II plus saralasin had no effects. These observations indicate that angiotensin II formed in the postglomerular capillary and/or interstitial environment can gain access to, and enhance the sensitivity of, the vascular elements that respond to signals from the macula densa cell. Considering recent morphological observations of the juxtaglomerular apparatus [44], it is also possible that the enhanced sensitivity of the tubuloglomerular feedback mechanism is due to the alteration of the interstitial fluid balance of the juxtaglomerular apparatus, caused by angiotensin II.

Thus, it can be concluded that the amount of angiotensin II formed intrarenally is enough to significantly contribute to the regulation of intrarenal hemodynamics and, indeed, it is probable that most of the effects of angiotensin on kidney function are due to the effects of intrarenally formed angiotensin II. According to experimental data, intrarenally formed angiotensin II may have effects on renal circulation which are basically similar to those of circulating angiotensin II; however, there are also some subtle, but significant, differences.

Conclusions

In this presentation, recent studies on (1) the effects of angiotensin on renal hemodynamics, (2) direct assessment of the effects of angiotensin II on renal vascular segmental diameter, and (3) the effects of locally formed angiotensin II on renal hemodynamics have been reviewed.

It has been demonstrated, in whole kidney and micropuncture studies, that angiotensin II, either delivered systematically or formed locally, has a crucial role in the regulation of both afferent and efferent arteriolar resistances throughout the cortex. Angiotensin-induced constriction of preglomerular arterioles has been further confirmed by direct assessment of segmental vascular responses during systemic or topical administration of the peptide. The preglomerular vasoconstrictor effects of the peptide are not restricted only to the afferent arteriole. Angiotensin II, formed even beyond the glomerular circulation in the postglomerular capillary and/or interstitial environment, can reduce glomerular and proximal tubular function. Recent findings on intrarenal angiotensin formation, e.g., the existence and response of angiotensinogen mRNA to different experimental and clinical conditions, the high intrarenal conversion of angiotensin I to II, the higher concentration of angiotensin I than angiotensin II in the blood, etc., all support the idea that the effects of angiotensin II on renal hemodynamics may be due mainly to the effects of the locally formed peptide. Therefore, it is especially important to emphasize that there are some observed differences between the effects of intrarenally formed angiotensin II versus systemically delivered angiotensin II on renal hemodynamics.

Acknowledgments. We are grateful to S. Adamkó for technical assistance. This study was supported by a Grant: OTKA/207 from the Hungarian Research Foundation.

References

1. Bohr DF (1974) Angiotensin on vascular smooth muscle. In: Page IH, Bumpus FM (eds) Angiotensin. Springer, New York, pp 424–440 (Handbook of experimental pharmacology, vol 37)

2. Fagard RH, Cowley AW, Navar LG, Langford HG, Guyton AC (1976) Renal responses to slight elevations of renal arterial plasma angiotensin II concentration in dogs. Clin Exp Pharmacol Physiol 3:531–538
3. Rosivall L, Navar LG (1983) Effects on renal hemodynamics of intrarenal infusions of angiotensins I and II. Am J Physiol 245:F181–F187
4. Göransson A, Sjöquist M, Ulfendahl HR (1986) Superficial and juxtamedullary nephron function during converting enzyme inhibition. Am J Physiol 251:F25–F33
5. Navar LG, Gilmore JP, Joyner WL, Steinhausen M, Edwards RM, Casellas D, Carmines PK, Zimmerhackl LB, Yokota SD (1986) Direct assessment of renal microcirculatory dynamics. Fed Proc 45:2851–2861
6. Steinhausen M, Sterzel RB, Fleming JT, Kühn R, Weis S (1987) Acute and chronic effects of angiotensin II on the vessels of the split hydronephrotic kidney. Kidney Int 31:S1–S10
7. Lohmeier TE, Cowley AW Jr (1979) Hypertensive and renal effects of chronic low level intrarenal angiotensin infusion in the dog. Circ Res 44:154–160
8. Kiil F, Kjekshus J, Loyning E (1969) Renal autoregulation during infusion of noradrenaline, angiotensin, and acetylcholine. Acta Physiol Scand 76:10–23
9. Casellas D, Carmines PK, Dupont M, Redon P, Moore LC (1990) Arteriolar renin and vascular effects of angiotensin II in juxtamedullary nephrons. Kidney Int 38:suppl 30:65–68
10. Blantz RC, Konnen KS, Tucker BJ (1976) Angiotensin II effects upon the glomerular microcirculation and ultrafiltration coefficient of the rat. J Clin Invest 57:419–434
11. Rosivall L, Carmines PK, Navar LG (1984) Effects of renal arterial angiotensin I infusion on glomerular dynamics in sodium replete dogs. Kidney Int 26:263–268
12. Schor N, Ichikawa I, Brenner BM (1980) Glomerular adaptations to chronic dietary salt restriction or excess. Am J Physiol 238:F428–F436
13. Navar LG, Jirakulsomchok D, Bell PD, Thomas CE, Huang WC (1982) Influence of converting enzyme inhibition on renal hemodynamics and glomerular dynamics in sodium-restricted dogs. Hypertension 4:56–68
14. Hall JE (1986) Regulation of glomerular filtration rate and sodium excretion by angiotensin II. Fed Proc 45:1431–1437
15. Olsen ME, Hall JE, Montani JP, Cornell JE (1987) Interaction between renal prostaglandins and angiotensin II in controlling glomerular filtration in the dog. Clin Sci 72:429–436
16. Heller J, Horácek V (1990) The effect of converting enzyme inhibitor, angiotensin II, and Saralasin on glomerular haemodynamics in the dog. Kidney Int 38:suppl 30:74–76
17. Keyeraas KJ, Aukland K (1987) Interlobular arterial resistance: influence of renal arterial pressure and angiotensin II. Kidney Int 31:1291–1298
18. Källskog Ö, Lindbom LO, Ulfendahl HR, Wolgast M (1976) Hydrostatic pressures within the vascular structures of the rat kidney. Pflugers Arch 363:205–210
19. Ericson A, Sjöquist M, Ulfendahl HR (1982) Single glomerular filtration rate in superficial and deep nephrons in rat kidneys. Acta Physiol Scand 114:201–209
20. Göransson A, Sjöquist M (1985) The effect of a converting enzyme inhibitor on autoregulation and intrarenal distribution of glomerular filtration in the rat. Acta Physiol Scand 124:515–523
21. Sjöquist M, Göransson A, Hansell P, Ulfendahl HR (1985) Regulation of filtration rate and blood flow in juxtamedullary nephrons of the rat kidney. Acta Physiol Scand 123:4A
22. Hansell P, Sjöquist M, Ulfendahl HR (1988) Effect of a converting-enzyme inhibitor on vasa recta blood flow in rat kidney. Am J Physiol 254:F492–F499
23. Click RL, Joyner WL, Gilmore JP (1979) Reactivity of glomerular afferent and efferent arterioles in renal hypertension. Kidney Int 15:109–115
24. Edwards RM (1983) Segmental effects of norepinephrine and angiotensin II on isolated renal microvessels. Am J Physiol 244:F526–F534
25. Yuan BH, Robinette JB, Conger JD (1990) Effect of angiotensin II and norepinephrine on isolated rat afferent and efferent arterioles. Am J Physiol 258:F741–F750

26. Casellas D, Carmines PK, Navar LG (1985) Microvascular reactivity of in vitro blood perfused juxtamedullary nephrons from rats. Kidney Int 28:752–759

27. Carmines PK, Morrison TK, Navar LG (1986) Angiotensin II effects on microvascular diameters of in vitro blood-perfused juxtamedullary nephrons. Am J Physiol 251:F610–F618

28. Carmines PK, Navar LG (1989) Disparate effects of Ca channel blockade on afferent and efferent arteriolar responses to ANG II. Am J Physiol 256:F1015–1020

29. Okamura T, Okunishi H, Ayajiki K, Toda N (1990) Conversion of angiotensin I to angiotensin II in dog isolated renal artery: role of two different angiotensin II-generating enzymes. J Cardiovasc Pharmacol 15:353–359

30. Rosivall L, Narkates J, Oparil S (1987) De novo intrarenal formation of angiotensin II during control and enhanced renin secretion. Am J Physiol 252:F1118–F1123

31. Campbell DJ (1985) The site of angiotensin production. J Hypertens 3:199–207

32. Admiraal PJJ, Derkx FHM, Danser AHJ, Pieterman H, Schalekamp MADH (1990) Metabolism and production of angiotensin I in different vascular beds in subjects with hypertension. Hypertension 15:44–55

33. Rosivall L, Rinder DF, Champion J, Khosla MC, Navar LG, Oparil S (1983) Intrarenal angiotensin I conversion at normal and reduced renal blood flow in the dog. Am J Physiol 245:F408–F415

34. Bührle CP, Rosivall L, Taugner R (1987) Intrarenal generation of angiotensin II evaluated by an electrophysiological technique. Am J Physiol 252:F635–F644

35. Wintroub BU, Klickstein LB, Dzau VJ, Watt KWK (1984) Granulocyte-angiotensin system. Identification of angiotensinogen as the plasma protein substrate of leukocyte cathepsin G. Biochemistry 23:227–232

36. Kawamura M, Yoshida K, Akabane S, Matsushima Y, Kawano Y, Kojima S, Takahashi N, Shimamoto K, Ito K, Omae T (1987) A sensitive method for precise measurement of endogenous angiotensins I, II and III in human plasma. Clin Exp Theory Practice A9: 687–691

37. Ludwig G, Ganten D, Murakami K, Fasching U, Hackenthal E (1987) Relationship between renin mRNA and renin secretion in adrenalectomized, salt depleted, or converting enzyme inhibitor-treated rats. Mol Cell Endocrinol 50:223–229

38. Dzau VJ, Ingelfinger JR (1989) Molecular biology and pathophysiology of the intrarenal renin-angiotensin system. J Hypertens 7:S3–S8

39. Gomez RA, Lynch KR, Chevalier RL, Everett AD, Johns DW, Wilfong N, Peach MJ, Carey RM (1988) Renin and angiotensinogen gene expression and intrarenal renin distribution during ACE inhibition. Am J Physiol 254:F900–F906

40. Britton SL (1981) Intrarenal vascular effects of angiotensin I and angiotensin II. Am J Physiol 240:H914–H919

41. Carmines PK, Rosivall L, Till MF, Navar LG (1983) Renal hemodynamic effects of captopril in anesthetized sodium-restricted dogs. Renal Physiol 6:281–287

42. Mitchell KD, Navar LG (1987) Superficial nephron responses to peritubular capillary infusions of angiotensins I and II. Am J Physiol 252:F818–F824

43. Mitchell KD, Navar LG (1988) Enhanced tubuloglomerular feedback during peritubular infusions of angiotensins I and II. Am J Physiol 255:F383–F390

44. Rosivall L (1990) Morphology and function of distal part of the afferent arteriole. Kidney Int 38:suppl 30:10–15

Dietary Factors and Progression of Chronic Renal Failure

Chair: Giuseppe Maschio (Italy)
William E. Mitch (USA)

Effects of Lipid Manipulations in Chronic Renal Failure

WILLIAM F. KEANE, BERTRAM L. KASISKE, MICHAEL P. O'DONNELL, PAUL G. SCHMITZ, and YOUNGKI KIM[1]

SUMMARY. Experimental results have demonstrated that a number of effects of hyperlipidemia are involved in the initiation and progression of glomerular injury. First, hyperlipidemia has been associated with the development of progressive mesangial expansion. This expanded mesangium is constituted, in part, by an accumulation of laminin, fibronectin and collagen. These changes in the mesangial region preceded the development of focal glomerulosclerosis (FGS). Similar changes in the mesangium have been observed in clinical and experimental studies, lending credence to the hypothesis that changes in mesangial matrix contribute to the development of FGS. The mechanisms whereby lipid-induced expansion of the mesangial region occur are poorly understood. A second effect of hyperlipidemia is to increase the number of glomerular Ia+ macrophages. This influx of macrophages into glomeruli is reminiscent of the influence of hyperlipidemia on macrophage subendothelial localization seen in large vessels during the development of atherosclerosis. Macrophages have also been implicated in glomerular injury in a variety of experimental renal diseases. However, the role that the macrophage or macrophage derived products may play in the development of lipid-induced glomerular injury is at present unknown. Finally, lipid-induced glomerular injury may ultimately lead to altered glomerular hemodynamics, specifically glomerular hypertension, a factor that may contribute to glomerular injury. Indeed, experimental data suggest that an interaction between hypertension and hyperlipidemia may occur, resulting in additive glomerular damage. This interaction between risk factors for glomerular injury may be similar to the interaction between risk factors seen in patients with atherosclerosis.

Introduction

It has been established that once a critical number of functioning nephrons have been injured progressive loss of renal function may ensue, even though the original cause

[1]Department of Medicine, Division of Nephrology, Hennepin County Medical Center, and Division of Pediatric Nephrology, University of Minnesota Hospital, University of Minnesota Medical School, Minneapolis, MN 55415, USA

of injury is no longer present [1]. The mechanisms involved in progressive renal injury have been extensively investigated during the past decade, and it has been found that a number of physiologic and metabolic changes that occur in the course of progressive renal disease may contribute to glomerular destruction [2,3]. Based on pharmacological and dietary intervention studies, it has been postulated that hemodynamic factors, particularly glomerular hypertension, are important in the pathogenesis of progressive renal injury [1–4]. Additionally, experimental studies have demonstrated that genetic and metabolic factors, specifically abnormal lipid metabolism, may modulate glomerular damage [2,3,5–7]. The possibility that abnormal lipid metabolism could be important in the development and progression of renal injury has intrigued investigators for well over a hundred years. Support for the notion that lipids are involved in renal injury can be derived from three areas of experimental investigation. First, high cholesterol diets are associated with albuminuria and glomerular injury in different animal species. Second, pharmacological agents, including bile acid sequestrants, 3-hydroxy 3-methyl coenzyme A (HMG-CoA) reductase inhibitors, and fibrate derivatives have reduced circulating lipids and ameliorated glomerular injury in different experimental models of renal disease associated with hyperlipidemia. Third, the intake of large amounts of dietary polyunsaturated fatty acids of the omega-3 and omega-6 classes has also decreased circulating lipids and reduced glomerular injury in a variety of models of renal disease.

Dietary Induced Hypercholesterolemia

It is well established that feeding a high cholesterol diet to different animal species leads to focal glomerulosclerosis (FGS). Interestingly, the extent of glomerular injury has usually correlated with the circulating cholesterol level. The mechanism for these glomerular effects is, however, not completely understood. Glomerular hypercellularity and expansion of the mesangial matrix were demonstrated as early morphologic changes in animals fed a high cholesterol diet [8,9]. For example, in rats fed a diet of increased cholesterol content, significant albuminuria and, ultimately, FGS was observed [9]. Glomerular enlargement, mesangial expansion, and hypercellularity were evident after only one month of increased circulating cholesterol. These changes in the glomerular mesangium preceded the appearance of FGS. Immunocytochemical studies have demonstrated that glomerular hypercellularity was, in part, a result of an increase in Ia+ macrophages [8]. A diet high in cholesterol has also led to an increased cortical content of cholesteryl esters [8,9]. In addition, a significant reduction in cortical arachidonic acid and an increased linoleic acid content were found in the cortical phospholipid fraction, suggesting an inhibitory effect of elevated cholesterol levels on desaturation and elongation of this essential fatty acid [9]. These changes in cholesteryl esters and fatty acids were also found to correlate significantly with the presence of glomerular injury [9]. Thus, high dietary cholesterol induced cellular, morphological, and biochemical changes in glomeruli similar to the changes, induced by hypercholesterolemia in large vessels, which were associated with the development of atherosclerosis. The precise role that these glomerular changes play in the development of FGS remains to be defined.

Recently, physiological studies in cholesterol fed rats have also been reported [9]. Micropuncture studies were performed after 6–8 weeks of a high cholesterol diet when albuminuria was minimal (> 5mg/24h), and glomeruli demonstrated mesangial expansion but no FGS [9]. In these studies single nephron glomerular filtration rate and plasma flow were maintained. However, an increase in glomerular capillary pressure (P_{GC}) and an increase in the transcapillary hydraulic pressure were observed. This increment in hydraulic pressure occurred, in part, because of an increase in colloid osmotic pressure, and a trend toward an increase in efferent arteriolar resistance [9]. These changes in osmotic pressure are unique to this model of hypercholesterolemia. In addition to changes in osmotic pressure and arteriolar resistance, diet-induced hypercholesterolemia may alter blood rheologic properties and these effects could also contribute to changes in glomerular hemodynamic function. Thus, in this model of diet-induced hypercholesterolemia both hemodynamic and structural abnormalities have been described that could contribute to progressive glomerular injury. In addition, it has been demonstrated that unilateral nephrectomy, clip hypertension, chemically induced diabetes and the nephrotic syndrome exaggerated the degree of glomerular injury in cholesterol-fed animals [6,7,10]. Thus, it would appear that experimentally induced hemodynamic stresses, as well as direct glomerular injury, may also interact with hyperlipidemia to exaggerate nephron damage.

Although hypercholesterolemia is associated with glomerular injury, the mechanism whereby this occurs is unknown. Recent advances in our understanding of the metabolism of lipoproteins have suggested that modifications in the structure of lipoproteins may affect their potential for vascular injury. In this regard, probucol, an antilipemic agent with anti-oxidant activity, has been shown to modify diet-induced hypercholesterolemic glomerular injury independent of changes in circulating cholesterol levels [11]. These data suggested the possibility that the local glomerular deposition of lipoproteins and their oxidation might be important in lipid-induced glomerular injury. In support of this concept, mesangial cells have been shown to express receptors for low-density lipoproteins (LDL) [12]. In addition, LDL cholesterol induced a biphasic effect on mesangial cell proliferation. At lower concentrations (< 200 μg/ml), LDL stimulated proliferation, while at higher concentrations of LDL (2000 μg/ml) inhibition of mesangial cell growth was observed and frank cytotoxicity was demonstrated [12–14]. The inhibition of mesangial cell growth at the higher LDL concentrations was associated with a tenfold increase in LDL malonaldehyde, a measure of lipid peroxidation [14]. Since mesangial cells are known to generate reactive oxygen molecules [15], we assessed whether scavengers of reactive oxygen molecules would be effective in preventing their peroxidation of lipoprotein and thus, their cytotoxicity. In these studies, both superoxide dismutase and butylated hydroxytoluene, scavengers of reactive oxygen molecules, decreased formation of malonaldehyde and abrogated the cytotoxic effects of oxidized LDL [14]. Thus, reactive oxygen molecules derived from mesangial cells might be important in altering lipids and rendering them cytotoxic. The possibility that mesangial cells can oxidize LDL is of more than passing interest. Oxidized LDL has recently been demonstrated to be present in atherosclerotic lesions in experimental models of atherosclerosis [16]. In addition, oxidized LDL is a chemo-attractant and is also endocytosed by macrophages and mesangial cells, through a scavenger receptor mechanism, at a more rapid rate than normal LDL [16]. This ultimately leads to increased formation of cholesteryl esters and foam cells. The biochemical demonstration of increased cholesteryl esters and the appearance of macrophages and foam cells in the glomerulus of cholesterol-fed rats [9] lends credence to the notion that oxidized LDL could participate in the glomerular injury seen in models of lipid-induced renal disease.

Pharmacological Treatment of Hyperlipidemia and the Pathogenesis of Glomerulosclerosis

In the obese Zucker rat, hyperlipidemia and microalbuminuria are present at 10–12 weeks of age [17,18]. Hypercholesterolemia becomes more pronounced as albuminuria increases. Mesangial matrix expansion and an increase in mesangial cellularity accompany the development of albuminuria. At 6 months of age, FGS is evident and subsequently progresses. Mild systemic hypertension and reduced renal function become manifest as glomerular and tubular interstitial injury evolve [17,18]. Immunohistochemical studies to define the changes which occurred in mesangial matrix in obese Zucker rats before the development of FGS have demonstrated that, at 24–28 weeks of age, obese rats have increased mesangial deposition of fibronectin, laminin, and type IV collagen, compared to lean Zucker rats. Glomerular staining for types I and III collagen was also increased in obese rats, but to a lesser extent. Thus, these studies indicated that the morphologic changes in the mesangial matrix by light microscopy are associated with an increase in accumulation of specific matrix proteins. In addition, we have demonstrated increased apolipoprotein (Apo) B deposits in glomerular sclerotic areas and in segmental areas of mesangial expansion. Since Apo B is the principal apolipoprotein of very low density lipoproteins in rats this observation may have important implications with respect to lipid-mesangial cell interactions. Characterization of the increased glomerular cellularity by immunocytochemical techniques demonstrated that obese rat glomeruli contain a three-fold increase in the number of Ia$^+$ macrophages in the mesangial region. These glomerular cellular changes were similar to those reported by us in dietary-induced hypercholesterolemic rats [9].

Micropuncture studies in obese and lean Zucker rats demonstrated normal glomerular function at 10–12 weeks of age, when only mild glomerular matrix expansion and minimal albuminuria (<5 mg/24h) were present [18]. We have recently studied older obese Zucker rats at 22–26 weeks of age when albuminura was increased (>50mg/24h), glomerular mesangial expansion was marked, but FGS was minimal [19]. In these studies, single nephron filtration rate was maintained by an increased P_{GC}. The mechanism responsible for the development of glomerular hypertension in older obese Zucker rats is unknown. Alterations in glomerular production of vasoactive substances or changes in blood rheology could have participated in the development of these hemodynamic changes. Thus, in this experimental model, glomerular hypertension developed late in the course of glomerular injury and may play a role in further amplifying renal injury.

Since hyperlipidemia was an early change in obese Zucker rats and preceded not only FGS, but also hemodynamic changes, we hypothesized that hyperlipidemia contributed to glomerular injury [20]. To test this thesis, we reduced circulating lipids with clofibric acid, the pharmacologically active form of clofibrate, or with lovastatin, an HMG-Co A reductase inhibitor. These therapies decreased serum lipids, reduced albuminuria, and prevented FGS [20]. In addition, with each of these therapies a decrease in mesangial cellularity and matrix expansion was observed. Micropuncture assessments performed after 4 weeks of antilipemic therapy failed to demonstrate alterations in glomerular hemodynamic function that could explain these beneficial effects [20].

The importance of systemic and glomerular hypertension in modulating progressive renal injury has been described [1–4]. In the remnant kidney model, for example, removal of 80%-90% of renal mass was accompanied by hypertension, proteinuria, uremia, and death. In addition, abnormal circulating lipids were found soon after ablative surgery, and secondary hypercholesterolemia developed as albuminuria worsened. We have shown that therapy with clofibrate or lovastatin effectively prevented secondary hypercholesterolemia in the remnant kidney model; this was associated with a reduction in proteinuria and decreased glomerular damage [21]. The effect of these agents appeared independent of effects on systemic or glomerular pressures [21].

The Dahl salt-sensitive rat is a model of systemic hypertension in which albuminuria and progressive glomerular damage are present [22]. Interestingly, hyperlipidemia was evident before many of the structural and functional changes developed in these rats [23]. Therapy with lovastatin has recently been shown to prevent the progressive increase in cholesterol levels and to have dramatically reduced albuminuria and FGS [24]. Thus, in two experimental models of systemic and glomerular hypertension associated with hypercholesterolemia, therapy with lipid lowering agents reduced the degree of proteinuria and the extent of glomerular injury. Finally, in studies of the nephrotic syndrome induced by the aminonucleoside of puromycin, a reduction in circulating lipids by cholestyramine or lovastatin has been shown to decrease glomerular injury and to preserve renal function [25,26]. Thus, in models of experimental disease in which hypercholesterolemia is a primary abnormality (obese Zucker rat), or in models in which abnormalities of lipids occur as a consequence of renal disease, pharmacologic modification of circulating lipids resulted in amelioration of glomerular injury and preservation of renal function.

The Effects of Polyunsaturated Fatty Acids in Glomerular Injury

The influence of dietary polyunsaturated fatty acid (PUFA) supplementation on the progression of glomerular injury has been evaluated in a number of immune and nonimmune models of renal disease [27]. In these studies, dietary supplementation with either the omega-3 or the omega-6 class of PUFAs has been evaluated and the results have shown that both PUFAs reduced proteinuria and decreased glomerular damage (Table 1). Recently, we have investigated the effects of PUFA supplementation in the obese Zucker rat. These studies were motivated by the observation that reduced cortical contents of omega-3 and omega-6 PUFAs were present in obese Zucker rats and that these changes correlated with glomerular injury [28]. We used diets containing sunflower and menhaden oils (diets enriched in omega-6 and omega-3 PUFA, respectively), and diets containing coconut oil or beef tallow (enriched in medium and long chain saturated fatty acids, respectively) and compared these to rats fed standard rodent chow. All rats were pair-fed and grew normally during the six-month study. Throughout the experiment, comparable blood pressures were measured in all groups. At the conclusion of the study, the PUFA diet rats demonstrated lower lipids

Table 1. Effects of polyunsaturated fatty acids on renal injury

Model	↑Linoleic acid (ω-6)	↑Eicosapentanoic acid (ω-3)
Murine lupus models	No change	↓
Murine immune-mediated models	↓	↓
5/6 Nephrectomy model	↓	↑/↓
Obese zucker model	↓	↓

↑, increase; ↓, decrease

and lower urine albumin excretion rates. In both the sunflower and menhaden oil supplemented groups of obese Zucker rats, there was a significant reduction in FGS and mesangial matrix expansion. Similar effects of a fish oil (Max EPA) supplemented diet in obese Zucker rats has also been recently reported [29]. The mechanisms whereby PUFA supplemented diets may ameliorate glomerular injury in obese Zucker rat are at present unknown. However, in addition to their lipid lowering effects, these fatty acids may influence renal hemodynamics, alter macrophage function, change eicosanoid production, and alter cell membrane biophysical properties [27]. Since many of these effects may modify renal injury, further investigations to define the role of these potential beneficial effects of PUFAs are necessary.

Acknowledgments. The authors acknowledge the assistance of Lee Schroeder and Ellen Davis in preparing this manuscript. Supported, in part, by grants received from the National Institutes of Health and the Baxter Extramural Grant Program.

References

1. Brenner BM (1985) Nephron adoption to renal injury. Am J Physiol 249:324–337
2. Keane WF, Anderson S, Aurell M, deZeeuw D, Narins RG, Povar G (1989) Angiotensin converting enzyme inhibitors and progressive renal insufficiency. Ann Intern Med 111:503–516
3. Klahr S, Schreiner G, Ishikawa I (1988) The progression of renal disease. N Engl J Med 318:1657–166
4. Anderson S, Rennke HG, Brenner BM (1986) Therapeutic advantage of converting enzyme inhibitors in arresting progressive renal disease associated with systemic hypertension in the rat. J Clin Invest 77:1993–2000
5. Moorhead JF, Chan MK, El-Nahas M, Varghese Z, et al. (1982) Lipid nephrotoxicity in chronic progressive glomerular and tubulointerstitial disease. Lancet I:1309–1311
6. Keane WF, Kasiske BL, O'Donnell MP (1988) Lipids and progressive glomerulosclerosis: A model analogous to atherosclerosis. Am J Nephrol 8:261–271
7. Diamond JR, Karnovsky MJ (1988) Focal and segmental glomerulosclerosis: Analogies to atherosclerosis. Kidney Int 33:917–924
8. Al-Shebeb T, Frohlich J, Magil AB (1988) Glomerular disease in hypercholesterolemic guinea pigs: a pathogenetic study. Kidney Int 33:498–507
9. Kasiske BL, O'Donnell MP, Schmitz PG, Kim Y, Keane WF (1990) Renal injury of diet induced hypercholesterolemia in rats. Kidney Int 37:880–891
10. Kasiske BL, O'Donnell MP, Cowardin W, Keane WF (1990) Lipids and the kidney. Hypertension 15:443–450

11. Kaplan R, Aynedjian HS, Bank N, Schlondorff D (1990) Cholesterol feeding causes renal vasoconstriction via oxidized lipoprotein activation of thromboxane. Kidney Int 37:371A.

12. Wasserman J, Santiago A, Rifici V, Holthofer H, Scharschmidt L, Epstein M, Schlondorff D (1989) Interactions of low density lipoprotein with rat mesangial cells. Kidney Int 35: 1168–1174

13. Wheeler DC, Persaud JW, Fernando R, Sweeny P, Varghese Z, Moorhead JF (1990) Effects of low density lipoproteins on mesangial cell growth and viability in vitro. Nephrol Dial Transplant 5:185–191

14. Keane WF, Phillips J, Kasiske BL, O'Donnell MP, Kim Y (1990) Injurious effects of low density lipoprotein on human mesangial cells. Kidney Int 37:509A.

15. Baud L, Hagege J, Sraer J, Rondeau E, Perez J, Ardaillou R (1983) Reactive oxygen production by cultured rat glomerular mesangial cells during phagocytosis is associated with stimulation of lipoxygenase activity. J Exp Med 158:1836–1852

16. Steinberg D, Parthasarthy S, Carew TE, Khoo JC, Witztum JL (1989) Modifications of low density lipoprotein that increase its atherogenicity. N Engl J Med 320:915–924

17. Kasiske BL, Cleary MP, O'Donnell MP, Keane WF (1985) Effects of genetic obesity on renal structure and function in the Zucker rat. J Lab Clin Med 106:598–604

18. O'Donnell MP, Kasiske BL, Cleary MP, Keane WF (1985) Effects of genetic obesity on renal structure and function in the Zucker rat II: Micropuncture studies. J Lab Clin Med 106:605–610

19. Schmitz PG, O'Donnell MP, Kasiske BL, Keane WF (1990) Glomerular capillary pressure is increased in old obese Zucker rats and is unchanged with enalapril. Kidney Int 37:520A.

20. Kasiske BL, O'Donnell MP, Cleary MP, Keane WF (1988) Treatment of hyperlipidemia reduces glomerular injury in obese Zucker rats. Kidney Int 33:667–672

21. Kasiske BL, O'Donnell MP, Garvis WJ, Keane WF (1988) Pharmacologic treatment of hyperlipidemia reduces glomerular injury in rat 5/6 nephrectomy model of chronic renal failure. Circ Res 62:367–374

22. Raij L, Azar S, Keane WF (1984) Mesangial immune injury, hypertension, and progressive glomerular damage in Dahl rats. Kidney Int 26:137–143

23. O'Donnell MP, Kasiske BL, Keane WF (1989) Risk factors for glomerular injury in rats with genetic hypertension. Am J Hypertens 2:9–13

24. O'Donnell MP, Kasiske BL, Schmitz PG, Katz SA, Keane WF (1990) Contrasting effects of lovastatin and enalapril and glomerular injury in Dahl salt-sensitive rats. Kidney Int 37:391A.

25. Hanchak NA, Karnovsky MJ, Diamond JR (1988) Cholestyramine resin lowers acute and recurrent proteinuria in chronic puromycin aminonucleoside necrosis. Kidney Int 33:376A.

26. Harris KPG, Purkerson ML, Yates J, Klahr S (1990) Lovastatin ameliorates the development of glomerulosclerosis and uremia in experimental nephrotic syndrome. Am J Kidney Dis 15:16–23

27. Schmitz PG, Kasiske BL, O'Donnell MP, Keane WF (1989) Lipids and progressive renal injury. Semin Nephrol 9:354–369

28. Kasiske BL, O'Donnell MP, Cleary MP, Keane WF (1989) Effects of reduced renal mass on tissue lipids and renal injury in hyperlipidemic rats. Kidney Int 35:40–48

29. Moorhead JF, Wheeler DC, Varghese Z (1989) Glomerular structures and lipids in progressive renal disease. Am J Med 87 (Suppl 5):12N–20N

Which Diet and When to Start It, in Patients with Chronic Renal Disease

Lamberto Oldrizzi, Carlo Rugiu, Vincenzo De Biase, and Giuseppe Maschio[1]

Summary. The effects of both early and late prescriptions of low-protein diets on the clinical course of chronic renal failure have been reviewed.

Many statistical tests showed that the clinical course of chronic renal failure was significantly worse in those patients to whom late conservative treatment was given.

This evaluation was carried out in an overall patient population of ($n = 450$) and in subjects with progressively declining renal function over time.

An analysis of the pros and cons of unsupplemented and supplemented low-protein diets is included in the second part of this review.

Introduction

Dietary treatment has been part of the conservative management of chronic renal failure (CRF) since the early 1960s. However, a renewed interest in the role of reduced protein intake has been shown in the last 10 years, mainly due to its regulating action on renal function when the nephron mass is reduced [1]. Nowadays, some important questions still remain to be answered regarding dietary treatment: when to use diets and how to use diets with CRF patients?

The presence in the early stages of CRF of well established functional and morphological damage [2] represents a valid motivation for early initiation of dietary protein restriction. Experimental evidence [3–7] exists that dietary treatment exerts the most positive effects when applied in the early stages of renal disease. Similarly, clinical studies [8] indicate a key role, at least as far as the progression of CRF is concerned, of early dietary treatment.

---

[1]Division of Nephrology, University of Verona, 37126 Verona, Italy

When to Diet

In line with these suggestions, we were looking for a value of renal function (we may call it "the point of no return") beyond which the positive effects of a low protein diet progressively decrease.

In general, we might discuss a zone, rather than a point, of no return; according to our 15-year clinical experience, we believe that such a zone should be identified within serum creatinine (SCreat) values ranging from 1.8 to 2.0 mg/dl.

This assumption is supported by a step-by-step statistical evaluation [9] performed on clinical data obtained from 450 patients with chronic renal failure, all kept on low protein diets.

Renal Survival Curves

Assuming a SCreat equal to or higher than 10 mg/dl to be "renal death," renal survival probability was computed by the Kaplan Meier method.

In the overall patient population, renal survival probability at 120 months was 62.4%. After stratifying the patients according to their initial SCreat values, two groups were identified regarding progression: patients with SCreat lower at the start than 1.8 mg/dl (EARLY group) and patients with SCreat higher at the start than 1.8 mg/dl (LATE group).

Renal survival probability at 120 months was found to be 79.1% in the EARLY group, whereas it was almost halved (48.4%) in LATE group patients. No overlapping in the relative survival trends was observed. The statistical comparison between the two curves was highly significant (Log Rank 33.96, Mantel 34.56, Wilcoxon 35.47, Prentice Peto 36.29 − P 0.0000).

General Characteristics

The follow-ups were, on average, nearly identical (57.9 vs 61.0 months) and there was no imbalance between the two groups regarding the underlying renal diseases.

Besides initial SCreat values (1.489 ± 0.198 vs 2.941 ± 1.135 mg/dl, t 18.81, P 0.000), the two groups differed in the duration of hypertension (22.8 ± 35.1 vs 32.1 ± 40.7 months − P 0.03), and duration of chronic renal failure (6.46 ± 15.01 vs 18.5 ± 25.6 months − P 0.000) before conservative treatment was started.

Clinical Course of CRF

The absolute increase in SCreat (1.623 ± 3.0 vs 3.176 ± 3.47 mg/dl, t 4.90, P 0.000), the monthly increase in SCreat (0.033 ± 0.07 vs 0.085 ± 0.114 mg/dl/month− t 5.77, P 0.000), and the percentage of patients requiring regular dialysis treatment (RDT) during follow-up (8.1% vs 30.6%, chi square 33.2, P 0.000) were significantly lower in the EARLY than in the LATE group.

The 95% confidence intervals of the mean monthly increase in SCreat in the two groups were 0.025–0.041 mg/dl per month (EARLY group) and 0.0725–0.0975 mg/dl per month (LATE group), respectively. As to the need for RDT, the outcome odds ratio between EARLY and LATE groups was 4.779; in other words, the risk of RDT within a 6-year follow-up was 5 times higher if conservative treatment had been delayed to a far advanced stage of CRF.

Multivariate Analysis

A statistical standardization (by dividing each single value for the SD of the mean) of all variables was required.

We plotted the monthly increase in SCreat (as an independent variable) against 35 variables, recorded at the start of follow-up on the low protein diet.

Multiple Regression Analysis

By means of a step-down procedure, we were able to identify two significantly independent variables: "entry" Screat (b 0.316, F 31.927) and duration of hypertension before conservative therapy (b 0.309, F 31.241) (r 0.482, P 0.000)

Cox Proportional Hazard Model

At variance with multiple regression, the Cox model pointed out one more prognostic factor: in addition to "entry" Screat (exp beta 1.81) and the duration of hypertension (exp 1.393), proteinuria (exp beta 1.66) was identified to negatively influence the course of CRF.

Selection of Patients with Proven Progressive CRF

It has been suggested that a definite percentage of patients with CRF may not experience any change in their renal function, regardless of conservative treatment [10]. In other words, there could be a population of patients affected with various renal diseases of a non progressive nature.

In order to eliminate this biasing factor, we decided to carry out the statistical analysis described above after removing from the sample those patients with no progression at all during follow-up (monthly increase in Screat lower than or equal to 0). This preliminary step cut out 116 of the 450 initial patients (60 from the EARLY and 56 from the LATE group).

Following the same procedural steps as those described above, we found that a preeminent influence on the history of CRF is the degree of functional deterioration present when dietary restriction is started.

Renal Survival Curves

Renal survival probability at 120 months was two times higher in the EARLY group, when compared with that observed in LATE group patients (69.2% vs 38.4% – Log

Rank 26.456, Mantel 27.00, Wilcoxon 28.273, Prentice Peto 28.94 – overall P 0.0000).

Clinical Course of CRF

Among the 334 selected patients, 72.6% of those in the EARLY group showed a very slow progression (monthly increase in Screat < 0.05 mg/dl per month), whereas only 36% of those in the LATE group had the same trend. The average monthly increase in Screat was significantly lower in EARLY (0.05 ± 0.08 mg/dl per month) than in LATE patients (0.114 ± 0.112 mg/dl per month) (t 5.76; P 0.000).

The 95% confidence intervals of the two means were 0.39–0.062 (EARLY) and 0.100–0.128 (LATE), respectively.

Seventeen patients in the early (12.8%) and 68 patients in the LATE group (39%) required RDT during follow-up. The outcome odds ratio was 4.377, a value quite close to that observed in the overall patient population and with the same prognostic implication as previously described.

Multivariate Analysis

Multiple regression analysis of standardized variables (step-down procedure) highlighted the influencing role of both "entry" Screat and duration of hypertension (F 31.3 and 22.49, respectively – r 0.476; P 0.000) on monthly increase in SCreat.

The Cox proportional hazard model confirmed the results obtained in the overall ($n = 450$) population (Scr exp beta: 1.774, U prot exp beta 1.554, hypertension exp beta 1.461).

The synopsis of this second statistical round may allow us to state that a positive role for an early dietary treatment is not overestimated by the presence of a hypothetical subgroup of non progressive patients.

Actually, a rough analysis of figures of survival rates, multivariate analysis, and odds ratios indicates the same risk of progression of CRF in the LATE group, either in the global or in the progressive patients' population.

Review

Clinical evidence exists to show that the natural history of patients with chronic renal failure is influenced by many factors, including conservative treatment of CRF.

Actually, this treatment means not only diet, but also administration of pharmacologic agents, more accurate and frequent clinical check-ups and, perhaps, significant changes in patients' life-style and mental habits [8,11]. But among the influencing factors, a critical one is the value of serum creatinine at which conservative treatment, namely a low protein diet, is prescribed. Thus, it appears useless or even dangerous for the patient to wait for a level of serum creatinine exceeding 1.8–2.0 mg/dl in order to make daily protein intake adequate to the reduced renal function. These conclusions, reached on a statistical basis, but also supported by daily empirical routine, put forward the second question. Which diet do we advise for patients with early CRF?

Which Diet?

In order to optimize the dietary treatment and thus the patients' compliance, two preliminary considerations have to be kept in mind: the characteristics of the diet and the patient's attitude toward the diet, this depending, in turn, on his/her psychosocial profile [11]. General guidelines for the dietary treatment of CRF must satisfy the following criteria: the diet must reduce the nitrogen intake, maintain nitrogen balance, cover essential aminoacid requirements, give a sufficient energy intake, and be palatable [11–13].

In line with these requirements, nephrologists face three possibilities: the unsupplemented low nitrogen diet with protein of high biologic value (HBV), the essential aminoacid supplemented diets and keto-acid supplemented diets.

Our experience with dietary treatment has been largely obtained with the use of the unsupplemented low-protein diet (LPD), mainly because we are convinced that this diet has some characteristics—namely palatability, simplicity, cheapness, long-term safety—which make it easy to follow, and therefore, well compliable. Thus its use appears suitable for early CRF patients [11].

However, we mustn't forget that the supplemented diets have been shown to be quite useful in renal patients, mostly in more advanced stages of CRF. Many positive effects have been obtained with these diets; however, a careful balance between the pros and cons suggests that their use in the very early stages of CRF is hardly suitable [14–18].

Pros	Cons
Slow progression rate	High Cost
No surface factor	Monotony
Improvement in metabolic state	Decreasing family support with time
Improvement of uremic neuropathy	Negative psychologic impact
Nitrogen sparing effect	Risk of malnutrition
Decrease in proteinuria	Careful and long lasting dietary education
Well-being of patients	Revolution in dietary habits
Decrease in S-PTH	Unknown effects on osteodystrophy

Turning to the LPD; this diet provides 35 KCal/kg body weight, 0.6 g/kg of proteins, 108 g/day of lipids, 320 g/day of carbohydrates, and 615 mg/day of phosphate. The requirements of trace elements and vitamins are satisfied [19].

With respect to proteins, 75% are HBV proteins. A quite peculiar characteristic of this diet is represented by the fact that 64% of the protein is of vegetable origin. The plant/animal protein ratio is 1.77, considerably higher than that recorded for current eating habits in European countries (< 1.0) [20]. Such a typical protein profile allows a low cholesterol and saturated fatty acid intake. While vegetable proteins have a slightly lower nutritive value than animal proteins, they might play a more effective protective role on the surviving nephrons, as already clinically and experimentally described [21,22].

The energy intake aims at well-established nutritional guidelines. As suggested by Kopple [23], patients with CRF who ingest 0.55–0.60 kg/kg of protein may have a neutral nitrogen balance and a reduced net urea generation only when the energy intake is above 30 KCal/kg per day.

The caloric support is given mainly by lipids (40%) and carbohydrates (53%). This division of energy supplies might arouse some controversy, since the fat and carbohydrate amounts are quite high. However, in the LPD, lipids are mostly of non-animal origin, the polyunsaturated to saturated fatty acid ratio is higher than 1, and the cholesterol intake is small. Moreover, there is no evidence that abnormalities of lipid metabolism in patients with CRF limit the usefulness of fat as an energy source.

Carbohydrates are provided as complex carbohydrates. The most likely metabolic effect of a high percentage of such substances in the diet is a direct effect on trygliceride levels. Actually, the mean trygliceride level did not increase during follow-up in our patients, either in the EARLY or in the LATE groups.

At variance with some other more restricted low-protein diets [13], the essential aminoacid requirements are satisfied by this diet, which provides nearly 32 g/day of high biologic value proteins. A negative aspect might be, on the other hand, the quite high amount of sulfur-containing aminoacids, especially because of their acidotic effect [13].

Finally, we have to support our hypothesis that 0.6 g/kg (body weight i.b.w.), no more and no less, is the optimum protein intake for patients with early CRF.

Many previous studies have clearly demonstrated that the daily protein requirement in patients with CRF is close to 0.6 g/kg per day. In 1958 Herndorn demonstrated that to maintain a patient in nitrogen balance nearly 0.5 g/kg of protein was required, with the high/low quality protein ratio as high as 70%. These results were confirmed in the following years, by Giordano, Kerr, Ford, and Kopple [24].

On the other hand, in a self-controlled study [25] we have previously shown that patients with early CRF switched from 0.6 g/kg to a protein intake of 0.8–0.9 g/kg, under strict metabolic and dietary control, experienced a decrease in GFR and an increase in proteinuria over a 9-month period.

A diet providing less than 0.6 g/kg per day of protein and the same energy supply as the LPD, would probably have problems concerning negative nitrogen balance and would require, in order to be nutritionally adequate, some supplement with artificial foods. This latter fact might be linked with a progressively worsening compliance. Such a possibility seems, to some extent, supported by some data from the literature [26,27]: patients advised to have a protein intake of 0.4–0.5 g/kg showed, when urinary urea was checked, a daily protein intake averaging 0.6 g/kg. In our patients, compliance with the LPD is quite satisfactory and lasting over time. In this respect, we cannot sincerely deny that these results are improved by the similarity which exists between Italian dietary habits and the LPD scheme; the global figure, however, is impressive.

Moreover, nutritional data in a group of our patients [28] show that the supplies of the LPD are adequate for maintaining nutritional indices within normal ranges after a 5-year follow-up. On the other hand, the data also suggest that, if no care is paid to the caloric intake of patients, some nutritional parameters may worsen.

An unsupplemented low-protein diet is not like a panacea. Many problems are related to its use and the good results we showed you were not achieved as easily as it might appear. The following problems should be considered before starting a LPD program:

a) The scheme is fairly monotonous and implies a surface factor, due to the relatively small quantity of foods of animal origin.

b) Frequent clinical and dietary checks are required.

c) A careful survey of caloric intake is required, especially in younger patients.

d) As with supplemented diets, mental stress might arise over time due to some social limitations.

e) No information is available on the aminoacid muscle pattern in patients on long-term LPDs.

f) No protective effects have been shown in patients with nephrotic syndrome.

References

1. Mitch WE (1988) Nutritional therapy and the progression of renal insufficiency. In: Nutrition and the kidney, Mitch WE (ed) Little, Brown, Boston, pp 154–179

2. Diamond JR (1990) Effects of dietary interventions on glomerular pathophysiology. Am J Physiol 258:F1–F8

3. Ibels LS, Alfrey AC, Haut L (1978) Preservation of function in experimental renal disease by dietary restriction of phosphate. N Engl J Med 298:122–126

4. Friend PS, Fernandes G, Good RA, Michael AF, Yunis EJ (1978) Dietary restriction early and late. Effects on the nephropathy of the NZB × NZW mouse. Lab Invest 38: 629–632

5. Motomura K, Okuda S, Sanai T, Ando T, Onoyama K, Fujshima M (1988) Importance of early initiation of dietary protein restriction for the prevention of experimental progressive renal disease. Nephron 49:144–149

6. Nath KA, Hostetter M, Hostetter M, Hostetter TH (1986) Dietary protein restriction in established renal injury in the rat. J Clin Invest 78:1199–1205

7. Remuzzi G, Zoja A, Remuzzi A (1985) Low protein diet prevents glomerular damage in adryamicin treated rats. Proc Eur Dial Transplant Assoc 22:927–931

8. Maschio G, Oldrizzi L, Rugiu C (1989) Early dietary and nondietary intervention in chronic renal failure. Contrib Nephrol 70:163–171

9. Kramer MS (1988) Clinical epidemiology and biostatistics. Springer, Berlin, chapters 4–18

10. El Nahas AM, Coles GA (1986) Dietary treatment of chronic renal failure: ten unanswered questions. Lancet I:597–600

11. Oldrizzi L, Rugiu C, De Biase V, Maschio G (to be published) Factors influencing dietary compliance in patients with chronic renal failure on unsupplemented low-protein diet. Contrib Nephrol 81

12. Giovannetti S (1989) The purposes and rationale of nutritional treatment of chronic renal failure. In: Giovannetti S (ed) Nutritional treatment of chronic renal failure. Kluwer, Boston, pp 163–172

13. Gretz N, Lasserre JJ, Jerabek A, Strauch M (1989) Protein/aminoacid composition of low-protein diets. Contrib Nephrol 72:11–20

14. Lucas PA, Meadows JH, Roberts DE, Coles GA (1986) The risks and benefits of a low protein-essential amino acid -ketoacid diet. Kidney Int 29:995–1003

15. Druml W, Mitch WE (1988) Protein-restricted diets and progression of renal failure. Blood Purif 6:285–298

16. Persichetti S, Sagliaschi G, Clemenzia G, Bolletta A (1988) Considerazioni di psiconefrologia sulla dieta nella insufficienza renale cronica. Mienrva Med 79:1075–1078

17. Giovannetti S (1989) Supplemented diet for severe chronic renal failure: some controversial points. Contrib Nephrol 75:147–154

18. Strauch M, Gretz N (1988) Aminoacid and ketoacid supplements. In: Giovannetti S (ed) Nutritional treatment of chronic renal failure. Kluwer, Boston, pp 191–198

19. Maschio G, Oldrizzi L, Rugiu C (1986) The effects of protein restriction on the course of chronic renal failure. In: Mitch WE, Brenner BM, Stein JH (eds) The progressive nature of renal disease. Churchill and Livingstone, New York, pp 203–218

20. Strauch M, Lasserre JJ, Jerabek A, Gretz N (1989) The normal food intake. Contrib Nephrol 72:1–10

21. Wiseman MJ, Hunt R, Goodwin A, Gross JL, Keen H, Viberti GC (1987) Dietary composition and renal function in healthy subjects. Nephron 46:37–42

22. Williams AJ, Baker F, Walls J (1987) Effect of varying quantity and quality of dietary protein intake in experimental renal disease in rats. Nephron 46:83–90

23. Kopple JD, Monteon FJ, Shalb JK (1986) Effect of energy intake on nitrogen metabolism in nondialyzed patients with chronic renal failure. Kidney Int 29:734–742

24. Ford J, Phillips ME, Toye FE, Luck VA, de Wardener HE (1969) Nitrogen balance in patients with chronic renal failure on diets containing varying quantities of protein. Br Med J [Clin Res] 1:735–740

25. Oldrizzi L, Rugiu C, Maschio G (1989) Different protein diets in renal failure: a self-controlled study. Am J Nephrol 9:184–189

26. Rosman JB, Langer K, Brandl M, Piers-Becht TPM, van Derhem GK, ter Wee P, Donker AJM (1989) Protein restricted diets in chronic renal failure: a four years follow-up shows limited indications. Kidney Int 3(Suppl 27):S96–S102

27. Bergstrom J, Alvestrand A, Bucht H, Gutierrez A (1989) Stockholm clinical study on progression of chronic renal failure. An interim report. Kidney Int 36(Suppl 27):S110–S114

28. Guarnieri GF, Toigo G, Situlin R, Carrao M, Tamaro G, Lucchesli A, Oldrizzi L, Rugiu C, Maschio G (1989) Nutritional state in patients on long-term low-protein diet or with nephrotic syndrome. Kidney Int 36(Suppl 27):S195–S200

Low Protein Diet and Progression of Chronic Renal Failure: Results of Controlled Clinical Trials

N. Gretz[1], S. Giovannetti[2], and M. Strauch[1]

SUMMARY. As indicated by results from small scale trials, performed mostly in single centers, a low protein diet seems to delay the progression of chronic renal failure. Data from large scale controlled clinical trials, i.e., prospective randomized trials, are largely missing. Currently, quite a number of such trials are being conducted or are awaiting final evaluation. Preliminary data from the North Italian Trial seem to indicate that patients on a low protein diet display a much slower progression to end-stage renal failure than do patients on a free diet. This trial has a sufficient number of patients enrolled and thus exhibits considerable statistical value. The crucial point with all clinical trials is that due to the high number of patients needed they have to be multi-center trials. However, in such trials comparable degrees of compliance are difficult to achieve in the individual centers. Thus, with respect to this variable, a considerable center effect is a major confounding variable. Other problems in these trials are statistical in nature: a high rate of drop-outs has to be handled and the standard deviation of results has to be reduced by adequate stratification. A serious logistic problem arises in that it is difficult to recruit an adequate number of patients. In our opinion, however, it makes no sense to develop excellent statistical designs, to use refined methods of GFR determination, and to recruit an adequate number of patients, if sufficient dietary compliance cannot be achieved.

Introduction

Today, low protein diets (LPDs) are more and more frequently used in order to delay the progression of chronic renal failure (CRF). It is of note that earlier this century, Volhard [1] demonstrated that it was possible to postpone the increase of serum urea

[1]Clinic of Nephrology, Klinikum Mannheim, D-6800 Mannheim 1, Federal Republic of Germany
[2]1ª Clinica Medica, Università di Pisa, I-56100 Pisa, Italy

concentrations for a prolonged period by restricting protein intake to 20 g, and allowing energy intake of at least 2000 kcal, per day. Thus, he was able to prevent uremic symptoms. When Kluthe, in 1974, pointed out for the first time that a LPD considerably delayed the progression of chronic renal failure, a new era in the use of these diets arose [2]. Subsequently, quite a number of studies have been performed. There has been, however, considerable criticism with respect to statistics, especially design problems and small sample size; there has also been criticism of the way GFR was determined and, recently, recognition of the fact that only poor compliance can be achieved. Despite that, most small single center trials have demonstrated that LPDs have a fair to excellent efficiency in delaying progression of CRF.

The aim of this paper is to survey observations on the impact of LPDs on the progression of CRF in controlled clinical trials. Before doing so, summarizing the results achieved so far from small scale trials seems to be warranted.

Results from Single Center Trials

In order to evaluate the results from single center trial, we introduced the so-called factor of delay (FD) [3]. The underlying idea was to have a comparable measure for all studies. Usually, different studies use quite different outcome measures, such as

Table 1. Summary of results obtained with different diets

Ref.	Diet		FD
	Protein	Phosphorus	
Early renal failure:			
[4]	C:free 95–125 g	1–1.8 g	1.5
	D:0.6 g/kg bw	12 mg/kg	
[4]	C:free 95–125 g	1–1.8 g	12.9
	D:0.6 g/kg bw	6 mg/kg	
[5]	C: 70 g	0.9 g	11.2
	D:0.6 g/kg bw	0.7 g	
Late renal failure: no supplement:			
[6]	C:free	?	2.3
	D:0.6 g/kg bw	0.6–0.7 g	
Late renal failure: eaa supplements			
[7]	C:40–60 g	?	10.5
	D:15–20 g	0.3–0.4 g	
[8]	C:0.5–0.7 g/kg bw	?	1.6
	D:0.5–0.7 g/kg bw	?	
Late renal failure: ka supplements:			
[9]	C:free	?	2.0
	D:0.4–0.5 g/kg bw	?	
[10]	C:0.6 g/kg bw	?	1.7
	D:0.4 g/kg bw	?	
[10]	C:0.4 g/kg bw	0.6–0.8 g	3.5
	D:0.4 g/kg bw	0.6–0.8 g	
[11]	C:0.3 g/kg bw	7–9 mg/kg bw	5.6
	D:0.3 g/kg bw	7–9 mg/kg bw	
[12]	C:1.2–1.4 g/kg bw	15–20 mg/kg bw	46.0
	D:0.2–0.6 g/kg bw	5–12 mg/kg bw	

Ref., reference number; Protein, protein intake; C, control; D, diet; FD, factor of delay

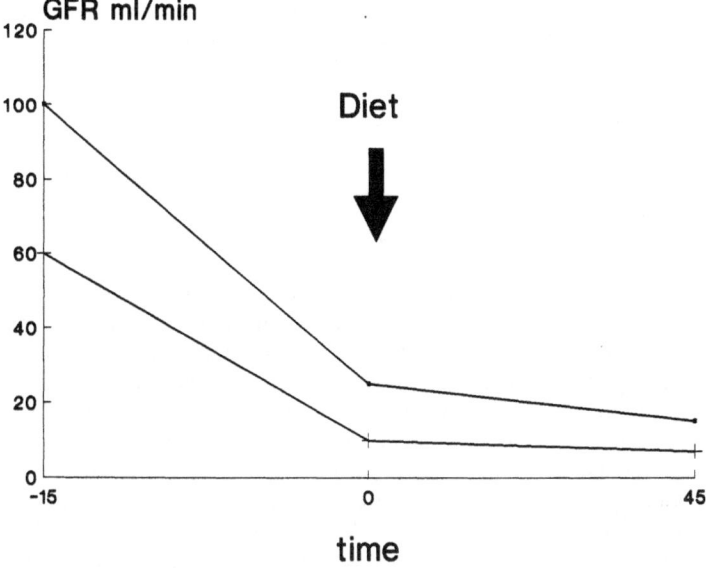

Fig. 1. Schematic drawing of the cross over of patients from free diet to LPD

1/SCR, creatinine clearance, or survival time, for the assessment of treatment efficiency. The FD is calculated as progression measure with diet, divided by progression measure without diet. Thus, the FD is the delay achieved with a LPD as a multiple of the progression in the control group. A list of studies providing data for control and treatment groups, thus allowing calculation of the FD, is shown in Table 1. From the table it is obvious that a wide scattering of FDs exists. It can, however, be concluded that at least an average FD of 2 can be achieved [4–12]. The trials presented, however, may be criticized for not being rigidly controlled clinical trials.

What is a "Controlled Clinical Trial?"

By definition the prerequisites for a controlled clinical trial are [13] that the study:

- is prospective,
- is randomized,
- contains a control group, and
- is double blind.

By definition, these trials are large scale, of necessity enrolling hundreds of patients. As it is impossible to recruit an adequate number of patients in a single center, controlled clinical trials are usually multicenter trials. Friedman et al. [13], however, noted that in some controlled clinical trials compromise was unavoidable. Thus, for example, a trial on dietary interventions can never be double-blind.

Cross Over Design in the Assessment of the Efficiency of LPDs

In some cases a cross-over design is used, thus the patient is his or her own control (Fig. 1). When applying such a design, the patient's decline in GFR is monitored before the start of a LPD and afterwards. Thereafter the rates of loss of GFR before and afterwards are calculated and compared. This cross over design, however, implies that all parameters influencing the progression of renal failure, e.g., blood pressure, hyperphosphatemia, hyperlipidemia, acidosis, etc., do not change while the disease progresses. This assumption, however, is highly improbable. On the other hand, such an analysis also implies that, as a linear regression analysis is used for the assessment of the slope of GFR, the decline in GFR is linear and an adequate and equal timing of blood sampling before and after start of LPD treatment is used. This, however, has only rarely been the case, as found when checking the literature. Despite these considerations, the cross-over approach is frequently used as the ensuing test statistics are reduced to a paired t-test and usually the sample size thought to be needed is fairly small. The significant P-values thus obtained, however, do not compensate for the inadequate design of studies. Thus, a cross over design is not suitable for assessment of the efficiency of a LPD in delaying the progression of CRF.

Stratification and Subgroups in Controlled Clinical Trials

From the statistical point of view, there is no way around the use of a prospective randomized trial, i.e., a controlled clinical trial, if the efficacy of a LPD in delaying the progression of CRF is to be analyzed. Thus, patients have to be randomly allocated to different types of treatment, e.g., no protein restriction, moderate protein restriction, or severe protein restriction. In order to reduce the often large standard deviation (SD) in these studies, adequate stratification before randomization is of utmost importance, as with larger SDs the size of sample needed increases (Fig. 2). As in patients with CRF different diets are used at different levels of renal function, it seems ethical to compare a LPD (e.g., 0.6 g/kg bw) in patients with good renal function versus patients with no protein restriction; while in the group with poor renal function, reducing protein intake in all subgroups seems to be warranted. Thus, the control group might be on a 0.6 g protein restricted diet while being compared with a group on a more restricted LPD with different amino acid or keto acid supplements. In addition to the stratification for renal function, in order to reduce SD, it seems appropriate to stratify for the underlying renal disease, as different renal diseases exhibit different progression rates [2,3,5]. Gender and age [14] are unsuitable as stratifying variables. This is underlined by the fact that in their final evaluation Rosman et al. [14] collapsed their initial strata into one group. It is, however, evident that the underlying renal disease, which to a certain extent is age and gender dependent, has a major impact on the average progression rate and differs from one renal

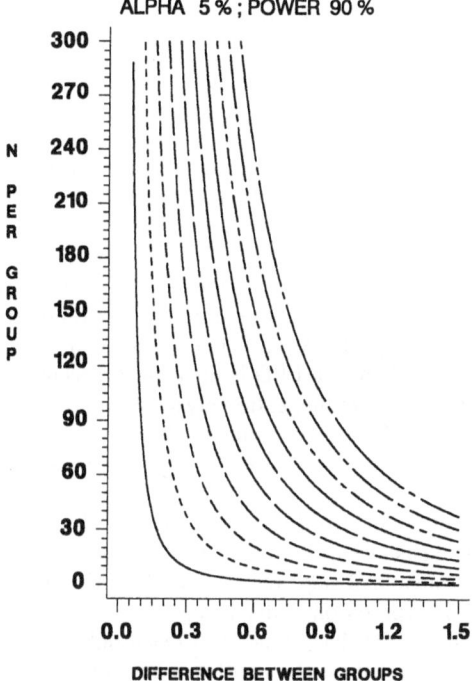

Fig. 2. Sample size calculation for given differences and standard deviations.

disease group to the other. Thus, ignoring this fact results in a considerable increase in the SD of the subgroups, or even results in missing an existing difference between groups.

Sample Size in Controlled Clinical Trials

The SD, however, is a major determinant for the sample size required in the study. Figure 2 shows the required sample size per subgroup on the y-axis, and the monthly difference in GFR (ml/min per month), between the groups on the x-axis. The individual curves represent the different SDs, starting from 0.1 (left curve) to 1 (right curve) in 0.1 steps. The diagram was calculated according to the formula given by Friedman et al. [13]. The assumptions used in this formula were also used for the calculation of the sample size in controlled clinical trials currently being conducted (see below).

Figure 2 may be used to recalculate whether, in a study, a difference between two groups of a given sample size really had the chance of being detected. The figure may also be used for the calculation of sample size in designing new trials. From the diagram it is obvious that in a trial where the impact of different LPDs on the progression of CRF is to be analyzed, sample sizes of at least 50–100 patients per subgroup are needed. Otherwise, the beta error, i.e., non detection of a difference between the groups, will be higher than ten percent.

Results from Multicenter Trials

Today, quite a number of controlled clinical trials are being conducted or are awaiting final evaluation. The 4 year follow up of the socalled Groningen Study [14] seems to provide a moderately optimistic view of the efficiency of the LPD in delaying the progression of CRF. It can be demonstrated, using survival analysis, that a significant difference between the control and the treatment group exists in the subgroup with poor renal function (P=0.025). Furthermore, the data seems to provide evidence that males benefit from LPDs, in contrast to females. As underlying renal disease influences progression rate, and the distribution of renal diseases is different in males and females, relating efficiency to gender seems inappropriate. The sex distribution in the different disease groups, however, is not given. Also the statement that only glomerular diseases benefit from a LPD is difficult to accept, as in this subgroup analysis, the sample size is sometimes extremely small. It is of note that in the analysis presented the problem of multiple testing might have confounded the results, as no adjustments for this problem were made, e.g., by using analysis of variance (ANOVA).

The preliminary results of the Northern Italian Trial, with a total enrollment of 456 patients, when evaluated using survival analyses, indicate that patients on 0.6 g protein restricted diets come to end-stage renal failure later than patients on a free protein intake [15]. This interpretation of the data presented seems to be valid, despite the fact that the calculated P-values sometimes reach only borderline significance. An analysis of the loss of renal function with respect to GFR slopes, however, it is still missing, as is the analysis of confounding factors.

None of the three ongoing trials: the French Cooperative Trial, the NIH-sponsored Modification of Diet in Renal Disease (MDRD) Trial, or the trial of the European Study Group for the Conservative Management of Chronic Renal Failure (ESG), can provide any data on progression. They will probably need some years to come to their projected end. In the meantime, the trial of the Medical Research Council of the United Kingdom has been cancelled, as the number of patients available for the study was too small.

Thus, there are only hints from one single center and from one multicenter trial that patients with chronic renal failure might benefit from low protein diets, insofar as progression to endstage renal failure is concerned. Final conclusions from large multicenter controlled clinical trials are still not available.

Major Problems in Ongoing Controlled Clinical Trials

The achievement of adequate compliance is probably the major difficulty found in ongoing controlled clinical trials. This is revealed by a survey of the literature (Table 2). In the ESG and MDRD trials an improvement of compliance, in the range of 0.2 g protein/kg body weight, has been noted over time. Rosman et al. [14] have also observed improved compliance over time. From the ESG and French Cooperative Study it became obvious that there was a considerable center effect with respect to compliance, indicating that the number of centers in a multicenter trial has to be as small as possible. This center effect also proves that it makes no sense to start dietary

Table 2. Compliance data from the literature

| Ref. | Renal function | Protein intake (g/kg bw) | | Time of assessment |
		Projected	Achieved[d]	
[16]	Good	Free	0.76 ± 0.47	Whole trial
		0.6	0.72 ± 0.66	
	Poor	0.6	0.68 ± 0.64	
		0.3[a]	0.63 ± 0.80	
[17]		Free	0.86[b] ± ?	18 months
		0.4	0.72[b] ± ?	
[18]	Good	1–1.4	1.04 ± 0.04	Whole trial
		0.58	0.91 ± 0.06	
		0.28[a]	0.69 ± 0.05	
	Poor	0.58	0.72 ± 0.03	
		0.28[a]	0.69 ± 0.03	
		0.28[a]	0.72 ± 0.03	
[14]	Good	Free	1.00[b] ± ?	18 months
		0.6	0.75[b] ± ?	
	Poor	Free	0.98[b] ± ?	
		0.4	0.86[b] ± ?	
[19]		Free	1.13 ± 0.26[c]	Whole trial
		0.55	0.67 ± 0.13[c]	

[a]Different amino/keto acid supplements
[b]Recalculated from figures in the paper, using Maroni's formula [19]
[c]Recalculated from SEM
[d]Means ± SD
Ref., reference number

management and a trial on the efficiency of a LPD at the same time in a center. This would result only in documentation of the process of learning dietary management.

Another problem is the recruitment of an adequate number of patients. The reader should be very concerned about results from small scale trials (see Fig. 2).

Acknowledgment. The authors appreciate the skillful help of Mrs. S. Redies in preparing the manuscript. Parts of this paper were made possible by grants from: Bundesministerium fuer Forschung und Technologie, FRG (Nr. 0704743).

References

1. Volhard F, Suter F (1931) Nieren und ableitende Harnwege. In: Mohr und Staehelin (eds) Handbuch der inneren Medizin, vol 5/1. Springer, Berlin, pp 804–811
2. Kluthe R, Oechslen D, Quirin H, Jesdinsky HJ (1972) Six years' experience with a special low-protein diet. In: Kluthe R, Berlyne G, Burton B (eds) Uremia. Thieme, Stuttgart, pp 250–256
3. Gretz N, Korb E, Strauch M (1983) Low-protein diet supplemented by keto acids in chronic renal failure: a prospective controlled study. Kidney Int 24(Suppl 16):S263–S267
4. Barsotti G, Giannoni A, Morelli E, Lazzeri M, Vlamis I, Baldi R (1984) The decline of renal function slowed by very low phosphorus intake in chronic renal patients following a low nitrogen diet. Clin Nephrol 21:54–59
5. Oldrizzi L, Rugiu C, Valvo E, Lupo A, Loschiavo C, Gammaro L, Tessitore N, Fabris A (1985) Progression of renal failure in patients with renal disease of diverse etiology on protein-restricted diet. Kidney Int 27:553–557

6. Bennet SE, Russel GI, Walls J (1983) Low protein diets in uraemia. Br Med J [Clin Res] 287:1344–1345

7. Alvestrand A, Ahlberg M, Bergstrøm J (1983) Retardation of the progression of renal insufficiency in patients treated with low-protein diets. Kidney Int 24(Suppl 16):268–272

8. Ando A, Orita Y, Nakata K, Fukuhara Y, Mikami H, Fujii M, Nakajima Y, Ueda N (1981) The effect of essential amino acid supplementation therapy on prognosis of patients with chronic renal failure estimated on the basis of the Markow process. Med J Osaka Univ 32:31–37

9. Gretz N, Meisinger E, Strauch M (1986) Influence of the underlying renal disease on the rate of progression. Contr Nephrol 53:92–101

10. Schmicker R, Frühling PT, Goetz KH, Kaschube I, Rakette I, Vetter K (1986) Influence of low protein diet supplemented with amino acids and keto acids on the progression of chronic renal failure. Contrib Nephrol 53:121–127

11. Walser M, LaFrance ND, Ward L, VanDuyn MA (1987) Progression of chronic renal failure in patients given ketoacids following amino acids. Kidney Int 32:123–128

12. Barsotti G, Ciardella F, Morelli E, Cupisti A, Mantovanelli A, Giovannetti S (1988) Nutritional treatment of renal failure in type 1 diabetes nephropathy. Clin Nephrol 29:280–287

13. Friedman LM, Furberg CD, DeMets DL (1982) Fundamentals of clinical trials. John Wright, PSG, Boston

14. Rosman JB, Langer K, Brandl M, Piers-Becht TPM, van der Hem G, ter Wee PM, Donker AJM (1989) Protein-restricted diets in chronic renal failure: A four year follow-up shows limited indications. Kidney Int 36(Suppl 27):S96–S102

15. Locatelli F (1989) Controlled study of protein-restricted diet in chronic renal failure. Contrib Nephrol 75:141–146

16. Giovannetti S, Gretz N, Attman PO, D'Amico G, Frühling PT (1990) Dietary compliance in the trial of the European Study Group: a preliminary analysis. Contrib Nephrol 81:61–70

17. Ihle BU, Becker GJ, Whitworth JA, Charlwood RA, Kincaid-Smith PS (1989) The effect of protein restriction on the progression of renal insufficiency. N Engl J Med 321:1773–1777

18. Kopple JD, Berg R, Houser H, Steinman TI, Teschan P (1989) Nutritional status of patients with different levels of chronic renal insufficiency. Kidney Int 36(Suppl 27):S184–S194

19. Walker JD, Bending JJ, Dodds RA, Mattock MB, Murrells TJ, Keen H, Viberti GC (1989) Restriction of dietary protein and progression of renal failure in diabetic nephropathy. Lancet II:1411–1415

Dietary Protein Restriction Retards Progressive Renal Failure in Type I Diabetes

KATHLEEN ZELLER[1], ELAINE WHITTAKER, LYNN SULLIVAN,
PHILIP RASKIN, and HARRY R. JACOBSON[2]

Introduction

Diabetes mellitus is currently the leading cause of end-stage renal disease in the United States. Approximately 50% of patients with Type I (or insulin-dependent) diabetes mellitus develop progressive renal insufficiency, despite attempts to vigorously control blood sugar and treat co-existing hypertension [1–6]. Data accumulated from a number of studies in experimental animal models of diabetes, as well as data from models of other forms of progressive renal failure, have suggested that, despite different underlying disorders, the progression of renal disease may have a significant hemodynamic component and may be slowed by a reduction in dietary protein, and possibly phosphorus, intake [7–19]. Glomerular micropuncture studies performed in a number of models, but most commonly in rats subjected to subtotal nephrectomy or rats rendered diabetic with streptozotocin treatment, reveal that single nephron glomerular plasma flow is increased, as is glomerular capillary hydrostatic pressure. While some controversy exists, it is felt that these hemodynamic changes contribute to the progressive renal damage seen in these animal models. Dietary protein restriction has been shown to not only slow the progression of glomerular sclerosis and renal failure in these animal models, but also to normalize the elevated glomerular plasma flow and capillary hydrostatic pressure. Based on these observations, a number of clinical studies on humans have been performed [20–24].

Many reports have suggested that there is a beneficial effect of dietary protein and phosphorus restriction in humans with various forms of renal disease. The rates of progression of renal failure have been reduced from 2 to 10-fold in patients on a low protein diet [20–24]. Most of these studies, however, have been retrospective and uncontrolled and have dealt with patients exhibiting a variety of renal diseases. To

[1]Department of Internal Medicine, Center for Human Nutrition, University of Texas Southwestern Medical Center, Dallas, TX 75235, USA
[2]Division of Nephrology, Vanderbilt University Medical Center, Nashville, TN 37232, USA

address a potential beneficial role for dietary protein restriction in renal disease, we elected to study a single disease entity, namely Type I diabetes mellitus, which is known to cause progressive renal insufficiency in approximately 50% of patients with this disorder. We performed a prospective, randomized, controlled study, evaluating dietary protein restriction on the progression of renal failure in 35 subjects with Type I diabetes mellitus.

Methods

Patient Selection

Patients between the ages of 18 and 60 years, who had documented Type I diabetes mellitus with onset before the age of 30, were recruited for this study. Patients required evidence of diabetic nephropathy, manifested by significant proteinuria, concurrent retinopathy, and the absence of other potential causes for renal failure. All patients had initial glomerular filtration rates between 15% and 85% of predicted norms, as measured by ^{125}I iothalamate clearance. Patients who had a contraindication to a low protein diet, such as severe infection, malignancy, or pregnancy, and patients who had brittle, difficult to control diabetes, were excluded. All patients required a follow-up of at least 12 months for inclusion in the analysis.

We originally enrolled 47 patients with Type I diabetes mellitus in the study. Out of this initial group, 35 patients were able to comply with the study requirements and have been followed for a minimum of 12 months. A total of 6 patients were dismissed from the study for inability to comply; 2 of these were in the control group and 4 were in the low protein intake group. Two additional patients, one from each group, were dropped from the study subsequent to their move from the Dallas area. An additional control patient was excluded from the study after development of severe congestive heart failure, secondary to a myocardial infarction, and an additional patient on the low protein diet died suddenly and unexpectedly shortly after enrollment. Finally, 2 patients randomized to the low protein diet, on repeated occasions during which dietary protein intake was calculated from urine area nitrogen measurements, were shown to be non-compliant with the diet, i.e., they were consuming in excess of the 0.8 gm/kg per day cutoff. These patients were excluded from analysis with the remaining patients on the low protein diet. However, their results were analyzed separately. Baseline characteristics for the patients in both groups are summarized in Table 1. The groups did not differ with respect to mean age, initial glomerular filtration rate, or initial 24 hour urine protein excretion.

Table 1. Patient characteristics

	Control (15)	Low protein (20)	P
Age (years)	35 ± 2	33 ± 2	NS
Initial GFR (ml/min per 1.73m²)	48.8 ± 7.1	46.3 ± 4.8	NS
Initial proteinuria (mg/24 h)	4266 ± 715	3144 ± 417	NS

Study Diet

Subjects were randomized to one of two diets. The low protein group consumed a diet containing 25–40 kcal/kg ideal body weight (IBW) per day with 0.6 gm/kg IBW per day protein, which was 70%–80% of high biologic value. The urinary losses of albumin were replaced gram for gram by increasing dietary protein intake. The diet also contained 2 grams of sodium, 500–1000 mg phosphorus and 1000 mg calcium. All subjects received a standard multi-vitamin preparation. Patients in the control group consumed their pre-study diet, with the stipulation that it contained 2 gms of sodium, 1000 mg of phosphorus, and $\geq$ 1 gm/kg IBW per day protein.

Measurements

Upon enrollment into the study, all patients underwent a complete history and physical examination, baseline renal function studies, dietary histories, determination of nutritional status, and measurement of glycemic control. Glomerular filtration rate was estimated by a number of parameters, including measurement of serum creatinine, collection of 24 hour urine for creatinine clearance, and measurement of radioisotopic tracer glomerular filtration rate, using ^{125}I iothalamate. Dietary protein intake was calculated by adding non-urea nitrogen losses (estimated at 31 mg/kg real body weight) to the measured urine urea nitrogen (UUN) and was adjusted for proteinuria [25]. A 24 hour urine collection was also made for measurement for sodium, potassium, calcium, and phosphorus. Nutritional status was evaluated by anthropometric measurements, determination of complete blood count, total protein and albumin. Diabetic control was assessed by measurements of glycosylated hemoglobin (HbA_{1c}), using high performance liquid chromatography [26] and lipid status was determined by measurements of serum cholesterol, triglycerides, and lipoproteins, via spectrophotometric analysis [27]. The laboratory measurements were performed monthly for three months and at three month intervals thereafter. Iothalamate determinations of glomerular filtration rate were performed at enrollment and at 3–6 month intervals. Iothalamate clearance determination was a standard procedure in our Renal Clinic and was performed as described previously [28]. Subjects were given an oral water load of 20 ml/kg and 10 drops of saturated solution of potassium iodine was administered to prevent thyroid uptake of radiolabelled iodine. Subsequently, ^{125}I labelled iothalamate was injected subcutaneously; clearance determinations were begun 60 minutes later. Three 30 min urine collections were obtained and were bracketed by collection of plasma samples for determinations of ^{125}I iothalamate. Urine and plasma were counted in an Abbott Autologic Gamma Counter and iothalamate clearances were calculated using the standard clearance formula. In some patients, significant scattering of clearance values between collection periods was observed, suggesting a problem with bladder emptying. In these patients, clearances were repeated after the insertion of a Foley catheter. The overall coefficient of variation for the iothalamate clearances was 8.4%.

At every visit, blood pressure was measured in the supine, sitting, and upright position, in the same arm. Every effort was made to maintain systemic blood pressure at a value of 140/85 mm/Hg or lower and patients were seen as often as weekly to obtain good blood pressure control. The use of angiotensin-converting enzyme (ACE) inhibitors was specifically avoided whenever possible, and only 2 patients received ACE inhibitors. As stated earlier, compliance with the prescribed dietary protein intake was assessed by repeated dietary history and measurement of UUN. Patients in the low protein group with protein intakes persistently > 0.8 gm/kg per day, or control patients with protein intakes persistently < 1 gm/kg per day were excluded from analysis.

Statistical Analysis

Data were analyzed, using ISP Software developed by the staff of the Academic Computering Services and by the General Clinical Research Center's statistician, using CLINFO and BMDP. The rate of decline of glomerular filtration rate was analyzed by three methods. First, regression lines for 1/serum creatinine were generated. Second, creatinine and iothalamate clearances over time were determined and mean slopes were calculated by regression analysis. Finally, initial renal function and final renal function, as assessed by creatinine clearance and iothalamate clearance, were determined and divided by the time interval between the measurements. When multiple values for a given parameter were obtained within a three month interval, the values were meaned to provide a single three month data point. The Student's two-tail t test was used to compare data between treatment groups if the variances were the same, and the Mann Whitney (MW) u test was used if they were not. Stepwise regression was performed, using data from the total study population, with the dependent variable being a change in glomerular filtration rate and the independent variables being protein intake, blood pressure, and hemoglobin A_{1c}.

Results

Progression of Renal Failure

The iothalamate clearances for the treatment and control groups are depicted in Fig. 1. The mean regression line for the groups is indicated by the "dashed" line. Those patients ingesting a low protein diet exhibited a rate of decline in renal function approximately four times slower than that exhibited by patients ingesting a normal protein diet. Numerical data are summarized in Table 2, where the reciprocal serum creatinine, the rate of decline of GFR with creatinine clearance, and the rate of decline of GFR with iothalamate clearance are depicted. The rate of decline of renal function was significantly slower in the low protein group, as assessed by iothalamate clearance (P = 0.02 by MW u test). Also, the rate of decline of renal function, as assessed by creatinine clearance, reached significance by t-test (P = 0.03). The rate of decline of renal function, as assessed by the reciprocal serum

Table 2. Decline in renal function assessed by linear regression analysis

	Control (15)	Low protein (20)	P
1/Cr ($1\mu Mol^{-1}mo^{-1} \times 10^6$)	-0.97 ± 0.27	-0.39 ± 0.15	NS
Creatinine clearance (ml/min per month)	-0.81 ± 0.20	-0.33 ± 0.12	<0.05
Iothalamate clearance (ml/min per month)	-1.01 ± 0.31	-0.26 ± 0.10	<0.05
Mean follow-up (months)	31.4 ± 2.5	37.1 ± 3.1	

Table 3. Changes in 24 h urinary protein excretion (mg/24 h)

	Control	Low protein
Initial	4266	3144
3 Months	5194	2384
Final	5290	2948

creatinine, was not statistically significant. When the data were expressed as a difference between initial and final clearances divided by time, the results were essentially the same. Of note, the two patients originally randomized to the low protein intake group, but whose mean protein intakes averaged 0.86 and 0.80 grams/kg per day were excluded from the overall data analysis, but had very stable renal function over a mean follow-up period of 44.5 months.

We subjected the data to analysis according to sub-groups of patients with initial glomerular filtration > or < 45 ml/min per 1.73 meters^2. In patients with GFR > 45 ($n = 18$, mean GFR 66.1 $\pm$ 4.1), the rate of decline of renal function, as assessed by the linear regression analysis of iothalamate clearances, was 0.003 $\pm$ 0.1 ml/min per month in patients ingesting the low protein diet. However, in patients ingesting the control diet, the rate of decline of GFR was 0.67 $\pm$ 0.22 ml/min per month (P = < 0.05). The data were not different when expressed as the difference between initial and final iothalamate clearances divided by time. In patients with an initial glomerular filtration rate < 45 ml/min per 1.73 meters^2 ($n = 15$, mean GFR 27.5 $\pm$ 2.0), the rate of decline of renal function was 0.51 $\pm$ 0.13 ml/min per month for patients in the low protein group and 1.41 $\pm$ 0.62 ml/min per month in patients ingesting the control diet. The difference between these two values, while large, did not quite make statistical significance.

Proteinuria

Approximately three months after initiation of the diet, urinary protein excretion in the protein restricted patients had fallen by a mean of 760 mg/24 h, whereas 24 h urine protein excretion in the control group had increased by 928 mg/24 h. At the conclusion of the study, the low protein intake patients had a mean 24 h urine protein excretion rate that was 196 mg/24 h less than their initial value, whereas the control group had a significantly elevated 24 h urine protein excretion rate that was 1024 mg/24 h above their initial value (Table 3).

Dietary Compliance

Protein intake over the entire study period was calculated for each patient from the UUN and was normalized for IBW. Control patients ingested a mean of 1.08 $\pm$ 0.10 gm/kg per day of protein, while protein restricted patients consumed a mean of 0.72 $\pm$ 0.06 gm/kg per day. Compliance, when expressed as the % intake in excess of that prescribed for each patient, came to 11% $\pm$ 2.3% over a mean follow-up of 37.1 months.

Sodium and potassium intake were estimated by 24 h urine collections and were not significantly different between the two dietary groups. However, in both groups the 24 h urine sodium excretion exceeded the prescribed 2000 mg/day.

Table 4. Effects of low protein diet on nutritional status

	Body weight (Kg)	Mid-arm muscle circumference (cm)	Albumin (g/l)
	+ 0.40 ± 0.77	+ 0.04 ± 0.30	+ 0.80 ± 0.90
P	NS	NS	NS

Diabetes Control

The hemoglobin A_{1c} in control patients throughout the study was 8.0% ± 0.4% and was not significantly different from the mean value on the low protein intake of 7.8% ± 0.2% (normal < 5.1%). There was no significant adjustment in the insulin requirements in either group.

Blood Pressure Control and Patient Visits

The average mean arterial pressure for control patients was 105.5 ± 0.9 mm/mercury, compared to 102.5 ± 1.2 mm/mercury in the protein restricted patients. This very small difference was significant at the P = 0.05 level. However, the contribution of this small blood pressure difference to the rate of progression of renal disease is likely to be minor.

Previous investigators have suggested that there is an inverse relationship between the number of patient visits with the physician and the rate of progression of chronic renal disease [30]. In the present study, the patients on the low protein diet were seen 10.6 ± 1.0 x/year, whereas control patients were seen 13.0 ± 1.8 x/year. This difference in patient visits was not significant.

Nutritional Parameters

Whether or not the prolonged intake of a low protein diet has adverse nutritional effects in subjects with Type I diabetes has not been evaluated. The results of those parameters followed in the present study—body weight, mean mid-arm circumference, and serum albumin—are listed in Table 4. The data are presented after one year follow-up because all patients were followed for a minimum of 12 months. It should be noted that in patients on low protein intake there were no significant changes in these parameters throughout the length of the study.

Listed in Table 5 are the lipid parameters, again after a follow-up period of 12 months. There were no significant changes in the serum cholesterol, triglycerides, or the LDL to HDL ratio.

Table 5. Effects of low protein diet on lipid status

	Initial	1 Year	P
Cholesterol (mMol/L)	5.1 ± 0.3	5.3 ± 0.3	NS
Triglycerides (g/l)	1.83 ± 0.33	2.05 ± 0.35	NS
LDL/HDL	2.91 ± 0.27	2.85 ± 0.25	NS

Discussion

A number of studies, in a number of experimental models of renal disease, have evaluated the efficacy of dietary protein restriction in preventing progressive renal failure and the associated hemodynamic changes thought to induce progression, (i.e., hyperfiltration) [7–16]. These experimental models include hypertension [10], renal mass ablation [8, 11–15], and diabetes [9]. A number of clinical trials in humans have suggested that there is a beneficial effect of protein and phosphorus restriction on the progression of renal failure, but the results of these trials have been challenged on several grounds [31,32]. Most studies have examined patient populations heterogeneous with respect to the cause of renal failure. In addition, in most studies, glomerular filtration rate has not been measured by what are currently the most acceptable and valid techniques, i.e., inulin clearance or radioisotopic tracer clearance, such as that of ^{125}I iothalamate. Indeed, many of these studies have relied on measurements of serum creatinine or on the determination of reciprocal serum creatinine, neither of which are accurate measures of glomerular filtration rate, especially when there is reduced intake of protein [33]. In addition, most of these studies have not reported anthropometric data to provide evidence for or against adequate maintenance of muscle mass and, presumably, nitrogen balance. While some studies have reported creatinine clearances, it is well known that this measurement may over-estimate GFR in patients with advanced renal insufficiency or decreasing muscle mass [34]. This is the first study which has assessed the impact of dietary protein intake on renal function, as determined by a well accepted technique for measuring GFR.

An additional advantage of the present study over previous reports is that compliance with the dietary protein intake was closely monitored by urine urea nitrogen measurements. In most previous studies, dietary compliance has been assessed predominantly by dietary history, which method is known to be inaccurate.

Finally, it is apparent that in the retrospective studies which have been reported previously, other uncontrolled variables may have played significant contributory roles in the progression of renal failure. This is especially true of blood pressure and, possibly, of sodium intake. The present study, because of its prospective design, paid attention to equally aggressive blood pressure control in both groups, as well as to equalization of dietary sodium intake.

The present study was specifically designed to address the effect of dietary protein intake on a single disease entity, namely, Type I diabetes mellitus. It was felt that choosing a single disease would increase the sensitivity of the study and, of course, the selection of diabetes is appropriate, since it is a major contributor to end-stage renal disease in the United States. The results of our study clearly demonstrate that a low protein diet can significantly influence the course of progressive diabetic nephropathy. The patients in the treatment group exhibited a four-fold decrease in the rate of progression of their chronic renal failure when compared to control patients. At the same time, nutrition has been well maintained and there has been no evidence of any dietary-related complications in nutritional status, diabetes control, or blood lipid control.

Previous studies [1,2] have shown that blood pressure control can reduce the progression of renal failure in Type I diabetic patients with clinical nephropathy. We observed a slight, but significant, difference in mean arterial pressure, of 3 mm/

mercury, between the treatment and control groups in the present study. While this may contribute somewhat to the difference in the rate of progression of renal failure, if one extrapolates from previous studies, where significant slowing of the decline of renal function was seen with reductions of mean arterial blood pressure of 12–14 mm/mercury, it is clear that the small differences in blood pressure cannot account for the major difference in the rate of renal function decline between the two groups.

While the present study clearly shows a beneficial effect of reduced dietary protein intake on progressive nephropathy of Type I diabetes, it cannot address the mechanism responsible for this beneficial effect. While the popular theory of hyperfiltration as the cause of progression, and the prevention of hyperfiltration by the low dietary protein intake, could explain our findings, we have no data to support this. Also, it is important to point out that while we are quite confident about our results, a tremendous amount of physician, nurse, and dietician effort is required to maintain a population of patients on such a dietary regimen. Thus, the practical and cost implications of such an approach should be considered. Also of importance is the fact that our subgroup analysis revealed that a beneficial effect of dietary protein restriction could be seen in patients with a mean initial glomerular filtration rate of 66 ml/min. Whether a beneficial effect can be seen in patients with even higher GFRs is unknown. Finally, we feel that a more complete understanding of the mechanisms responsible for the beneficial effect of dietary protein restriction will be important in helping to design possible alternative approaches, i.e., pharmacologic approaches, which can mimic the functional effects of low dietary protein intake.

References

1. Mogensen CE (1982) Long-term antihypertensive treatment inhibiting progression of diabetic nephropathy. Br Med J [Clin Res] 285:685–688
2. Parving HH, Anderson AR, Smidt UM, et al. (1983) Early aggressive antihypertensive treatment reduces rate of decline of kidney function in diabetic nephropathy. Lancet I:1175–1178
3. Knowles HC Jr (1974) Magnitude of the renal failure problem in diabetic patients. Kidney Int 6:1–7
4. Deckert T, Poulsen JE, Larsen M (1978) Prognosis of diabetics with diabetes onset before the age of thirty-one. Diabetologia 14:363–370
5. Dorman JS, LaPorte RE, Kuller LH, et al. (1984) The Pittsburgh insulin-dependent diabetes mellitus (IDDM) morbidity and mortality study. Diabetes 33:271–276
6. Anderson AR, Sandahl-Christiansen J, Anderson JK, Kreiner S, Deckert T: Diabetic nephropathy in type I (insulin-dependent) diabetes (1983) An epidemiological study. Diabetologia 25:496–501
7. Farr LE, Smadel JE (1939) The effect of dietary protein on the course of nephrotoxic nephritis in rats. J Exp Med 70:615–627
8. Hostetter TH, Olson JL, Rennke HG, Venkatachalam MA, Brenner BM: Hyperfiltration in remnant nephrons (1981) A potentially adverse response to renal ablation. Am J Physiol 241:F85–F93
9. Wen SF, Huang TP, Moorthy AV (1985) Effects of low-protein diet on experimental diabetic nephropathy in the rat. J Lab Clin Med 106:589–597
10. Dworkin LD, Feiner HD (1986) Glomerular injury in uninephrectomized spontaneously hypertensive rats. A consequence of glomerular capillary hypertension. J Clin Invest 77:797–809

11. Kenner CH, Evan AP, Blomgren P, Aronoff GR, Luft FC (1985) Effect of protein intake on renal function and structure in partially nephrectomized rats. Kidney Int 27:739–750

12. Kleinknecht C, Salusky I, Broyer M, Gubler MC (1979) Effect of various protein diets on growth, renal function and survival of uremic rats. Kidney Int 15:534–541

13. Laouari D, Kleinknecht C, Gubler MC, Broyer M (1983) Adverse effect of protein on remnant kidney. Dissociation from that of other nutrients. Kidney Int 24(Suppl 16):S248–S253

14. El-Nahas AM, Paraskevakou H, Zoob S, Rees AJ, Evans DJ (1983) Effect of dietary protein restriction on the development of renal failure after subtotal nephrectomy in rats. Clin Sci 65:399–406

15. Kikuchi H, Matsushita T, Hirata K (1983) Improved dietary treatment with low protein and phosphorus restriction in uremic rats. Kidney Int 24(Suppl 16):S254–S258

16. Neugarten J, Feiner HD, Schacht RG, Baldwin DS (1983) Amelioration of experimental glomerulonephritis by dietary protein restriction. Kidney Int 24:595–601

17. Ibels LS, Alfrey AC, Haut L, Huffer WE (1978) Preservation of function in experimental renal disease by dietary restriction of phosphate. N Engl J Med 298:122–126

18. Karlinsky ML, Haut L, Buddington B, Schrier NA, Alfrey AC (1980) Preservation of renal function in experimental glomerulonephritis. Kidney Int 17:293–302

19. Lumlertgul D, Burke TJ, Gillum DM, et al. (1986) Phosphate depletion arrests progression of chronic renal failure independent of protein intake. Kidney Int 29:658–666

20. Maschio G, Oldrizzi L, Tessitore N, et al. (1982) Effects of dietary protein and phosphorus restriction on the progression of early renal failure. Kidney Int 22:371–376

21. Barsotti G, Morelli E, Giannoni A, Guiducci A, Lupetti S, Giovanetti S (1983) Restricted phosphorus and nitrogen intake to slow the progression of chronic renal failure: A controlled trial. Kidney Int 24(Suppl 16):S278–S284

22. Mitch WE, Walser M, Steinman TI, Hill S, Zeger S, Tungsanga K (1984) The effect of a keto acid-amino acid supplement to a restricted diet on the progression of chronic renal failure. N Engl J Med 311:623–629

23. Rosman JB, ter Wee PM, Meijer S, Piers-Becht TP, Sluiter WJ, Donker AJ (1984) Prospective randomized trial of early dietary protein restriction in chronic renal failure. Lancet II:1291–1296

24. Evanoff GV, Thompson CS, Brown J, Weinman EJ (1987) The effect of dietary protein restriction on the progression of diabetic nephropathy. A 12-month follow-up. Arch Intern Med 147(3):492–495

25. Maroni BJ, Steinman TI, Mitch WE (1985) A method for estimating nitrogen intake of patients with chronic renal failure. Kidney Int 27:58–65

26. Nathan DM, Raskin P (1984) A convenient automated method for high performance liquid chromatography measurement of glycated (glycosylated) hemoglobin. Clin Chem 30:813–814

27. Petri A, Dunn FI, Raskin P (1980) The effect of improved diabetic control on plasma lipid and lipoprotein levels: A comparison of conventional therapy and continuous subcutaneous insulin infusion. Diabetes 29:1001–1005

28. Israelit AH, Long DL, White MG, Hull AR (1973) Measurement of glomerular filtration rate utilizing a single subcutaneous injection of ^{125}I-iothalamate. Kidney Int 4:346–349

29. Diabetic Retinopathy Study Research Group. Diabetic Retinopathy Study Report number 6. Design, methods, and baseline results. (1981) Invest Ophthalmol Vis Sci 21(1, pr2):149–209

30. Bergstrom J, Alvestrand A, Bucht H, Guttierrez A (1986) Progression of chronic renal failure in man is retarded with more frequent clinical follow-ups and better blood pressure control. Clin Nephrol 25:1–6

31. Zeller KR, Jacobson HR (1989) Reducing dietary protein intake to retard progression of diabetic nephropathy. Am J Kidney Dis 13(1):17–19

32. El Nahas AM, Coles GA (1986) Dietary treatment of chronic renal failure: Ten unanswered questions. Lancet I:597–600
33. Mitch WE (1984) Nutritional therapy in renal failure. Annu Rev Med 35:249–264
34. Schuster VL, Seldin DW (1985) Renal clearance. In: Seldin DW, Giebisch G (eds) The kidney: physiology and pathophysiology, vol 1. Raven, New York, pp 365–395
35. Walser M, Drew HH, LaFrance ND (1988) Creatinine measurements often yield false estimates of progression in chronic renal failure. Kidney Int 34:412–418

Proposed Mechanisms for Changes in Progression by Dietary Manipulation

WILLIAM E. MITCH[1]

SUMMARY. It has been known for at least 50 years that manipulation of the diet of rats with chronic renal disease slows progression of the disease. Understanding the mechanism for this effect could lead to modifications that would amplify any benefit proven effective in humans with renal disease. Proposed mechanisms can be divided into 1) nephrotoxicity of a constituent of the diet, including phosphate and lipids and 2) damage resulting from adaptive changes which occur in response to renal failure. The latter include hemodynamic, hypertrophic, and metabolic changes. Extensive investigation in rats has not yielded consistent results. In humans, even less is known, but tempting hypotheses include nephrotoxicity from excess dietary protein, plus a link to hypertension and hormonal responses.

Introduction

More than 50 years ago, it was shown that manipulation of the diet could affect the severity of progressive kidney damage, chronic renal failure (CRF), in rats subjected to subtotal nephrectomy or other types of experimental renal disease [1]. The mechanism for this effect remains obscure, but over the last several years growing evidence indicates that dietary manipulation can exert a similar beneficial effect in humans with progressive renal failure. Understanding the mechanism is important because the protective effect could be magnified by making more specific changes in the diet. Unfortunately, there is controversy surrounding the cause of progressive renal damage in even the most simple model: rats with renal failure after subtotal nephrectomy (the remnant kidney model). There is no uniform agreement about which nutrient(s) promotes progressive renal damage. It is not difficult to understand, therefore, why there is no uniform agreement about the cause of progressive damage in humans or about the way in which changing the diet could ameliorate the

---

[1]Renal Division, Emory University School of Medicine, Atlanta, GA 30322, USA

loss of renal function. I will assess the evidence that mechanisms proposed from studies in rats apply to humans with CRF.

Proposed mechanisms for the effect of dietary manipulation can be divided into groups: those related to a toxic effect of specific components of the diet; those related to adaptive responses to loss of kidney function; and those not obviously related to the diet.

Nephrotoxicity of the Dietary Constituents

In early studies of normal rats, it was noted that long-term feeding of a diet rich in liver, meat, or casein was associated with pathological damage to the kidney and loss of renal function. Moise and Smith documented that a high-casein diet (and hence, excess phosphorus) was associated with the development of glomerular and tubular lesions in uninephrectomized rats [1]. Chanutin and Ludewig showed that the severity of renal pathology, hypertension, and loss of renal function was related to the percentage of dried meat fed to remnant-kidney rats [2]. Subsequently, the opposite was noted, namely that restriction of dietary protein limited proteinuria and histological damage, preserved renal function, and prolonged survival even when renal damage was produced by immunologic methods [2,3]. Similar results have been obtained more recently. Since protein was restricted, one conclusion is that dietary protein led to accumulation of a nephrotoxin arising from metabolism of the protein. Another hypothesis was that the "work" required to excrete metabolites of excess protein led to kidney damage. To date, no nephrotoxin has been identified, nor is there persuasive evidence for the "renal work" hypothesis.

The only dietary nephrotoxin that has been manipulated experimentally is phosphate intake. The link with a high-protein diet is that such diets are almost invariably associated with a high phosphate intake. It has been suspected for many years that precipitation of calcium phosphate causes progressive deterioration of renal function and would account for interstitial rather than glomerular damage in experimental renal disease [4,5]. In 1937, Donohue and associates reported that excessive calcium deposition in residual renal tissue of remnant-kidney rats could be blocked by parathyroidectomy [6]. Ibels et al. reported that restriction of dietary phosphorus (plus aluminum hydroxide) in remnant-kidney rats preserved renal function and histology as well as survival [7]. One problem was that renal function was monitored by changes in serum creatinine, but low-phosphate diets induce weight loss so serum creatinine may not have accurately reflected renal function. To circumvent this problem, Lumlertgul et al. fed a normal diet plus a phosphate binder to remnant-kidney rats and found that rats receiving the phosphate binders exhibited less proteinuria and histologic damage and had improved renal function and survival [8]. In another manipulation, 3-phosphocitrate (an inhibitor of calcium phosphate precipitation and tissue calcification) dramatically limited calcium disposition and interstitial disease [9]. Collectively, the results suggest a prominent role for dietary phosphorus in progressive renal insufficiency in rats. However, the importance of dietary phosphate has been questioned. Critics argue that any benefit of low dietary phosphorus is due to reduced food and/or protein intake. Tapp and associates studied remnant-kidney rats, which were carefully pair-fed, in order to examine the influence of protein and food intake independently [5]. Note that pair-feeding has not been routine in many studies of progression in rats, hence interpretation of results is suspect. It was concluded that restriction of food intake prevented the development of end-stage renal pathology, regardless of whether dietary protein was restricted and it was concluded that mediators of growth might play an important role in this response.

In humans with CRF, it has been difficult to test the influence of dietary phosphate for two reasons: firstly, it is virtually impossible to restrict dietary phosphate without restricting protein, since foods rich in phosphate are generally rich in protein; and secondly, it is difficult to add phosphorus to the diet because of concern about inducing secondary hyperparathyroidism. Barsotti et al. fed the same low-protein diet to two groups of patients who also received either 6.5 or 12 mg phosphorus/kg per day [10]. Patients who had a low urinary phosphorus had no change or an improvement in creatinine clearance while those with values above 400 mg/day had a decrease in clearance. Although these results are impressive, they need to be confirmed.

Hyperlipidemia and Progression

Manipulation of the diet to avoid excess dietary protein (or phosphorus) could change the intake of other important nutrients such as lipids. Similarities between mesangial and smooth-muscle cells, which are so important in the pathogenesis of atherosclerosis, have led to the proposition that lipid accumulation in mesangial cells could stimulate proliferation and could ultimately induce focal glomerulosclerosis [11]. A central theme is that persistent proteinuria stimulates production of abnormal lipoproteins which perpetuate the proteinuria and promote glomerular damage.

Attempts to test the hypothesis by manipulating dietary lipids in rats have shown variable and sometimes conflicting results. A high-cholesterol diet has been associated with focal glomerulosclerosis in guinea pigs and in the obese Zucker rat; such a diet also seems to aggravate glomerular sclerosis in rats treated with puromycin. Other evidence for a nephrotoxic effect of dietary lipids includes decreased focal glomerulosclerosis in the remnant kidney model of rats treated with antihyperlipidemic drugs [11]. Exercise training of partially nephrectomized rats lowers serum lipids and decreases proteinuria and focal glomerulosclerosis.

Fatty acid metabolites could be mediators of progressive renal damage. Administration of a thromboxane synthesis inhibitor to remnant-kidney rats was associated with functional and histologic improvement [11]. However, a diet enriched with the arachidonic acid precursor, linoleic acid, had variable effects; in mice with immune complex nephritis [12] and in remnant-kidney rats, linoleic acid-enriched diets were reported to preserve renal function; other investigators report no beneficial effect of the regimen [13]. In mice genetically predisposed to develop immune-mediated nephropathy, a diet enriched with fish oils prevented proteinuria and increased survival, yet the same diet was associated with functional and histologic deterioration in remnant-kidney rats [14]. The mechanism for these conflicting effects induced by different types of polyunsaturated fatty acids is unknown.

For humans with renal disease, evidence that dietary lipids play an important pathogenetic role is lacking. Renal insufficiency is not a prominent feature of diseases associated with hypercholesterolemia. It is also disturbing to note that addition of specific lipids to the diet of rats has yielded such conflicting results.

Adaptive Responses and the Loss of Renal Function

The Hyperfiltration Hypothesis

In the 1980s it was proposed that the progressive loss of renal function in remnant-kidney rats was caused by the adaptive increase in glomerular perfusion which increased the function of less severely affected nephrons. Glomerular capillary hydrostatic pressure was associated with glomerulosclerosis. A link to the diet was provided when it was shown that protein restriction largely prevented glomerular capillary hypertension, proteinuria, and glomerular sclerosis [15]. Angiotensin II has been studied most intensively as a mediator of efferent arteriolar vasoconstriction. For example, remnant-kidney rats treated with an angiotensin converting enzyme inhibitor (CEI) had less systemic hypertension, nearly normal glomerular capillary hydrostatic pressure, and importantly, less proteinuria and glomerular damage than rats treated with a combination of reserpine, hydralazine, and hydrochlorothiazide [16]. A low-protein diet and CEI therapy has also been reported to benefit remnant-kidney rats given high doses of glucocorticoids and rats with diabetes mellitus.

In spite of the attractiveness of these experiments, other conditions have been studied in which glomerular sclerotic changes can be dissociated from glomerular hemodynamics. In rats given aminonucleoside drugs to induce proteinuria and sclerosis, administration of CEI reduced the degree of glomerular sclerosis without affecting intraglomerular pressure [17]. These studies employed a novel and technically demanding method of making serial measurements of glomerular hemodynamics in a single nephron, in order to analyze the relationship between glomerular hypertension and sclerosis; however the studies yielded no correlation between glomerular sclerosis and single nephron GFR (SNGFR) or glomerular pressure. These investigators also reported that enalapril and standard antihypertensive therapy (reserpine, hydralazine and hydrochlorothiazide) were equally effective at reducing glomerular sclerosis following subtotal nephrectomy, despite the more impressive reduction in glomerular pressure with enalapril [18]. In their view, glomerular hypertrophy appeared to be the primary determinant of sclerosis, hence growth stimuli cause progressive loss of renal function. Finally, a thromboxane synthesis inhibitor reduced systemic blood pressure, but markedly increased renal plasma flow and SNGFR in remnant-kidney rats [11]. Yet, in spite of hyperfiltration, treated rats had less proteinuria and glomerular damage than untreated rats, so stimuli other than glomerular capillary hypertension seemed to cause renal damage.

Besides these inconsistencies, there is the important question of how closely the subtotal nephrectomy model mimics the pathophysiology of CRF in humans. Many of the experiments have been performed in strains of rats with a high incidence of spontaneous glomerular sclerosis. Moreover, when dogs were subjected to 75% nephrectomy and followed for four years, renal pathology was minimal. Preliminary results from adult baboons fed high- vs low-protein diets and followed for one year after subtotal nephrectomy, showed no difference in progression despite a modest increase in proteinuria [19]. This raises the possibility that there may be important species differences with respect to the influence of dietary protein on renal function and morphology.

To assess the influence of adaptive changes in glomerular hemodynamics on progressive kidney damage in humans, normal subjects or CRF patients were fed a high-protein meal and changes in renal blood flow and GFR were measured. Bosch and associates concluded that CRF patients had little or no response because glomerular hemodynamics were maximally stimulated even in the resting state [20]. There have been a plethora of these studies, but few show such striking results. Hostetter evaluated the response to a meal consisting of 3.5 g protein/kg body weight and found that 4 of 10 patients had no increase in GFR above basal values [21]. Chan and associates performed an even more extensive analysis of the renal response to a high-protein meal and reached similar conclusions [22]. It should be emphasized that period to period measurements of GFR in humans have inherent variability (as expected with any biologic measurement). This fact raises questions about conclusions based on comparing baseline with the "peak" value following a high-protein meal.

The second method of assessing the influence of glomerular dynamics has been to evaluate renal function in patients with a unilateral nephrectomy. In kidney donors (who develop a compensatory increase in single kidney GFR and who are, presumably, eating a normal diet), there seems to be a slightly higher incidence of hypertension but little evidence for progressive renal failure [23].

Glomerular Hypertrophy

Following subtotal nephrectomy, there is a hypertrophic response and the development of glomerulosclerosis [11]. The diet could participate in the hypertrophic response because dietary protein modulates glomerular size in normal animals; high- or low-protein diets increase or decrease, respectively, the renal hypertrophy which occurs after nephrectomy or experimental diabetes. Although glomerular hypertrophy has been linked to abnormal glomerular hemodynamics, experimental support for this theory is lacking [18]. Administration of CEI to remnant-kidney rats markedly reduces glomerular hypertrophy which, according to some authors, is the primary determinant of sclerosis. In rats, Yoshida et al. performed a left nephrectomy, and either diverted the right ureter into the peritoneal cavity or performed a 2/3 right nephrectomy [24]. Despite a comparable degree of glomerular hypertension in both groups, glomerular hypertrophy and sclerosis was greater in remnant-kidney rats, suggesting that the loss of nephrons, and not simply the loss of excretory function, stimulates glomerular hypertrophy.

Nephron Hypermetabolism

Another hypothetical mechanism is based on the increase in cellular metabolism stimulated by loss of renal function. Remnant-kidney rats had increased oxygen consumption, which could not be accounted for by sodium reabsorption; the difference was eliminated in rats treated by verapamil or dietary phosphate restriction [4]. It was suggested that "nephron hypermetabolism" increases free radicals and membrane lipid damage, resulting in tubulointerstitial nephritis. The beneficial effect of verapamil suggested that changes in intracellular calcium, and hence abnormal signaling processes, are involved in the development of progressive renal damage. However, others find verapamil does not protect against progressive damage in the remnant-kidney model [25].

Intraglomerular Coagulation

A proposed mechanism that has little apparent relationship to the diet involves intraglomerular coagulation. Intraglomerular thrombosis is present in the remnant kidney and in glomeruli after immunologically-mediated nephritis is induced in rats. In similar models, anticoagulants or inhibitors of platelet aggregation can be shown to reduce glomerular injury and progression, suggesting that coagulation may contribute to loss of glomerular capillaries [11]. Fibrin deposits are found in glomerular capillaries of some patients with rapidly progressive glomerulonephritis and, apparently, the survival of platelets in subjects with membranoproliferative glomerulonephritis is shortened [26].

It is, therefore, interesting that heparin, independently of its anticoagulant properties, limits glomerulosclerosis in the remnant-kidney model. Since heparin also has antiproliferative properties [11], the beneficial effect may be due to suppression of mesangial growth and expansion.

Progression in Patients with Chronic Renal Failure

From the foregoing discussion, it should be obvious that the cause of progressive renal insufficiency in humans is not known. Two potential mechanisms have been suggested: damage from hypertension and damage from excess glucocorticoids. There is evidence that hypertension reduced GFR in experimental glomerulonephritis, even though glomerular morphology was unaffected [27]. In spite of these experimental results and results from patients with diabetic nephropathy, there is scarce evidence that hypertension exerts an important influence on the progression of renal disease in humans. Lindeman and associates found that hypertension was significantly correlated with the decline in creatinine clearance in elderly patients with evidence of renal dysfunction [28]. The association was weak, however, since only about 9% of the decline in clearance could be attributed to variation in mean blood pressure. Recently, Brazy et al., in a retrospective analysis of dialysis patients, reported that blood pressure was related to changes in renal function [29]. They found that patients with more rapid rates of progression had higher levels of systolic and diastolic blood pressure. Importantly, they also found that control of diastolic pressure below 90 mmHg was associated with slowing of the loss of renal function. The role of diet in these changes is unclear. Dietary restriction could limit intake of salt or some other factor causing hypertension. Alternatively, attention to the diet, with more frequent visits to the physician, could influence blood pressure control (and hence deterioration of renal function).

Finally, Walser and Ward reported that changes in GFR in CRF patients were related to the rate of excretion of glucocorticoid which in turn, was related to the type of diet; a ketoacid regimen was associated with the most benefit [30]. It seems unlikely that these results can be explained by the same factors shown to cause nephropathy in remnant-kidney rats, because the steroid dose used experimentally was quite high [31].

In summary, the exciting possibility that the diet can slow the loss of renal function in CRF patients has been widely studied in rat models, primarily in the remnant-kidney model. Several mechanisms have been proposed, but experiments in humans have lagged far behind. At present, there is no widely accepted explanation for the effect of dietary manipulation on preservation of renal function.

Acknowledgment. This work was supported by NIH grant DK 37175 and DK 40907.

References

1. Moise TS, Smith AH (1927) Effect of high protein diet on the kidneys. Arch Pathol Lab Med 4:530–560
2. Chanutin A, Ludewig S (1936) Experimental renal insufficiency produced by partial nephrectomy. V. Diets containing whole dried meat. Arch Intern Med 58:60–80
3. Farr LE, Smadel JE (1940) The effect of dietary protein on the course of nephrotoxic nephritis in rats. Am J Pathol 16:615–627
4. Schrier RW, Harris DCH, Chan L, Shapiro JI, Caramelo C (1988) Tubular hypermetabolism as a factor in the progression of chronic renal failure. Am J Kidney Dis 12:243–249
5. Tapp DC, Wortham WG, Addison JF, Hammonds DN, Barnes JL, Venkatachalam MA (1989) Food restriction retards body growth and prevents end-stage renal pathology in remnant kidneys of rats regardless of protein intake. Lab Invest 60:184–195
6. Donohue W, Springarn C, Pappenheimer AM (1937) The calcium content of the kidney as related to parathyroid function. J Exp Med 66:697–701
7. Ibels LS, Alfrey AC, Haut L, Huffer W (1978) Preservation of function in experimental renal disease by dietary restriction of phosphate. N Engl J Med 298:122–126
8. Lumlertgul G, Burke TJ, Gillum DM, Alfrey AC, Harris DC, Hammond WS, Schrier RW (1986) Phosphate depletion arrests progression of chronic renal failure independent of protein intake. Kidney Int 29:658–666
9. Gimenez L, Walker WG, Tew WP, Hermann JA (1982) Prevention of phosphate-induced progression of uremia in rats by 3-phosphocitric acid. Kidney Int 22:36–41
10. Barsotti G, Giannoni A, Morelli E (1984) The decline of renal function slowed by very low phosphorus intake in chronic renal patients following a low nitrogen diet. Clin Nephrol 21:54–59
11. Klahr S, Schreiner G, Ichikawa I (1988) The progression of renal disease. N Engl J Med 318:1657–1666
12. Kher V, Barcelli U, Weiss M, Pollak VE (1985) Effects of dietary linoleic acid enrichment on induction of immune complex nephritis in mice. Nephron 39:261–267
13. Keane WF, Kasiske BL, O'Donnell MP (1988) Hyperlipidemia and the progression of renal disease. Am J Clin Nutr 47:157–160
14. Scharschmidt LA, Gibbons NB, McGarry L, Berger P, Axelrod M, Janis R, Ko YH (1987) Effects of dietary fish oil on renal insufficiency in rats with subtotal nephrectomy. Kidney Int 32:700–709
15. Hostetter TH, Olston JL, Rennke HG, Venkatachalam MA, Brenner BM (1981) Hyperfiltration in remnant nephrons. Am J Physiol 241:F85–F93
16. Anderson S, Rennke HG, Brenner BM (1986) Therapeutic advantage of converting enzyme inhibitors in arresting progressive renal disease associated with systemic hypertension in the rat. J Clin Invest 77:1993–2000
17. Fogo A, Yoshida Y, Glick AD, Homma T, Ichikawa L (1988) Serial micropuncture analysis of glomerular function in two rat models of glomerular sclerosis. J Clin Invest 82:322–330
18. Yoshida Y, Kawamura T, Ikoma M, Fogo A, Ichikawa L (1989) Effects of antihypertensive drugs on glomerular morphology. Kidney Int 36:626–635

19. Bourgoignie JJ, Gavellas G, Hwang KH, Disbrow MR, Sabnis SG, Antonovych TT (1989) Renal function of baboons (*papio hamadryas*) with a remnant kidney, and impact of different protein diets. Kidney Int. 36:S86–S90

20. Bosch JP, Lauer A, Glabman S (1984) Short-term protein loading in assessment of patients with renal disease. Am J Med 77:873–879

21. Hostetter TH (1986) Human renal response to a meat meal. Am J Physiol 19:F613–F618

22. Chan AYM, Cheng ML, Keil LC, Myers BD (1988) Functional response of healthy and diseased glomeruli to a large, protein-rich meal. J Clin Invest 81:245–254

23. Bay WH, Hebert LA (1987) The living donor in kidney transplantation. Ann Intern Med 106:719–727

24. Yoshida Y, Fogo A, Ichikawa I (1989) Glomerular hemodynamic changes vs hypertrophy in experimental glomerular sclerosis. Kidney Int 35:654–660

25. Brunner FP, Thiel G, Hermle M, Bock HA, Mihatasch MJ (1989) Long-term enalapril and verapamil in rats with reduced renal mass. Kidney Int 36:969–977

26. Donadio JV, Anderson CF, Mitchell JC, Holley KE, Ilstrup DM, Fuster V, Chesebro JH (1984) Membranoproliferative glomerulonephritis: A prospective clinical trial of platelet-inhibitor therapy. N Engl J Med 310:1421–1426

27. Blantz RC, Gabbai F, Gushwa LC, Wilson CB (1987) The influence of concomitant experimental hypertension and glomerulonephritis. Kidney Int 32:652–663

28. Lindeman RD, Tobin JD, Shock NW (1984) Association between blood pressure and the rate of decline in renal function with age. Kidney Int 26:861–868

29. Brazy PC, Stead WW, Fitzwilliam JF (1989) Progression of renal insufficiency: Role of blood pressure. Kidney Int 35:670–674

30. Walser M, Ward L (1988) Progression of chronic renal failure is related to glucocorticoid production. Kidney Int 34:859–866

31. Garcia DL, Rennke HG, Brenner BM, Anderson S (1987) Chronic glucocorticoid therapy amplifies glomerular injury in rats with renal ablation. J Clin Invest 80:867–874

Renal Diseases in Asia

Chair: Visith Sitprija (Thailand)
Wan-Yu Chen (Taipei, China)

Hepatitis B Virus Infection and Primary Glomerular Disease

LEISHI LI, JINHONG ZHANG, and ZHIHONG LIU[1]

SUMMARY. Since the first report of a possible pathogenetic association between persistent antigenemia and membranous Australian glomerulonephritis (GN) in 1951, the implications of hepatits B virus (HBV) on the pathogenesis of primary glomerular disease, particularly in the Asian region, have been extensively discussed.

Now the association of the HBV infection with membranous nephropathy (MN) in children is well established. There is a close relationship between the frequency of the HBsAg carrying state in MN and the underlying prevalence of HBsAg carriage in the general population. The HBV-MN in children is also unique in its clinical presentation, serology, and immunopathology, with HBeAg as the dominant type of HBV antigen deposited in glomeruli.

However, the investigation of HBV-GN relied mainly upon the demonstration of HBV specific antigens in the glomeruli which was subject to many technical errors and discrepancies. Opinions about the pathogenetic association between HBV and other types of primary GN (PGN) are still controversial.

Introduction

Since the first report of a possible pathogenetic association between persistent Australian antigenemia and membranous GN in 1951 [1], many studies have demonstrated the presence of HBsAg, HBeAg, and HBcAg in glomerular deposits of various morphological patterns [2,3]. The implications of HBV on the pathogenesis of PGN, particularly in the Asian region, have been extensively discussed.

In this review, we will briefly appraise the association of HBV infection with PGN, its incidence and salient features, and in particular, the experience obtained from China, in order to re-evaluate the significance of HBV infection on the immunopathogenesis of PGN [4-6].

[1]Department of Nephrology, Jinling Hospital, Nanjing University Medical School, Nanjing 210002, People's Republic of China

Evidence for the Etio-Pathogenetic Association of HBV Infection with PGN

Frequency of HBV Carriers among Patients with PGN

Statistics have shown that there is a greater than expected incidence of chronic HBsAg carriers among patients with MN, mesangio-capillary GN (MCGN) and, less frequently, mesangio-proliferative GN (MsPGN) (Fig. 1). Although the total positive rate of HBsAg antigenemia among PGN patients is not different from that in the general population, yet interestingly, HBV carriage in children with MN is in mutual relationship with the underlying prevalence of HBsAg carriage in the local region (Table 1). Also, the prevalence of MN among different types of PGN in children increases in relation to the rising frequency of HBV antigenemia in the local population. For instance, in Poland and China, where HBV antigenemia prevails, 86.7%–91.3% of children with MN are HBV carriers and MN accounts for 22%–28% in the whole group of PGN, values much higher than those in U.S.A. [3,5] (Table 2). This indicates a strong association between childhood MN and HBV infection. However, the frequency of HBsAg carriage in adults with MN is still significant but of a less magnitude (Table 3).

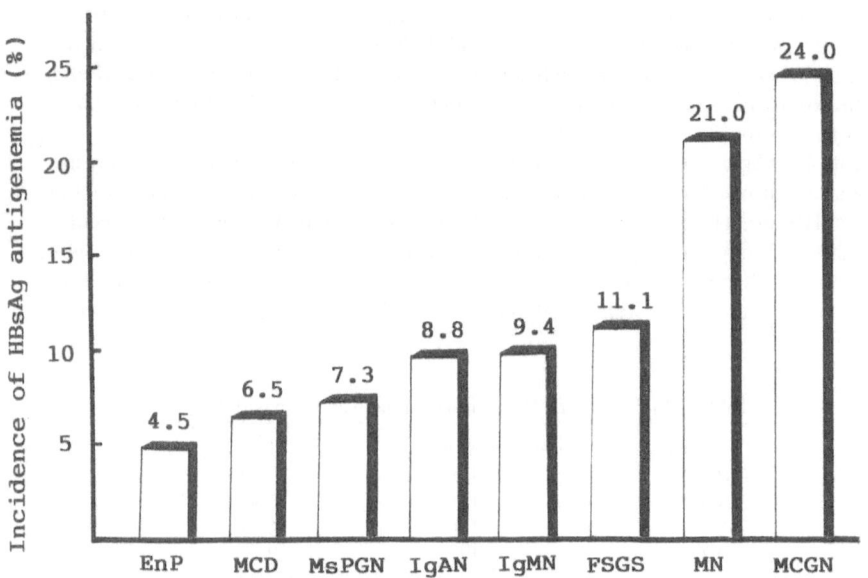

Fig. 1. Incidence of HBs antigenemia in 1375 Chinese patients with various types of PGN. EnP, endocapillary proliferative GN; MCD, minimal change disease; MsPGN, mesangio-proliferative GN; IgAN, IgA nephropathy; IgMN, IgM nephropathy; FSGS, focal segmental glomerular sclerosis; MN, membranes nephropathy; MCGN, mesangiocapillary glomerulonephritis

Table 1. Incidence of MN and HBV-MN in children

Country	Incidence of MN among PGN	Frequency of HBV-MN among children with MN
USA		
(Southwest Pediatric Nephrol Study Group, 1985)	5.5%	20%
China (Gou, 1989)	14.6%	86.7%
Poland (Slusarczyk, 1989)	23.5%	91.3%

MN, membranous nephropathy; HBV, hepatitis B virus; PGN, primary glomerular diseases

Regarding the types of serum HBV markers in PGN, there seem to be no significant differences between the positive rates of various HBV markers. Practically speaking, HBsAg is the type of serum marker most commonly recorded in the literature [7].

Demonstration of HBV Antigens in Glomerular Immune Deposits

Based on collective data in the literature, up to 1989 a total of 1578 patients with various GN with HBsAg antigenemia had been examined for HBV antigens in their glomerular immune deposits, among whom 497 patients (31.5%) showed positive results.

Three distinct antigens, HBsAg, HBcAg, and HBeAg were detected by immunofluorescence (IF) or immunoperoxidase (IP) techniques in renal biopsies from these patients. Different authors had conflicting reports on the nature and frequency of the glomerular HBV antigens which were identified in various glomerulopathic entities. Data are shown collectively in Figs. 2 and 3. More sophisticated assays, and the application of monoclonal antibodies have led to the strong suggestion that HBeAg is the dominant type of HBV antigen deposited in HBV-MN, and that HBsAg is common in MCGN [8,9,10].

Both HBeAg and HBsAg are large (10^6 daltons) in size and are anionic. They are of a size that is unlikely to penetrate the basement membrane into the subepithelial space. HBeAg, a part of viral nucleoprotein, was found in two forms, with molecular weights of 19000 and 300000. These two forms are also anionic, but induce anti-HBeAg, which are largely cationic (PI 5.8–10.2), that can shift the pI of HBeAg from 4.3–4.8 to the 6.4–8.4 range (bound to anti-HBe). HBeAg circulating immune

Table 2. Incidence of HBsAg antigenemia in children with MN

Country	General carrier rate (%)	HBsAg +ve (%)
USA	0.1–1.0	20
France	0.1–1.0	42
Italy	0.1–1.0	64
Poland	5–10	91–92
Japan	2–20	57–81
South Korea	10–15	80
China	10–15	86
South Africa	10–20	89–100
Hong Kong	10–20	94–100
Taiwan	10–20	100

MN, membranous nephropathy

Table 3. Incidence of HBsAg antigenemia in adults with MN

Country	Author		General carrier rate	n	+ve (%)
Great Britain	Rashid	(1981)	1%	28	1(4.0)
Scotland	Mactier	(1986)	1%	54	0(0)
France	Cahen	(1989)	1%	69	0(0)
Hungary	Nagy	(1979)	1–5%	17	3(18.0)
Hong Kong	Lai	(1982)	5–10%	23	10(43.0)
Taiwan	Chen	(1990)	20%	28	3(10.7)
South Korea	Lee	(1988)	2–20%	49	10(20.4)
China	Li	(1990)	10–15%	105	22(21.0)

MN, membranous nephropathy

complexes (CICs) are also small (2.5×10^5 daltons) and thus might be capable of localizing in the subepithelial space. HBeAg CICs have been identified in 44% of children with HBV-MN, and appear to correlate with disease activity. The potential importance of HBeAg in HBV-MN is further supported by observations that circulat-

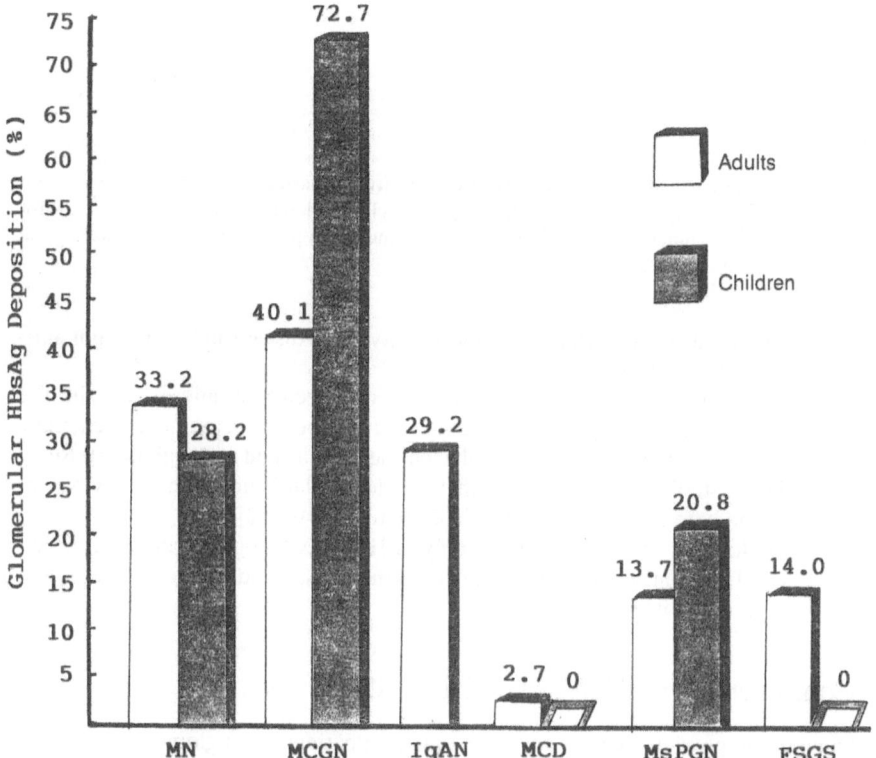

Fig. 2. Cumulative data on glomerular HBsAg deposition in various types of PGN. MN, membranous nephropathy; MCGN, mesangiocapillary glomerulonephritis; IgAn, IgA nephropathy; MsPGN, mesangio-proliferative GN; FSGS, focal segmental glomerular sclerosis

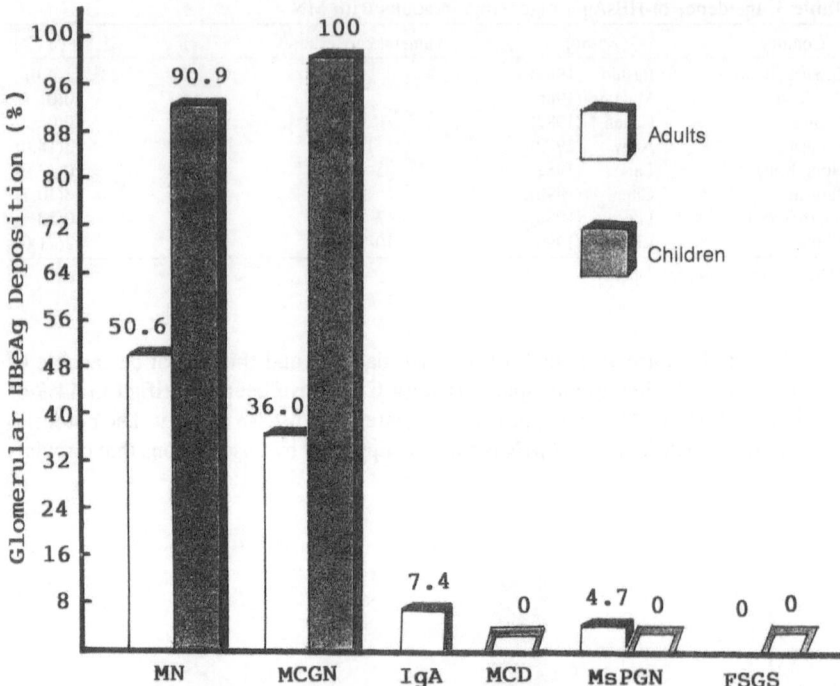

Fig. 3. Cumulative data on glomerular HBeAg deposition in various types of PGN. MN, membranous nephropathy; MCGN, mesangiocapillary glomerulonephritis; IgAN, IgA nephropathy; MCD, minimal change disease; MsPGN, mesangio-proliferative GN; FSGS, focal segmental glomerular sclerosis.

ing HBeAg frequently correlates with the activity of the disease and is the major antigen in the immune deposits [6,7,8,11].

Viral-like particles have been identified on electronic microscopy in the subepithelial and subendothelial areas of the glomerular basement membrane (GBM) as well as within endothelial cells, epithelial cells and mesangium [3]. Renal tissue elution studies have also shown that the glomerular bound Ig in HBV-MN contained antibody to HBV antigens, particularly to HBeAg [12].

The results of in situ hybridization study of HBV-DNA in glomeruli are conflicting. Lai et al. [6] confirmed its presence in 2 of the 6 cases studied, but Zhang [9] and Yu failed to prove its presence.

Controversies on HBV Associated GN

Some of the previous reports emphasized that in patients with glomerular diseases there is a significantly higher incidence of HBs antigenemia than that in the general population or in hospitalized patients, suggesting that HBsAg carriers were predisposed to glomerular disease. But survey statistics of large series collected from HBV endemic areas including China, Korea, and Taiwan did not confirm this phenomenon. In other words, the prevalence of GN in HBV carriers is not higher than that in the general population [10,13].

Although a number of authors reported that HBsAg or HBcAg could be identified by direct or indirect IF or IP techniques in the glomeruli of GN patients associated with HBV antigenemia, others could not confirm such observations [13]. Furthermore, the presence of HBsAg was demonstrated in the glomeruli of patients who had no detectable HBsAg in the serum [9]. Such conflicting results made many researchers doubt the specificity of fluorescent staining for HBsAg within the deposits [14].

In contrast to the accepted strong association of HBV with MN in children, opinions on the causal relationship between HBV infection and adult patients with MN are controversial; in particular, the reports from Taiwan and Korea did not favor such a concept. Chen et al. concluded that there was no significant association of HBV infection and PGN in adults except in MCGN [13]. Using a direct IF technique with monoclonal antibodies, they did not find any case showing immune deposits of HBV related antigens in renal biopsy specimens of PGN in adults.

Lai and others emphasized a significantly higher HBV carrier rate among patients with IgA nephropathy [8]. HBsAg and/or HBcAg were the chief type of HBV markers found in the glomeruli. Yet reports from China and Japan (Chen [13] and Iida [19]) respectively, failed to confirm this phenomenon [19].

Divergence of findings may be due, at least partly, to differences in staining techniques and quality of antisera, and may even be due to the methods of processing specimens [9,14,15].

Maggiore et al. found that the glomerular deposits contained immunoglobulin with antiglobulin activity which bound the Fc part of the anti-HBsAg antibody, thus the results described in the earlier studies may have been falsely positive [14].

Zhang et al. [9] compared results of HBV antigen deposition in adult GN patients with and without virus antigenemia. Not much difference was found between the groups, which included MN and lupus nephritis, while HBsAg could be more commonly detected in patients with virus antigenemia with MCGN and MsPGN. As far as technique factor is concerned, a series of studies using McAb to HBsAg, HBeAg, and HBcAg have shown that the 4-layer peroxidase antiperoxidase (PAP) method is too sensitive to identify HBV deposition in the kidney with some false positive findings. Indirect IP or IF and the avidin-biotin-complex (ABC) methods are fairly good techniques, although nonspecific staining is not entirely excluded.

Antibodies to HBV might have some false positive staining due to the contamination of antibodies to plasma proteins (Goodman et al. [15]). Besides, HBsAg may also bind horseradish peroxidase nonimmunologically and these entities may cause false positive staining. It is therefore essential to have well qualified antiserum and standard technique during the detection of HBV markers in glomeruli.

Theoretically, in order to ascertain whether a particular glomerular disease is etiologically associated with chronic HBV infection, it has to fulfill the following criteria:

1. Demonstration of HBV specific antigen(s) in the glomeruli.
2. Disappearance of the glomerular pathology with the eradication of the microorganism.
3. Experimental reproducibility of the morbidity in an animal model.

Unfortunately, at present the evidence for the presence of so-called "HBV associated GN" is founded basically on the demonstration of HBV specific antigen(s) in the glomeruli. Solid research work to confirm causal relationship between the therapeutic result and the effort to eradicate the HBV virus is still lacking although in anecdotal cases clearance of HBeAg was reported to be associated with resolution of the nephrotic syndrome [7].

For the purpose of staining glomerular HBeAg deposits more specifically, F(ab')$_2$ fragments of McAb raised against HBeAg were introduced into the study carried out by Hirose et al. [16]. In our laboratory, results obtained from a detailed comparison between the glomerular staining of McAb against HBsAg and its F(ab')$_2$ fragments in 12 cases with GN did show a marked difference between the two types of anti-sera being used. The positive rate of McAb against HBsAg was 75%; in contrast, the McAb-F(ab')$_2$ was only 33.3%.

Currently, the diagnosis of HBV-GN depends mainly on the demonstration of HBV specific antigens in the glomeruli. However, due to the different antibodies and various techniques used in histopathologic studies different authors reported wide variations in positive rates of glomerular deposition of HBV antigen. Investigators have pointed out that the glomerular staining of HBV antigens might be artifact, cross reactivity, or non-specific trapping [9,14,15]. Discrepancies between the HBV antigenemia and glomerular HBV deposits were also noticed in some reports.

Salient Features of HBV Associated MN in Children

Children with HBV-MN generally have no history or clinical evidence of ongoing liver disease. With rare exceptions, the liver pathology in children with HBV-MN usually shows chronic persistent hepatitis or minimal abnormality [4,7,17,18].

Despite a negative history for hepatitis, liver function tests and serum transaminases are usually mildly abnormal, in contrast to such values in idiopathic MN [4]. It is generally agreed that as many as 80%–100% of childhood HBV-MN patients are males [4,17]. Nephrotic syndrome or non-nephrotic proteinuria and microscopic hematuria are the common clinical presentations. Clinical remission, which mimics minimal change nephropathy, is quite common. HBV-MN in children usually follows a benign course. Only rarely do children with HBV-MN manifest renal insufficiency.

HBsAg and anti-HBc can almost always be demonstrated in the circulation [3,17]. Approximately 60%–80% of children will also have HBeAg, and the remainder will have anti-HBe antibody in their sera.

Serum C3 and C4 levels may be normal or depressed [17,18]. CICs have been reported in up to 80% of cases of childhood HBV-MN. Staining of the glomerular capillary wall is usually positive for IgG (100%), C3 (75%), IgM (50%), and IgA (10%) [4,7]. In contrast to idiopathic MN, where deposits are seen in an exclusively subepithelial location, HBV-MN is characterized by the presence of subepithelial immune deposits in association with subendothelial and/or mesangial deposits. HBeAg has been identified to be the predominant type of HBV antigen deposited in the glomeruli of HBV-MN [7,17].

Clinical manifestations of adult HBV-MN tend to differ. Frequently there is a history of acute hepatitis, usually 6 months to several years prior to the onset of the kidney disease, and the typical liver pathology of chronic active hepatitis is common.

The nephrotic syndrome in adult HBV-MN patients usually does not respond to steroids and may progress to renal insufficiency.

Possible Immunopathogenesis of HBV-Associated GN

Several potential mechanisms for the development of HBV-MN have been suggested.

Immune Complex Formation

The observation that all 3 major HBV antigens, including HBsAg, HBeAg, and HBcAg have been identified in the glomeruli of patients with HBV-MN supports a mechanism involving HBV antigen-containing immune deposit formation either as a result of passive trapping of CICs or due to local IC formation.

CICs containing HBV antigens have been demonstrated in many patients with HBV-MN. However, CICs rarely result in subepithelial deposits, unless the CICs are very small and cationic. HBeAg CICs are small (2.5×10^5 daltons) and thus might be capable of localizing in the subepithelial space [6,7,20]. Immune complex-mediated GN requires a continuous supply of antigen and a maintained antibody response. Apparently, these requirements seem to be met in chronic HBV carriers. Thus, it is conceivable that MN, a GN with subepithelial deposits of HBeAg and antibody, could result from passive trapping of small cationic preformed CICs. The fact that HBeAg is the dominant type of HBV antigen deposited in HBV-MN also supports the above hypothesis [6,11].

Lai et al. [6] reported that HBeAg, rather than HBcAg, may play a pathogenetic role in the mesangial and subendothelial immune deposits commonly seen in MsPGN or MCGN associated with chronic HBV infection. However, there is currently little experimental evidence to support a preformed CIC trapping mechanism in the pathogenesis of HBV-MN.

A local mechanism of immune deposit formation in HBV-MN is also suggested. As anti-HBe antibodies are cationic, sequential localization of cationic antibody, followed by anionic HBeAg, could result in subepithelial IC formation in situ. The persistence of free antigen or antibody in the circulation may also favor this mechanism.

PGN and HBV Infection are Associated on the Basis of Genetic Predisposition

The association of PGN and HBV infection may not be caused by either HBV virus or by secondary liver disease, but rather may result from genetic predisposition or an underlying immunologic abnormality that increases the likelihood of these patients to develop both diseases independently of each other. Conditions associated with defective cell-mediated immunity do predispose HBV infected patients to become chronic HBsAg carriers, and defective cellular immunity has also been observed in cases with MN. Thus the possibility cannot be ruled out that MN and chronic HBV infection are not causally related, but rather are due to an inherent susceptibility of a subset of patients to develop both diseases. However, studies of human leucocyte antigen (HLA) patterns of patients with HBV-MN have not been reported [7].

Autoimmune Mechanism

Another possible pathogenetic mechanism for HBV-PGN involves the induction of autoantibodies to intrinsic glomerular antigens. Immunopathogenesis involving autoantibodies directed against glomerular antigens in MN has been established by both experimental and clinical studies. It was reported that many autoantibodies were demonstrated in patients with chronic HBV infection. Autoantibodies may contribute to some of the liver injuries in HBsAg positive chronic active hepatitis. Autoantibodies against glomerular antigens have also been identified. Thus, an autoimmune etiology for HBV-PGN should not be excluded.

Conclusions

The association of HBV infection with MN in children is now well established. There is a close relationship between the frequency of the HBsAg carrying state in MN and the underlying prevalence of HBsAg in the general population. The HBV-MN in children is also unique in its clinical presentation, serology, and immunopathology.

However, there is still controversy about the pathogenetic association in other types of PGN, even including HBV-associated MN in adults.

Currently, diagnosis and clinical research of HBV-associated PGN depends mainly on the demonstration of HBV specific antigens in the glomeruli, which demonstration is subject to many technical discrepancies. Improving the techniques and qualifying the immune reagents are mandatory to furthering the future understanding of these conflicting results.

References

1. Combes B, Stastny P, Shorey J, Eigenbrodt EH, Barrera A, Hull AR, Carter NW (1951) Glomerulonephritis with deposition of Australia antigen-antibody complexes in glomerular basement membrane. Lancet II:234
2. Brzosko WJ, Krawczynski K, Nazarewicz T, Morzycka M, Nowoslawski A (1974) Glomerulonephritis associated with hepatitis-B surface antigen immune complexes in children. Lancet II:477
3. Slusarczyk J, Michalak T, Mezer Teresa-Nazarewicz-de, Krawxzynski K, Nowostawski A (1980) Membranous glomerulopathy associated with hepatitis B core antigen immune complexes in children. Am J Pathol 98:29
4. Hsu HC, Lin GH, Chang MH, Chen CH (1983) Association of hepatitis B surface (HBs) antigenemia and membranous nephropathy in children in Taiwan. Clin Nephrol 20:121
5. Zhang YE (1986) An immunopathological study of hepatitis B immune complex glomerulonephritis in 33 cases. Chin J Nephrol 2:127
6. Lai KN, Lai FM, Chan KW, Chow CB, Tong KL, Vallance-Owen J (1987) The clinicopathologic features of hepatitis B virus-associated glomerulonephritis. Q J Med 18:411
7. Johnson RJ, Couser WG (1990) Hepatitis B infection and renal disease: immunopathogenetic and therapeutic considerations. Kidney Int 37:663
8. Lai KN, Lai FM, Tam JS, Vallance-Owen J (1988) Strong association between IgA nephropathy and hepatitis B surface antigenemia in endemic areas. Clin Nephrol 29:229

9. Zhang JH, Zhou H, Li LS (1990) Is there a hepatitis B virus (HBV)-associated GN? Identification of HBV in kidney with in situ hybridization and avidin biotin complex (ABC) methods (abstract). 4th Asian-Pacific Congress of Nephrology, 1990. Beijing, Peoples Republic of China p 165

10. Lee HS, Choi Y, Yu SH, Koh HI, Kim MJ, Ko KW (1988) A renal biopsy study of hepatitis B virus-associated nephropathy in Korea. Kidney Int 34:537

11. Anonymous (1987) HBV and glomerulonephritis. Lancet II:252 (editorial)

12. Hattori S, Furuse A, Matsuda I (1988) Presence of HBe antibody in glomerular deposits in membranous glomerulonephritis is associated with hepatitis B virus infection. Am J Nephrol 8:384

13. Chen WY, Chu TS, Chang CH, Chen YM, Tsal SL, Yen TS, Hsu HC, Lee SH (1989) Studies on adults primary glomerulonephritis and hepatitis B virus infection in Taiwan. The Eighth Asian Colloquium in Nephrology, 1989. Jakarta, Indonesia , p 263

14. Maggiore Q, Bartolomeo F, L'Abbate A, Misefari V (1981) HBsAg glomerular deposits in glomerulonephritis: Fact or artifact? Kidney Int 19:579

15. Goodman ZD, Langloss JM, Bratthauer GL, Ishak KG (1988) Immunohistochemical localization of hepatitis B surface antigen and hepatitis B core antigen in tissue sections. Am J Clin Pathol 89(4):533

16. Hirose H, Udo K, Kojima M, Takahashi Y, Miyakawa Y, Miyamoto K, Yoshizawa H, Mayumi M (1984) Deposition of hepatitis B e antigen in membranous glomerulonephritis: identification by F(ab')2 fragments of monoclonal antibody. Kidney Int 26:338

17. Southwest Pediatric Nephrology Study Group (1985) Hepatitis B surface antigenemia in North American children with membranous glomerulonephropathy. J Pediatr 106(4):571

18. Lin C-Y (1990) Hepatitis B virus associated membranous nephropathy: clinical features, immunological profiles and outcome. Nephron 55:37

19. Iida H, Izumino K, Asaka M, Fujita M, Takata M, Sasayama S (1990) IgA nephropathy and hepatitis B virus. IgA nephropathy unrelated to hepatitis B surface antigenemia. Nephron 54:18

20. Takekoshi Y, Tanaka M, Shida N, Sataka Y, Saheki Y, Matsumoto S (1978) Strong association between membranous nephropathy and hepatitis-B surface antigenaemia in Japanese children. Lancet II:1065

Snake Bite Induced Renal Disease

K.S. Chugh and V. Sakhuja[1]

SUMMARY. A variety of renal lesions have been documented following bites by viper, hydrophid, and colubrid snakes. Acute renal failure is the most frequent manifestation and complicates the course in 5–30% of victims of snake bite. The commonly encountered histological renal lesions are of acute tubular and acute cortical necrosis. Fibrin thrombi are often seen in the renal microvasculature in these cases. Less frequently, proliferative glomerulonephritis, interstitial nephritis and renal papillary necrosis are observed. The consistent presence of several hemostatic abnormalities in patients and animals, of which disseminated intravascular coagulation (DIC) is the most prominent, has focussed attention on the latter playing a significant role in the causation of renal failure. Other systemic effects including bleeding, hypotension, shock, and intravascular hemolysis could play a contributory role. Glomerular changes such as mesangiolysis, mesangial proliferation, and occasional crescent formation are most likely related to the toxic action of the "hemorrhagin" fraction of the venom on the glomerular capillaries. However, these lesions are inconsequential in most patients with renal failure. Severe glomerulonephritis has been documented in a few patients, but appears to be related to hypersensitivity to venomous or anti-venomous proteins. Myoglobinuria is the major factor in the pathogenesis of renal failure in sea snake and Australian land snake envenoming. A consensus has not yet been reached on the precise role of the nephrotoxicity of venom in producing acute tubulo-interstitial lesions.

Introduction

Of the 2700 species of snake recognized the world over, fewer than 450 are venomous; the majority of these are distributed in the tropical and subtropical regions.

[1]Department of Nephrology, Postgraduate Institute of Medical Education and Research, Chandigarh-160012, India

The most frequent targets are farmers and fishermen, making snake bite a professional hazard. Less commonly, amateur collectors, cult followers, and others are affected. The world mortality from snake bites has been assessed to be around 40,000 per year.

Renal Lesions

Relatively recently, renal lesions following bites by venomous snakes have attracted attention; these lesions have been primarily associated with viperid, hydrophid, and colubrid snakes. Clinical reports on venom-induced renal disease have therefore appeared from geographical regions where snakes of these families are prevalent. The reported renal manifestations include acute renal failure, nephrotic syndrome, acute glomerulonephritis, necrotizing vasculitis, and papillary necrosis.

Acute Renal Failure (ARF)

The most frequently reported and devastating effect of envenomation on the kidney is the development of acute renal failure [1,2]. In Burma, where more than 1000 (3.3/100000) deaths occur annually from snake bite, Russell's viper envenomation constitutes 44%–70% of all cases of acute renal failure requiring dialysis and carries a mortality of 35% [3]. In Thailand, ARF has been recorded in 5% of patients bitten by Russell's viper and by sea snakes [4]. In Nigeria, ARF has been observed in 10% of puff adder bites [5] and in less than 1% of *Echis carinatus* envenoming [6]. In Israel, 6% of patients bitten by Palestinian viper [7] and in Sri Lanka, 26% of snake bite victims develop this complication [8]. In India, Russell's viper and *Echis carinatus* cause ARF in 13%–32% of those bitten by these two species [2,9,10]; patients bitten by these two species constitute nearly 3% of the total cases of ARF in our center. In some hospitals in Kerala [South India], snake poisoning accounts for 0.32%–1.4% of total hospital admissions and is responsible for 23% of cases of ARF amongst adults and children [11,12].

The histological entities encountered in envenomed patients with acute renal failure are:

Acute Tubular Necrosis

Cumulative data from several studies have shown that histological changes consistent with acute tubular necrosis [ATN] are seen in 60%–80% of envenomed patients [2,13]. On light microscopy, tubules appear dilated and lined by flattened epithelium. Severe cases exhibit cell necrosis and desquamation of necrotic cells from the basement membrane. Hyaline, granular, and pigment casts are seen in tubular lumina. Varying degrees of interstitial edema, hemorrhage, and inflammatory cell infiltration are seen. Later biopsies show regenerating tubular epithelium [1,2,9]. Fibrin deposits are seen in the glomerular capillaries in some cases [14].

Electron microscopy reveals dense intracytoplasmic bodies in the proximal tubules, which represent degenerating organelles or protein resorption droplets, distal tubular apoptosis, severe vascular lesions, and the presence of mast cells, eosinophils, and active fibroblasts in the interstitium, not observed in tubular necrosis due to other causes [14,15].

Acute Cortical Necrosis

Acute diffuse or patchy cortical necrosis has been reported in 20%–25% of patients bitten by *Echis carinatus* [1,2,10] and Russell's viper [1,2,16,17]. *Agkistrodon hypnale* [18] and *Bothrops* species [19,20] have also been associated with cortical necrosis. For reasons which are still not clear, cortical necrosis is observed more frequently among Indian patients than among Thais [2].

Under light microscopy, glomeruli and tubules appear necrotic and only their outlines can be discerned. Fibrin thrombi are present in the glomerular capillaries in 10%–25% of cases. The deeper cortical and medullary tissue shows changes of extensive tubular necrosis [1,2,13]. Calcification of necrotic areas may occur at a later stage [21]. In patchy cortical necrosis, varying numbers of glomeruli may be spared. With healing, fibroblastic proliferation and organization of the thrombi are seen [2,9].

Electron microscopy reveals collapsed capillary basement membrane denuded of foot processes. No viable mesangial or endothelial cells are seen, but capillary lumina may show swollen rounded cells, possibly of endothelial origin. Tubular basement membrane shows thickening and is lined by flattened epithelium. Fibroblastic proliferation is seen in the interstitium. Endothelial swelling of small arterioles and necrosis of peritubular capillaries is also seen [22].

Glomerular Lesions

Ballooning of the capillaries, mesangial proliferation, thickening and splitting of the basement membrane, swelling of endothelial cells, and crescent formation have been documented in some patients with renal failure. Seedat et al. [23] reported two patients with puff adder bite who developed oliguric renal failure soon after the bite; the renal histology showed changes consistent with crescentic glomerulonephritis. The authors suspected hypersensitivity to the venom as the basis for the renal lesions. Renal failure attributable to severe glomerulonephritis has also been reported in one case of Mamushi bite [24] and in four patients following Russell's viper or green pit viper bites [19]. IgM and C_3 deposits were seen in 63% of envenomed patients, C_3 alone was seen in 8% and no deposits were seen in 29% of patients.

Though other glomerular lesions are commonly seen in association with acute tubular necrosis, their precise contribution to the development of acute renal failure is not defined. Only an occasional patient has presented with evidence of overt glomerular disease.

Acute Interstitial Nephritis

In isolated renal failure patients, renal histology has shown a diffuse and intense mononuclear cell infiltration in the interstitium, suggesting the occurrence of acute interstitial nephritis. This has been observed in two patients bitten by Russell's viper [25,26] and in one bitten by *Echis carinatus* [9].

Acute Necrotizing Vasculitis

Necrotizing arteritis of the interlobular arteries has been observed in association with acute renal failure in two cases of Russell's viper bite. Other changes included thrombophlebitis of the arcuate veins and their tributaries. Immunofluorescence showed C_3 deposits in the afferent and efferent arterioles, but the significance of this finding is not clear [27].

Papillary Necrosis

A recent report has documented occurrence of papillary necrosis following snake bite, but the species was not identified [28].

Nephrotic Syndrome

A single case of nephrotic syndrome developing after an Australian snake bite has been reported by Steinbeck [29]. However, the renal histology was not studied in this case.

Pathogenesis of Renal Failure

One of the unresolved problems in snake venom research is the precise mechanism by which renal failure develops in envenomed patients. Several investigators have attempted to answer the question of whether or not the severe hemodynamic changes resulting from the vasculotoxic, hemotoxic, or myotoxic actions of the venom play a crucial role, or whether it is the nephrotoxic action of the venom on the glomeruli, interstitium, and the tubules which is vital to the development of acute renal failure. The available evidence is summarized.

Hemodynamic Changes

Significant hemodynamic changes result from the occurrence of several concurrent abnormalities in envenomed patients [1,2,6] and in animals [9]. These include bleeding, hypotension, shock, disseminated intravascular coagulation, hemoglobinuria, myoglobinuria, and hypersensitivity to venomous or anti-venomous proteins which are all known to cause acute renal failure individually or in combination.

Bleeding

Bleeding is a striking feature of most viperine bites and results from the direct vasculotoxic effect of the hemorrhagin component of the venom [30,31], which is caused by either a direct lytic action on the capillary endothelium [31,32], or by a widening of the intercellular junctions through which the erythrocytes and the plasma may escape [33]. The hemorrhagin component of *Echis carinatus* venom is ten times more potent than Russell's viper venom and has no effect on the coagulation cascade. Thrombocytopenia and consumptive coagulopathy, which are frequently present in viper-envenomed patients, enhance the tendency to bleeding initiated by hemorrhagin, and thus the tendency to produce ischemic tubular injury.

Hypotension and Shock

Hypotension and shock could be the consequences of bleeding or loss of plasma into the bitten extremity or could be due to hemodynamic effects directly attributable to the presence of certain enzymes such as bradykinin in Russell's viper or *Echis carinatus* venoms [34,35]. Puff adder (*Bitis arietans*) venom causes hypotension by causing myocardial depression, arteriolar dilatation, and increased vascular permeability [36].

Disseminated Intravascular Coagulation (DIC)

The consistent presence of several abnormalities in viper envenomed patients and animals [1–3,6,9,37–44], of which DIC is the most prominent, has focused attention on the latter playing a major pathogenetic role in the causation of renal lesions of acute tubular and cortical necrosis. The procoagulants in Russell's viper venom are known to cause a massive intravascular coagulation within minutes of the bite. Though the injected dose of the venom in human victims is generally insufficient to cause a rapid catastrophe, the deposition of microthrombi in the microvasculature may contribute significantly to the causation of acute renal failure. Carefully conducted histological studies have confirmed the presence of fibrin thrombi in the renal vasculature and occlusion of the glomerular capillaries in viper-envenomed patients and animals [1,3,14]. Intravascular coagulation and fibrin thrombi in the glomeruli are also a hallmark of the cortical necrosis associated with abruptio placentae, amniotic fluid embolism, and septic abortion [45,46]. Intra-glomerular fibrin deposition of lesser degree has been suspected to cause acute tubular necrosis by temporary interruption of the tubular blood supply [47]. In a recent study from our own center, acute disseminated intravascular coagulation was demonstrated in 56% of envenomed patients who developed acute renal failure [2].

Intravascular Hemolysis

Evidence of intravascular hemolysis was present in 50% of patients following bites by Russell's viper and *Echis carinatus* snakes [2,16]. The observation has been confirmed in Rhesus monkeys following administration of the venom of these two species of snakes [43,44]. In a study reported from Burma, hemolysis was absent in patients bitten by Russell's viper [3]. Hemolysis results from the action of phospholipase A2, which is present in almost all snake venoms. The occurrence of micro-angiopathic hemolytic anemia has also been documented in human victims of Russell's viper [1,2], puff adder [5], and gwardar snake [48], and also in animals given Malayan pit viper venom [49]. Intravascular hemolysis is known to be associated with acute renal failure [50].

Myoglobinuria

Sea snakes [51,52] and Australian land snakes [48,53,54] are myotoxic and renal failure may occur due to rhabdomyolysis and myoglobinuria.

Venom Nephrotoxicity

Glomerular Lesions

Current understanding of the pathogenesis of glomerular lesions is based on experimental studies which have been carried out with the venom of the Habu snake which is indigenous to Japan [55–59]. Habu venom contains a vasculotoxic factor "hemorrhagin" which has also been demonstrated in *Echis carinatus*, *Vipera palestinae*, *Agkistrodon halys*, and *Bothrops jararaca*. Within 6–24 h of administration of Habu venom, destruction of mesangium (mesangiolysis) occurs, resulting in segmental ballooning of capillaries. The capillaries become packed with red cells and fibrin, giving the appearance of "blood cysts." Within 3 days, proliferation of mesangial cells occurs which fills up the entire ballooned capillaries, giving an appearance resembling segmental proliferative glomerulonephritis. Rarely, crescents are also noted. Depending upon the period of envenomation, the histological lesions may resemble glomerular aneurysms or a focal proliferative glomerulonephritis.

In human victims of snake bite, mesangiolysis, which represents the earliest glomerular changes, has been documented in only one instance following *Agkistrodon halys* (Mamushi) bite [24]. This patient had presented with acute renal failure. Since renal histology is seldom studied in the first 24–48 hours, mesangiolysis is likely to be missed and this could account for the infrequent documentation of this lesion in snake-bite patients. These experimental studies have further suggested that the frequently observed proliferative changes in human biopsy and autopsy specimens of the kidney (which generally become available days or weeks after envenoming), are likely to represent a late stage in the evolution of glomerular changes. To what extent these changes contribute to acute renal failure is uncertain.

Tubulo-Interstitial Lesions

Despite several clinical and experimental studies, a consensus has still not been reached on the exact role of the nephrotoxicity of the venom in producing the tubular and interstitial lesions which are commonly seen in patients with renal failure. At least three experimental studies have supported a direct toxic action of the venom as an important factor in the causation of acute tubular necrosis. Schmidt et al. [60] observed proximal tubular damage in mice on electron microscopy after administration of rattlesnake venom, although the proximal tubular epithelium remained unaffected following administration of sea snake venom. Raab and Kaiser [61] attributed the increase in urinary alkaline phosphatase and aminopeptidase activity, following *Agkistrodon piscivorus* venom, to a direct effect of the venom on tubular epithelium. Ratcliffe et al. [62] documented characteristic changes, suggestive of acute tubular necrosis, in the urinary indices following exposure of isolated perfused kidney to Russell's viper venom.

Some studies have documented equivocal results, e.g., Hadler and Brazil [63] considered tubular damage following injection of crude *Crotalus terrificus* venom to be primarily due to shock and renal ischemia and partially due to the effect of lysolcithin formed by phospholipase A. Experimental studies with I^{125} labelled *Echis carinatus* venom and demonstration of venom antigen in envenomed patients using ELISA technique, have clearly shown that the venom may be excreted in urine without causing damage to the kidneys [64]. In two other studies carried out in rhesus monkeys, administration of lethal doses of *Echis carinatus* and Russell's viper venom was followed by acute tubular necrosis in only 20% of the animals, whereas following sublethal envenomation, more than 50% of animals showed significant renal lesions [2,9]. Fibrin thrombi were demonstrated in 50%–70% of glomeruli. The coagulation abnormalities and the histological changes were similar to those seen in human victims. The paucity of renal lesions in monkeys given lethal doses of viper venoms argues against a direct toxicity of the venom as a major factor contributing to the pathogenesis of acute renal failure.

Other Factors

At least three acute glomerulonephritis patients reported in the literature—two following puff adder bite [65] and one following Russell's viper bite [66]—appear to be examples of hypersensitivity to venomous or anti-venomous protein. Though significant complement abnormalities have been documented by us [66] and others [67], the role of these abnormalities in causing renal damage is far from clear.

Conclusions

Most of the studies have failed to provide convincing evidence in favor of a direct toxic action of the venom on the kidney as the predominant cause of the histological lesions of acute tubular and cortical necrosis which are frequently observed in human victims of snake bite. Instead, it has been found that hemodynamic changes, particularly DIC, resulting from systemic effects of envenoming, are likely to play a major role in the pathogenesis of acute renal failure. Mesangiolysis and proliferative changes in the glomeruli noted in some patients are likely to be due to the toxic action of the "haemorrhagin" fraction of the venom, but do not appear to play a significant role in the causation of acute renal failure. Efforts to solve the mysteries of this venomous disorder are continuing.

References

1. Chugh KS, Aikat BK, Sharma BK, Dash SC, Mathew T, Das KC (1975) Acute renal failure following snake bite. Am J Trop Med Hyg 24:692–697
2. Chugh KS (1989) Snake bite induced acute renal failure in India. Kidney Int 35:891–907
3. Myint-Lwin, Warrell DA, Phillips RE, Tin-Nu-Swe, Tun-Pe, Maung-Maung-Lay (1985) Bites by Russell's viper (*Vipera russelli siamensis*) in Burma: Hemostatic, vascular and renal disturbances and response to treatment. Lancet II:1259–1264
4. Sitprija V, Boonpucknavig V (1979) Snake venoms and nephrotoxicity. In: Lee CY ed, Snake Venoms. Springer, Berlin, pp 997–1018
5. Warrell DA, Ormerod D, Davidson N McD (1975) Bites by the puff adder (*Bitis arietans*) in Nigeria and value of anti venom. Br Med J [Clin Res] 4:697–700
6. Warrell DA, Davidson N McD, Greenwood BM, Omerod LD, Pope HM, Watkins BJ, Prentice CRM (1977) Poisoning by bites of the saw scaled or carpet viper in Nigeria. Q J Med 46:33–62

7. Efrati P, Reif L (1953) Clinical and pathological observations on 65 cases of viper bites in Israel. Am J Trop Med Hyg 2:1085–1108
8. Visuvaratram M, Vinayagamoorthy C, Balakrishnan S (1970) Venomous snake bites in North Ceylon—Study of fifteen cases. J Trop Med Hyg 73:9–14
9. Chugh KS, Pal Y, Chakravarty RN, Datta BN, Mehta R, Sakhuja V, Mandal AK, Sommers SC (1984) Acute renal failure following poisonous snake bite. Am J Kidney Dis 4:30–38
10. Mittal BV, Kinare SG, Acharya VN (1986) Renal lesions following viper bites. Indian J Med Res 83:642–651
11. Mathai TP, Date A (1981) Acute renal failure in children in snake bite. Ann Trop Pediatr 1:73–76
12. Jayarajan PM, Vijyakumar T, Leena Devi KR, Mathew MT (1979) Renal involvement in ophidism. J Assoc Physicians India 27:619–624
13. Chugh KS, Sakhuja V (to be published) Renal disease due to snake venom: In: AT Tu (ed) Handbook of natural toxins. Marcel Dekker, New York
14. Aung-Khin M (1977) Histological and ultrastructural changes of the kidney in renal failure after viper envenomation. Toxicon 16:71–75
15. Date A, Shastry JCM (1982) Renal ultrastructure in acute tubular necrosis following Russell's viper envenomation. J Pathol 137:225–241
16. Jeyarajah R (1984) Russell's viper bite in Sri Lanka—A study of 22 cases. Am J Trop Med Hyg 33:506–510
17. Sarangi A, Patnaik BC, Das GC, Tripathy N, Misra G, Swain AK, Das GK (1980) Renal involvement in viper snake bite. Indian J Med Res 71:918–923
18. Varagunam T, Panabokke RG (1970) Bilateral cortical necrosis of the kidneys following snake bite. Postgrad Med J 46:449–451
19. Sitprija V, Boonpucknavig V (1983) Glomerular changes in tropical viper bite in man. Toxicon 16:71–75
20. DaSilva OA, Lopez M, Godoy P (1979) Bilateral cortical necrosis and calcification of the kidney following snake bite: a case report. Clin Nephrol 11:136–139
21. Oram S, Ross SG, Pell L, Winteler J (1963) Renal cortical calcification after snake bite. Br Med J [Clin Res] 1:647–648
22. Date A, Shastry JCM (1981) Renal ultrastructure in cortical necrosis following Russell's viper envenomation. J Trop Med Hyg 84:3–8
23. Seedat YK, Reddy J, Edington DA (1974) Acute renal failure due to proliferative nephritis from snake bite poisoning. Nephron 13:455–463
24. Otsuji Y, Irie Y, Ueda H, Yotsueda K, Kitahara T, Yokoyama K, Higashi Y (1978) A case of acute renal failure caused by Mamushi (*Agkistrodon halys*) bite. Med J Kagoshima Univ (Jpn) 30:129–135
25. Sitprija V, Suvanpha R, Pochanugool C, Chusil S, Tung-sanga K (1982) Acute interstitial nephritis in snake bite. Am J Trop Med Hyg 31:408–410
26. Indraprasit S, Boonpucknavig V (1986) Acute interstitial nephritis after a Russell's viper snake bite. Clin Nephrol 25:111
27. Sitprija V, Benyajati C, Boonpucknavig PV (1974) Further observations of renal insufficiency in snake bite. Nephron 13:396–403
28. Mathew MT, Rajaratnam K (1987) Renal papillary necrosis in ophitoxemia (abstract). J Assoc Physicians India 35:20
29. Steinbeck AW (1960) Nephrotic syndrome developing after snake bite. Med J Aust 1:543–545
30. Taylor J, Mallick SMK (1935) Observations on poisoning with the venom of *Echis carinatus* and its treatment with a heterologous antivenom. Indian J Med Res 23:141–146
31. McKay DG, Moroz C, DeVries A, Csavossy J, Cruse V (1970) The action of hemorrhagin and phospholipase derived from *Vipera palestinae* venom on the micro-circulation. Lab Invest 22:387–399

32. Ownby CL, Bjarnason J, Tu AT (1978) Hemorrhagic toxins after rattle snake (*Crotalus atrox*) venom. Am J Pathol 93:201-218
33. Tsuchiya M, Ohshio C, Ohashi M, Ohsaka A, Suzuki K, Fujishiro Y (1974) Cinematographic and electron microscopic analyses of the hemorrhage induced by the main hemorrhagic principle HRI isolated from venom of *Trimeresurus flavoviridis*. Platelets, Thombosis, and inhibitors. In: Didisheim P, Shimamato T, Yamazaki H, Stuttgart FK (eds) F.K. Schattauer, pp 439-446
34. Chopra RN, Chowhan JS (1934) Action of the Indian daboia venom on the circulatory system. Indian J Med Res 23:493-506
35. Chopra RN, Chowhan JS, De NN (1935) An experimental investigation into the action of the venom of *Echis carinatus*. Indian J Med Res 23:391-405
36. Osman OH, Gumma KA (1974) Pharmacological studies of snake (*Bitis arietans*) venom. Toxicon 12:569-575
37. Than-Than, Hutton RA, Myint-Lwin, Khin-Ei-Han, Soe-Soe, Tin-Nu-Swe, Phillips RE, Warrell DA (1988) Hemostatic disturbances in patients bitten by Russell's viper in Burma. Br J Haematol 69:513-520
38. Shastry JCM, Date A, Carman RH, Johny KV (1977) Renal failure following snake bite. Am J Trop Med Hyg 26:1032-1038
39. Warrell DA, Pope HM, Prentice CRM (1976) Disseminated intravascular coagulation caused by the carpet viper: Trial of heparin. Br J Haematol 33:335-342
40. Lakier B, Fritz VU (1969) Consumptive coagulopathy caused by a boomslang bite. S Afr Med J 43:1052-1055
41. Nicolson IC, Ashby PA, Johnson ND, Versey J, Slater L (1974) Boomslang bite with hemorrhage and activation of complement by the alternate pathway. Clin Exp Immunol 16:295-300
42. Simon TL, Grace TG (1981) Envenomation coagulopathy in wounds from pit vipers. N Engl J Med 305:443-447
43. Chugh KS, Mohanthi D, Pal Y, Das KC (1979) Coagulation abnormalities induced by Russell's viper venom in the Rhesus monkey. Am J Trop Med Hyg 28:763-769
44. Chugh KS, Mohanthy D, Pal Y, Das KC, Ganguly NK, Chakravarty RN (1981) Hemostatic abnormalities following *Echis carinatus* (saw scaled viper) envenomation in the rhesus monkey. Am J Trop Med Hyg 30:1116-1120
45. Chugh KS, Singhal PC, Sharma BK, Pal Y, Mathew MT, Dhall K, Datta BN (1976) Acute renal failure of obstetric origin in Indian patients. Obstet Gynecol 48:642-646
46. Chugh KS, Singhal PC, Kher VK, Gupta VK, Malik GH, Narayan G, Datta BN (1983) Spectrum of acute cortical necrosis in Indian patients. Am J Med Sci 286:10-20
47. Clarkson AR, Macdonald MK, Fuster V, Cash JD, Robson JS (1970). Glomerular coagulation in acute ischemic renal failure. Q J Med 39:585-599
48. Harris ARC, Hurst PE, Saker BM (1976) Renal failure after snake bite. Med J Aust 2:409-411
49. Rubenberg ML, Bull BS, Regoeczi E, Dacie JV, Brain MC (1967) Experimental production of microangiopathic hemolytic anemia in vivo. Lancet II:1121-1123
50. Chugh KS, Singhal PC, Sharma BK, Mahakur AC, Pal Y, Datta BN, Das KC (1977) Acute renal failure due to intravascular hemolysis in North Indian patients. Am J Med Sci 274:139-146
51. Reid HA (1961) Myoglobinuria and sea-snake bite poisoning. Br Med J 1:1284-1289
52. Sitprija V, Sribhibhadh R, Benyajati C (1971) Hemodialysis in poisoning by sea snake venom. Br Med J 3:218-219
53. Rowlands JB, Mastaglia FL, Kakulas BA, Hainsworth D (1969) Clinical and pathological aspects of a fatal case of mulga [*Pseudechis australis*] snake bite. Med J Aust 1:226-230

54. Hood VL, Johnson JR (1979) Acute renal failure with myoglobinuria after tiger snake bite. Med J Aust 2:638–641
55. Suzuki Y, Churg J, Grishman E, Mautner W, Dachs S (1963) The mesangium of the renal glomerulus. Electron microscopic studies of pathologic alterations. Am J Pathol 43:555–578
56. Kitamura H, Hashiguchi T, Hamada R, Oyama M, Ikeda T, Inamori S, Mori T (1958) The pathological study of "Habu" (*Trimeresurus flavoridis*) venom II. The histopathological study of rabbit renal lesions caused by intravenous inoculation of "Habu" venom. Med J Kagoshima Univ (Jpn) 9:1586–1593
57. Sakaguchi H, Kawamura S (1963) Electron microscopic observations of the mesangiolysis. The toxic effects of "Habu snake" venom on the renal glomerulus. Keio J Med 12:99–106
58. Cattell V, Bradfield JWB (1977) Focal mesangial proliferative glomerulonephritis in the rat caused by Habu snake venom. A morphological study. Am J Pathol 87:511–524
59. Morita T, Kihara I, Oite T, Yamamoto T, Suzuki Y (1978) Mesangiolysis. Sequential ultrastructural study of Habu venom induced glomerular lesions. Lab Invest 38:94–102
60. Schmidt ME, Abdelbaki YZ, Tu AT (1976) Nephrotoxic action of rattle and sea snake venom: An electron microscopic study. J Pathol 118:75–81
61. Raab W, Kaiser E (1966) Nephrotoxic action of snake venoms. Mem Inst Butantan 33:1017–1020
62. Ratcliffe PJ, Purkittayakamee S, Ledingham JGG, Dunnill MS (1985) Acute renal failure in the isolated perfused kidney, induced by Russell's viper venom. Clin Sci 68(Suppl II):39–40
63. Hadler WA, Brazil OV (1966) Pharmacology of crystalline crotoxin nephrotoxicity. Mem Inst Butantan 33:1001–1008
64. Greenwood BM, Warrell DA, Davidson NMcD, Ormerod ED, Reid HA (1974) Immuno-diagnosis of snake bite. Br Med J 4:743
65. Sitprija V, Boonpucknavig V (1980) Extracapillary proliferative glomerulonephritis in Russell's viper bite. Br Med J 2:1417
66. Chugh KS, Pal Y, Ganguly NK (1977) Complement depletion following envenomation by Russell's viper and *Echis carinatus* (saw scaled viper) in the Rhesus monkey. Am J Trop Med Hyg 26:1039–1043
67. Warrell DA, Greenwood BM, Davidson NMcD, Ormerod LD, Prentice CRM (1976) Necrosis, hemorrhage and complement depletion following bites by the spitting cobra. Q J Med 45:1–22

Acute Renal Failure in Asia

M. RAHMAN and M. HOSSAIN[1]

Introduction

Acute renal failure (ARF) is an important nephrological disorder in most Asian countries, causing significant morbidity and mortality. Over the years the etiology of ARF has undergone considerable changes, particularly in Europe and developed Asian nations like Japan. In these developed countries ARF due to infection and septic abortion has practically disappeared, whereas, even today, infections of one kind or another, caused by bacteria, parasites, viruses, various toxins, and septic abortion remain as the major causes of ARF in most Asian countries. In addition, ARF following hypersensitivity reactions due to drugs, ARF due to immunological disorders such as primary glomerulonephritis and systemic lupus erythematosus (SLE) nephritis, and ARF due to hematological disorders such as myelomatosis etc. is as common in Asian countries as it is in Europe and in the United States. In this communication, we will briefly review different aspects of ARF in relation to Asia.

Definition and Prevalence

Acute renal failure is defined as deterioration of renal function, resulting in the rise of nitrogenous waste products, i.e., urea and creatinine, in blood [1]. Acute renal failure may occur in a previously healthy person; in such a person more than 50% deterioration in renal function is necessary to produce a rise in serum creatinine, whereas in a person with diseased kidneys (acute or chronic) a 10%–50% reduction of glomerular filtration will produce a rise in serum creatinine. Acute renal failure may progress slowly or rapidly (hypercatabolic) and may be associated with complete anuria, oliguria, or even with normal to high urine volume.

---

[1]Department of Nephrology and Paediatrics, Institute of Postgraduate Medicine and Research, Dhaka, Bangladesh

Prevalence of acute renal failure is variable, not only from one country to the other, but also in different parts of the same country and in different periods of the year [2]. In Bangladesh 4%–8% of admissions to nephrology units (dealing with adult patients) are due to acute renal failure [3,4]. In the years 1981–1989 children between the ages of 1–12 years were admitted to the Pediatric Nephrology unit of the Institute of Postgraduate Medicine and Research in Dhaka at the rate of 5–6 admissions a day. All these children presented with hypovolemic/ischemic acute renal failure with complete anuria of 1–13 days duration [5–8]. In most Asian countries the prevalence of acute renal failure due to gastroenteritis, septic abortions, malaria, leptospirosis, and snake bites, etc. is very common.

Specific Types of ARF in Asia

Acute renal failure is traditionally classified into (a) Pre-renal/Ischemic, (b) Renal due to intrinsic renal disease and various toxins, and (c) Post-renal/Obstructive groups. In the following chapters a brief description of specific types of ARF prevalent in Asia and due to various causes will be made.

Hypovolemic or Acute Ischemic Renal Failure (AIRF)

Fluid and electrolyte loss (producing hypovolemia), due to infective diarrhea, pyrexial illness, vomiting, and acute dysentery, remains the major causes of acute ischemic renal failure both in adults and children in countries like Bangladesh, India, Pakistan,

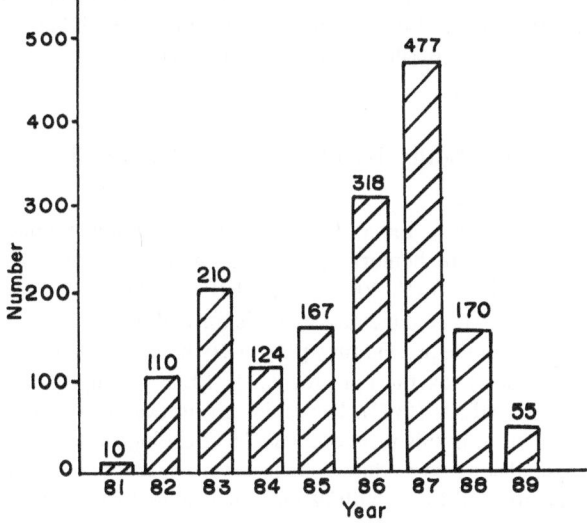

Fig. 1. Acute anuric non-obstructive renal failure in children of Bangladesh

Table 1. ARF in Bangladeshi children 1981–1989 (n = 1941)

Age range	Preceed illness	Duration of anuria	S. creat mean ±SD	Mortality
1–10 years	Pyrexia of unknown origin (PUO) 62% Diarrhea 28% Misc 10%	1–13 days	701±267.98 Micromol/l	87%

Indonesia, and Malaysia [9–13]. This form of acute renal failure is common in the densely populated developing countries of Asia which have mass poverty and illiteracy. Most of the patients are children and usually because of inadequate replacement of fluid and electrolytes, they develop oliguria, which usually goes unnoticed by illiterate parents; the children are generally brought to physicians after anuria has set in. During the period 1981–1989 in Bangladesh, there was almost an epidemic of ARF following pyrexial/diarrheal illness. In the year 1987 alone 477 children with ARF were admitted to the Paediatric Renal Unit of the Institute of Postgraduate Medicine and Research, Dhaka (Fig. 1). These children came with high serum creatinine and were treated with peritoneal dialysis; details are shown in Table 1. Overall mortality in this group of children suffering from AIRF was 87%–90%, compared to only 15% mortality in children suffering from ARF due to hemolytic uremic syndrome (HUS) [14,15].

Renal hypoperfusion is the mechanism responsible for producing acute renal failure in these cases. It seems likely that hypoperfusion which persists because of continued fluid and electrolyte loss may produce graded renal morphological changes, from none in pre-renal to acute or even cortical necrosis, depending on the severity of the insult and the delay in institution of corrective therapy. Therefore, it is reasonable to assume that this form of acute renal failure, which claims so many lives in Asian countries, is largely preventable. The pathogenic mechanisms, histological lesions, and methods of protection from this form of ARF have been the subject of extensive study in experimental animals [16–19].

Pregnancy Related Acute Renal Failure (PR-ARF)

In countries like Bangladesh, India, Thailand, Singapore, and Indonesia, ARF in pregnancy following severe hemorrhagic shock, with or without overwhelming infection, makes up about 15%–20% of all AIRF in adults [21–24], whereas in Western European countries the incidence of this form of AIRF has shown a ten-fold decrease, to about 3%, at the present time [25]. ARF during pregnancy occurs during the first trimester, due to toxemias of pregnancy (PE-E), abruptio placentae (AP), and post-partum hemorrhage (PPH). Disseminated intravascular coagulation (DIC) is a common association in this form of ARF. The histological lesion in PR-ARF is generally acute tubular necrosis; however, in severe cases there can be patchy or diffuse cortical necrosis. Patients with patchy cortical necrosis are usually left with renal insufficiency and those with diffuse cortical necrosis develop chronic renal failure, requiring dialysis for survival.

In most Asian countries PR-ARF patients are brought to hospital very late with severe manifestations, e.g., DIC with cerebral symptoms. The use of heparin is controversial, but recently, the use of fresh blood and fresh frozen plasma along with proteinine (antiprotiolytic agent) within 24–48 hours has been found to be beneficial. This group of ARF has a 30% mortality rate in Bangladesh. Legalization of abortion and institution of proper ante- and perinatal care would certainly reduce this form of ARF in Asian countries.

ARF Associated with Hemolysis

Acute renal failure due to severe hemolysis occurs following (1) *Plasmodium falciparum* malaria, (2) in G6 PD deficiency individuals when exposed to certain drugs, and in the (3) hemolytic uremic syndrome, etc.

Falciparum Malaria

Acute renal failure is a common complication of *Plasmodium falciparum* infection. In Thailand this infection is responsible for about 30% of ARF cases. Acute renal failure occurs in patients with partial loss of immunity and heavy parasitic infections. These patients are acutely ill with high pyrexia and jaundice; renal failure is generally hypercatabolic. Acute intravascular hemolysis may occur, which may be induced by antimalarial durgs, e.g., chloroquin, quinine, and pyrimethamine in patients with or without G6 PD deficiency. Black water fever is another possible cause of ARF due to severe hemolysis and can be diagnosed after drug-induced hemolysis has been excluded [26–28].

The pathogenic mechanism of ARF due to falciparum malaria has been extensively studied. The following factors: hypovolemia, hyponatremia, acute intravascular coagulation and hemolysis, hyperviscosity, activation of the renin-angiotensin system, and hyperbilirubinemia, have all been implicated [26,29]. These seriously ill patients need careful management with dialytic therapy. In places where hemodialysis facilities are not available, continuous equilibration peritoneal dialysis (CEPD) can be used [30,31]. With the return of malaria this form of ARF is becoming a potentially real threat in countries like Bangladesh and Burma.

G-6 PD Deficiency

Acute renal failure due to G-6 PD deficiency-associated hemolysis has been reported mostly from India. The incidence of G-6 PD deficiency has been variable among Asian nations: from the highest incidence, in Kurdish Jews (60%), to between 2%–15% in China and on the Indian subcontinent. In India this incidence constitutes about 20% of all patients with ARF needing dialytic therapy, who come to certain centers [32]. These patients usually have a history of febrile illness and have been exposed to analgesics and antimalarial drugs. The patients present with abrupt onset of hemolysis, anemia, reticulocytosis, jaundice, and hemoglobinuria. There are fragmented red cells in peripheral blood film. It is necessary to differentiate these patients from those with the hemolytic uremic syndrome.

Hemolytic Uremic Syndrome (HUS)

Hemolytic uremic syndrome is one of the common causes of ARF in children not only in developed countries, but also in certain Asian countries, including Bangladesh. It is characterized by sudden severe hemolysis with development of anemia and acute renal failure. This disease may precede diarrheal illness (Typical HUS) or may follow upper respiratory tract infection or vague non-specific symptoms (Atypical HUS). In Bangladesh, HUS has also been reported in children with shigellosis. The pathogenesis is not clear. However, it has been shown that intravascular platelet activation is associated with both typical and atypical forms of HUS [33,34].

This condition is also associated with fragmented and crenated red cells in the peripheral blood, anemia (at times very severe), thrombocytopenia, and reticulocytosis. This picture is consistent with that of micro-angiopathic hemolytic anemia and renal failure. Among Bangladeshi children, the recovery rate from HUS-caused ARF following fresh blood transfusion and peritoneal dialysis has been found to be 85%, in contrast to the recovery rate in acute ischemic renal failure, which was only 10%-13%. In certain cases, particularly in atypical HUS, relapse may occur and the patient may ultimately develop chronic renal failure.

Leptospirosis

Acute renal failure following leptospirosis is found in Bangladesh, Sri-Lanka, Philippines, Singapore, and Thailand [35,36]. The most prevalent serotype in The Philippines is L-autumnalis and in Thailand it is L-batavia. Acute renal failure occurs in 20%-66% of leptospirosis cases. The patients may have mild renal failure and may also develop severe renal failure requiring dialysis; this is found particularly in The Philippines and in Singapore [37,38]. Those patients with mild renal failure are anicteric; patients with severe renal failure are usually jaundiced, with thrombocytopenia, bleeding diathesis, and hepatic encephalopathy. In many cases there may be intravascular hemolysis with features of HUS.

In leptospirosis the predominant changes involve proximal tubules and interstitium. The glomerular and vascular changes are usually mild. The pathogenic mechanism is renal ischemia and direct nephrotoxicity. The overall mortality rate is around 10%.

Snake Bites

Acute renal failure is found in 5%-25% of patients following snake bite. The incidence of ARF among hospitalized snake bite patients has been highest in Sri Lanka, with 49% [39,40], about 28% in India, 5% in Thailand [41], and less than 1% in Bangladesh. In India, between 1965 and 1986, 3% of a total of 1962 ARF cases were due to snake bite. The snakes responsible for causing ARF were generally either Russell's viper or *Echis carinatus*. Following snake bite, ARF may be protracted, hypercatabolic, and often associated with jaundice and disseminated intravascular coagulation and bleeding manifestations. In this symposium a separate chapter has been devoted to this topic.

Rhabdomyolysis and ARF

Rhabdomyolysis and myoglobinuria (resulting from hyperpyrexia, heat stroke, multiple wasp stings, and crush syndrome) which cause ARF have been found in almost all countries of Asia. Extreme heat has been known to produce direct toxicity, causing dehydration, increased blood viscosity, disseminated intravascular coagulation, muscle damage, myoglobinuria, and in turn, acute renal failure [42,43]. Initially, hypokalemia is a predisposing factor for rhabdomyolysis; once muscle damage has been produced, intractable hyperkalemia is a feature. Tubular obstruction by myoglobin casts is regarded as the principal mechanism for producing ARF. Acute renal failure due to rhabdomyolysis can be diagnosed, apart from the history, by the elevation of creatinine phosphokinase and aldolase levels in the blood. In this condition hypocalcemia and calcium deposition in the damaged muscles during the oliguric/ anuric phase, and hypercalcemia during the diuretic phase, have been described as characteristic features [44].

Acute Renal Failure in Epidemic Hemorrhagic Fever

Epidemic hemorrhagic fever is characterized by sudden high temperature, hemorrhagic manifestations, and renal dysfunction, ranging from transient to established acute renal failure. This disease is due to a RNA virus (Hanta virus) and is found in Japan, Korea, and China [45]. The risk of Hanta virus infection is high among farmers in rural areas. Two to three weeks after contact with the infection the clinical syndrome, which can be divided into 5 phases as follows begins: febrile, hypotensive, oliguric, diuretic, and convalescent.

The acute febrile illness may be accompanied by abdominal pain and conjunctival hemorrhage. During this stage, leucocytosis, thrombocytopenia, raised serum GOT, GPT, and LDH are found. Urinalysis may show proteinurea and hematuria. The stage of hypotension may be associated with shock; the majority of deaths occur in this phase.

The renal lesion may be: (1) Mild glomerular alteration with mesangial cell proliferation, (2) Degeneration and necrosis of tubular epithelium, and (3) Lastly, congestion and hemorrhage into the renal tissue. Immunofluorescent studies show deposition of IgA, IgM, C3,C4 and C_{1q} along capillary basement membrane, indicating activation of both complement pathways [46,47].

The diagnosis is confirmed by demonstrating the rising titer of antibodies against Hanta viruses in two blood samples collected at intervals of one week. Recently, specific IgM antibodies have been more helpful in making the diagnosis possible quite early in the disease process in about 95% of cases. The introduction of peritoneal dialysis has reduced the mortality in this disease to about 10%.

Acute Renal Failure Due to Glomerular Nephritis (GN) and Toxic Agents

Acute renal failure due to intrinsic renal disease is the second most common cause of ARF in Asia. All forms of secondary glomerulonephritis, due to streptococcal infection [48,49], hepatitis β virus (HBV) infection [50], and primary glomerulonephritis, including even minimal change disease [57], have been reported to produce ARF in Asia. Rapidly progressive GN due to SLE [52] and Goodpasture's syndrome is also common. Acute renal failure due to malignant lymphoma [34] and myelomatosis [54] has also been reported. Acute renal failure due to various toxins, e.g., the raw bile of the grass carp [55], wasp stings [56,57], and toxins/infections of an undetermined nature has produced acute renal failure with, at times favorable outcome [58,59], and at other times the very unfavorable outcome of 100% mortality, which occurred in ARF presenting with anuria and intern developing neurological manifestations, involving the brain stem, causing death [60]. Acute renal failure due to copper sulphate has been reported, mostly from India [61]. Apart from this, drug-induced ARF, due to acute interstitial nephritis induced by drugs such as NSAIDs, aminoglycosides, and, currently, cyclosporin, is also not uncommon [62]. But the ARF of this group is relatively milder, having a comparatively better prognosis than AIRF.

Post-Renal ARF

Acute renal failure due mostly to bilateral ureteric obstruction, and, to a lesser extent, to lower urinary tract obstruction is quite common in countries like Bangladesh, India, and Pakistan [63]. This form of ARF makes up about 5%–9% of all cases of acute renal failure. The result of treatment, even in those patients with the most severe disease in this group are very rewarding.

Treatment Constraints

It is the experience of almost all Asian countries that patients come to hospital severely ill, in an advanced state of established ARF. In a few advanced countries like Japan, this pattern may be an exception. Most of these patients require dialytic forms of therapy immediately; with the introduction of peritoneal dialysis, the prognosis has greatly improved, even in hypercatabolic acute renal failure patients. But in remote areas of developing Asian countries the hospitals may not have the necessary biochemical facilities and even the facilities for peritoneal dialysis may be lacking; these factors coupled with poor referral systems and bad communication, may result in only conservative therapy, which leads to fatality in most of these cases. However, in most reported series, the mortality rate of ARF (18%–30%) has been comparable to that of the West.

Prevention and Mitigation

The acute renal failure which occurs in Asian countries due to infective causes, e.g., the ARF which is caused by diarrhea, malaria, leptospirosis, Hantaviruses, hepatitis viruses, and pregnancy-related septicemia, is no doubt mostly preventable. In addition, exposure to drugs and toxins can also be controlled to reduce this form of ARF.

This type of prevention can be called "Macroprevention" and is obviously dependent on the overall socioeconomic conditions in the country. Pretreatment with mannitol or furosemide of patients at high risk for development of ARF, e.g., those at risk for post-operative ARF, has been found to reduce its incidence, or at least lessen its severity [64–66]. Various agents, e.g., clonidine [67], Ca-antagonists [68], and ATP [69] used to prevent/mitigate ARF in experimental animals may be called "Microprevention" and as yet have no role in human disease.

Conclusion

The various types of acute renal failure prevalent in most Asian countries are largely preventable. Yet due to the developing nature of these countries and due to limited dialytic facilities a large proportion of these ARF cases prove to be fatal. It will be quite some time, probably even the twenty-first century before Asian nephrologists will be faced with the kind of ARF patients currently being faced by their Western counterparts. This difference in disease pattern has been clearly shown by Chugh et al. in their Chandigarh study [70].

References

1. Brezis M, Rosen S, Epstein FH (1986) Acute renal failure. In: The kidney, 3rd edn. W.B. Saunders, pp 735–779
2. Chugh KS, Singhal PC (1981) Acute renal failure in the Tropics. Asian Man Nephrol, SEAMIC, 181–194
3. Rahman M, Roy AC, Chowdhury D, Hossain M (1985) Clinicopathological spectrum of renal diseases in IPGMR. An analysis of 2000 cases in 11 years. J of BCPS III(No. 1)
4. Rashid HU, Azhar MA, Rahman A, et al. (1989) Pattern of acute renal failure in Bangladesh adults. Bang Ren J 6(1):16–20
5. Hoque M, Rashid HU (1982) Acute renal failure in children. Bang Ren J 1(2):12–15
6. Hoque M, Chowdhury D, Rahman M, Rashid HU, Talukder MQK, Khan MR (1985) Clinical course and outcome of acute anuric renal failure in children—A study of 275 cases. Bang J Child Health 9(1):5–9
7. Chugh KS, Narang A, Kumar L, Sakhuja V, Narayanan Unni V, Prizada R, Singh N, Pereira BJG, Singhal PC (1987) Acute renal failure amongst children in a tropical environment. Int J Artif Organs 10(2):97–101
8. Pereira BJG, Narang A, Pereira S, Gupta A, Sakhuja V, Chugh KS (1989) Acute renal failure in infants in the tropics. Nephrol Dial Transplant 4:535–538
9. Razzaque A, Ahmed S, Rahman M (1983) Profile of acute renal failure in adults. Bang Ren J 2(2):5–6
10. Malhotra UK (1989) Renal problems in India: Most prevalent kidney diseases and related problems. Proceedings of the eighth Asian colloquium of nephrology, Nov 17–21, 1989. pp 289–302
11. Sumanggar PS, Jose Roesma, Roemiati Oesman, Markum MS Gambaran gagal akut dibagian ilmu penyakit dalam FKUI/RSCM, Jakarta, (in Indonesian)
12. Herriyati S, Sukandar E Tinjauan Kasus Kegagalan ginjal mendadak disubagian ginjal-hipertensi bagianilmupe nyakit dalam RS hasan sadikin (in Indonesian) bandung SE lama 3 tahun (1977–79)

13. Azhar MA, Rahman MA, Rashid HU (1985) Acute renal failure following copper intoxication and its reversal after dialysis. 4(1):19–20

14. Rahman M, Chowdhury D, Hoque M, et al. (1982) Acute anuric renal failure in children.
Bang Ren J 1(2):3–5

15. Rahman M, Chowdhury D, Islam KMN, Hoque M (1984) Acute anuric renal failure in children (abstract). IXth International Congress of Nephrology, Jun 11–16, 1984. p 120A

16. Schrier RW, Shapiro JI (1985) Current concepts in ischaemic acute renal failure. Proceedings of the sixth Asian colloquium of nephrology, Kuala Lumpur. pp 1–8

17. Raymond KH, Stein JH (1988) Acute renal failure: In vitro experimental models. Proceedings of the Xth international congress of nephrology, vol 2. pp 964–974

18. Fried TA, Stein JH (1984) Experimental acute renal failure: pathophysiology and methods
of protection. Proceedings of the IXth international congress of nephrology, vol 1. pp
731–747

19. Himes HD, Hunt DA, Clark MJ, White MP, Weinberg JM (1984) Cellular mechanism of
protection in nephrotic and ischemic acute renal failure. Proceedings of the IXth international congress of nephrology, vol 1. pp 770–783

20. Chugh KS, Singhal PC, Sharma BK, Yash P, Thomas MM, Kamla D, Datta Bn (1976) Acute
renal failure of obstetric origin. 48(6)

21. Pravin C, Singhal VK, Kher, Gian I, Dhall, RL, Mehta, Kasi Visweswaran R, Narayanan
Nampory MR, Kirpal S, Chugh (1982) Conservative vs surgical management of septic
abortion with renal failure. Int J Gynaecol Obstet 20:189–194

22. Rakachanaran S, Jayatissa SK, Herath CA, Salgado M (1990) Aetiology and mortality of
acute renal failure (ARF) in Sri Lanka (abstract). Conference, Beijing, China

23. Suleiman AB (1982) Clinical review of acute renal failure (1982) A 5 years experience at
Kuala Lumpur. 11(1)

24. Suleiman AB, Morad S, Prasad S Prospective study of acute renal failure: In a general
hospital Kuala Lumpur

25. Stratta P, Canavese C, Dogliani M, et al. (1989) Pregnancy related acute renal failure. Clin
Nephrol 32:14–20

26. Boon PV, Sitprija V (1979) Renal disease in acute plasmodium falciparum infection in
man. Kidney Int 16:44–52

27. Rahman H, Biswas GC, Rouf MA, Rashid HU (1988) Reversible acute renal failure following malaria—A case report. Bang Ren J 7(1):24–27

28. Sitprija V (1985) Acute renal failure in malaria and leptospirosis. Proceedings of the sixth
Asian colloquium of nephrology, Kuala Lumpur. pp 15–40

29. Sitprija V (1989) Tropical diseases and acute renal failure: jaundice model. Proceedings of
the eighth Asian colloquium of nephrology, Nov 17–21, 1989. pp 347–350

30. Hossain M, Chowdhury D, Rahman M (1986) Continuous equilibration peritoneal dialysis
in hypercatabolic acute renal failure. Bang Ren J 5(2):63–65

31. Lanjona IA, Neidus OD, Daysog A Jr, et al. (1986) Continuous equilibration peritoneal
dialysis (CEPD) in acute renal failure. Phil J Nephrol 1:90–96

32. Chugh KS, Singhal PC, Sharma BM, Mahakur AC, Pal Y, Datta BN, Das KC (1977) Acute
renal failure due to intravascular hemolysis in North Indian patients. Am J Med Sci
274(2):139–146

33. Walters MDS, Levin M, Smith C, et al. (1988) Intravascular platelet activation in the
hemolytic uremic syndrome. Kidney Int 33:107–115

34. O'Regan S, Blais N, Russo P, et al. (1989) Hemolytic uremic syndrome glomerular filtration rate, 6-10 years later measured by 99 MTC DTPA plasma slope clearance. Clin
Nephrol 32:217–220

35. Sitprija V (1986) Acute renal failure due to tropical diseases. Phil J Nephrol 1:35–39

36. Ismael AE, Naidas OE, Daysog JA, et al. (1986) Acute renal failure in Leptospirosis. Phil
J Nephrol 1:54–58

37. Estrada DR, Naidus OD, Daysog JA, et al. (1986) Nonoliguric acute renal failure. Its clinical features as observed at the Saint Thomas University Hospital. Phil J Nephrol 1:71-78
38. Ramachandran S, Rajapakse CNA, Perera MVF, Yoganathan M (1976) Patterns of acute renal failure in Leptospirosis. J Trop Med Hyg 158-160
39. Ramachandran S (1987) Renal failure: profiles and challenges. Ceylon Med J 32:59-74
40. Ramachandran S, Perera MVF (1974) Survival renal cortical necrosis due to snake bite. Postgrad Med J 50:314-316
41. Chugh KS (1989) Snake bite induced acute renal failure in India. Kidney Int 35:891-907
42. Honda N (1983) Acute renal failure and rhabdomyolysis. Kidney Int (Nephrology Forum) 23:888-898
43. Chugh KS, Singhal PC, Nath IVS, Pareek SK, Ubr HS, Sarker AK (1979) Acute renal failure due to non-traumatic rhabdomyolysis. Postgrad Med J 55:386-392
44. Han WH, Shieh S-D, Chen W (1983) A prospective study of soft tissue calcification in rhabdomyolysis induced acute renal failure. Taiwan I Hsueh Hui Tsa Chih 82:1139-1149
45. Lee HW (1988) Hantavirus infection in Asia. Proceedings of the Xth international congress of nephrology, vol 2. pp 816-830
46. Li LS (1986) Renal disease in China: An overview. Proceedings of the 3rd Asian Pacific congress of nephrology, Oct 5-10, 1986. pp 292-296
47. Kim MJ (1989) Hanta virus infection in Korea. Proceedings of the eighth Asian colloquium of nephrology, Nov 17-21, 1989. pp 303-313
48. Rahman M, Rahman H, Chowdhury D (1988) Post streptococcal acute glomerulonephritis in Bangladesh. A follow up study of 250 patients. Bang Ren J 7:46-51
49. Chugh KS, Malhotra HS, Sakheja V, et al. (1986) Prognosis of post-streptococcal GN-Chandigarth study. Proceedings of 3rd APCN, B 272-285
50. Rahman MA, Azhar MA, Rahman MH, Rashid HU (1985) Reversible acute renal failure associated with uncomplicated viral hepatitis – report of two cases. Bang Ren J 4(2):52-55
51. Haque A, Rahman M, Islam MN (1982) Reversible renal failure in minimal change neprhotic syndrome. Bang Ren J 1(1):1-3
52. Sultan M, Bari R, Rashid HU (1983) A case of acute renal failure following introgenic infection from a dextrose infusion. Bang Ren J 2(2):14
53. Roy AC, Rahman M (1983) Acute renal failure in malignant lymphoma. Report of a case. Bang Ren J 2(2):12-13
54. Dun-Lin Chen, Jong-Da Lian, Yun-Fu Yang, Kuo-Hsiung Shu, Chi-Hung Cheng, Lai-Ping Chen (1989) Acute renal failure in patients with multiple myeloma. J Nephrol ROC 3:221-226
55. Wan Yu Chen, Tsan Shin Yen, Jen Tse Cheng, Bor Shen Hsieh, Hey Chi Hsu (1976) Acute renal failure due to ingestion of raw bile of grass carp (*Clenopharyngodon Idellus*). Taiwan I Hsueh Hui Tsa Chih 75:149-157
56. Chiu-Ching Huang, Chi AU, Leung Chen, Swei Hsueh (1983) Acute renal failure and hepatic injury following multiple wasp stings – Report of 2 cases. Taiwan I Hsueh Hui Tsa Chih 82:623-628
57. Sakhuja V, Bhalla A, Pereira BJG, Kapoor MM, Bhusmurmath SR, Chugh KS (1988) Acute renal failure following multiple hornet stings (abstract). Nephrol 49:319-321
58. Chowdhury D, Kawser CA, Talukder MQK, Rashid HU, Rahman M (1982) Favourable outcome in four cases of anuric acute renal failure in children. Bang Paed J 6(1):31-33
59. Fatmi LE, Hoque M, Mannan MA (1985) Acute renal failure complicating Stevens-Johnson syndrome in a six year old child. Bang J Child Health 9(3):192-195
60. Rahman H, Chowdhury D, Rashid NU, Rahman M (1987) Acute renal failure in adults with central nervous system involvement—A new entity. Bang Ren J 6(2):53-58
61. Chugh KS, Sharma BK, Singhal PC, Das KC, Datta BN (1977) Acute renal failure following copper sulphate intoxication. Postgrad Med J 53:18-25

62. Schrier RW, Shapiro JI (1985) Drug-induced acute renal failure. Proceedings of the sixth Asian colloquium of nephrology, Kuala Lumpur, pp 9–14

63. Nagvi SAJ (1989) Regional problems in Pakistan–Most prevalent kidney diseases and related problems. Proceedings of the eighth Asian colloquium of nephrology, Nov 17–21, 1989. pp 283–288

64. Dawson JI (1965) Post-operatiave renal function in obstructive jaundice: Effect of mannitol diuresis. Br Med J [Clin Res] 1:82–86

65. Old CW, Lehrner LM (1980) Prevention of radio contrast induced acute renal failure with mannitol. Lancet I:885

66. Nuutimen LS, Kairabwoma M, Ruoonen S, et al. (1978) The effect of furosemide on renal function in open heart surgery. J Cardiovasc Surg (Torino) 19:471–479

67. Solez K, Racusen LC, Wheltoln A (1984) Clonidine, propranolol and the prevention of acute renal failure. Proceedings of the IXth international congress of nephrology, vol 1. pp 784–790

68. Burke TJ, Arnold PE, Schrier RW (1984) The role of calcium channel blockers. Proceedings of the IXth international congress of nephrology, vol 1. pp 791–799

69. Siegel NJ, Gandio KM, Mashgarian M (1984) Adenine nucleotides in the prevention of ischemic acute renal failure. Proceedings of the IXth international congress of nephrology, vol 1. pp 800–806

70. Chugh KS, Kjellstrand CM (to be published) The changing epidemiology of acute renal failure. Patterns in economically advanced and developing countries. In: International year book of Nephrology in press

Renal Stone Disease in the Middle East

WILLIAM G. ROBERTSON, VALERIE R. WALKER, HERBERT HUGHES[1],
IMTIAZ HUSAIN, and SALAH AL-FAQIH[2]

SUMMARY. The pattern of urinary stone disease varies widely throughout the Middle East in terms of prevalence, site of formation, stone composition, diet, and urinary risk factors. In the developing countries, whose economies are still largely based on agriculture, ammonium urate-containing bladder stones in children are still a frequent finding, although this form of the disorder is decreasing with improving nutritional standards. In the more affluent Gulf states upper urinary tract stones in adults are extremely common—the life-time prevalence in men over the age of 60 being greater than 20%, the highest in the world. In these patients, the stones are composed mainly of calcium oxalate and/or uric acid. Calcium phosphate-containing calculi and infection stones are relatively uncommon. The high prevalence of calcium oxalate and uric acid stones can be attributed to the low urine volumes, more acid urines, hyperuricosuria, hypocitraturia, and extensive mild hyperoxaluria which are common in the region. These urinary abnormalities are due to the consumption of a diet over-rich in animal protein, purine, and oxalate but low in calcium. Addition of 1g/day calcium to the diet reduces urinary oxalate to normal without any major increase in urinary calcium.

Introduction

The pattern of stone disease in the Middle East is complex, but basically consists of two main themes which may be closely interwoven through different sections of society within the same country. Firstly, as a relic of the past history of the disease as it was known in the West in the last century, there is the formation of ammonium urate-containing stones in boys living in the developing countries of the region whose economies are still highly dependent on agriculture, e.g., Iraq, Jordan, and Egypt [1,2]

[1]Department of Biological and Medical Research, King Faisal Specialist Hospital and Research Centre, P.O. Box 3354, Riyadh 11211, Saudi Arabia
[2]King Khalid University Hospital, Riyadh, Saudi Arabia

and, secondly, there is the formation of calcium- and uric acid-containing upper urinary tract stones in adults (mainly men) in the more affluent, oil-rich states of the Arabian Peninsula, such as Kuwait, the United Arab Emirates (UAE), and the Kingdom of Saudi Arabia [3,4]. These forms of the disorder often occur together in the same country but, as nutritional standards improve, the incidence of bladder stones in children decreases [1,2] and that of upper urinary tract stones in adults increases [5,6].

Prevalence of Stones

There are few data on the actual prevalence of urolithiasis in the population and many studies have had to rely on hospital admission rates for stone disease as an indication of prevalence. Table 1 shows the data from various countries for adults and children. In general, these support the contention that stone-formation in adults is most common in affluent countries, but that its prevalence may be further aggravated by a number of environmental factors, such as living and/or working in a hot dry environment [5,6]. This factor, however, may only be of importance once the indigenous population concerned has reached a moderate level of affluence, as evidenced by data from various tropical countries in Africa and Asia where the climate is as hot as that in the more affluent countries of the Middle East but the prevalence of stones is considerably lower [6].

Table 1 shows that the Middle Eastern countries fall into three groups: (a) countries such as Iraq, Sudan, Turkey, Egypt, and Iran where bladder stones in children are still a frequent finding; (b) countries such as Jordan and Syria where bladder stones have largely disappeared and upper tract stone-formation in adults is now the predominant form of the disorder; and (c) countries such as Kuwait, the UAE, and Saudi Arabia where there are no bladder stones in children but where the occurrence of upper tract stones in adults and children is now of epidemic proportions.

In the few countries of the world where true prevalence studies have been carried out the pattern of the life-time risk of stones in men over the age of 60 (Table 2) is similar to that indicated in Table 1. Table 2 also contains data on the percentage of patients attending General Hospital Urology Clinics who have urolithiasis as their primary diagnosis. In general, they fit the pattern shown in Table 1, with the highest percentages occurring in the countries of the Arabian Peninsula.

The questions now arise — why do bladder stones in boys predominate at the lower end of the affluence scale, why do upper urinary tract stones in adults take over as the dominant form of the disorder as countries become industrialized, and why does the prevalence of upper tract stones continue to increase as these countries become more and more affluent?

Affluence and Stone-Formation

As a country develops and becomes more affluent, at least three factors are known to change which might influence the risk of stone-formation in the population. Firstly, both the standard of hygiene and supply of safe drinking water increase; secondly, the level of nutrition changes from one poor in energy to one richer in protein, refined carbohydrate, fat, and purine; and thirdly, the average level of physical

Table 1. Annual rate of hospitalization for urinary stone disease per 10000 population

Region	Annual hospital admissions in adults per 10000 adults in the population	Annual hospital admissions in children per 10000 children in the population
Thailand	1.0	8.0
India	1.0	7.0
Iraq	1.6	5.5
Sudan	2.1	5.4
Turkey	nd	5.0
Egypt	1.7	4.1
Iran	1.3	2.5
Indonesia	0.7	1.0
Pakistan	0.6	nd
South Africa (Bantu)	0.1	nd
Jordan	1.7	0.5
Sicily (1955)	2.5	0.5
Sicily (1970)	4.0	0.1
Syria	2.9	0.4
Czechoslovakia	1.6	nd
Nigeria	1.1	0.2
E. Mediterranean	2.0	nd
Japan	2.2	nd
Eire	3.0	nd
Austria	4.1	nd
Norway	4.3	nd
Italy	4.8	nd
UK	4.9	0.1
Finland	4.9	nd
Holland	5.0	nd
Australia	6.2	nd
W. Germany	6.3	nd
Denmark	7.0	nd
Sweden	7.5	nd
New Zealand	7.6	nd
Canada	10.1	nd
Kuwait	12.5	0.2
USA	15.0	0.1
United Arab Emirates	20.6	0.2
Saudi Arabia	22.1	0.2

nd, not determined

activity associated with the daily work routine decreases as people move from a rural to an urban lifestyle [1,2,5].

Hygiene and Drinking Water

One of the major changes in a country undergoing development is the increase in the overall standard of hygiene, including a safe supply of drinking water. The incidence of chronic diarrhea decreases and with it, probably, the risk of forming ammonium urate stones. Prior to the improvement in the level of hygiene the situation is analogous to that in cases of laxative abuse, as reported by Dick et al. [7], where ECF volume

Table 2. Occurrence of urolithiasis in various countries

Country	Urology patients with stones (%)	Life-time stone prevalence in men over 60 years (%)
China	–	1.5
Japan	–	5.4
UK	5–10	7.8
W Germany	–	8.0
Sweden	–	8.6
Canada	10–15	12.0
USA	10–20	13.0
United Arab Emirates	15–30	18.0
Saudi Arabia	20–50	20.1

depletion and intracellular acidosis produce a urine with a low volume and low sodium content and markedly reduced levels of potassium and citrate. Ammonia secretion into urine, in order to buffer hydrogen ions, is increased and the resulting high concentration of ammonium ions combines with urate to form ammonium urate crystals.

Nutrition

In children in many developing countries, where the level of hygiene is changing only slowly, this situation is aggravated by the consumption of a diet which is poor in meat protein, calcium, and phosphate and where rice is the staple constituent at an early age. The low intake of phosphate leads to a low urinary excretion of the ion which is normally required as a buffer. This promotes the production of ammonia and of a urine with a pH greater than 6. The combination of a high ammonium ion concentration in conjunction with a urinary pH between 6 and 7 is an unusual situation, which may be accentuated by the effects of chronic diarrhea, as described above. Furthermore, the total excretion of uric acid tends to be high in children, as result of rapid tissue turnover, and this will exist entirely in the form of urate in urine at pH values > 6. The resultant high ammonium and urate ion concentrations may lead to excessive supersaturation of urine with respect to ammonium urate.

In some countries, particularly in SE Asia, the addition of certain leaves which have a high content of oxalate to the diets of young children may lead to mild hyperoxaluria. This is often accentuated by the low intake of calcium. The resulting high concentrations of urinary oxalate may lead to calcium oxalate being deposited along with ammonium urate in the stones. As the level of hygiene and nutrition both improve, the risk of children forming ammonium urate-containing stones decreases and this form of the disorder may well disappear completely, as it has done previously in all developed countries, by the end of the century.

Why ammonium urate-containing stones should form mainly in the bladder and why only in boys is still a matter of conjecture. One possibility is that ammonium urate can exist as a colloid and only crystallizes relatively slowly, so that it is generally cleared from the kidney before crystalluria can develop. In the bladder, urine has a longer residence time in which to form abnormal crystals. These may occur in the urines of both boys and girls but, because of the wider urethra of the latter, the particles may be more readily expelled before they become large enough to be trapped and form the nucleus of a stone.

As countries develop and become more affluent, dietary composition changes quite markedly. Initially there is an increase in calcium intake as more dairy produce is consumed and this is accompanied by increases in the intakes of oxalate, refined carbohydrates, fats, purines, and animal protein. There is a concomitant decrease in dietary fiber. The strongest correlation at several demographic levels is between the consumption of animal protein (and purine) and affluence [6].

The effect of these dietary changes within a given population is to produce urine which is, on average, acidic and which is high in calcium, oxalate, and uric acid and low in citrate. Chemically this combination of urinary abnormalities increases the risk of calcium oxalate and uric acid crystalluria and stones. Most of these changes in urinary composition are attributable to the high consumption of animal protein and purine [8]. If, in addition, there are increases in the intakes of refined carbohydrates and oxalate, as mentioned above, then some of the effects on urine composition may be exaggerated, particularly in stone-formers, who appear to respond more sensitively to some of these dietary stimuli.

Conversely, it has been noted that if the consumption of animal protein and purine is reduced, the excretions of calcium, oxalate, and uric acid are also decreased and the biochemical risk of stones is low [8]. Vegetarians have a low predicted risk of stone-formation and a lower prevalence of the disorder than that in the general population [9].

Level of Physical Activity

One other factor which is influenced by increasing affluence in a given population is the average level of physical activity among the workforce. The movement away from the more active types of occupation associated with an agricultural economy and an increasing reliance on automation, office work, and more managerial types of activities, together lead to a reduction in the level of physical activity in the population. It has been considered for a number of years that stone disease is more prevalent among sedentary workers than among more physically active workers. Unfortunately, because individuals who have sedentary occupations are often more highly paid than those who perform more manual types of work, it is difficult to distinguish whether the higher prevalence of stones among the former is due to their more affluent lifestyle or to their less active occupations.

In this connection it has been suggested that the much lower prevalence of stones in women in developing countries (where the male/female ratio among stone-formers is about 5:1) than in their counterparts in the industrialized countries (where the male/female ratio is 2:1 or less) is due to the fact that the former lead much more physically active lives than the latter [2]. Again, however, the reasons are not clear-cut since the women from the industrialized countries are generally more affluent than those from the developing countries and this will affect the diets of the two groups.

Stone-Formation in the Arabian Peninsula

As indicated in Tables 1 and 2, the prevalence of stones in the populations of the oil-rich countries of the Arabian Peninsula is extremely high. The projected life-time

Table 3. Percentage occurrence of main constituents of stones

Stones containing	UK (1984)	USA (1964)	KSA (1989)
Uric acid	4.0	9.4	21.3
Calcium oxalate	77.7	72.1	73.1
Calcium phosphate	47.9	40.0	28.5
MAP	9.6	9.2	3.3
Cystine	1.6	0.9	2.1
Others	0.1	0.1	0.7

KSA, Kingdom of Saudi Arabia

risk of stone-formation in men over the age of 60 is at least 50% higher than the highest corresponding figures in the West.

In terms of stone composition, there is a considerable shift toward calculi containing calcium oxalate and/or uric acid, compared with data from the United Kingdom (Table 3). There are fewer calcium phosphate-containing stones and infection stones but more of the rare types of calculi which result from inborn errors of metabolism, such as cystinuria, xanthinuria and 2,8-dihydroxyadeninuria. Data from the United States lie between those of the United Kingdom and Saudi Arabia, but more recent figures suggest that the pattern in the United States over the past 25 years has shifted closer to that in Saudi Arabia (LH Smith, personal communication). Apparently there are now more uric acid-containing and fewer calcium phosphate-containing stones in the United States than in 1964.

The different patterns of stone composition between the Middle East and the West correlate well with the average composition of urine in the two regions (Table 4). Urine from men in the Arabian Peninsula has a lower volume, a lower pH, a lower calcium and citrate content, and a much higher oxalate and uric acid content than urine from men in the West. This leads to Middle Eastern men having generally higher levels of supersaturation of urine with respect to calcium oxalate and uric acid and lower levels of supersaturation with respect to calcium phosphate. This would explain the higher percentage of uric acid-containing stones and the lower proportion of calcium phosphate-containing stones in that part of the world.

In turn, the differences in urine composition can be accounted for by the differences in dietary intakes of the main nutrients influencing the excretion of stone-

Table 4. Comparison of 24-hour urine biochemistry in normal and stone-forming Middle Eastern and Western men

Constituent	Normals				Stone-formers			
	UK	USA	UAE	KSA	UK	USA	UAE	KSA
Volume (1)	1.60	1.55	1.44	1.25	1.76	1.70	1.68	1.56
pH	6.04	5.95	5.90	5.82	6.00	5.90	5.70	5.68
Calcium (mmol)	6.0	5.8	4.2	3.2	8.8	7.9	5.2	4.6
Oxalate (mmol)	0.33	0.41	0.46	0.53	0.43	0.49	0.63	0.69
Uric acid (mmol)	2.9	4.0	4.6	4.7	3.3	4.3	4.7	4.8
Citrate (mmol)	3.3	2.9	–	1.0	3.1	1.9	–	–

UAE, United Arab Emirates; KSA, Kingdom of Saudi Arabia

Table 5. Daily dietary intakes in male calcium stone-formers

Constituent	UK	USA	UAE	KSA
Animal protein (g)	61	85	"High"	87
Calcium (mmol)	24.5	25.0	23.0	13.0
Oxalate (mmol)	1.4	2.4	5.5	3.8
Purine (mg)	190	257	"High"	268
Oxalate/calcium (mmol/mmol)	0.06	0.10	0.24	0.29

UAE, United Arab Emirates; KSA, Kingdom of Saudi Arabia

forming minerals in urine. Table 5 shows that in the Arabian Peninsula male stone-formers consume more meat (i.e., a higher animal protein and purine intake), more oxalate, and less calcium than do their counterparts in the West.

Table 6 summarizes the data on normal men available from a number of countries. This shows that the life-time risk of stones rises in parallel with the ratio of oxalate/calcium in the diet and with the daily intake of animal protein. Diets high in oxalate and low in calcium have been shown to markedly increase the urinary excretion of oxalate, the most potent biochemical risk factor for stone disease next to a persistently low urine volume. Diets high in animal protein (and purine) have been shown to acidify urine, to increase the excretions of calcium, oxalate, and uric acid and to decrease the excretion of citrate. Where both dietary aberrations occur together, as in the affluent countries of the Arabian Peninsula, the risk of stone-formation explodes exponentially.

Table 6 also supports the observation that there is no relationship between the risk of calcium stone-formation and the urinary excretion of calcium [10]. Conversely, there is a high correlation between the prevalence of the disorder and the urinary excretion of oxalate [10].

Table 6. Relationship between life-time prevalence of urolithiasis in 60 to 70-year-old men and urinary and dietary composition in normal men in various countries

Country	Life-time stone prevalence in men > 60 years (%)	Urinary Ox (mmol/day)	Urinary Ca (mmol/day)	Diet Ox/Ca (mmol/mmol)	Diet AP (g/day)
China	1.5	–	3.5	–	21
Japan	5.4	0.31	4.1	–	39
UK	7.8	0.33	6.0	0.05	53
W Germany	8.0	0.36	5.8	0.06	59
Sweden	8.6	0.35	5.0	0.06	60
Canada	12.0	0.38	5.5	–	66
USA	13.0	0.41	5.8	0.10	76
United Arab Emirates	18.0	0.46	4.2	0.33	"Very high"
Saudi Arabia	20.1	0.53	3.2	0.29	82

Ox, oxalate; Ca, calcium; AP, animal protein

Treatment of Stone Disease in the Middle East

As indicated in Table 6, hypercalciuria is an uncommon finding in the Middle East. The reasons for this are two-fold—firstly, dietary calcium is lower than in the West (Table 5) and, secondly, hyperabsorption of calcium from a given oral load is rare [11]. The latter may be due to the paradoxically low vitamin D levels in Middle Eastern men. In terms of treatment, therefore, any measures designed to reduce urinary calcium excretion below the already low values are not likely to succeed.

Utilizing the above observations that calcium intake and absorption are low, a pilot study was carried out to determine the effects of adding 1g/day, extra calcium (in the form of calcium citrate) to the diets of 12 recurrent idiopathic stone-formers. This regimen reduced the urinary oxalate excretions of all the patients. Only one value remained slightly above the normal range for urinary oxalate in the West. Since there was no major rise in urinary calcium, the biochemical risk of forming calcium oxalate stones was reduced. It is now the intention to extend this form of treatment by adding potassium citrate to the calcium citrate in order to alkalinize urine and increase the excretion of citrate. By this means it ought to be possible to further reduce the risk of calcium oxalate stones and, at the same time, to eliminate the risk of uric acid stones.

References

1. Andersen DA (1973) Environmental factors in the aetiology of urolithiasis. In: Cifuentes Delatte L, Rapado A, Hodgkinson A (eds) Urinary calculi. Karger, Basel, pp 130-144
2. Asper R (1984) Epidemiology and socioeconomic aspects of urolithiasis. Urol Res 12:1-5
3. Husain I, Badsha SA, Al-Ali IH, Walton M, Saheb A, Jafree S (1979) A survey of urinary stone disease in Abu Dhabi. Emirates Med J (Suppl) 1:17-33
4. Robertson WG, Nisa M, Husain I, Al-Faqi S, Chakrabarty A, Qunibi W, Taher S, Hughes H, Barkworth SA, Holbrow G, Louis S (1989) The importance of diet in the aetiology of primary calcium and uric acid stone-formation—the Arabian experience. In: Walker VR, Sutton RAL, Cameron ECB, Pak CYC, Robertson WG (eds) Urolithiasis. Plenum, New York, pp 735-739
5. Blacklock NJ (1979) Epidemiology of renal lithiasis. In: Wickham JEA (ed) Urinary calculous disease. Churchill Livingstone, Edinburgh, pp 21-39
6. Robertson WG (1982) Urolithiasis: epidemiology and pathogenesis. In: Husain I (ed) Tropical urology and renal disease. Churchill Livingstone, Edinburgh, pp 143-164
7. Dick WH, Lingeman JE, Preminger GM, Smith LH, Wilson DM, Shirrell WL (1989) Laxative abuse as a cause for ammonium urate renal calculi. In: Walker VR, Sutton RAL, Cameron ECB, Pak CYC, Robertson WG (eds) Urolithiasis. Plenum, New York, pp 303-305
8. Robertson WG, Peacock M, Heyburn PJ, Hanes F, Rutherford A, Clementson E, Swaminathan R, Clark PB (1979) Should recurrent, calcium-containing stone-formers become vegetarians? Br J Urol 51:427-431
9. Robertson WG, Peacock M, Marshall DH (1982) Prevalence of urinary stone disease in vegetarians. Eur Urol 9:334-339
10. Robertson WG, Peacock M (1980) The cause of idiopathic calcium stone disease: hypercalciuria or hyperoxaluria? Nephron 26:105-110
11. Walker VR, Bissada N, Qunibi W, Hughes H, Barkworth SA, Holbrow G, Phillips R, Robertson WG, Russell RGG (1989) Urinary calcium excretion in Saudi Arabia. In: Walker VR, Sutton RAL, Cameron ECB, Pak CYC, Robertson WG (eds) Urolithiasis. Plenum, New York, pp 717-719

Environmental Studies in Man in the Dead Sea Region

ORI S. BETTER[1]

SUMMARY. The Dead Sea contains a hyperconcentrated solution and is an example of the salt lakes which abound along geological fault lines. It is important to study human exposure to such media because of intentional or accidental immersion in these lakes. The present communication reviews the effect of (1) experimental, neck out immersion (NI); and (2) accidental near drowning (ND) in the Dead Sea.

1) NI in Dead Sea water failed to produce the expected natriuresis, diuresis and hypotension that is seen during NI in fresh water. The reason is probably the tourniquet-like effect of the venous system in the lower limbs, due to the high head of pressure of Dead Sea water. Such an increased pressure head may prevent the rise in venous return from the lower body seen during immersion in fresh water.

2) ND in the Dead Sea causes much greater fatality and morbidity than ND in sea water. The reason for this increased danger is, at least partly, due to the augmented load of solutes on ND victims in the Dead Sea. Such an increased solute load may lead to extreme hypercalcemia and hypermagnesemia.

The Dead Sea is a lake that lies at the bottom (minus 400 m below sea level) of the hot, arid area of the Syrian-African Rift. Due to its geographic peculiarities and high rate of evaporation, its solute content is extremely high (specific gravity 1.2). Somewhat similar salt lakes abound along the entire length of the Syrian-African Rift and along other geological rifts, such as those found in the Western United States of America (including the Great Salt Lake of Utah). Many of these lakes are located in scenic environments and are used as recreation and resort areas as well as open mining regions for minerals. Man may be exposed to the water of these salt lakes either intentionally or accidentally. It is therefore important to learn the effects of immersion and of near drowning in hyperconcentrated solutions. The purpose of this communication is to review: (a) the effects of experimental immersion to the neck (NI)

[1]Department of Nephrology, Rambam Hospital, and Faculty of Medicine, Technion, Israel Institute of Technology, Haifa, 35254, Israel

on volume control; (b) plasma electrolyte disturbance during near drowning (ND) in
the Dead Sea.

Immersion Studies

The extensive, pioneering studies of Gauer and Henry [1] and Epstein [2] have shown
that NI in thermoneutral (34°C) fresh water is associated with natriuresis and diuresis, leading to negative salt and water balance. The mechanism of these changes was
secondary to centripetal redistribution of body fluids with central (intrathoracic)
hypervolemia. We decided to extend these experiments by comparing the effects of
NI in Dead Sea water, (which is a hyperconcentrated medium) at 34°C, on volume
regulation with those of NI in fresh water [3]. Our results, partially summarized in
Fig. 1, show that NI in fresh water for 4 h did indeed produce the expected natriuresis, diuresis and weight loss (1.4 ± 0.4 kg). In marked contrast, and somewhat unexpectedly, NI in Dead Sea water failed to cause diuresis, natriuresis or change in body
weight. Surprisingly, NI in Dead Sea water caused an increase in systolic and
diastolic blood pressure, whereas NI in fresh water caused a decrease in systolic and
diastolic blood pressure. The differences between the means of the blood pressure
changes in the two immersion media were statistically significant.

We speculate that the absence of natriuresis and diuresis during NI in Dead Sea
water is due to the following hydrostatic conditions: NI in the Dead Sea provides a
20% greater head of pressure on the body (specific gravity 1.2) than fresh water
would. It may be calculated that the pressure on the body 1 m below the neck would
be 91.2 mm Hg in Dead Sea water, compared with 76 mm Hg in fresh water. At 91.2
mm Hg external pressure, venous return from the lower limbs to the heart would be
obliterated, and hemodynamic effects negated.

Information on the effect of immersion on arterial blood pressure is scant and conflicting. Epstein stated, in 1978, that "Immersion in fresh water was associated with
significant, albeit slight, decrease in mean arterial blood pressure" [4]. A later study
by the same author [5] also showed a decrease in mean arterial pressure during
immersion in fresh water in, at least, certain individuals. Arborelius et al. [6], utilizing intraarterial manometry, found that immersion caused a mean increase in arterial
pressure of 10 mm Hg. This was, however, less than the increase of pressure of 15 to
20 mm Hg in the ambient water surrounding the immersed arm in which the brachial
artery was cannulated for the manometry. Moreover, their study was short and
did not last for 100 min of immersion, which is when hypotension was seen in the
present study.

Other independent studies have confirmed that NI in fresh water will lower blood
pressure in the pregnant woman [7], in the normal man [8], and in patients with
cirrhosis [9].

The cause of the hypotension of immersion appears to be the suppression, by NI,
of at least three vasoconstrictor systems (AVP, catecholamine, and renin-angiotensin
II), and the stimulation of the vasodilator system (atrial natriuretic factor). It is possible that minor changes in immersion medium temperature (± 0.5° C) could affect
blood pressure determination, thus explaining the controversy on this matter.

In summary, the specific gravity of the medium in which NI is performed has
profound effects on the resulting hemodynamic influences. A high specific gravity

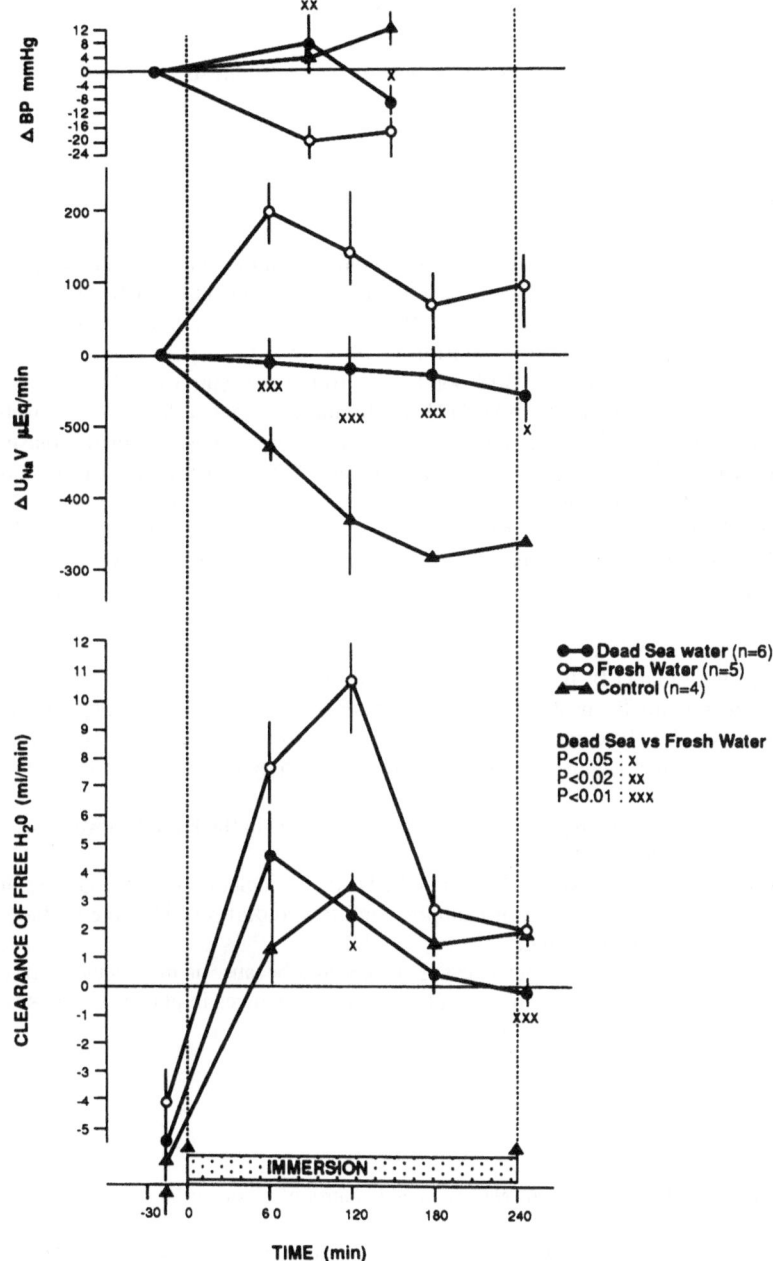

Fig. 1. Influence of neck-out immersion on systolic blood pressure (*BP*) (*top panel*), rate of urinary sodium excretion (*UNaV*) (*middle panel*), and clearance of free water (*bottom panel*). Note a fall in blood pressure and an increase in natriuresis and diuresis during immersion in fresh water. In contrast, immersion in Dead Sea water results in an increase in blood pressure not associated with increased natriuresis, and is associated only with moderately increased diuresis. Quiet sitting is not associated with changes in blood pressure or with increased natriuresis. Results are expressed as mean ± SD

medium may negate the hypotension, natriuresis and diuresis seen in NI in fresh water.

Near-Drowning (ND) in the Dead Sea

Drowning is defined as death due to submersion in water or other media. ND refers to at least temporary survival after asphyxia due to submersion [10]. Of patients with ND in fresh water or sea water, 91% survive; there are only minor changes in plasma electrolytes due to aspiration of fluids [9]. In marked contrast, ND in the Dead Sea (approximately 30% solutes, $\times$ 10 the concentration of the oceans), carries a mortality of at least 40% [11]. Such fatality is due, at least in part, to the load of solutes, which causes striking changes in the composition of the plasma, particularly in the concentration of divalent ions. The Dead Sea has extreme concentrations of calcium and magnesium. The hypercalcemia and hypermagnesemia after ND in the Dead Sea may reach 28.8 and 33.0 mg/dl (!) [12], respectively, values which separately, in other circumstances, are incompatible with life. Most patients, following ND in the Dead Sea, presented with disturbed sensorium, adult respiratory distress syndrome, tachyarrhythmia, and conduction disturbances. Surprisingly, the QTc interval in their ECG was normal in the face of extreme hypercalcemia and hypermagnesemia [12]. It is speculated that this co-intoxication with these divalent cations was mutually protective, since calcium and magnesium are physiological antagonists [13]. Moreover, intravenous calcium infusion was used as an emergency measure to protect against the otherwise refractory hypotension of extreme hypermagnesemia [14].

In general, the best single predictor of survival in ND in the Dead Sea was a serum calcium level below 15.5 mg%.

The recommended treatment of ND in the Dead Sea includes on-scene gastric suction for alert patients, respiratory support, and forced diuresis. The role of dialysis in ND is still being evaluated.

In summary, ND in the Dead Sea is dangerous, because it may cause extreme changes in plasma divalent ion concentration. Such changes in plasma composition are usually not seen in ND in the sea or in fresh water lakes.

References

1. Gauer OH, Henry JP (1976) Neurohumoral control of plasma volume. Int Rev Physiol 9:145–190
2. Epstein M (1978) Renal effects of head-out water immersion in man: implications for an understanding of volume homeostasis. Physiol Rev 58:529–581
3. Ish-Shalom N, Better OS (1984) Volume regulation in man during neck-out immersion in a medium with high specific gravity (Dead Sea water). Isr J Med Sci 20:109–112
4. Epstein M, Preston S, Weitzman RE (1981) Isoosmotic central blood volume expansion suppresses plasma arginine vasopressin in normal man. J Clin Endocrinol Metab 52:256–262
5. Epstein M (1978) Studies of volume homeostasis in man utilizing the model of head-out water immersion. Nephron 22:9–19

6. Arborelius M Jr, Balldin UI, Lilja B, Lundgren CEG (1972) Hemodynamic changes in man during immersion with the head above water. Aerospace Medicine 43:592–598

7. Kokot F, Ulman J, Cekauski A (1983) Influence of head out water immersion on plasma renin activity, aldosterone, vasopressin and blood pressure in late pregnancy and toxemia. Proc Eur Dial Transplant Assoc 20:557–561

8. Leung WM, Logan AG, Campbell PJ (1987) Role of ANP and urinary cGMP in the natriuretic and diuretic response to central hypervolemia in normal human subjects. Can J Physiol Pharmacol 65:2076–2080

9. Skorecki KL, Leung WM, Campbell P, Warner LC, Wong PY, Bull S, Logan AG, Blendis LM (1988) Role of atrial natriuretic peptide in the natriuretic response to central volume expansion induced by head-out water immersion in sodium retaining cirrhotic subjects. Am J Med 85:375–382

10. Modell JH, Graves SA, Ketover A (1976) Clinical course of 91 consecutive near drowning victims. Chest 70:231–238

11. Yagil Y, Stalinkowicz R, Michaeli J, Mogle P (1985) Near drowning in the Dead Sea. Electrolyte imbalances and therapeutic implication. Arch Intern Med 145:50–53

12. Porath A, Masseri M, Harman I, Ovsyshecher I, Keinan A (1989) Dead Sea poisoning. Ann Emerg Med 18:187–191

13. Levin BS, Coburn JW (1984) Magnesium, the mimic/antagonist of calcium (editorial). N Engl J Med 310:1523–1524

14. Mordes JP, Swartz R, Arky RA (1975) Extreme hypermagnesemia as a cause of refractory hypotension. Ann Intern Med 83:657–658

Progression and Chronicity of Acute Post-Streptococcal Glomerulonephritis (APSGN)

Nobuyuki Yoshizawa[1] and Inge Sagel[2]

Summary. In a follow-up study of 33 patients who had had overt acute post-streptococcal glomerulonephritis (APSGN), 11 patients had intermittent or persistent hematuria and/or proteinuria with or without hypertension 2–15 years after onset.

In a prospective survey conducted in two separate areas of Japan, onset of asymptomatic APSGN after infection with β hemolytic streptococci was observed in 25% of the subjects studied. A follow-up of not less than two years was carried out on these patients. Progression of the disease into chronicity, as defined by persistent or intermittent hematuria, was observed in three of 10 patients. Repeat renal biopsies were performed in seven patients (three asymptomatic and four overt). Proliferative glomerulonephritis without deposition of IgA (non-IgA nephropathy) was diagnosed in all of these cases. Antibody titers were measured in 73 patients with non-IgA nephropathy detected as chance hematuria, using a streptococcal protein which we believe is the nephritogenic antigen. Titers against this antigen were, in our experience, uniformly elevated in patients with asymptomatic and overt APSGN. It was found that 14 of the patients (19%) had elevated levels as compared with normal subjects. These findings suggest that many of the non-IgAN patients may have progressed from asymptomatic APSGN.

Asymptomatic APSGN [1,2]

The author wishes to describe the results of a survey conducted in New York [3]. In the survey, 248 children with streptococcal infection were followed on a weekly basis with urinalysis and CH50 for at least 6 weeks. Of the 248 children, 194 developed no abnormal findings and were no longer followed. The remaining 54 children

[1]Department of Medicine, National Defense Medical College, 3-2 Namiki, Tokorozawa, 359 Japan
[2]Department of Pediatrics, New York Medical College, NY, USA

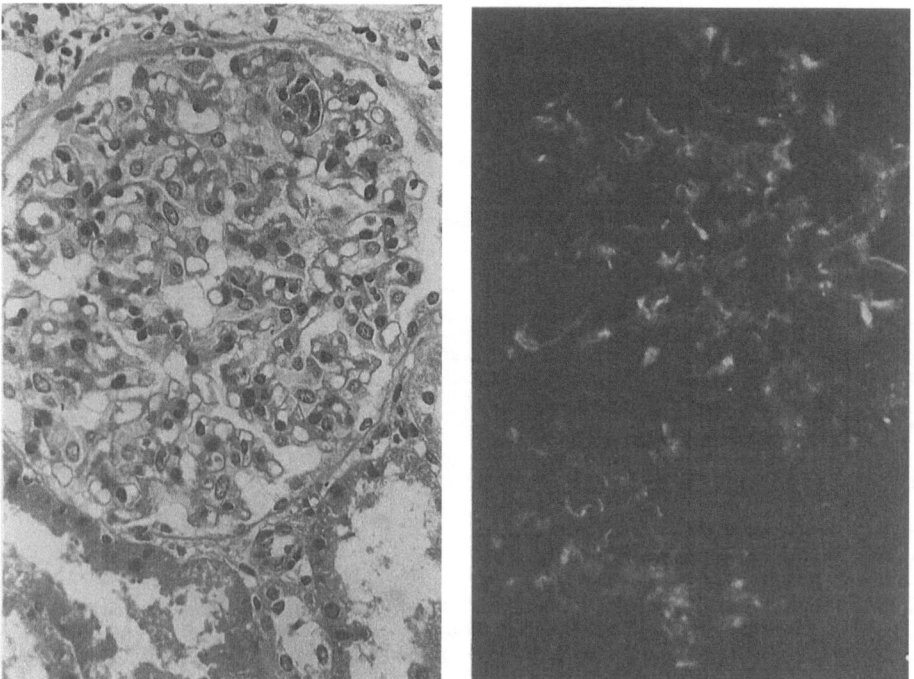

Fig. 1. a Acute glomerulonephritis (AGN) (PAS), **b** AGN (C3)

showed one of the following abnormalities: 1] proteinuria and/or hematuria (15), 2] transient decrease in CH50 (19), 3] both of the above (20).

Renal histology in patients with both disorders showed that one was normal, seven had mild proliferative (+AGN), and nine had moderate proliferative change (++AGN). Three patients showed the classical pathology seen in APSGN (+++AGN). By immunofluorescence (IF) test five were negative, while the remainder showed positive segmental or diffuse granular deposition of IgG and C3 (Figs. 1,2). The infecting strains of group A, β hemolytic streptococci were mostly T type 4, 12, and Impetigo 19. All children were asymptomatic, except one who had mild periorbital edema.

These data indicate that the incidence of glomerular pathology among children infected by group A, β hemolytic streptococci is much higher than the reported incidence, and glomerulonephritis, even in the asymptomatic cases, is morphologically quite evident. In these asymptomatic APSGN cases, serum complement level decreased transiently at the early stage of the disease, together with the appearance of the urinary findings, suggesting development of nephritis subsequent to the streptococcal infection.

From 1978–1979 and from 1982–1984, a prospective survey was conducted, in the same manner as the survey in New York, in the Takanedai area of Funabashi City and

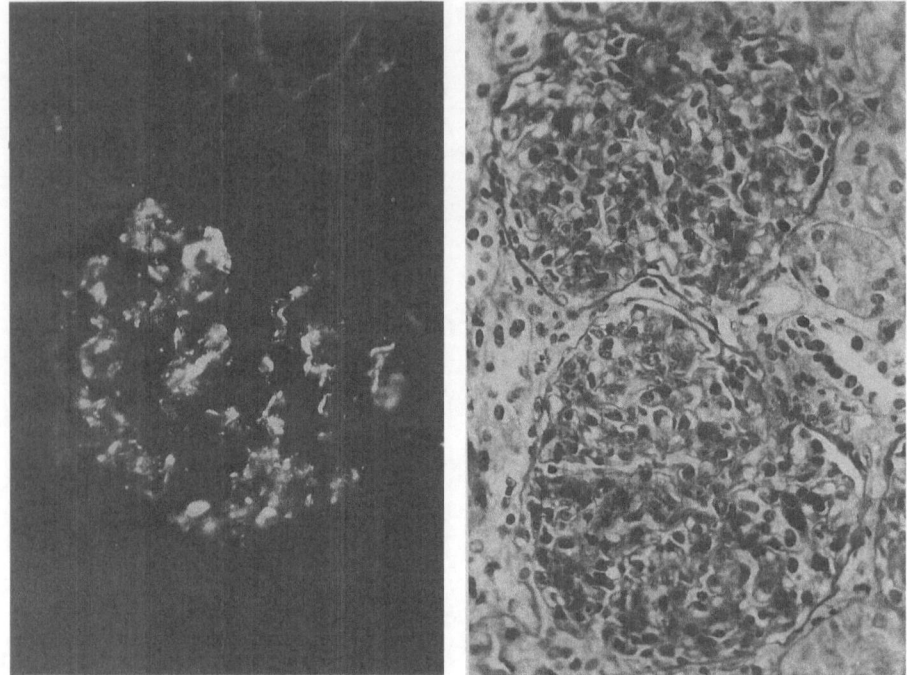

a   b

Fig. 2. a AGN (PAS), **b** AGN (C3)

the Kanayamacho area of Tokorozawa City in Japan. Proteinuria and/or hematuria
with or without decrease in CH50 were detected in 25% of the 44 patients with streptococcal upper respiratory infection (URI) in both groups [4] and all were asymptomatic. Table 1 shows the laboratory findings for our patients. In all cases, the
presence of proliferative changes was confirmed by renal biopsy. The severity of
these lesions varied, ranging from +AGN or mild, to classical +++AGN.

Incidence of Chronicity Following Asymptomatic and Overt APSGN

APSGN is considered to be a "curable nephritis" in most cases and is reported to
progress into chronicity in only 5% of affected children and in about 20%–30% of
affected adults. According to the diagnostic criteria published by the Ministry of
Health and Welfare in Japan, chronic glomerulonephritis is defined as abnormal urinary findings or hypertension persisting over one year after onset of nephritis. As
shown in Fig. 3, patients with overt APSGN may have normal urinary findings within
one to two years after onset of the disease, therefore, we regard abnormal urinary
findings of at least two years duration as progression into chronicity. Furthermore,
as shown in Fig. 3, some patients, after an interval with normal urine, showed recur-

Table 1. Clinical and laboratory data of 13 patients with asymptomatic APGN

Patients		Latent period (W)	ASO	CH50	Urinalysis			Biopsy	Follow-up period	Outcome
					Protein	RBC	WBC			
1. S.M.	11F	3	500	24.5	+	0–1	0–1	+ AGN	2 Y	Recovered
2. U.H.	5F	7	1250	23.2	+	0–1	1–2	+ AGN	2 Y	Recovered
3. H.M.	26F	8	500	22.8	–	1–2	0–1	+ AGN	2 Y	Recovered
4. A.N.	11F	4	625	20.6	–	0–2	1–2	+ AGN	2 Y	Recovered
5. I.M.	34F	1	333	22.0	–	10–15	1–3	++ AGN	5 Y	Chronic
6. K.M.	11F	4	333	13.5	+	2–3	1–2	++ AGN	6 Y	Chronic
7. N.H.	11M	9	833	22.8	+	1–2	1–2	+ AGN	6.5 Y	Recovered
8. K.H.	16F	?	833	24.0	–	15–20	1–2	++ AGN	6.5 Y	Chronic
9. N.M.	13M	1	625	24.2	+	0–1	0–2	+ AGN	7 Y	Recovered
10. B.S.	8F	7	1250	<5	+	14–17	0–1	+ AGN	8 Y	Recovered
11. S.T.	13F	5	625	20.4	–	0–3	0–1	+ AGN	8 Y	Recovered
12. T.Y.	7M	2	625	17.5	+	0–1	1–2	+ AGN	8 Y	Recovered
13. S.M.	12F	2	625	<12	–	20–25	1–2	⧣ AGN	8 Y	Recovered

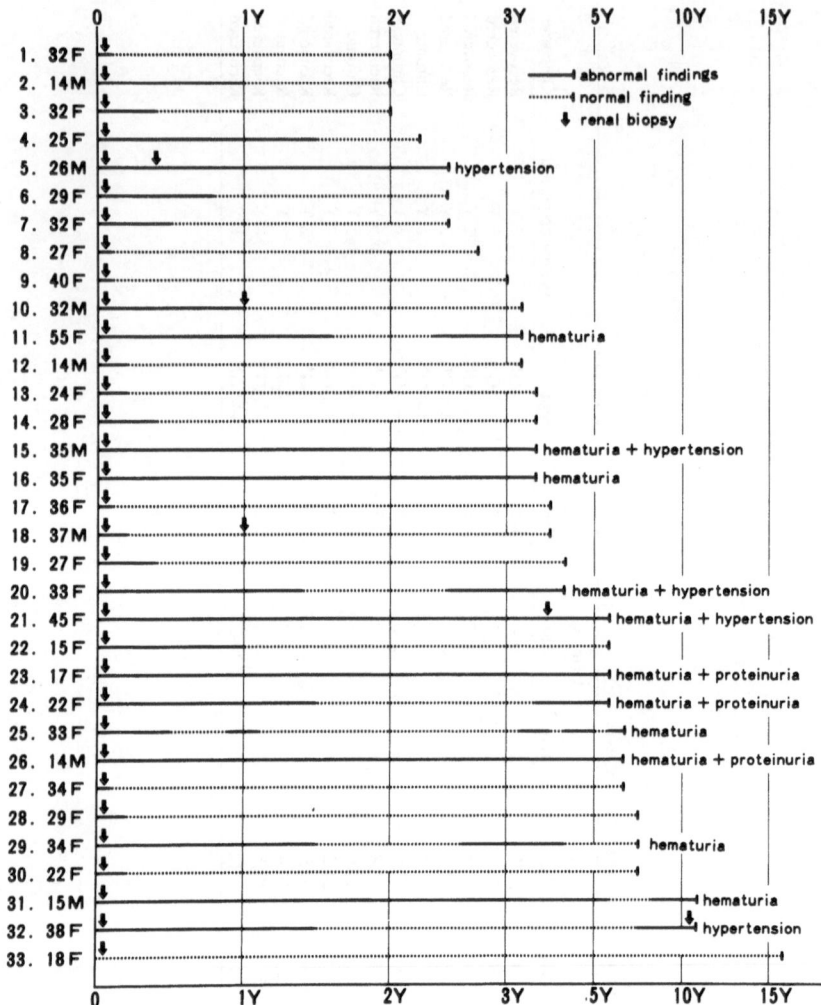

Fig. 3. Clinical course of 33 patients with overt APSGN

rence of abnormal urinary findings two–three years after the disease appeared to have
healed, thus, the definition of chronicity is not easy.

The clinical course of thirteen Japanese patients with asymptomatic APSGN was
followed up for 8 years. Three were lost to follow-up and three of the remaining 10
patients followed for at least 2 years had persistent or intermittent hematuria (Fig. 4).
Of 33 patients with biopsy-proven overt APSGN, 11 (33.3%) progressed into "chronicity" by presenting with hematuria and/or proteinuria with or without hypertension (Fig. 3). Table 2 summarizes the results of renal biopsies in seven of these
patients. Histology showed mild to moderate mesangial proliferative glomerulonephritis without IgA deposits, which is classified as Non-IgA nephropathy. The

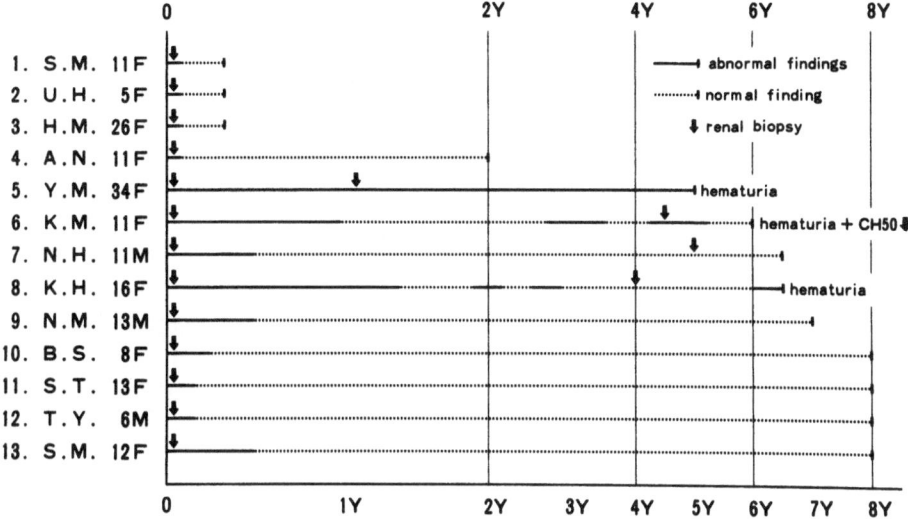

Fig. 4. Clinical course of 13 patients with asymptomatic APSGN

above-mentioned findings suggest that many patients with initially undetected streptococcal infections may present with chance hematuria and/or proteinuria in school
or corporate physical examinations.

Non-IgA nephropathy is not an established entity; however, in Japan, 30%–40% of
patients with chronic glomerulonephritis are of this type; this nephropathy along
with IgA nephropathy, constitutes a principal type of nephritis, in the etiology of
chance hematuria and/or proteinuria. Asymptomatic APSGN may develop insidi-

Table 2. Follow-up biopsies of 7 patients with chronic PSGN

Patient		Onset ↓ Biopsy	IF					LM
			C3c	G	A	M	Fib	
1. T.Y.	26M	20d	⧣	++	−	++	−	⧣ A G N
		110d	+	−	−	++	−	+ C G N
2. S.C.	38F	22d	++	+	(+)	−	−	++ A G N
		10y	−	−	−	−	−	+ C G N
3. W.K.	45F	31d	++	−	−	−	(+)	++ A G N
		4y	−	−	−	−	−	++ C G N
4. S.M.	39F	25d	++	−	−	−	−	++ A G N
		5y	−	−	−	−	−	+ C G N
*5. K.M.	11F	21d	+	+	−	+	(+)	++ A G N
		4.5y	+	+	−	±	(±)	+ C G N
*6. K.H.	16F	40d	+	±	(+)	±	(+)	+ A G N
		4y	+	±	(+)	±	(+)	+ C G N
*7. I.M.	34F	44d	++	+	(+)	+	(+)	++ A G N
		1.5y	+	−	(±)	±	(±)	+ C G N

*Asymptomatic
IF, immunofluorescence; LM, light microscopy
( ), focal

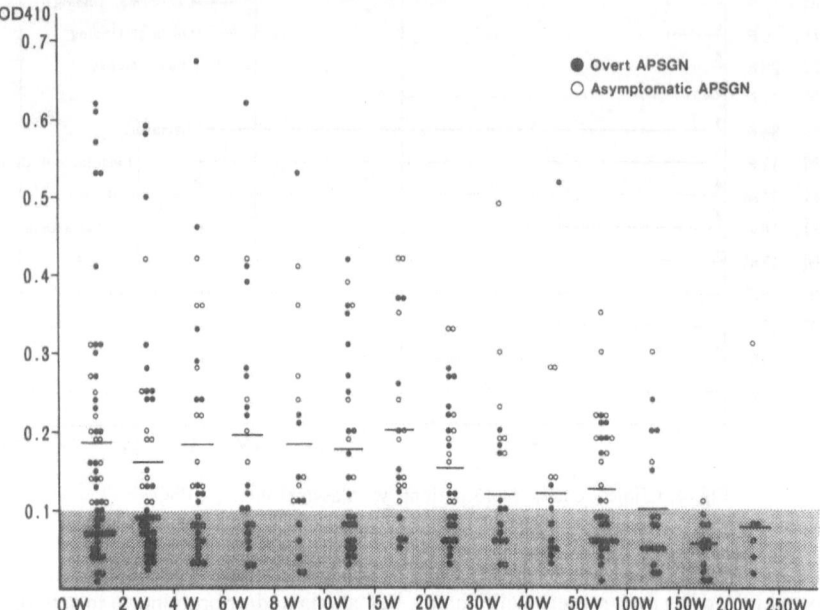

Fig. 5. Antibody to PA-Ag in APSGN (ELISA)

ously and may be detected accidentally as chance hematuria/proteinuria. For further clarification, we determined serum antibody titers against preabsorbing antigen (PA-Ag), using enzyme-linked immunoadsorbent assay (ELISA). In patients with asymptomatic and overt APSGN, mean titers of the antibody were significantly higher than those in normal adults and in patients with uncomplicated streptococcal infections. One third of the patients continued to have high titers for more than two years after onset (Fig. 5). Of 73 patients with Non-IgA nephropathy detected as chance hematuria, results were found to be positive in 14 (19%) patients (Fig. 6). This result suggests that streptococcal infection may have been the cause of the nephropathy detected as chance hematuria.

Preabsorbing antigen (PA-Ag) [5–7] is a protein fraction which we consider to have nephritogenic properties, isolated from nephritogenic streptococci. During the acute phase of APSGN this fraction was found to localize on the glomerular basement membrane and in the mesangium; the fraction is a purified form of endostreptosin [8,9] with a M.W. 43000 and pI 4.7.

Mechanism of Chronicity (Fig. 7)

Jennings and Earle [10] postulated that the severity of certain histologic lesions at disease onset was related to chronicity. According to these investigators, such lesions include (1) endothelial cell proliferation, (2) glomerular damage (lobular necrosis or

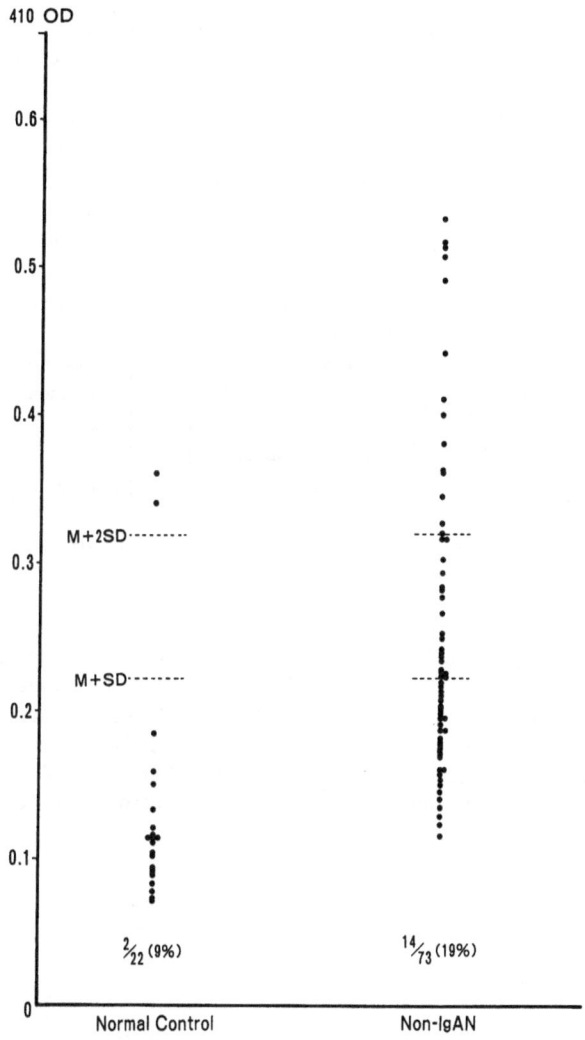

Fig. 6. Antibody titers to PA-Ag in patients with non-IgA nephritis detected by chance hematuria

scar, thrombosis, crescent, adhesion, or hyalinization), and (3) interstitial reaction. These authors postulated that the more severe and diffused these lesions, the more likely it would be that the disease would become chronic. Baldwin et al. [11] suggested that intrarenal vascular sclerosis can lead to glomerulosclerosis, and they proposed that ischemia might play an important pathogenetic role in the progression of APSGN to chronicity. In addition to the above, interstitial cellular infiltration [12,13] may also be an important factor in the development of chronic disease. We investigated interstitial cellular infiltration within the glomerulus and tubulointer-

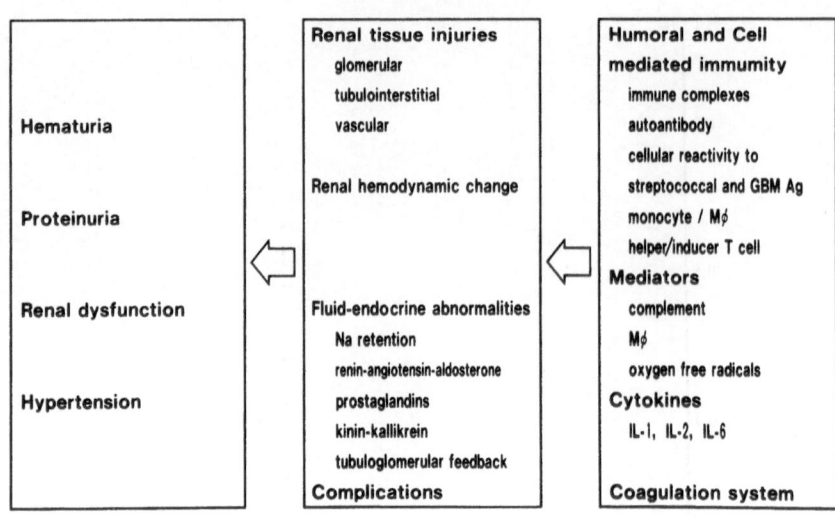

Fig. 7. Factors contributing to chronicity of APSGN

stitium (Fig. 8), using monoclonal antibody in various types of glomerulonephritis, and we found that there is little or no cellular infiltration in the glomerulus, except in APSGN. However, cellular infiltration, mostly of helper/inducer T cells and monocyte/Mφ (Fig. 9), was increased in the interstitial tissue, with no apparent difference in the pattern of infiltration among various glomerulonephritides [14]. In ddition, there was a significant positive correlation between the extent of cell

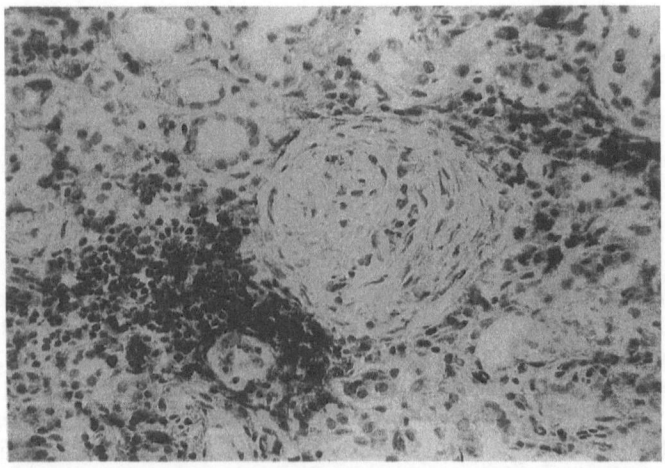

Fig. 9. Interstitial cellular infiltration (CD4 : helper/inducer T cell)

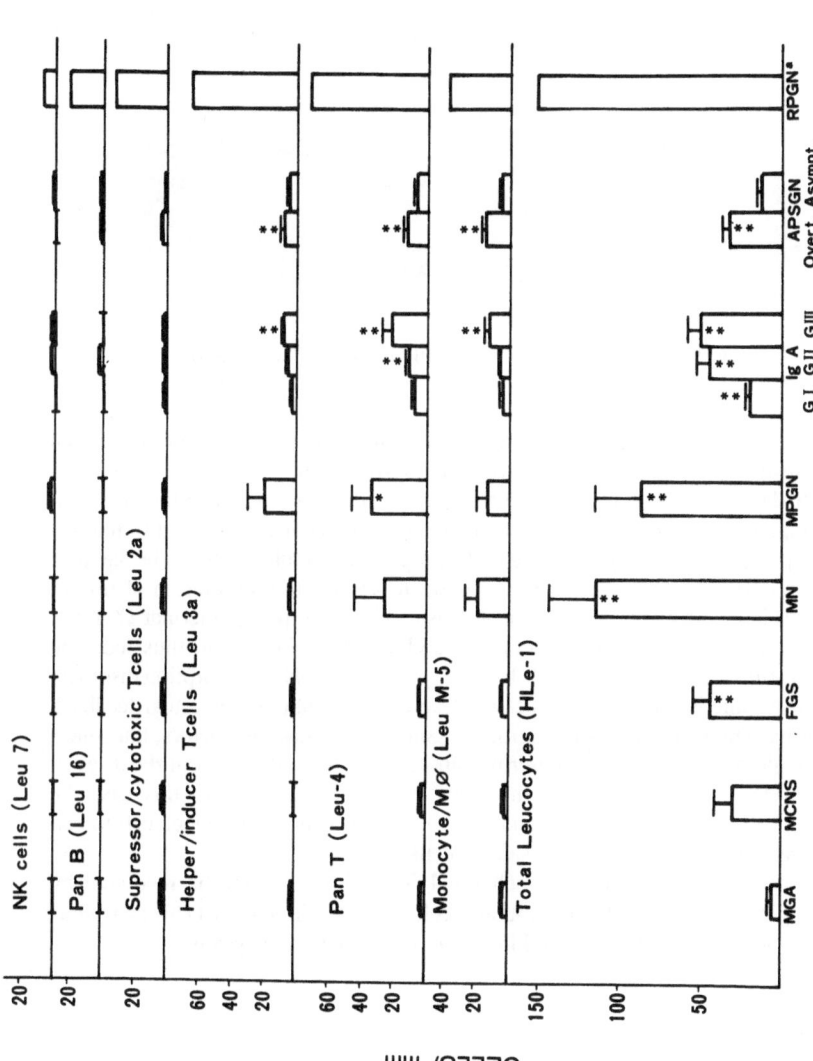

Fig. 8. Analysis of interstitial infiltrating leucocyte subpopulations in various glomerulonephritis. MGA, minor glomerular abnormalities; MCNS, minimal change nephrotic syndrome; FGS, focal glomerular sclerosis; MN, membranous nephropathy; MPGN, membranoproliferative glomerulonephritis; RPGN, rapidly progressive glomerulonephritis; * $P < 0.05$ as compared with MGA; ** $P < 0.01$

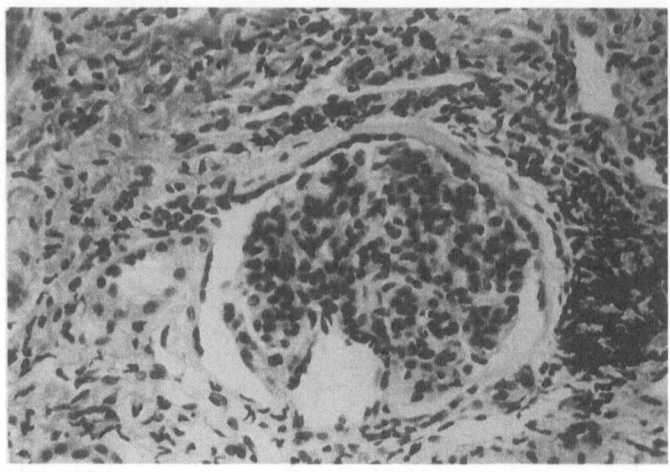

Fig. 10. Periglomerular cellular infiltration in APSGN (PAS)

infiltration and serum creatinine levels. That is, the more extensive the interstitial cellular infiltration, the more severe the renal dysfunction.

Tubular damage, caused by glomerular injury or other etiology, can unmask antigenic components of the tubules, thereby inducing antigenicity, which in turn induces delayed type hypersensitivity, resulting in the progression of tubulointerstitial damage. Interleukin-I (IL-1), released by Mφ, is known to accelerate proliferation of fibroblasts, and it is possible that interstitial fibrosis can increase postglomerular capillary resistance and can cause deterioration in the glomerular circulation, thus reducing glomerular filtration rate (GFR) [15]. It is also possible that Na reabsorption disorders caused by dysfunction of the tubules can reduce GFR via tubulo-glomerular feedback mechanisms. These are mainly interstitial responses to aggravating factors, but generally, if the glomerular damage as described above is severe at the onset of the disease, periglomerular cellular infiltration may have occurred (Fig. 10). In this case the infiltrating cells are mostly T cells and monocyte/Mφ, which can induce cell to cell interactions with infiltrating and mesangial cells.

Persistence and progression of such renal tissue injuries may be mediated by immunologic factors, namely humoral and cell-mediated immunity [16], as well as by complement, macrophages, cytokines, and the coagulation system.

References

1. Cohen JA, Levitt MF (1963) Acute glomerulonephritis with few urinary abnormalities. Report of two cases proved by renal biopsy. N Engl J Med 268:749–753
2. Freedman P, Meister HP, Co BS, Markowitz AS, Dubin A (1966) The subclinical renal response to streptococcal infection. New Engl J Med 275:795
3. Sagel I, Treser G, Yoshizawa N, Ty A, Kleinberger H, Yuceoglu M, Wasserman E, Lange K (1973) Occurrence and nature of glomerular lesions after group A streptococci infection in children. Ann Intern Med 79:492

4. Yoshizawa N, Oshima S, Takeuchi A, Sagel I, Treser G (1987) Occurrence of chronicity following asymptomatic and overt acute poststreptococcal glomerulonephritis (APGN). Proceedings of the Xth international congress of nephrology
5. Yoshizawa N, Treser G, Sagel I, Ty A, Ahmed U, Lange K (1973) Demonstration of antigenic sites in glomeruli of patients with acute poststreptococcal glomerulonephritis by immunofluorescein and immunoferritin techniques. Am J Pathol 70:131
6. Yoshizawa N, Oshima S, Takeuchi A, Takahashi K, Sagel I, Treser G (1985) Serological studies in poststreptococcal glomerulonephritis using streptococcal antigen (preabsorbing antigen, PA-Ag). In: Recent advances in streptococci and streptococcal diseases. Readbooks, Berkshire, p 251
7. Yoshizawa N, Oshima S, Takeuchi A, Takahashi K, Sagel I, Treser G (1985) A streptococcal antigen. (preabsorbing antigen, PA-Ag) causing in situ immune reaction in acute poststreptococcal glomerulonephritis (APGN). In: Recent advances in streptococci and streptococcal diseases. Readbooks, Berkshire, p 353
8. Lange K, Ahmed U, Kleinberger H, Treser G (1976) A hitherto unknown streptococcal antigen and its probable relation to acute poststreptococcal glomerulonephritis. Clin Nephrol 5:207
9. Lange K, Seligson G, Cronin W (1983) Evidence for the in situ of poststreptococcal glomerulonephritis: glomerular localization of endostreptotosin and the clinical significance of the subsequent antibody response. Clin Nephrol 19:3
10. Jennings RB, Earle DP (1961) Poststreptococcal glomerulonephritis: Histopathologic and clinical studies of the acute, subsiding acute and early chronic latent phases. J Clin Invest 40:1525
11. Baldwin DS, Melvin C, Gluck MC, et al. (1974) The long-term course of poststreptococcal glomerulonephritis. Ann Intern Med 80:342
12. Hooke DH, Gee DC, Atkins RC (1987) Leucocyte analysis using monoclonal antibodies in human glomerulonephritis. Kidney Int 31:964–972
13. Hotta O, Yoshizawa N, Oshima S, Takeuchi A, Kawamura O, Kondo S, Kubota T, Niwa H (1987) Significance of renal hyaline arteriolosclerosis and tubulointerstitial change in IgA glomerulonephritis and focal glomerular sclerosis. Nephron 47:262–265
14. Oda, T, Yoshizawa N, Takeuchi A, Kubota T, Akashi Y, Oshikawa Y, Hotta O, Ohshima S, Niwa, H (1988) Significance of tubulo-interstitial (T-1) change in IgAGN (abstract). Kidney Int 35:372
15. Bohle A, Gise HV, Mackensen HS, Stark JB (1981) The obliteration of the post-glomerular capillaries and its influence upon the function of both glomeruli and tubuli. Klin Wochenschr 59:1043–1051
16. Zabriskie JB, Utermohlen V, Read SE, et al. (1973) Streptococcus related glomerulonephritis. Kidney Int 3:100

Pathobiology of Glomerular and Tubular Basement-Membranes

Chair: Yashpal S. Kanwar (USA)
Mitsumasa Nagase (Japan)

High Resolution Ultrastructure of the Basement Membrane

Zensuke Ota, Hirofumi Makino, and Kenichi Shikata[1]

SUMMARY. The glomerular basement membrane (GBM) is thought to be a main filtration barrier in the glomerulus. However, its ultrastructure was unknown until recent years. In 1977, we were the first to demonstrate electron microscopically and by the negative staining method that the GBM is composed of a three-dimensional meshwork structure which has micropores approximately 3 nm in diameter. Since then, we have also found that alveolar basement membrane and other basement membranes exhibit a similar three dimensional meshwork structure, and we have advocated the molecular sieve theory of the basement membrane. In our subsequent studies, we established, by the ultrathin sectioning method, that type IV collagen forms the meshwork of the GBM. Since the diameter of micropores in the GBM is slightly smaller than the axis of albumin molecules, it is considered that GBM functions as a molecular sieve in the glomerulus. In the GBM of experimental nephrotic animals, it was observed that the meshwork was destroyed and the micropores were enlarged. Consequently, it is presumed that in nephrotic syndrome, the destruction of the molecular sieve is mainly responsible for the occurrence of proteinuria.

Introduction

Ultrafiltration takes place in the glomerulus, through which both water and low molecular weight solutes in blood are filtered nonselectively. On the other hand, however, substances of some magnitude, namely those larger than albumin molecules, are scarcely filtered through and remain in the blood. Human albumin has a molecular weight of 66248, which is the threshold value for the proteins; however, smaller proteins than this, such as β_2-microglobulin, are able to filter virtually completely through the glomerulus. If the glomerulus is observed under an electron

[1]The Third Department of Internal Medicine, Okayama University Medical School, Okayama, 700 Japan

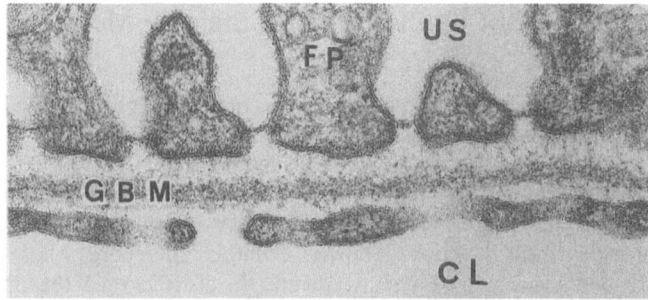

Fig. 1. Ultrathin section of the glomerular capillary wall from normal rat kidney GBM, glomerular basement membrane; FP, foot process; US, urinary space; CL, capillary lumen, ×80000

microscope by the standard ultrathin sectioning method, the ultrastructure of the glomerular basement membrane (GBM) can be observed as an amorphous substance [1] (Fig. 1), and, at the same time, if seen by the freeze etching replica method, its fine structure looks like microgranules approximately 4 nm in diameter [2]. For these reasons, the ultrastructure of the GBM remained controversial and was not understood until recent years, despite a large number of studies. In 1977, we demonstrated for the first time, under an electron microscope, that bovine GBM which had been treated by the negative staining method formed a three-dimensional structure and constituted a molecular sieve for blood components such as albumin [3]. In this paper we describe results obtained thereafter and the mechanism of the onset of proteinuria.

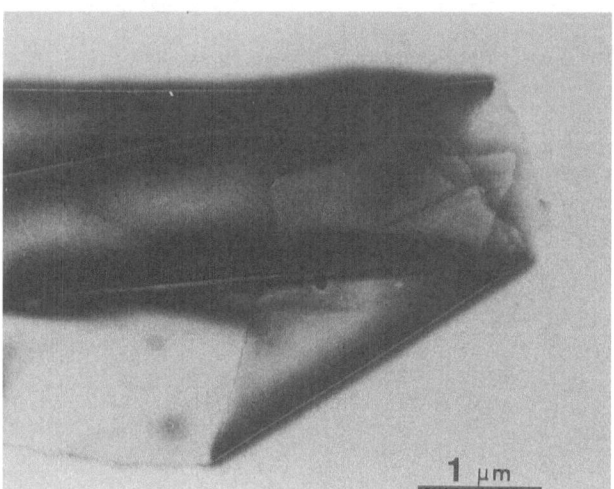

Fig. 2. Negative staining of unfixed rat glomerular basement membrane with 1% PTA. Note the broken folded paper-like appearance with felt-like surface, ×20000

Observation of GBM by the Negative Staining Method

We isolated GBM from bovine and rat kidney, according to Spiro's method [4]. The unfixed GBM thus isolated was observed, in 1% phosphotungstic acid (pH 7.3), electron microscopically by the negative staining method.

When observed at low magnification, the GBM appeared as felt-like paper pieces (Fig. 2). If seen at high magnification, the GBM showed a three-dimensional meshwork composed of fibrils in which there were countless micropores whose diameter was virtually identical (Fig. 3). Figure 4 indicates the distribution of the long dimensions and short dimensions of these micropores. Their mean long dimension was 3.1 ± 0.6 nm and their mean short dimension was 2.5 ± 0.3 nm [3,5–7]. We made further observations of GBM in the rat and human in the same fashion, and demonstrated that all the GBMs consisted of a three-dimensional meshwork composed of fibrils [5,8].

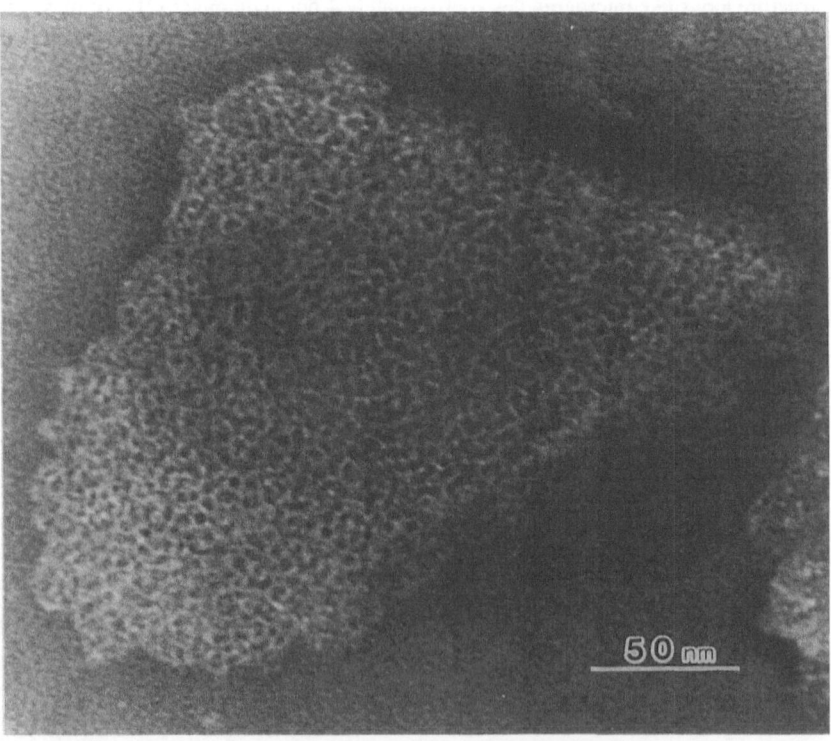

Fig. 3. Negative staining of unfixed bovine glomerular basement membrane at higher magnification. Note clearly discernible fibrils and micropores which form a meshwork structure, ×500000

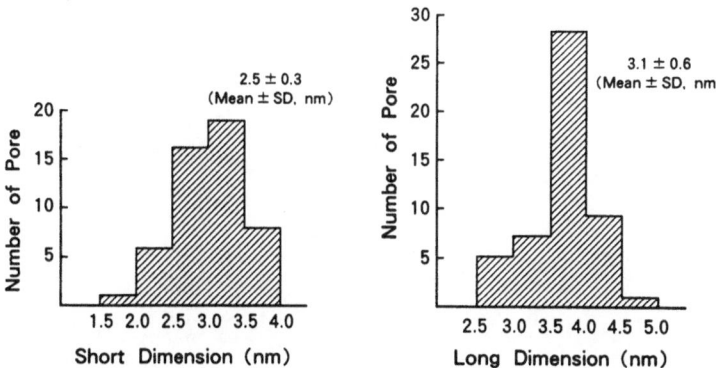

Fig. 4. Distribution of short and long dimensions in bovine glomerular basement membrane

Observation of Other Basement Membranes by the Negative Staining Method

When the unfixed tubular basement membrane (TBM) was isolated from the rat kidney and observed by the negative staining method, it was noted that in this membrane there was a meshwork structure composed of fibrils similar to that in the GBM [9,10] (Fig. 5). The micropores formed by the mesh had a larger diameter than did those in the GBM. This meshwork was also seen in the Descemet's membrane of bovine cornea and in alveolar basement membrane. Consequently, we proposed the molecular sieve theory of the basement membrane [11].

Observation of Chemically Treated GBM by the Ultrathin Sectioning Method

When an isolated GBM is untreated and observed by the ultrathin sectioning method, it is seen as amorphous and ribbon-like, and not as a meshwork structure. Because of this, in order to investigate the ultrastructure in more detail, we chemically treated GBM for observation and successfully demonstrated a meshwork structure even by the ultrathin sectioning method.

Observation by Treatment with Elastase

Rat GBM was isolated according to Spiro's method. The isolate was treated with 0.01% elastase (from porcine pancreas) at 37°C for 5 hours. The chemically treated GBM was fixed, embedded, and observed by the ultrathin sectioning method. In the specimen thus treated, there were fibrils that had disentangled from the GBM; they

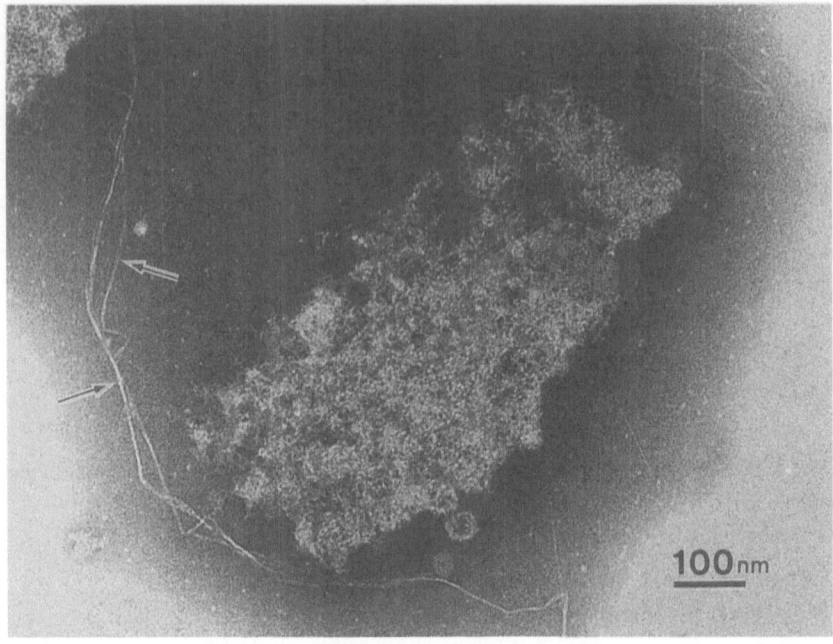

Fig. 5. An unfixed fragment of tubular basement membrane shows fine meshwork. Negative staining with 1% PTA. Note several long fine fibrils disentangling from around the fragment of basement membrane (*arrows*), ×120000

were approximately 3 nm in diameter. These fibrils were also seen in the interior of the GBM, forming a meshwork with micropores approximately 3 nm in diameter. Nodular structures, approximately 10 nm in diameter, were observed on the fibrils [12] (Fig. 6).

When the specimen was observed by immunoelectron microscopy, using anti-type IV collagen antibody obtained by the peroxidase labeled antibody method, the elastase-treated GBM was seen to be positively stained; thus indicating that the treated GBM consisted of type IV collagen [13].

Observation by Treatment with Elastase, Sodium Dodecyl Sulfate (SDS), and 2 Mercaptoethanol

Isolated GBM was treated with 0.01% elastase at 37°C for 24 hours, further treated with sodium dodecyl sulfate (SDS) and 2-mercaptoethanol at 37°C for 72 hours, and was observed by the ultrathin sectioning method. The treated specimen showed more clearly than did the previous method the structure of a meshwork, composed of fibrils over the GBM layer, along with nodular structures on the fibrils (Fig. 7). Stereographic observation revealed the three-dimensional form of this meshwork [14]. The micropores formed by the meshwork had a diameter of approximately 3–5 nm, which was very close to results obtained by the negative staining method.

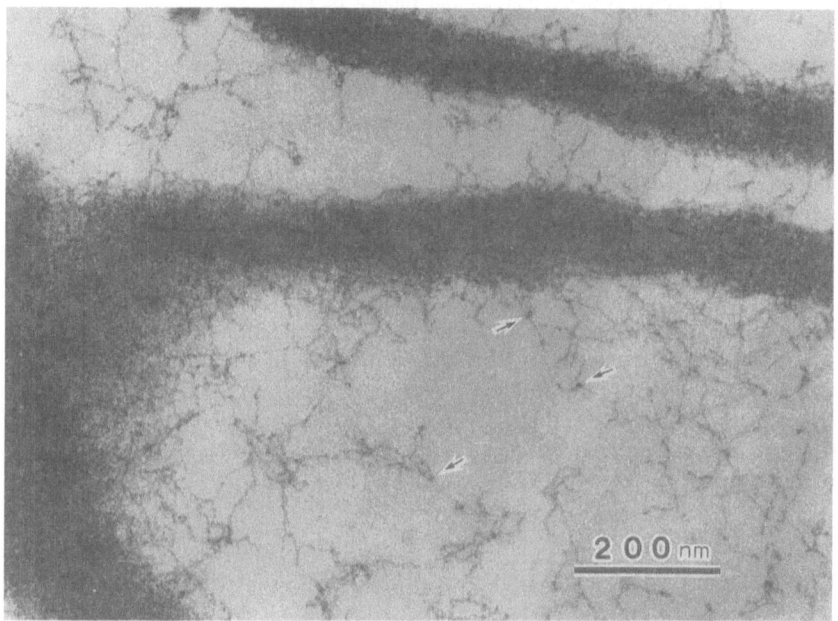

Fig. 6. An ultrathin section of isolated rat glomerular basement membrane (*GBM*) treated with elastase. Fibrils are drifting away from the surface of the GBM and nodular structures (*arrows*) are seen on the fibrils, ×120000

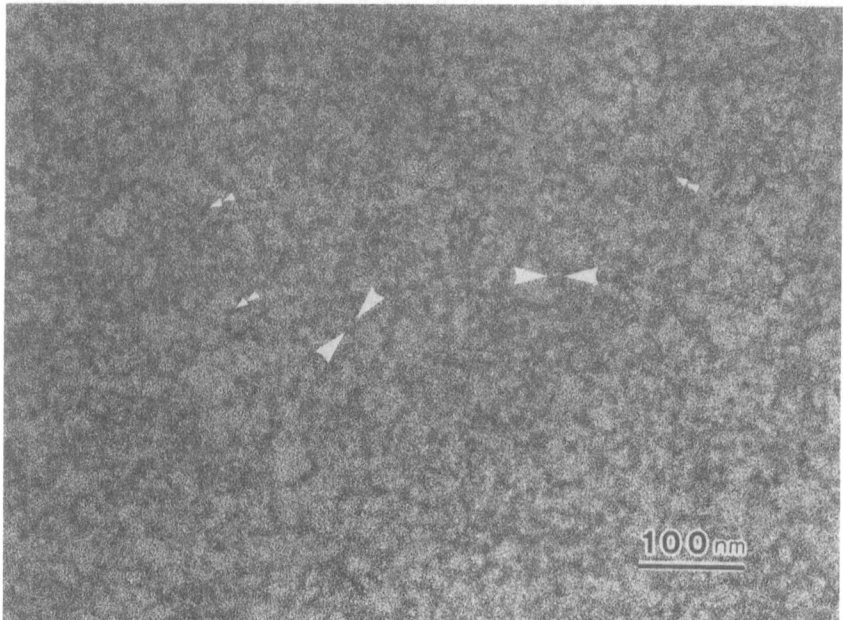

Fig. 7. An ultrathin section of bovine glomerular basement membrane treated with elastase, SDS, and 2-mercaptoethanol. Meshwork structure is composed of fibrils. Note the nodular structures (*double arrowheads*) and numerous micropores (*large arrowheads*), ×165000

These findings suggest that the GBM consists mostly of a three-dimensional mesh-work structure, composed of type IV collagen, which contains micropores approximately 3 nm in diameter. The findings also support observations made according to the negative staining method.

In 1981, Timpl et al. confirmed that type IV collagen, the main constituent of the basement membrane, is a fibril similar to the fibrils we had found and that it forms a meshwork [15]. The meshwork that they showed was very large. They failed to demonstrate the micropores of approximately 3 nm in diameter which we had found in our experiments. Nevertheless, their findings serve as supporting evidence of the characteristics of GBM ultrastructure that we demonstrated. Since then, Lawrie et al. have shown the existence of fibrils called "cords" in an electron-microscopic observation of the GBM [16]. Kubosawa et al. have described the GBM by the deep-etch replica method [17]. In addition, Yurchenco et al. observed the tumor matrix of EHS sarcoma and established its meshwork [18]. Their results appear to support our molecular sieve theory.

Observation of the GBM in Nephrotic Rats

In accordance with the method of Arisz et al., nephrotic rats were prepared by inducing chronic serum sickness by means of bovine serum administration. When the isolated GBM was observed under an electron microscope by the negative staining method, the meshwork in the nephrotic rats was seen to be destroyed and the diameter of the micropores had enlarged significantly when compared with the GBM of control animals [19] (Fig. 8 and Table 1).

We have previously shown in the same manner that there is also an enlargement of the diameter of micropores in Masugi nephritis [20], in aminonucleoside nephritis [21], and in diabetic nephropathy. It is thought that the enlargement of micropore diameter is chiefly responsible for the occurrence of proteinuria.

GBM as a Size Barrier

The diameter of the micropores of the GBM is approximately 3 nm. However, the albumin molecule is a prolate ellipsoid, whose major and minor axes are 15.0 nm and 3.8 nm, respectively. In other words, the diameter of the micropores of the GBM is slightly smaller than the minor axis of the albumin molecule (Fig. 9). GBM, therefore, is thought to function as a molecular sieve in the production of filtrate in the glomerulus.

Another factor that affects filtration is static electric force. Since both the basement membrane and albumin are negatively charged, because of heparan sulfate proteoglycan, etc., and an isoelectric point, respectively, a repellent force is considered to occur between the GBM and albumin molecules on filtration [22]. On the basis of results of an experiment with dextran sulfate, etc., clearance increases as its electric charge shifts from negativity through neutrality to positivity. For this reason, it appears that the Coulomb force between electric charges cannot be ignored in the

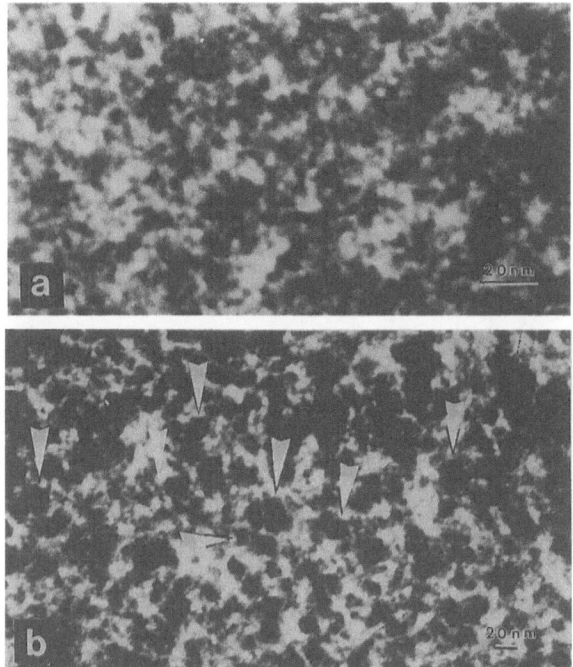

Fig. 8a,b. Negative staining of rat GBM with 1% PTA **a** control rat GBM, ×300000, **b** experimental rat GBM. Note enlarged micropores (*arrows*), ×125000

process of filtration [23]. Consequently, it follows that filtration involves two major barriers, namely the size barrier and the charge barrier.

When a massive amount of protein is filtered through in human nephrotic syndrome, which barrier would be involved more heavily? Based on the results of numerous studies of experimental nephritis, reduced charge of the GBM does not necessarily correlate with proteinuria. On the other hand, some results indicate an involvement of the size barrier [24]. Furthermore, our electron microscopic observations and results obtained from quantitative filtration experiments with ferritin

Table 1. Micropore and fibril diameters of glomerular basement membrane of rats with chronic serum sickness (CSS)

	Control	CSS
Long dimension, (nm)	4 ± 1	9 ± 5*
Short dimension, (nm)	3 ± 1	6 ± 3*
Diameter of fibrils, (nm)	3 ± 1	4 ± 1

a, Values are the means ± SD of 100 micropores or fibrils
*Statistically significant difference from controls ($P < 0.001$)

-Enlargement of Molecular Sieve-

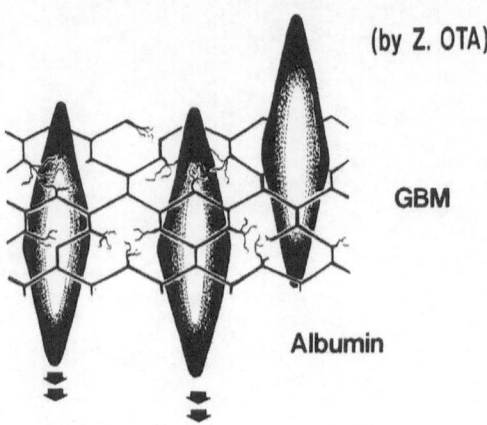

Fig. 9. Schematic representation of mechanism of proteinuria, from our studies (by Z. Ota)

monomers and polymers suggest that the size barrier is much more heavily involved in the filtration of proteins [25]. Therefore, it is presumed that the destruction of the molecular sieve of the basement membrane is chiefly responsible for such filtration.

Acknowledgment. This research was supported by a "Research Grant for Progressive Renal Disease" from diseases specially selected by the Ministry of Health and Welfare Research Project, the Ministry of Health and Welfare of Japan.

References

1. Farquhar MG, Palade GE (1961) Glomerular permeability. II Ferritin transfer across the glomerular capillary wall in nephrotic rats. J Exp Med 114:699–716
2. Ota Z (1975) Electron microscope studies on frozen kidney tissue (in Japanese). Cell 7:350–361
3. Ota Z, Makino H, Miyoshi A, Hiramatsu M, Takahashi K, Ofuji T (1977) Electron microscopic demonstration of meshwork structure in human and bovine glomerular basement membranes. Acta Med Okayama 31:339–342
4. Spiro RG (1967) Studies on the renal glomerular basement membrane. Preparation and chemical composition. J Biol Chem 242:1915–1922
5. Ota Z, Makino H, Miyoshi A, Hiramatsu M, Takahashi K, Ofuji T (1979) Molecular sieve in glomerular basement membrane as revealed by electron microscopy. J Electron Microsc (Tokyo) 28:20–28
6. Ota Z, Makino H, Takaya Y, Ofuji T (1980) Molecular sieve in renal glomerular and tubular basement membranes as revealed by electron microscopy. Renal Physiol 3:317–323
7. Ota Z, Makino H, Takaoka M, Soda K, Suzuki S (1985) Mechanism of proteinuria in rats with chronic serum sickness. In: Glomerular dysfunction and biopathology of vascular wall. Academic Press, Tokyo, pp 165–174

8. Makino H (1982) Molecular sieve in rat glomerular basement membrane as revealed by negative staining. Acta Med Okayama 36:371-382

9. Makino H, Ota Z, Takaya Y, Kida K, Miyoshi A, Hiramatsu M, Takahashi K, Ofuji T (1979) Ultrastructure of rat renal tubular basement membrane – meshwork structure demonstration by negative staining. Acta Med Okayama 33:133-136

10. Makino H, Ota Z, Takaya Y, Miyoshi A, Ofuji T (1981) Molecular sieve in rat tubular basement membrane as revealed by negative staining. Renal Physiol 4:180-190

11. Makino H, Toyofuku H, Mino Y, Takaoka M, Ota Z (1983) Molecular sieve in bovine Descemet's membrane as revealed by negative staining. Acta Med Okayama 37:155-157

12. Ichiyasu A, Takaoka M, Makino H, Takahashi K, Ota Z (1987) Fibrillar ultrastructure of the glomerular basement membrane of the rat kidney as revealed by digestive treatment. Acta Med Okayama 41:183-185

13. Ichiyasu M, Makino H (1988) Molecular sieve of the rat glomerular basement membrane: A transmission electron microscopic study of enzyme-treated specimens. Acta Med Okayama 42:317-325

14. Shikata K, Makino H, Ichiyasu A, Ota Z (1990) Three-dimensional meshwork structure of glomerular basement membrane revealed by chemical treatment. J Electron Microsc (Tokyo) 39:182-185

15. Timpl R, Wiedermann H, Van Delden V, Furthmayr H, Kuhn K (1981) A network model for the organization of type IV collagen molecules in basement membrane. Eur J Biochem 120:203-211

16. Laurie GW, Leblond CP, Inoue S, Martin GR, Chung A (1984) Fine structure of the glomerular basement membrane and immunolocalization of five basement membrane components to the lamina densa (basal lamina) and its extensions in both glomeruli and tubules of the rat kidney. Am J Anat 169:463-481

17. Kubosawa H, Kondo Y (1985) Ultrastructural organization of the glomerular basement membrane as revealed by a deep-etch replica method. Cell Tissue Res 242:33-39

18. Yurchenco PD, Ruden GC (1988) Type IV collagen lateral associations in the EHS tumor matrix—comparison with amniotic and in vitro networks. Am J Pathol 132:278-291

19. Makino H, Soda K, Komoda K, Ota Z (1988) Changes in the molecular sieve of the glomerular basement membrane of rats with chronic serum sickness. Acta Med Okayama 42:53-60

20. Makino H (1983) Changes in the molecular sieve of glomerular basement membrane in rats with Masugi nephritis. Renal Physiol 6:266-274

21. Takaya Y, Ota Z, Makino H, Kida K, Miyoshi A, Hiramatsu M, Takahashi K, Ofuji T (1980) Changes in the molecular sieve of glomerular basement membrane in rats with aminonucleoside nephrosis. Acta Med Okayama 34:67-70

22. Kanwar YS, Linker A, Farquhar MG (1980) Increased permeability of the glomerular basement membrane to ferritin after removal of glycosaminoglycans (heparan sulfate) by enzyme digestion. J Cell Biol 86:688-693

23. Bohrer MP, Deen WM, Robertson CR, Brenner BM (1977) Mechanism of angiotensin II-induced proteinuria in the rat. Am J Physiol 233:F13-F21

24. Kanwar YS (1984) Biology of disease. Biophysiology of glomerular filtration and proteinuria. Lab Invest 51:7-21

25. Ota Z, Kumagai I, Shikata K, Makino H (1989) Human liver ferritin as a new tracer for studying glomerular permeability. Act Med Okayama 43:363-365

Glomerular Basement Membrane: Molecular Structure of Type IV Collagen and Its Involvement in Diseases

BILLY G. HUDSON, SRIPAD GUNWAR, BILLIE J. WISDOM, JR., MARK D. HUDSON, and MILTON E. NOELKEN[1]

SUMMARY. Glomerular basement membrane is a specialized extracellular matrix that functions as a molecular sieve in the nephron. Its function is altered in three notable human diseases that affect the kidneys, Goodpasture syndrome, Alport syndrome, and diabetes mellitus. Over the past decade, great advances have been made in understanding the supramolecular structure of this membrane and its role in the pathogenesis of these diseases. The membrane's major constituent is type IV collagen which provides tensile strength to the matrix and serves as a scaffold for the binding and alignment of several other macromolecular constituents. Recently, three new chains (α3, α4, and α5) of type IV collagen have been discovered, and they have been implicated in the pathogenesis of Goodpasture and Alport syndromes and potentially in that of diabetic nephropathy. This review will briefly describe the molecular structure of type IV collagen and its involvement in these diseases.

Introduction

Basement membranes are complex extracellular matrices that play key roles in diverse biological processes. The processes include: molecular sieving [1]; orchestration of embryonic development; and maintenance of tissue architecture during remodeling and repair [2,3]. Basement membrane function is altered in three notable human diseases that affect the kidneys, *Goodpasture syndrome*, *Alport syndrome* and *diabetes mellitus*, leading to serious and often fatal consequences. In these diseases, the molecular sieving function of the glomerular basement membrane (GBM) is altered (Fig. 1), which often leads to end-stage renal disease.

---

[1]Department of Biochemistry and Molecular Biology, University of Kansas Medical Center, Kansas City, KS 66103, USA

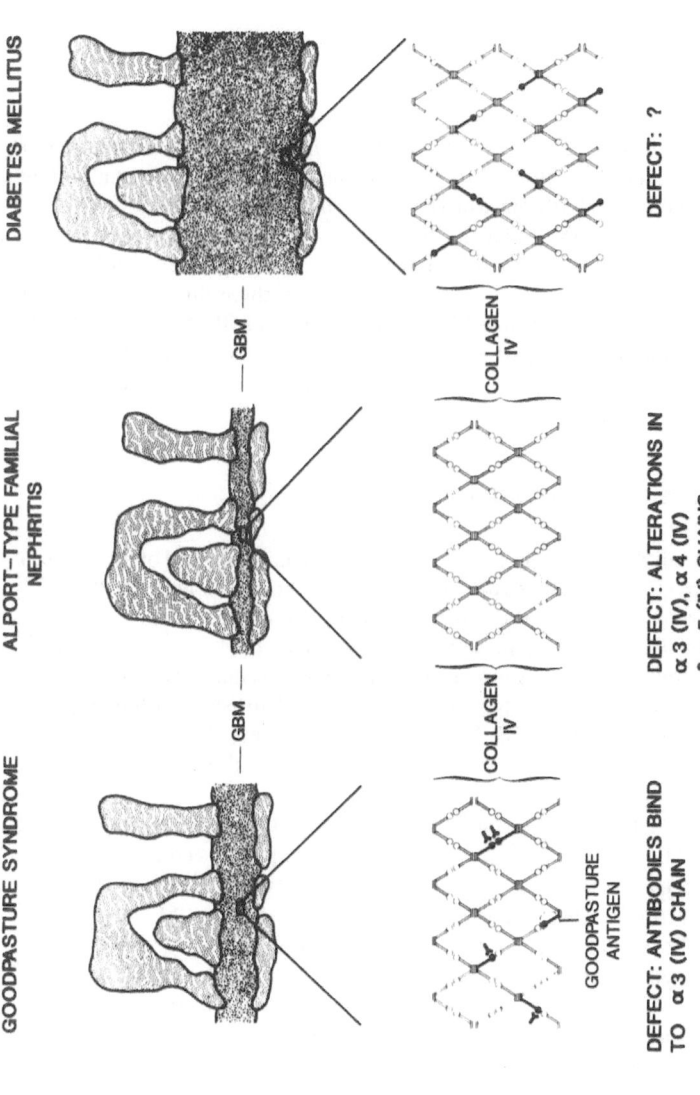

Fig. 1. Schematic illustration of the ultrastructural alteration and proposed molecular defect in GBM of 3 notable human diseases that affect the kidneys. In Goodpasture syndrome the autoantigen to which Goodpasture antibodies bind has been localized to the novel α3(IV) chain. In Alport-type familial nephritis (Alport syndrome) the GBM is characterized by thinning and some-times multilamination. Evidence has been presented which shows that the α3(IV), α4(IV), and α5(IV) chains are either absent or are present in reduced amounts. In diabetes the GBM is unusually thickened, however the molecular defect which correlates to altered ultrafiltration has not been elucidated, but may involve type IV collagen. (Adapted from [5] with permission)

Over the last decade, great advances have been made by numerous investigators in advancing the understanding of basement membrane structure, function, and dysfunction. Recently, three new chains (α3, α4, and α5) of type IV collagen have been discovered and they have been implicated in the pathogenesis of Goodpasture and Alport syndromes [4-16]. Potentially, they may play a role in the development of diabetic nephropathy.

Molecular Structure of GBM

The molecular structure of GBM is very complex. The membrane is composed of several macromolecular constituents: type IV collagen, laminin, heparan sulfate proteoglycan, entactin, and fibronectin (Fig. 2). These interact to form a supramolecular complex. Type IV collagen, the major constituent, provides tensile strength to the matrix and its supramolecular structure serves as a scaffold for the binding and alignment of the other constituents [17,18]. A three-dimensional model of this suprastructure has been proposed [19]. The structure of GBM varies from that of other basement membranes, particularly with regard to the chemical nature of type IV collagen. This structural variation may be of fundamental importance in conferring a distinct function to GBM.

Supramolecular Structure of Type IV Collagen

The protomer, or building block unit, of type IV collagen is comprised of three α(IV) chains and is characterized by three distinct structural domains. These are: the NC1 domain at the carboxy-terminus; the triple-helical domain in the middle region; and the 7S domain at the amino-terminus (Fig. 3, lower panel) [4,17,18]. Protomers interact through covalent associations to form a supramolecular structure (Fig. 3, upper panel). Protomers associate in a head-to-head (NC1-to-NC1) fashion to form dimers, and in a tail-to-tail (7S-to-7S) fashion to form tetramers. Although these fundamental ways of connecting protomers are known, the three-dimensional structure of the collagen matrix remains largely unknown.

Several protomer subtypes, differing in the chemical nature of the α chains, exist in GBM (Fig. 4). The classical protomer, designated subtype A, is comprised of two α1 chains and one α2 chain, and is common to all basement membranes. The complete primary structure of these chains has been determined [20-25]. At least one other, and possibly several, protomer subtypes, exist in GBM because of the existence of the newly discovered α3, α4, and α5 chains. These are designated subtypes B, C, and D (Fig. 4), and correspond to protomers that contain these respective chains; however, the chain compositions are unknown.

The existence of several protomer subtypes introduces the possibility of several distinct arrangements in which protomers are interconnected and distributed in the supramolecular structure (Fig. 5). Different subtypes can be interconnected through their NC1 domains, forming homo- or hetero-dimers, and through their 7S domains, forming homo- and hetero-tetramers. The subtypes can be distributed in a regional or random fashion within the suprastructure [4]. In the extracellular matrix of the

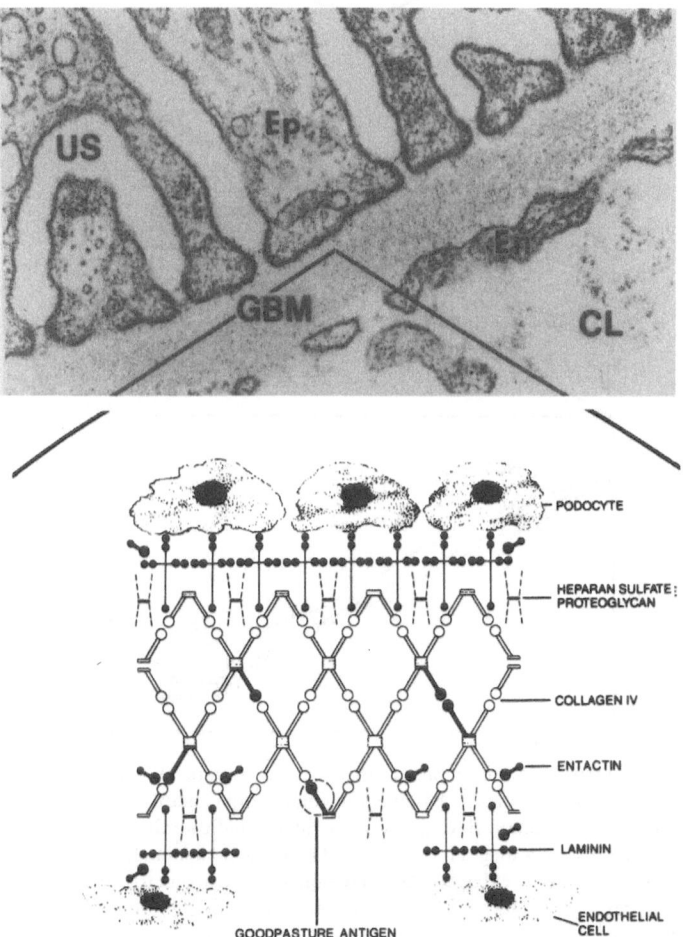

Fig. 2. The glomerular capillary wall and the intrinsic components of the GBM which form a functional matrix. The *upper panel* is an electron micrograph of the glomerular capillary wall. The *bottom panel* is a schematic depicting the arrangement of the macromolecular constituents of GBM. Type IV collagen serves as a scaffolding upon which the other components (laminin, heparan sulfate proteoglycan, and entactin) bind to form a functional matrix. Classical type IV protomer (Subtype A, see Fig. 4) contains one α2 and two α1 chains and is represented by the *undarkened protomers*. Protomers (Subtype B, see Fig. 4) containing the α3 chain (the Good-pasture antigen) are represented by the *darkened protomers*. Distribution of components represented within the matrix is preferential (but not exclusive). CL, capillary lumen; En, endothelium; Ep, epithelial podocytes; GBM, glomerular basement membrane; US, urinary space. (Adapted from [4] with permission)

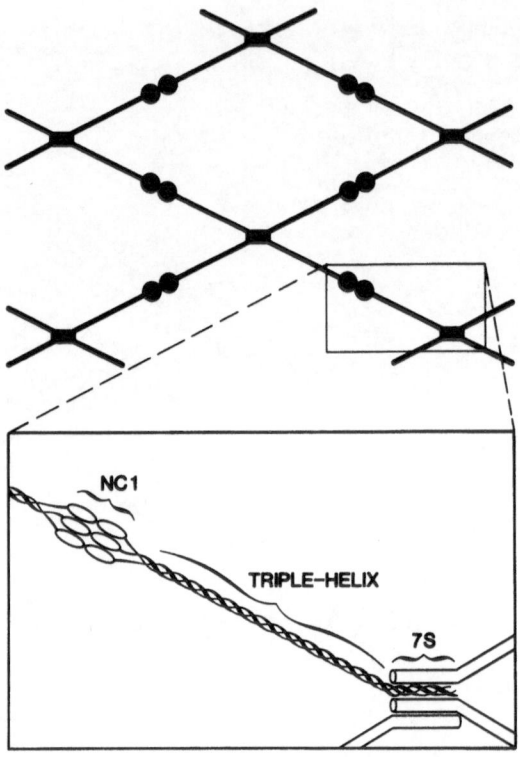

Fig. 3. Schematic drawing of the supramolecular structure of type IV collagen. The depicted model is based on studies of the basement membrane-like matrix produced by mouse Engelbreth-Holm-Swarm tumor. Several lines of evidence indicate that the model applies to GBM. The *upper panel* is a diagram of the type IV collagen supramolecular structure. The *boxed area* (*lower panel*) is an enlargement of a region of the structure to show the type IV collagen protomer and ways in which it is connected in the matrix. The protomer is a triple-helical molecule comprised of three polypeptide chains and has three distinct structural domains. These are the 7S domain at the amino-terminus, the triple-helical domain in the middle region, and the NC1 domain at the carboxy-terminus. Protomers are shown to associate in a head-to-head (*NC1-to-NC1*) fashion to form dimers and in a tail-to-tail (*7S-7S*) fashion to form tetramers. In addition to terminal interactions, helical or lateral interactions occur between type IV collagen protomers. (From [4] with permission)

glomerulus, subtype A appears to have a more endothelial/mesangial distribution, whereas subtype B is restricted to the GBM in the peripheral capillary loops [26]. The organization and function of these subtypes is unknown.

Evidence for the Existence of New Chains

Recently, we discovered the $\alpha 3$ and $\alpha 4$ chains of type IV collagen. The evidence is based on numerous chemical, physicochemical, and immunochemical studies of the NC1 domain (hexamer) of type IV collagen from GBM [4–9]. The chain identity was

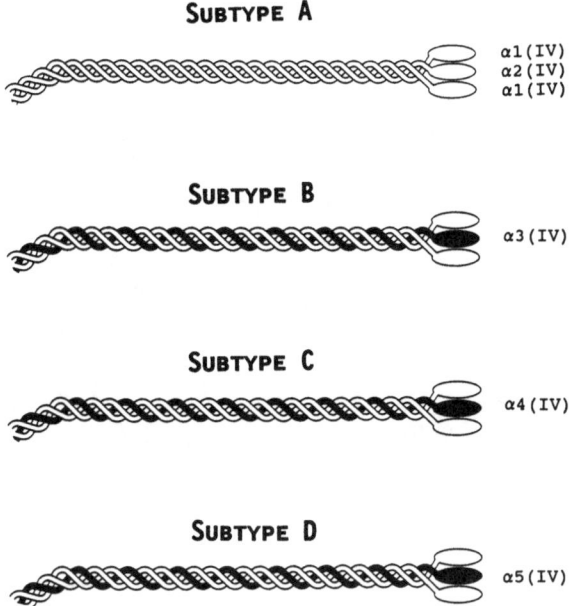

Fig. 4. Protomer subtypes of type IV collagen. The classical type IV collagen protomer (heterotrimer) is comprised of two α1 chains and one α2 chain (*undarkened chains*) and is designated as subtype A. Hypothetical type IV collagen protomers containing the α3, α4, or α5 chain (*darkened molecule*) are designated subtypes B, C, and D, respectively. (Adapted from [4] and [5] with permission)

deduced from amino-terminal sequences of NC1 monomers (Fig. 6) in which the sequences of α3 and α4 chains are highly related to, but distinct from, the collagenous-NC1 junctional regions of the classical α1 and α2 chains. Subsequently, we obtained chemical evidence for the collagenous domain of these chains [10]. The evidence is based on the molecular properties of a 60K collagenous component, extracted from GBM, that contains both a collagenous domain and the noncollagenous domain of the α3 chain (Fig. 7). The α5 chain was discovered by molecular cloning technologies and the primary structure of most of the chain has been elucidated [14–16].

Goodpasture Syndrome and Type IV Collagen

Goodpasture (GP) syndrome is an autoimmune disorder consisting of the triad of glomerulonephritis, lung hemorrhage, and anti-GBM antibody formation [27]. It includes a broad spectrum of clinical features, ranging from massive pulmonary hemorrhage with little overt evidence of renal disease to fulminant crescentic glomerulonephritis and little overt evidence of pulmonary hemorrhage. The nephritis is mediated by auto-antibodies that bind to the noncollagenous (NC1) domain of type IV collagen, and specifically to the NC1 domain of the α3 chain [4,6]. Many

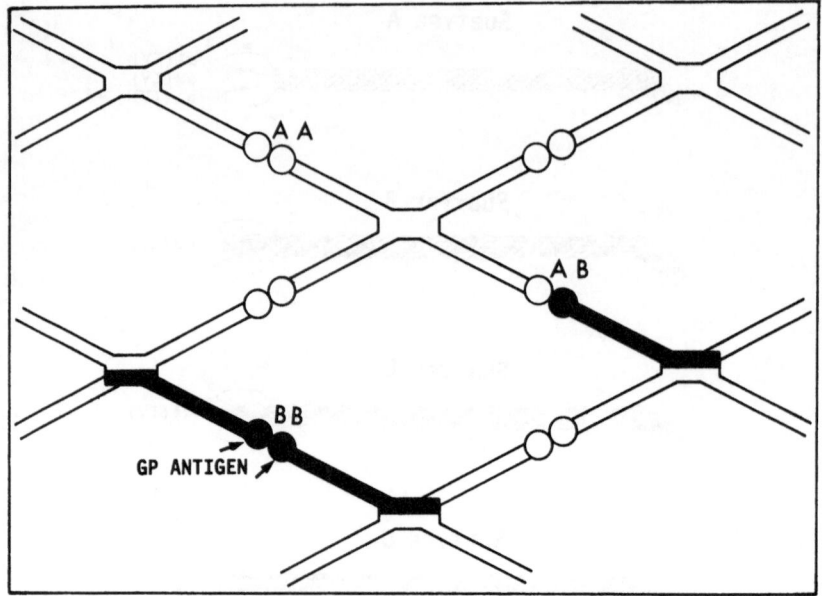

Fig. 5. End-to-end connections of protomer subtypes in type IV collagen supramolecular structure. Several different arrangements are possible, in which the subtypes are interconnected
through their NC1 domains forming homo- or hetero-dimers and through their 7S domains
forming homo- or hetero-tetramers in the type IV collagen matrix (see Fig. 3). *Undarkened
protomer*, classical type IV collagen protomer; *Darkened protomer*, subtypes B containing the
Goodpasture (*GP*) antigen. The darkened protomer also represents subtype C and D protomers
(Fig. 4). (Adapted from [4] with permission)

important questions remain unanswered about the $\alpha 3$ chain, also termed the GP-
antigen, with regard to its chemical nature, organization in the protomer, function,
and role in the pathogenesis of Goodpasture syndrome.

Alport Syndrome and Type IV Collagen

Classical Alport syndrome in human beings is a heritable disorder that eventually
causes kidney failure and deafness [28]. The nephritis is characterized by chronic
hematuria with progression to end-stage renal disease, and by ultrastructural abnormalities (thinning, diffuse splitting, and multilaminations of the lamina densa) in the
GBM (Fig. 1). The syndrome eventually leads to renal dialysis or transplantation
because there is no known treatment that alters the clinical course or affects the
underlying pathologic process. The ultrastructural abnormalities are widely accepted
to reflect the primary molecular defect causing nephritis in all phenotypes.

There are several lines of circumstantial evidence for the absence or diminished
quantity of one or more of the three new chains ($\alpha 3$, $\alpha 4$ and $\alpha 5$) of type IV collagen
in Alport GBM. The binding of GP-antibodies to Alport GBM is frequently absent,

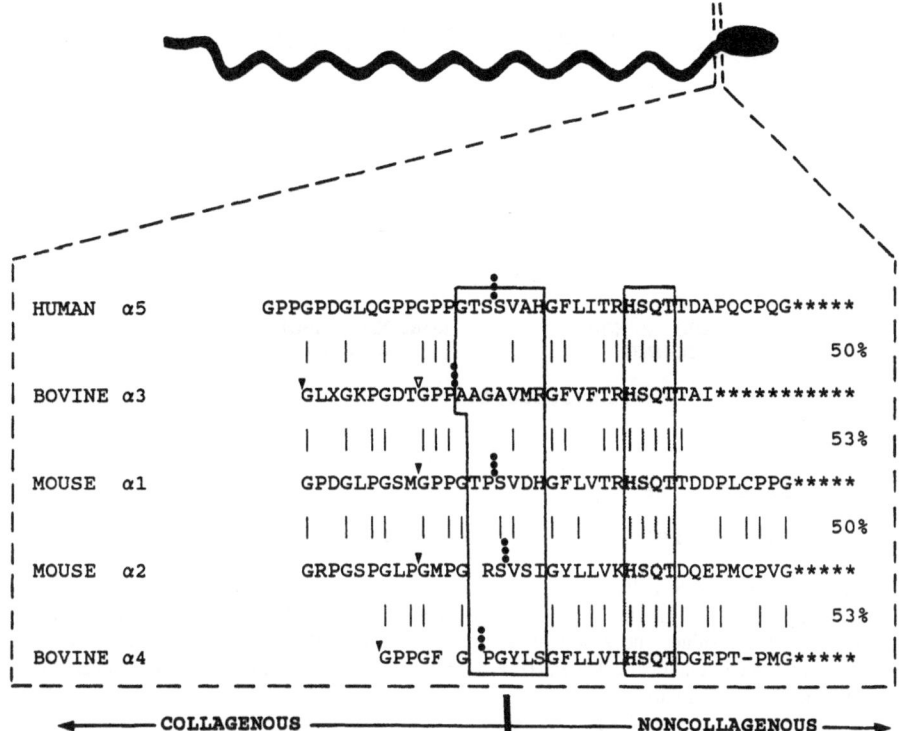

Fig. 6. Comparison of amino acid sequence of the collagenous-NC1 junction regions of the α1, α2, α3, α4, and α5 chains. The *darkened* α(IV) *chain* is drawn to show the region of sequence comparison. The five α(IV) chains have been aligned for maximal matching. The degree of homology between the upper and lower chains is given *at the right*. The *boxed areas* show positions of identity. The α1 and α2 sequences are taken from reference [22,25], the α3 and α4 are from reference [8,9], and the α5 is from reference [14]. *Lines* indicate identity of residues between sequences; *triangles* (*both undarkened and darkened*) represent collagenase cleavage sites; and *dots* indicate the junction region between the collagenous and NC1 domains. (Adapted from [5] with permission)

as determined by immunofluorescence of tissue sections [29–33]. The binding of a monoclonal antibody, directed to GP-antigen, to GBM is absent or diminished in 10 Alport patients [34]. Two components of the NC1 domain of collagen IV, M28+ and M28+++, which appear to correspond to the α3 and α4 chains [35], respectively, are absent from the GBM of three Alport patients [36]. Some Alport patients develop anti-GBM nephritis after renal transplantation, causing loss of allograft function. The alloantibodies show reactivity with unidentified dimer and monomer components of the NC1 domain of collagen IV [31,37–41]. A recent study reveals that genetic mutations in the α5 gene are present in kindred of Alport patients, which may relate to dysfunctional GBM [42]. Overall, these studies clearly implicate these new chains in the pathogenesis of the disease, particularly the α3 and α5 chains.

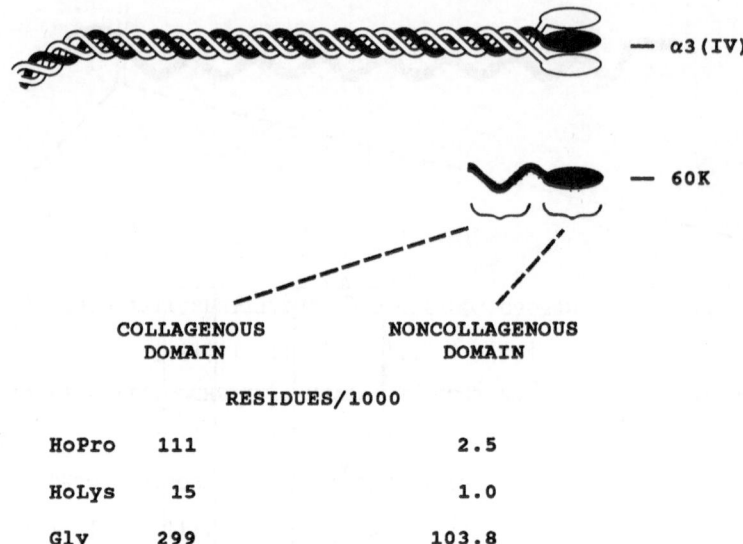

Fig. 7. Evidence for the collagenous domain of the α3 and α4 chains of type IV collagen. The 60K component was purified from a urea extract of GBM [10]. It contains a collagenous domain of 279 residues and a noncollagenous domain of 249 residues. Those amino acids indicative of a triple-helical collagen (HoPro, HoLys, Gly) are given for both the collagenous and noncollagenous regions

Conclusions and Perspectives

The structural knowledge of basement membrane constituents, particularly that of type IV collagen, has provided the necessary knowledge base from which we can begin to unravel the pathogenic mechanisms underlying the molecular sieving dysfunction of GBM in Goodpasture and Alport syndromes. Concurrent searches for the underlying mechanisms in these diseases have, in turn, provided deeper insights into the molecular complexity of this collagen, and into the molecular nature of GBM. A molecular commonality, which involves the new chains of type IV collagen, is emerging between the pathogenic mechanisms of Goodpasture and Alport syndromes. However, many questions about the molecular structure and assembly of this collagen, and its role in the pathogenic mechanism of these diseases, remain unanswered.

References

1. Farquhar MG, Courtoy PJ, Lemkin MC, Kanwar YS (1982) Current knowledge of the functional architecture of the glomerular basement membrane. In: Kuehn K, Schoene H, Timpl R (eds) New trends in basement membrane research. Raven, New York, pp 9–29
2. Hay ED (1984) Cell-matrix interaction in the embryo: cell shape, cell surface, cell skeletons, and their role in differentiation. In: Trelstad RL (ed) The role of extracellular matrix in development. Alan R Liss, New York, pp 1–32

3. Bernfield M, Banerjée SD, Koda JE, Rapraeger AC (1984) Remodeling of the basement membrane as a mechanism of morphogenic tissue interaction. In: Trelstad RL (ed) The role of extracellular matrix in development. Alan R Liss, New York, pp 545–572

4. Hudson BG, Wieslander J, Wisdom BJ, Noelken, ME (1989) Goodpasture syndrome: molecular architecture and function of basement membrane antigen. Lab Invest 61:256–269

5. Hudson BG, Wisdom BJ, Gunwar S, Noelken ME (to be published) Collagen IV: Role in Goodpasture syndrome, Alport-type familial nephritis, and diabetic nephropathy. In: Kang A (ed) Collagen, vol V: Pathobiochemistry. CRC, Boca Raton

6. Butkowski RJ, Langeveld JPM, Wieslander J, Hamilton J, Hudson BG (1987) Localization of the Goodpasture epitope to a novel chain of basement membrane collagen. J Biol Chem 262:7874–7877

7. Langeveld JPM, Wieslander J, Timoneda J, McKinney P, Butkowski RJ, Wisdom BJ, Hudson BG (1988) Structural heterogeneity of the noncollagenous domain of basement membrane collagen. J Biol Chem 263:10481–10488

8. Saus J, Wieslander J, Langeveld JPM, Quinones S, Hudson BG (1988) Identification of the Goodpasture antigen as the α3(IV) chain of collagen IV. J Biol Chem 263:13374–13380

9. Gunwar S, Saus J, Noelken ME, Hudson BG (1990) Glomerular Basement Membrane: Identification of a Fourth Chain, α4, of Type IV. Collagen. J Biol Chem 265:5466–5469

10. Fagg WR, Timoneda J, Schwartz CE, Langeveld JPM, Noelken M, Hudson BG (1990) Glomerular Basement Membrane: Evidence for Collagenous Domain of α3 and α4 Chains of Collagen IV. BBRC 170:322–327

11. Wieslander J, Langeveld J, Butkowski R, Jodlowski M, Noelken M, Hudson BG (1985) Physical and immunochemical studies of the globular domain of type IV collagen: Cryptic properties of the Goodpasture antigen. J Biol Chem 260:8564–8570

12. Butkowski RJ, Wieslander J, Wisdom BJ, Barr JF, Noelken ME, Hudson BG (1985) Properties of the globular domain of type IV collagen and its relationship to the Goodpasture antigen. J Biol Chem 260:3739–3747

13. Wieslander J, Barr JF, Butkowski RJ, Edwards SJ, Bygren P, Heinegard D, Hudson BG (1984) Goodpasture antigen of the glomerular basement membrane: Localization to noncollagenous regions of type IV collagen. Proc Natl Acad Sci USA 81:3838–3842

14. Hostikka SL, Eddy RL, Byers MG, Höyhtyä M, Shows TB, Tryggvason K (1990) Identification of a distinct type IV collagen α chain with restricted kidney distribution and assignment of its gene to the locus of X chromosome-linked Alport Syndrome. Proc Natl Acad Sci USA 87:1606–1610

15. Myers JC, Jones TA, Pohjolainen ER, Kadri AS, Goddard AD, Sheer D, Solomon E, Pihlajaniemi T (1990) Molecular cloning of α5(IV) collagen and assignment of the gene to the region of the X chromosome containing the Alport syndrome locus. Am J Hum Genet 46:1024–1033

16. Pihlajaneimi T, Pohjolanainen E-R, Myers JC (1990) Complete Primary Structure of the Triple-helical Region and the Carboxyl-terminal Domain of a New Type IV Collagen Chain, α5(IV). J Biol Chem 265:13758–17366

17. Martin GR, Timpl R, Kühn K (1988) Basement membrane proteins: molecular structure and function. Adv Protein Chem 39:1–50

18. Timpl R (1989) Structure and biological activity of basement membrane proteins. Eur J Biochem 180:487–502

19. Yurchenco PD, Schittny JC (1990) Molecular architecture of basement membranes. FASEB J 4:1577–1590

20. Brazel D, Oberbäumer I, Dieringer H, Babel W, Glanville RW, Deutzmann R, Kühn K (1987) Completion of the amino acid sequence of the α1 chain of human basement membrane collagen (type IV) reveals 21 non-triplet interruptions located within the collagenous domain. Eur J Biochem 168:529–536

21. Soininen R, Haka-Risku T, Prockop DJ, and Tryggvason K (1987) Complete primary structure of the α_1-chain of human basement membrane (type IV) collagen. FEBS Lett. 225: 188–194
22. Muthukumaran G, Blumberg B, Kurkinen M (1989) The complete primary structure for the α1-chain of mouse collagen IV: differential evolution of collagen IV domains. J Biol Chem 264:6310–6317
23. Brazel D, Pollner R, Oberbäumer I, Kühn K (1988) Human basement membrane collagen (type IV): The amino acid sequence of the α2(IV) chain and its comparison with the α1(IV) chain reveals deletions in the α1(IV) chain. Eur J Biochem 172:35–42
24. Hostikka SL, Tryggvason K (1988) The complete primary structure of the α2 chain of human type IV collagen and comparisons with the α1(IV) collagen. J Biol Chem 263: 19488–19493
25. Saus J, Quinones S, MacKrell A, Blumberg B, Muthukumaran G, Pihlajaniemi T, Kurkinen M (1989) The complete primary structure of mouse α2(IV) collagen: alignment with mouse α1(IV) collagen. J Biol Chem 264:6318–6324
26. Butkowski RJ, Wieslander J, Kleppel M, Michael AF, Fish AJ (1989) Basement membrane collagen in the kidney: regional localization of novel chains related to collagen IV. Kidney Int 35:1195–1202
27. Glassock RJ, Cohen AH, Adler SG, Ward HJ (1986) Secondary glomerular diseases. The Kidney 3:1014–1083
28. Atkin CL, Gregory MC, Border WA (1988) Alport syndrome. In: Schrier RW, Gottschalk CW (eds) Diseases of the Kidney, 4th edn. Little, Brown, Boston, pp 617–641
29. Jenis EH, Valeski JE, Calcagno PL (1981) Variability of anti-GBM binding in hereditary nephritis. Clin Nephrol 15:111–114
30. Jeraj K, Kim Y, Vernier RL, Fish AJ, Michael AF (1983) Absence of Goodpasture's antigen in male patients with familial nephritis. Am J Kidney Dis II:626–629
31. Kashtan C, Fish AJ, Kleppel M, Yoshioka K, Michael AF (1986) Nephritogenic antigen determinants in epidermal and renal basement membrane of kindreds with Alport-type familial nephritis. J Clin Invest 78:1035–1044
32. McCoy RC, Johnson HK, Stone WJ, Wilson CB (1982) Absence of nephritogenic GBM antigen(s) in some patients with hereditary nephritis. Kidney Int 21:642–652
33. Olson DL, Anand SK, Landing BH, Heuser E, Grushkin CM, Lieberman E (1980) Diagnosis of hereditary nephritis by failure of glomeruli to bind anti-glomerular basement membrane antibodies. J Pediatr 96:697–699
34. Savage COS, Pusey CD, Kershaw MJ, Cashman SJ, Harrison P, Hartley B, Turner DR, Cameron JS, Evans DJ, Lockwood CM (1986) The Goodpasture antigen in Alport's syndrome: studies with a monoclonal antibody. Kidney Int 30:107–112
35. Butkowski RJ, Shen G-Q, Wieslander J, Michael AF, Fish AJ (1990) Characterization of type IV collagen NC1 monomers and Goodpasture antigen in human renal basement membranes. J Lab Clin Med 115:365–373
36. Kleppel MM, Kashtan CE, Butkowski RJ, Fish AJ, Michael AF (1987) Absence of 28 kilodalton noncollagenous monomers of type IV collagen in glomerular basement membrane. J Clin Invest 80:263–266
37. Kashtan CE, Atkin CL, Gregory MC, Michael AF (1989) Identification of Variant Alport phenotypes using an Alport-specific antibody probe. Kidney Int 36:669–674
38. Shah B, First MR, Mendoza NC, Clyne DH, Alexander JW, Weiss MA (1988) Alport's syndrome: Risk of glomerulonephritis induced by anti-glomerular-basement-membrane antibody after renal transplantation. Nephron 50:34–38
39. Fleming SJ, Savage COS, McWilliam LJ, Pickering SJ, Ralston AJ, Johnson RWG, Ackrill P (1988) Anti-glomerular basement membrane antibody-mediated nephritis complicating transplantation in a patient with Alport's syndrome. Transplantation 46:857–859

40. Heuvel LPWJvd, Schröder CH, Savage COS, Menzel D, Assmann KJM, Monnens LAH, Veerkamp JH (1989) The development of anti-glomerular basement membrane nephritis in two children with Alport's syndrome after renal transplantation: characterization of the antibody target. Pediatr Nephrol 3:406–413
41. Savage COS, Noel LH, Crutcher E, Price SRG, Grunfeld JP, Lockwood CM (1989) Hereditary nephritis: immunoblotting studies of the glomerular basement membrane. Lab Invest 60:613–618
42. Barker DF, Hostikka SL, Zhou J, Chow LT, Oliphant AR, Gerken SC, Gregory MC, Skolnick MH, Atkin CL, Tryggvason K (1990) Identification of mutations in the COL4A5 collagen gene in Alport syndrome. Science 248:1224–1226

Relevance of Proteoglycans in Glomerular Matrix Pathology

Hirofumi Makino[1], Naoki Kashihara[1], Shuji Ikeda[1],
Brigitte Lelongt[2], and Yashpal S. Kanwar[2]

SUMMARY. Proteoglycans are one of the essential components of the extracellular matrices, i.e., glomerular basement membrane and mesangial matrix. Heparan sulfate-proteoglycan (HS-PG) appears to be the major proteoglycan present in the extracellular matrices, with small amounts of chondroitin sulfate-proteoglycans present in the mesangial matrix. The functions of the chondroitin sulfate-proteoglycans in the mesangium are unknown. The latter may play some role in glomerulosclerosis in various forms of nephritides, e.g., diabetes. The biologic relevance of HS-PG has been investigated extensively since its discovery a decade ago. Its biologic significance was first explored in glomerular permeability. Normally, anionic molecules such as plasma albumin are highly restricted during their passage across the glomerular capillary. With either the removal of or neutralization of the charge of HS-PG, the passage of albumin is greatly facilitated and the albumin appears in urine. Thus, the HS-PG imparts charge and size selectivity to the glomerulus. The loss of charge selectivity has been seen in several forms of glomerulonephritis, including diabetic nephropathy, where the synthesis of HS-PG has been found to be decreased. Moreover, intravenous administration of anti-HS-PG antibodies induces a proteinuric response and dramatically alters the extracellular matrices, thereby indicating that the HS-PG is nephritogenic. Another important role of HS-PG has been recently elucidated in renal morphogenesis. With the perturbation of proteoglycan metabolism, one finds failure in the development of the whole kidney in general, and also delayed maturation of the glomeruli as well as their extracellular matrices. Finally, several heparin binding domains on the laminin molecule have been described in in vitro systems, but their biologic significance is unknown.

---

[1]Third Department of Internal Medicine, Okayama University Medical School, 2-5-1 Shikata-cho, Okayama 700, Japan
[2]Department of Pathology, Northwestern University Medical, Chicago, IL, USA

Introduction

The glomerulus is comprised of three cell types: visceral epithelium, endothelium, and mesangium, and their two extracellular matrices: glomerular basement membrane (GBM) and mesangial matrix (MM). The visceral epithelium and endothelium cover the GBM from outside and inside, respectively; while the mesangial cell is embedded within its matrix. The GBM and MM, apparently synthesized by all the cell types of the glomerulus, are made up of various glycoproteins; these include: type IV collagen [1], laminin [2], entactin [3], heparan sulfate-proteoglycan (HS-PG) [4,5], chondroitin sulfate proteoglycan [6], nidogen [7], fibronectin [8], and amyloid P component [9]. The amyloid P component, fibronectin, and chondroitin sulfate-proteoglycan are exclusively located in the mesangium, while the remaining glycoproteins are present in both glomerular extracellular matrices. All these glycoproteins of the extracellular matrix play respective vital roles in various biologic and pathogenetic mechanisms involving the renal glomerulus. In this chapter certain mechanisms relevant to the pathobiology of the glomerular proteoglycans will be discussed.

What are Proteoglycans?

Proteoglycans are heterogeneous macromolecules distributed in most of the mammalian tissues, including extracellular matrices. A special type of proteoglycan, termed HS-PG, is found in the glomerular extracellular matrices. Its presence has been elucidated with the use of histochemical dyes (ruthenium red), selective binding with cationic proteins (cationized ferritin and lysozyme), and by labelling with isotopes, e.g., [^{35}S]-sulfate [5,6]. Evidence from several studies indicates that the molecular weight of proteoglycans varies greatly, depending upon the method of isolation and the source of the tissue. In general, they are made up of a core-protein to which glycosaminoglycan (GAG) chains are attached to the peptide via xylose-serine linkages. The GAG chains are made up of disaccharide units of glucuronic acid and glucosamine. The GAG chains are highly sulfated, which apparently imparts charge characteristics to the molecule. As ascertained by radiolabeling studies, the molecular weight of the intact HS-PG is 150–200,000 [10], while many other studies suggest that perhaps the de novo synthesized HS-PG is a smaller fragment of a relatively larger precursor macromolecule which has a molecular weight exceeding 1,000,000 [11,12]. Conceivably, the HS-PGs interact with one another by lateral or end to end associations; they also interact with other extracellular matrix macromolecules, thus forming the meshwork of the GBM. The mature GBM so assembled is endowed with charge and size-selective properties.

Role of Proteoglycans in Glomerular Ultrafiltration

The glomerular ultrafiltration unit is made of various strata. From the peripheral urinary space towards the inner capillary lumen they are: visceral epithelial foot processes with intervening diaphragms, GBM, and fenestrated endothelium. This

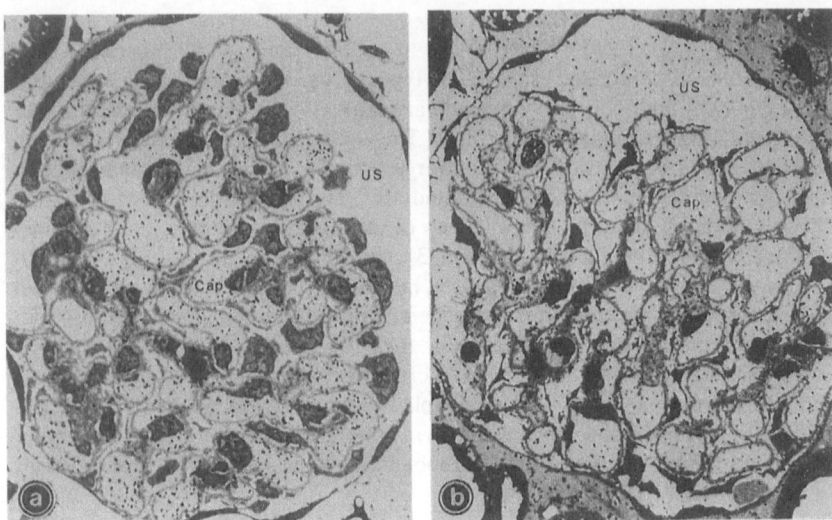

Fig. 1a-b. Light microscopic autoradiograms of glomeruli from control (a) and heparitinase-treated (b) kidneys that were subsequently perfused with ^{125}I-bovine serum albumin (*BSA*). Note that BSA molecules readily leaked into the urinary space (*US*) in glomeruli of the kidney treated with the heparitinase. Cap, capillary lumen

ultrafiltration unit is endowed with charge and size-selective properties which are partly due to the intrinsic presence of HS-PG in the GBM. Normally, the transcapillary passage of a given tracer with fixed molecular weight and varying degrees of charge would be as follows: cationic > neutral ≫ anionic. In in vivo situations, the anionic proteins such as plasma albumin have a highly restricted passage through the glomerular capillaries. With the removal of HS-PG from the GBM, the plasma albumin readily traverses into the urinary space [13] (Fig. 1). Similarly, the transcapillary passage of anionic ferritin is increased with the enzymatic digestion of HS-PG of the GBM. In the same manner, a proteinuric response is observed in rats with the constant intravenous infusion of hexadimethrine [14].

In addition to their critical role in ultrafiltration, the HS-PGs play an important role in protecting the GBM from assault by circulating plasma proteins [15]. They repulse the plasma proteins from the GBM by virtue of their electronegative charge. Also, they preserve the GBM matrix in a hydrated state by holding water molecules between the sulfate radicals. Thus, they prevent the non-specific adsorption of plasma proteins onto the GBM and do not allow it to become clogged by these proteins. In doing so, the HS-PGs allow a constant solute flow across the glomerular capillary, while keeping the GBM hydrophilic and keeping plasma proteins away from the GBM and in circulation. With the elimination of these anti-clogging functions of the GBM, one finds non-specific adsorption of anionic proteins, e.g., ferritin, albumin, and insulin, onto the GBM, resulting in an abrupt cessation of glomerular filtration (Fig. 2). Thus, it appears that under normal isoosmolar conditions, sulfated polyanionic macromolecules such as HS-PG act as anticlogging agents by preventing hydrogen bonding and adsorption of

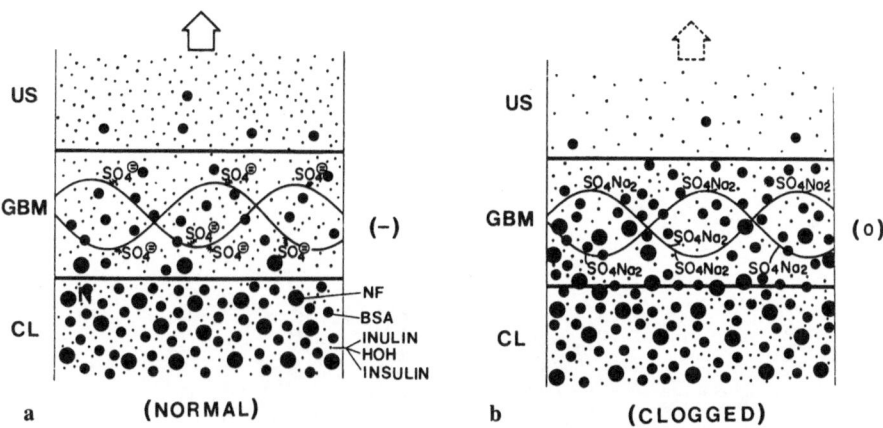

Fig. 2a,b. Schematic drawing of the phenomenon of clogging of glomerular basement membrane (*GBM*). Normally (**a**), anionic native ferritin (*NF*) and bovine serum albumin (*BSA*) do not adsorb onto the GBM, and small molecules like inulin or insulin or water pass through readily and reach the urinary space (*US*). With inactivation of sulfate radicals of proteoglycans (**b**), the NF and BSA adsorb onto the GBM and clog the filter; therefore, smaller molecules or plasma water do not pass through the glomerular capillaries readily. CL, Capillary lumen

plasma proteins onto the glycoproteins of the GBM; thereby a sustained transcapillary solute flow is maintained.

Proteoglycans in Diabetes Mellitus

Nonspecific adsorption of circulating plasma proteins, e.g., albumin and IgG, onto the GBM is seen in diabetic nephropathy. Such an adsorption has been attributed to the change in the biophysical/biochemical characteristics of the GBM. It has been shown that nonenzymatic glycation may interfere in the interaction of various glycoproteins of the GBM, but convincing data are not yet available in the literature. However, abnormalities in the metabolism of HS-PGs have been repeatedly demonstrated [16–20]. Usually, there is decreased incorporation of the precursor products (e.g., [35S]-sulfate) of HS-PGs into the GBM in experimental diabetic states (Fig. 3) [16,19,20]. Similar biochemical abnormalities have been observed in human tissues as well. Also, it appears that the decrease is usually proportional to the degree of proteinuria and excretion of urinary proteins in diabetes (personal observations). Thus, it appears that there is a decrease in the synthesis of HS-PGs of the GBM, and this reduction probably relates to the increased spillage of proteins into the urine, at least in the nephrotic stage of diabetic nephropathy. However, the nature of the biochemical lesion in the early stages of diabetes, i.e., the microalbuminuric stage, is unclear. It is possible that insulin or insulin-like growth factors may possibly play some role in the hyperplasia/hypertrophy of the mesangial cells, which occurs in the pathogenesis of the early stages of diabetic nephropathy. Certainly, it seems that insulin-like and transforming growth factors upregulate the functions of glomerular

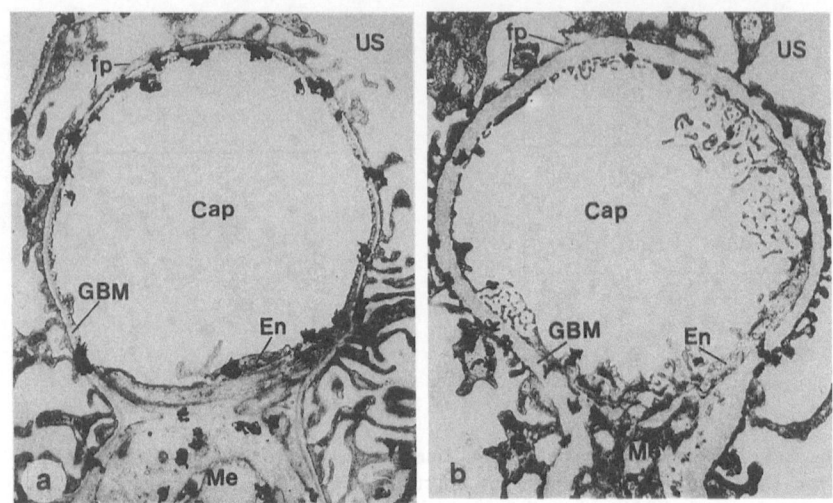

Fig. 3a,b. Electronmicroscopic autoradiograms of glomerular capillary loops of normal (**a**) and diabetic (**b**) rat kidneys radiolabelled with [^{35}S]-sulfate. Note the reduction in the autoradiographic grains overlying the glomerular basement membrane (*GBM*) of diabetic animal. US, urinary space; fp, foot processes; En, endothelium; Cap, capillary lumen; Me, mesangium

cells and increase the synthesis of proteoglycans specific to the mesangium [21,22]. At the moment, intensive investigatory efforts are being made in several laboratories to sort out various biochemical events which may shed some light on the pathogenesis of diabetic nephropathy.

Proteoglycans in Nephrotic Syndrome

Besides diabetes, the status of HS-PGs has been investigated in a wide variety of nephritides. Fractional clearance studies do provide the evidence of loss of charge-selectivity in various forms of glomerulonephritis. However, comparable histopathologic data are somewhat sparse. With the application of polyethylenemine, a dramatic decrease in the concentration of HS-PG was noted in patients with congenital nephrotic syndrome [23]. In regard to results obtained from experimental animals, there is much controversy. Aminonucleoside nephrosis in rats, a model of minimal change disease in man, has been exhaustively studied. The status of HS-PGs was investigated by the use of anti-HS-PG antibodies, and highly controversial results were obtained. The differences so observed can be reconciled if one takes into account the source of the antibody and the antigen. It is conceivable that in aminonucleoside nephrosis, certain antigenic epitopes, represented in a given antibody molecule, are lost while others remain preserved. This would likely be expected when the heterogeneous nature of the HS-PG macromolecule is taken into consideration during preparation of the antigens and antibodies.

Nephritogenicity of Anti-HS-PG Antibodies

The GBM as a whole is highly nephritogenic, i.e., anti-GBM antibodies, when administered intravenously, induce functional and structural alterations in the glomerulus which resemble those seen in Goodpasture's syndrome. Investigators have wondered about the glycoprotein or glycopeptide of the GBM which could be held responsible for the induction of the disease. Although the intact GBM is highly nephritogenic, the antibodies raised against its individual components, e.g., type IV collagen and laminin, evoke a weak proteinuric response. In view of these considerations, we investigated the nephritogenicity of proteoglycans in rats. Within a few hours of injection of anti-HS-PG antibodies, the animals showed a mild proteinuric response, minimal complement activation, and a transient influx of polymorphonuclear neutrophils (PMNs) into the glomerular capillaries. These changes regressed within a week. During the third week, tremendous ultrastructural alterations were observed, but without any proteinuric response. The changes included mesangial cell proliferation, irregular knob-like thickening of GBMs and occasional influx of monocytes and mesangial interposition (Fig. 4) [24]. The animals recovered completely 8 weeks after the administration of the antibodies. On the other hand, IgG-sensitized rats developed typical immune-complex nephritis within 7–10 days of injection of antibodies. After a week, subepithelial and subendothelial deposits were observed, along with complement activation. Subsequently, the subepithelial deposits enlarged in size and proteinuric response was accentuated (Fig. 4). The proteinuria was complement-dependent [25]. Finally, the deposits were reabsorbed by 3 months. Thus, it appears that the immune response and the formation of subepithelial immune-complex deposit is dependent upon the immune status of the animals. In this regard, we investigated the nephritogenicity of proteoglycans in various strains of mice and rats. The proteinuric response and ultrastructural alterations were dependent upon the genetically determined immune status of the animal. For example, Brown Norway rats and NZB/NZW (F1) mice exhibit maximal nephritogenic response as compared to other strains (unpublished work). Also, it appears that the degree of influx of monocytes into the glomerular capillaries is proportional to the severity of the disease; thereby indicating that inflammatory mediators somehow inflicted the damage to the glomerulus. In this regard, further investigatory efforts were made in order to delineate the nature of the mediator which could affect the HS-PGs of the GBM. The exposure of the glomerulus to interleukin-1 (IL-1) resulted in the degradation of the proteoglycan (unpublished work). In addition, a dramatic reduction in the incorporation of [^{35}S]-sulfate into the HS-PGs was observed, with the inclusion of reactive oxygen radicals in the medium (unpublished work). These experiments possibly suggest that a large number of inflammatory mediators can affect the integrity of the GBM HS-PG and that can result, conceivably, in a proteinuric response, which is observed in various forms of nephritides.

The other question which is relevant to the subject matter here pertains to the pathogenetic mechanisms involved in the formation of subepithelial immune-complex deposits. Recently, an attractive hypothesis has been advanced by Andres et al. [26]. According to this hypothesis, the antibodies bind to the antigenic epitopes present at the base of the visceral epithelial foot processes; this is followed by clustering of antigen-antibody complexes on the plasmalemma of the podocytes, with

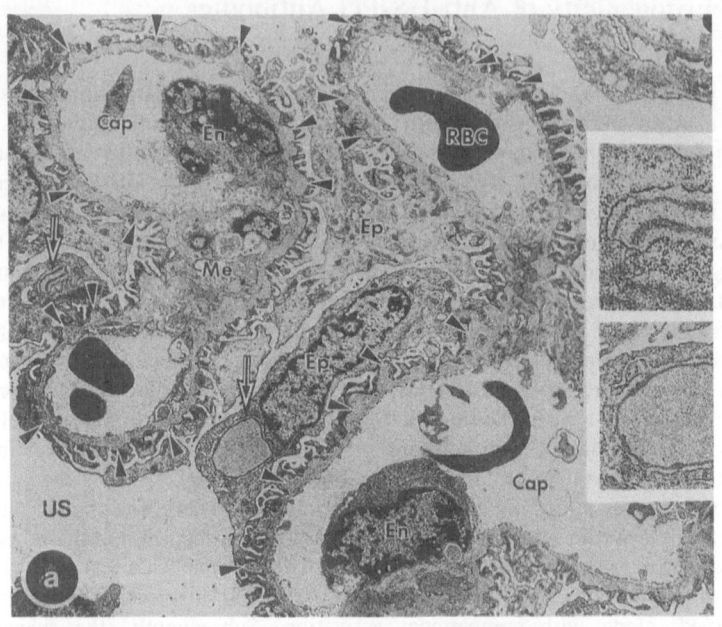

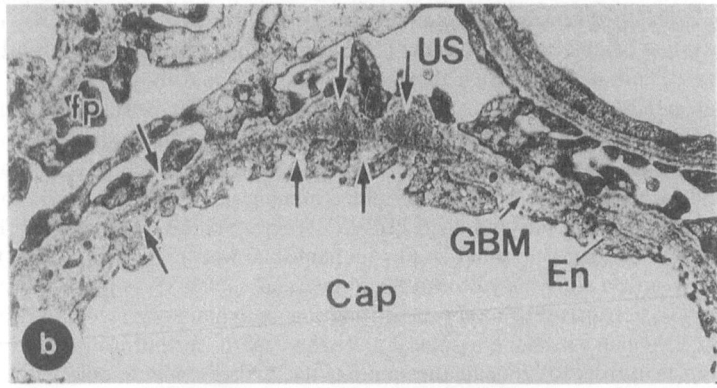

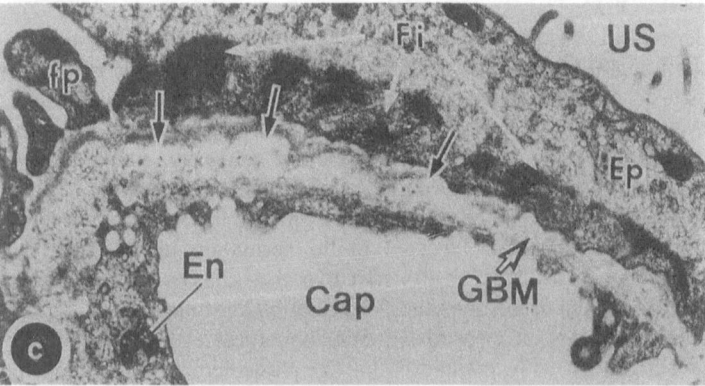

consequential capping and shedding of the complexes into the subepithelial space with eventual immune-deposit formation. The second hypothesis takes into account the intrinsic hemodynamics of the glomerulus. According to this, shear forces of relatively greater magnitude are prevalent in the inner layers of the GBM and the velocity of these sweeping plasma fluid currents is weak in the outer layers of the GBM (Fig. 5) [25]. Therefore, the ligands bound in the subepithelial space would have a delayed clearance and a prolonged residence in the peripheral layers of the GBM, and thus could serve as a core nidus for the formation of immune-deposits. In support of this contention, the intravenously injected ligands first accumulate in the inner layers of the GBM; after 12–24 h they equilibrate on both sides of the GBM, and by 7th day they are exclusively seen in the outer layers of the GBM (Fig. 5). The ligands localized in the peripheral layers of the GBM would evoke an immune-response and would ultimately lead to the formation of subepithelial deposits.

Role of Proteoglycans in Renal Development

Presumably, all components of the extracellular matrices regulate organogenesis/morphogenesis. However, proteoglycans have attracted most of the attention in this field. As they regulate organogenesis in many other organs, the proteoglycans possibly regulate renal organogenesis. Evidence for this came from the studies by Lelongt et al. [27]. It was noted that with the interference in the metabolism of proteoglycans, the metanephric tissues did not mature normally. The ureteric bud branches were disorganized and the number of nephrons seen was relatively less than the number seen in the control metanephric kidney (Fig. 6). In addition, the glomerular extracellular matrices were poorly assembled, lacked ruthenium red staining granules, and had a dramatic reduction in the incorporation of [^{35}S]-sulfate. This meant that indeed the perturbed proteoglycan metabolism had some relationship with metanephric development. The other glycoproteins of the extracellular matrices, i.e., laminin and type-IV collagen, were minimally affected. Further investigation of the renal development was conducted using puromycin aminonucleoside (PAN). Here too, dysmorphogenesis of the metanephric tissues was observed, in association with a dramatic decrease in the synthesis of proteoglycans [28]. It is interesting to note here that the proteoglycans synthesized in metanephric tissue are much larger ($\gg 2.5 \times 10^6$) than those isolated from the adult rat kidney. Also, the embryonic renal proteoglycans contain substantial amounts of chondroitin sulfate. The reasons for such variations are unclear, but may be related to the fact that the

---

◁

Fig. 4a-c. Electronmicrographs of glomerular capillary loops of kidneys from normal (a) and IgG-presensitized rats (b,c) injected with anti-HS-PG antibodies. Note the remarkable subepithelial thickening of the basement membrane (*arrow heads*) and basement membrane like material in the visceral epithelia (*arrows*) in glomeruli from normal rats. In the presensitized rats the immune-deposits are initially formed on both sides of the GBM (b); later on they are seen only in the subepithelial regions where they are being reabsorbed (c). US, urinary space; En, endothelium; Cap, capillary lumen; Me, mesangium; RBC, red blood cell; FP, foot processes; Ep, epithelium

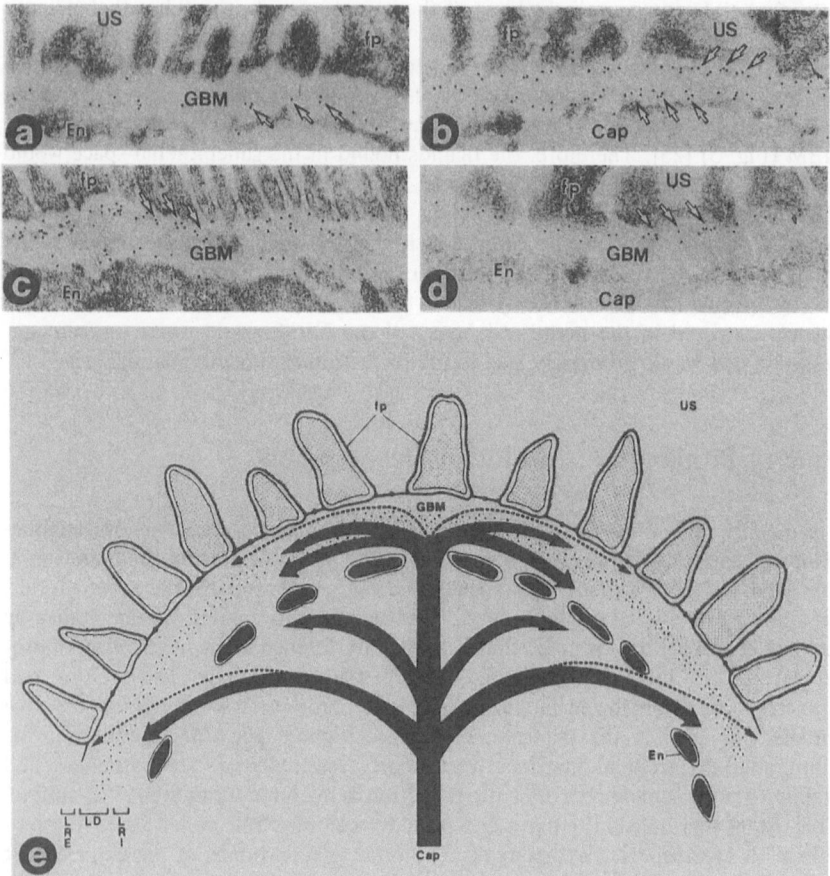

Fig. 5a-e. Electron micrographs of glomerular capillaries from kidneys of rats injected with anti-HS-PG antibody and sacrificed 1 h (**a**), 12 h (**b**), 3 days (**c**) and 7 days (**d**) later. The antibody was localized by immunogold method. Within one h the antibody localizes in the inner layers of the GBM (*arrows*); at 12 h it equilibrates on both sides of the GBM and remains there for three days; while on the 7th day the antibody molecules are exclusively localized in the outer layers of the GBM. **e** is a schematic drawing to indicate that the plasma fluid currents have relatively higher shear forces in the inner layers of the GBM than in the outer layers. This suggests that because of the higher shear forces the ligands present in the inner layers are easily cleared, while those in the outer layers remain localized and evoke a host immune-response and ultimately serve as a nidus for the formation of antigen-antibody immune complexes

US, urinary space; cap, capillary lumen; En, endothelium; FP, foot processes; LRE, lamina rara externa; LD, lamina densa; LRI, lamina rara interna

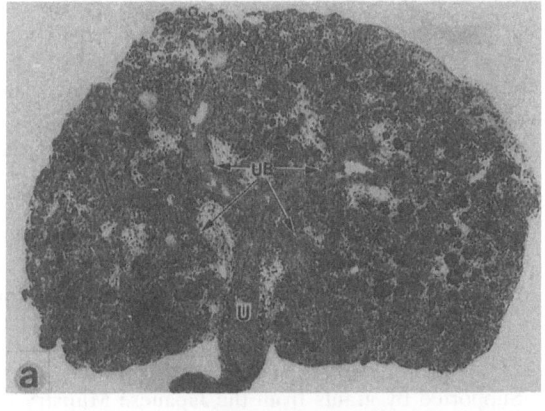

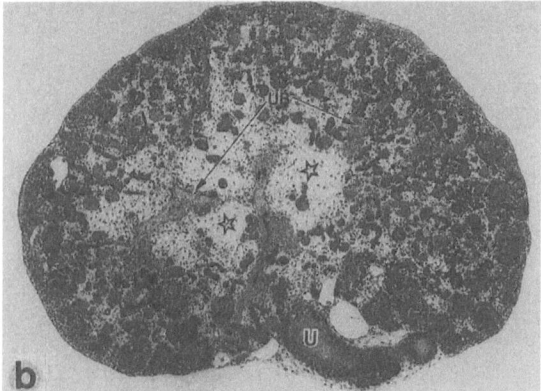

Fig. 6a,b. Light micrographs of normal (**a**) and beta-xyloside-treated (**b**) metanephric kidneys. Note in the xyloside-treated kidney the disorganization of the ureteric bud (*UB*) branches, looseness of the mesenchymal tissue (*) and reduction in the population of the nephrons as compared to the control metanephric kidney. U, ureter

embryonic tissues contain precursor proteoglycan macromolecules which later, in mature tissues, are modified to a smaller size via post-transcriptional or post-translational modifications.

Interactions of Proteoglycans with Other Glycoproteins

Several heparin binding domains have been localized on the various extracellular matrix proteins [29]. Presumably, these interactions may be relevant in the assemblage of the extracellular matrix. Proteoglycans, in general, accentuate the interactions among other matrix proteins. For instance, it has been shown that fibronectin bound to proteoglycans exhibits increased binding towards collagen. Similarly, the interactions of proteoglycans with other cell surface proteins have been investigated extensively. It appears that proteoglycans may serve as receptors which maintain communication between intracellular and extracellular matrix proteins [30]. Thus, it is possible that they may be responsible for some yet to be characterized transmembrane cellular signalling processes, and perhaps they also play a role in cell adhesion mechanisms. All these processes indicated above have been demonstrated in in vitro systems. Unfortunately, in vivo biologic proof, has so far yet to be elucidated.

In summary, we can say, with a certain degree of assurance, that proteoglycans play an essential role in regulating the morphogenesis and ultrafiltration of the renal glomerulus. Thus, derangements in the macromolecular structure of proteoglycans result in proteinuric responses which are seen in various forms of renal diseases.

Acknowledgments. Supported by grants from the Japanese Ministry of Education, Science and Culture (C-01570644) Japan, and NIH (DK28492) USA.

References

1. Keflides NA (1973) Int Rev Connect Tissue Res 6:63–104
2. Timpl R, Rohade H, Robey GP, Rennard SI, Foidart JM, Martin GR (1979) J Biol Chem 254:9933–9937
3. Carlin B, Jaffe R, Bender B, Chunh AE (1981) J Biol Chem 256:5209–5214
4. Kanwar YS, Farquhar MG (1979) Proc Natl Acad Sci USA 76:1303–1307
5. Kanwar YS, Veis A, Kimura JH, Jakubowski ML (1984) Proc Natl Acad Sci USA 81:762–766
6. Kanwar YS, Rosenzweig LJ, Jakubowski ML (1983) Lab Invest 49:216–225
7. Timpl R, Fujiwara S, Dziadek M, Aumailley M, Weber S, Engel J (1984) Ciba Foundation Symposium 108. London, Pitman, pp 25–43
8. Courtoy PJ, Kanwar YS, Hynes RD, Farquhar MG (1980) J Cell Biol 87:691–696
9. Houser MT, Scheinman JI, Basgen J, Steffes MW, Michael AF (1982) J Clin Invest 69:1169–1175
10. Kanwar YS, Hascall VC, Farquhar MG (1981) J Cell Biol 90:527–532
11. Hassell JR, Robey PG, Barrach HJ, Wilczek J, Rennard SI, Martin GR (1980) Proc Natl Acad Sci USA 77:4494–4498
12. Klein DJ, Brown DM, Oegema TR (1988) J Cell Biol 106:963–970
13. Kanwar YS (1984) Lab Invest 51:7–21
14. Hunsicker LG, Shearer TP, Shaffer SJ (1981) Kidney Int 20:7–17
15. Kanwar YS, Rosenzweig LJ (1982) J Cell Biol 93:489–494
16. Cohen MP, Surma ML (1981) J Lab Clin Med 98:715–720
17. Parthasarthy N, Spiro RG (1982) Diabetes 31:738–741
18. Rohrbach DH, Hassell JR, Kleinman HK, Martin GR (1982) Diabetes 31:185–188, 1982
19. Kanwar YS, Rosenzweig LJ, Linker A, Jakubowski ML (1983) Proc Natl Acad Sci USA 80:2272–2275
20. Klein DJ, Brown DM, Oegema TR (1986) Diabetes 35:1130–1142
21. Border WA, Okuda S, Languino LR, Ruoslahti E (1990) Kidney Int 37:689–695
22. Watanabe Y, Dalecki TM, Kanwar YS (to be published)
23. Vernier RL, Klein DJ, Sisson SP, Mahan JD, Oegema TR, Brown DM (1983) N Engl J Med 309:1001–1005

24. Makino H, Gibbons JT, Reddy MK, Kanwar YS (1986) J Clin Invest 77:142–156
25. Makino H, Lelongt B, Kanwar YS (1988) Kidney Int 34:195–219
26. Andres G, Brentjens JR, Caldwell PRB, Camussi G, Matsuo S (1986) Lab Invest 55:510–520
27. Lelongt B, Makino H, Dalecki T, Kanwar YS (1988) Dev Biol 128:256–276
28. Liu Z, Dalecki T, Kashihara N, Kanwar YS (to be published)
29. Ruoslahti E (1988) Annu Rev Cell Biol 4:229–255
30. Sanderson RD, Bernfield M (1988) Proc Natl Acad Sci USA 85:9562–9566

Pathobiology of Tubular Basement Membranes in Renal Cystic Disease

FRANK A. CARONE and YASHPAL S. KANWAR[1]

SUMMARY. The pathogenic role of the tubular basement membrane was studied in polycystic kidney disease (PKD) induced by diphenylthiazole (DPT) or its major urinary metabolite, phenol II, and in cyst-derived cells from human autosomal dominant PKD kidneys. DPT induced, in rats, progressive, but reversible cystic change of collecting tubules (CDs), characterized by thickening of the tubular basement membrane with marked reduction of the de novo synthesis of sulfated proteoglycans. The phenol II was administered for 4 days to determine the sequence of tubular cell and BM changes in the development of PKD. At day one, 12% of CDs were cystic and their BMs were altered. Over the 4 day interval, BMs remained structurally altered and cystic change increased progressively. Cell proliferation was not detected until day 2 and occurred both in cystic and in non-cystic renal zones; it did not increase as cystic change progressed. By immunofluorescence, there was a decrease in anti-heparin sulfate proteoglycan core protein reactivity and an increase in anti-fibronectin reactivity of the extracellular matrices of cystic tubules. In the in vitro studies, the growth rate, cell doubling time, and end cell number of cyst-derived autosomal dominant polycystic kidney disease (ADPKD) and normal human renal epithelial (NK) cells were the same; moreover, ADPKD cells did not exhibit any in vitro features of transformed cells. Post-confluent NK and ADPKD cells in vitro elaborated distinct BMs. By electron microscopy, BMs of NK cells were of uniform thickness with a regular pattern of ruthenium red (RR) binding sites indicative of proteoglycans. In contrast, BMs of ADPKD cells were less dense, thicker, and lacked RR sites; immunofluorescent reactivity to anti-HS-PG core protein was uneven and decreased while reactivity to anti fibronectin was increased. The findings suggest that BM components are in a dynamic metabolic state, capable of rapid modulation, and that PKD may be due to a defect in the synthesis/degradation of one or more basement membrane components, resulting in faulty tubular morphogenesis.

[1]Northwestern University Medical School, Chicago, IL, USA

Introduction

Polycystic kidney disease (PKD) presents as gigantic expansion of tubules and occasionally of glomeruli [1]. It is a localized, segmental event due to an aberration of one or more factors regulating tubular (or glomerular capsular) morphogenesis. PKD represents one of the most dramatic processes in biology, since some tubules increase in diameter from about 30 microns (not visible to the naked eye) to more than 5 centimeters. Furthermore, PKD is an excellent model to study the dynamics of transcellular fluid movement, cell growth, and the interactions and interdependence of tubular cells and their extracellular matrix. In some forms of PKD, cystic changes involve a specific segment of all nephrons, for example the collecting tubules in human autosomal recessive or infantile PKD. In other forms of PKD, cystic change involves random tubular sites of a small number of nephrons, for example in human autosomal dominant PKD, cystic change occurs only in a small percentage of nephrons where it can involve any segment of the nephron. Human PKD can pursue a rapid course with renal failure occurring early in life, or a benign course without renal failure developing during the natural life of the individual. Human acquired PKD develops in end stage kidneys that are atrophic and scarred. Clinical findings indicate that this form of PKD is reversible following renal transplantation with correction of the azotemic state [2]. Additionally, we have shown that PKD, induced experimentally by diphenylthiazole (DPT), reverses following withdrawal of the compound [3]. Whether other forms of human or experimental PKD are reversible remains to be determined. PKD occurs in the microenvironment of specific tubular segments. Baert microdissected two cases of ADPKD at an early stage of the disease [4]. Localized cystic dilatations were found in the proximal, distal, and collecting tubules and in Henle's loop. Many nephrons were normal. Cysts were localized distentions in otherwise normal tubules free of obstruction. Thus, expression of the gene defect in ADPKD is a localized event resulting in loss of tubular morphogenesis with extracellular matrix remodelling, tubular epithelial cell hyperplasia, and accumulation of tubular fluid.

Altered cell-BM interactions may be central to the pathogenesis of PKD. The epithelial cell is primarily responsible for synthesis/degradation of BM components, and the composition of the BM, in turn, plays a regulatory role in tissue morphogenesis and mobility, shape, differentiation, growth, and gene expression of the cell [5]. The tubular extracellular matrix is composed primarily of type IV collagen, laminin, sulfated proteoglycans (PGs), and fibronectin. These components have specific binding sites for each other and for structural components, both on the cell surface and in the underlying dense connective tissue [6]. Our studies on DPT or its hydroxylated metabolite phenol II and on autosomal dominant kidney disease (ADPKD) cells in vitro suggest that a faulty tubular extracellular matrix (basement membrane) plays a key role in the development of cystic change.

Materials and Methods

Two models of PKD were studies. 1. PKD was induced in rats by the oral administration of DPT [7] or its major urinary metabolite, 2-amino-4 hydroxyphenyl-5 phenyl thiazole, designated Phenol II [8]. Control animals were pair-fed. 2. In vitro methods

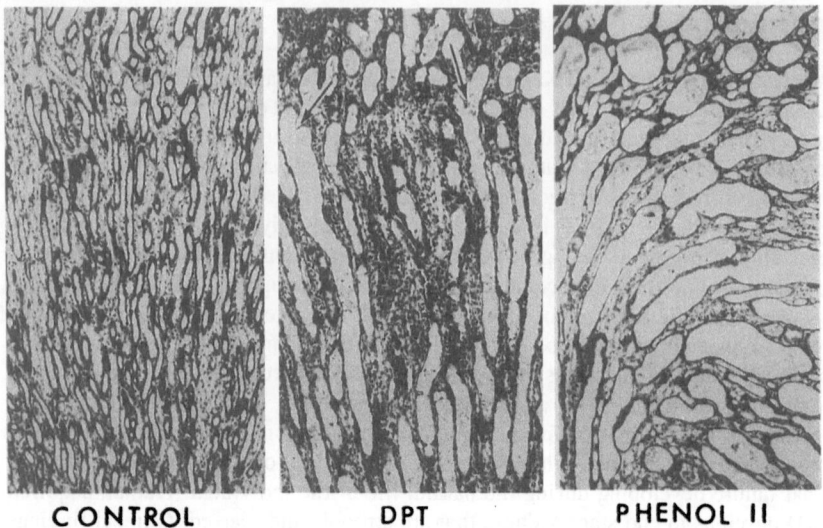

CONTROL   **DPT**   **PHENOL II**

Fig. 1. Outer medulla of control and 4 day *DPT* and *phenol II* treated (*PKD*) kidneys, X 66 DPT, diphenylthiazole; PKD, polycystic kidney disease

were developed to isolate and propagate large numbers of cells from cysts of ADPKD kidneys and from normal human kidneys (NK) [9].

Rat kidneys were perfusion fixed and examined by light microscopy. For electron microscopy ruthenium red (RR) was added to the fixative [3]. To study the de novo synthesis of proteoglycans (PGs) in DPT-induced PKD, renal PGs were labeled with [^{35}S]-sulfate in a recirculating kidney-perfusion system [10]. The reactivity of tubules, tubular cells and extracellular matrices to anti-heparin sulfate-proteoglycan, -type IV collagen, -laminin and -fibronectin were ascertained by indirect immunofluorescence [11]. Standard tissue culture methods were employed to study the biological behavior of human ADPKD and NK cells in vitro [9].

Results and Discussion

We found that administration of DPT induced PKD, involving collecting ducts, in rats (Fig. 1); it occurred in the presence of normal glomerular and tubular function and normal intratubular pressure, and in the absence of tubular obstruction [7]. These findings suggest that cystic transformation is due to an inherent alteration in the wall of the tubule. By electron microscopy, BMs showed progressive thickening and loss of ruthenium red staining (indicative of loss of proteoglycans) with progressive development of cysts. Biochemical analysis of isolated, and purified tubular basement membrane (TBM), revealed an overall increase in the concentration of low molecular weight glycoproteins [12]. Immunochemical studies revealed a normal concentration of laminin, entactin and type IV collagen but an increased concentration of type 1 collagen and fibronectin; the latter components are probably not intrin-

Table 1.

	Control	Phenol II treated			
		Day			
		1	2	3	4
% Cystic tubules	0	12*	21*	25*	30*
Basement membrane					
Thickness	N	3+	3+	3+	3+
RR Staining	N	N	N	LOSS	LOSS
Cell proliferation					
% Thymidine labeling					
Cortex	.11	.43	2.5*	2.6*	1.4*
Medulla	.24	.57	5.9*	8.0*	6.4*

*, Significant, N, normal, RR, ruthenium red

sic to the TBM. These morphological and chemical alterations in DPT-induced PKD suggest that cystic transformation may be due to a change in TBM compliance. However, the deformability and viscoelastic creep of BM lining cysts induced by DPT were not significantly different from normal TBMs [13]. Immunofluorescence studies of BMs of cystic tubules in DPT-treated animals showed the following compared to controls: uneven staining for type IV collagen and laminin, weak or absent staining for heparin sulfate proteoglycans (HS-PG), and intense staining for fibronectin [11]. Further studies demonstrated a decreased de novo synthesis of PGs in DPT-induced PKD in rats [10]. The PGs of normal and cystic kidneys were labelled with [^{35}S]-sulfate in an organ perfusion system. Total radioactivity in cellular, basement membrane, and media fractions of cystic kidneys was reduced 9, 7, and 3-fold, respectively. PGs from cystic and normal kidneys had similar molecular weight profiles. In addition to heparin sulfate, 15–20% of glycosaminoglycans (GAGs) synthesized by cystic kidneys were chondroitin sulfate; PGs synthesized by cystic kidneys had a lower charge density, possibly related to decreased sulfation of the PGs. Quantitative autoradiography revealed a 2 and 2.5-fold decrease of grain-densities over the cellular and extracellular compartments, respectively, in cystic kidneys. Collectively, these data suggest that DPT alters the biosynthesis/degradation of one or more BM components, particularly HS-PG and fibronectin, resulting in a defective BM.

The major urinary metabolite of DTP, 4-hydroxyphenyl-5 phenyl thiazole, (phenol II) was administered for 4 days to determine the sequence of tubular cell and BM changes in the development of PKD [8]. Following *only* 4 days of treatment, phenol II induced a significantly greater degree of impairment of concentrating ability and cystic transformation than DPT (Fig. 1). BMs remained structurally altered and cystic change increased progressively up to day 4 (Table 1). Significant cell proliferation (thymidine labeling) was not detected until day 2; it occurred both in cystic (outer medullary) and non-cystic (cortical) zones, and it did not increase as cystic change progressed (Table 1). At days 3 and 4, by immunofluorescence, there was an apparent decrease in anti-heparin sulfate proteoglycan core protein reactivity, and an increase in anti-fibronectin reactivity of the extracellular matrices of cystic tubules. The findings suggest that BM components are in a dynamic state capable of rapid modulation. Highly significant is the observation that TBM changes occurred in tandem with cystic transformation of the tubules and preceded the onset of tubular cell proliferation.

We obtained comparable findings from in vitro studies with normal human renal epithelial cells (NK) and cyst-derived cells (ADPKD) from kidneys of patients with autosomal dominant PKD [9]. Post-confluent NK and ADPKD cells grown on collagen matrices synthesized basement membranes. BMs elaborated by NK cells were uniformly dense, exhibited regularly spaced ruthenium red positive granules (Fig. 2), and displayed uniform intense reactivity to fluorescein-tagged antibodies to fibronectin, laminin, type IV collagen and HS-PG core protein (Fig. 3). In contrast, BMs elaborated by ADPKD cells were thicker, less distinct, lacked ruthenium red positive granules, (Fig. 2) and had diminished reactivity to anti-HS-PG core protein and increased reactivity to anti-fibronectin (Fig. 3). Immunofluorescence studies in human ADPKD kidneys similarly revealed a loss of reactivity to anti-HS-PG and a greatly enhanced reactivity to anti-fibronectin in cystic tissue [11]. Thus, there is an apparent altered synthesis/degradation of PGs and fibronectin in both models of PKD, namely DPT-induced and ADPKD cyst derived cells in vitro. Collectively, these findings provide strong evidence that BM alterations are a key factor in the development of cystic disease.

Relevant to this concept are the data of Ebihara et al., who report abnormal regulation of BM gene expression in a murine model of congenital PKD [14]. Levels of mRNA for the alpha 1 (IV) chain of collagen IV were half normal one week after birth and then increased, while mRNA levels for laminin B1 and B2 chains were 80% of normal at one week but were maintained at that level. Identification of the alpha 1 chain mRNA by in situ hybridization with a radiolabeled cDNA probe revealed highest expression in cystic regions, with localization mainly to interstitial cells adjacent to cyst walls, suggesting that these cells are the source of elevated alpha 1 (IV) chain mRNA. These observations may be unique to PKD since interstitial cells are not usually associated with BM synthesis. As cysts developed rapidly between 1 and 2 weeks after birth, immunostaining for collagen IV, laminin and HS-PG around cysts appeared reduced and discontinuous. There was an apparent discrepancy between mRNA levels and protein content of cystic BMs, possible due either to defective translation or post-translation events, or to altered turnover of BM components. These data indicate an abnormal regulation of BM gene expression in congenital (autosomal recessive) PKD.

It has been proposed that PKD is due to hyperplasia and/or preneoplastic transformation of renal epithelial cells [12,15]. Cell proliferation is a feature of human and experimental PKD and increase in tubular cell number is a requirement for the growth of cysts. It has been shown that several proto-oncogenes are significantly over-expressed in cystic kidneys [16]. Moreover, a model of PKD was produced in transgenic mice by deregulation of the c-myc proto-oncogene [17]. However, in a recent in vitro study we found that cyst-derived cells from human kidneys with ADPKD did not exhibit accelerated growth or possess the phenotypic features of transformed cells, compared to renal epithelial cells from normal human kidneys [9]. Moreover, in a chronic study (30 weeks), DPT induced progressive cystic change in the absence of a detectable increased rate of tubular cell proliferation [18]. Similarly, in newborn 1–3 week-old cpk mice, when diffuse PKD involvement of collecting tubules was progressing at an alarming rate, no increase in the mitotic index was detected, even though epithelial cellularity of collecting ducts was obviously increased [19]. Thus, cell growth may be a secondary rather than a primary event in the pathogenesis of PKD.

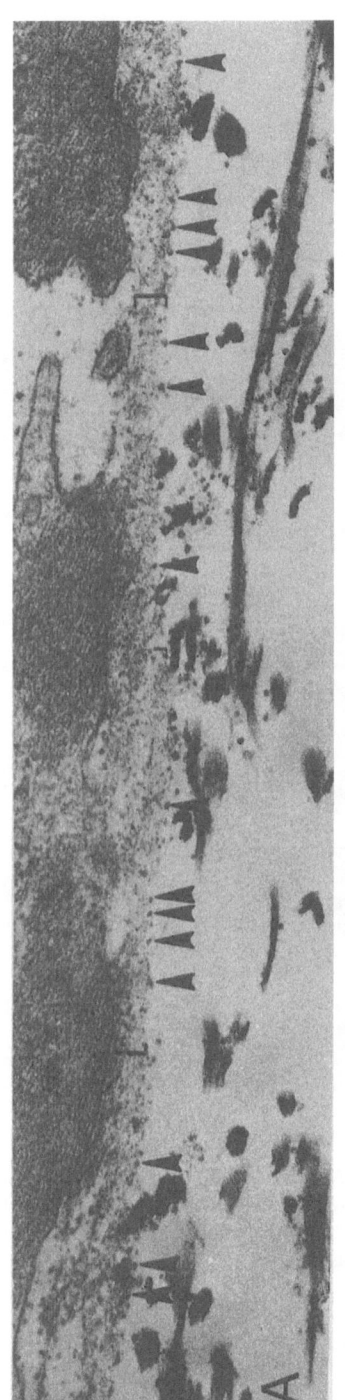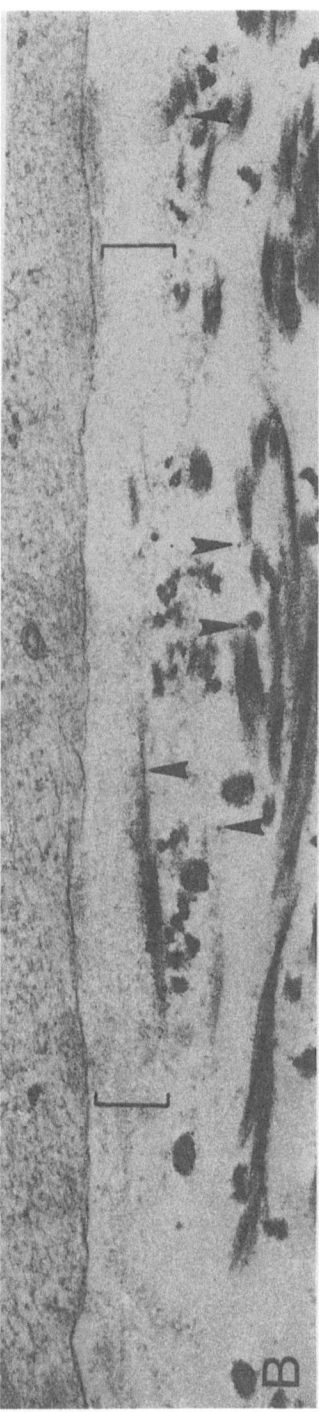

Fig. 2. Electron micrographs of basement membranes (*BM*) stained with ruthenium red (*RR*). *Panel A* shows *BM* of NK cells and *panel B* shows *BM* of ADPKD cells (*BM* delineated by brackets). *Arrow heads* indicate RR binding sites. X 45,000. NK, normal human renal epithelial cells; ADPKD, autosomal dominant polycystic kidney disease

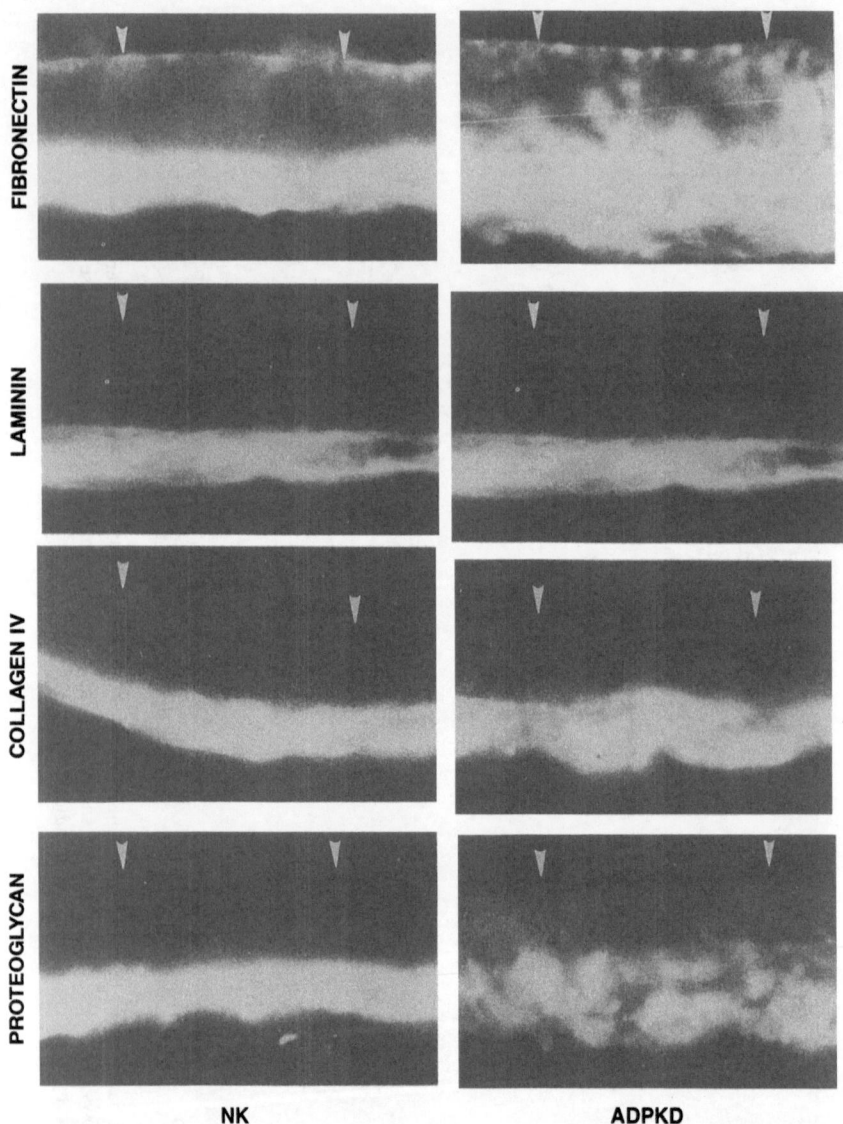

Fig. 3. Cell monolayers and basement membranes of *NK* and *ADPKD* cells stained with anti-fibronectin/laminin/collagen, type IV/HS-PG core protein (proteoglycan). (*Arrows* indicate the luminal membranes of the cell monolayers). X 500. NK, normal human renal epithelial cells; ADPKD, autosomal dominant polycystic kidney disease

Our findings support the concept that PKD may be due to a defect in the biosynthesis/secretion of one or more BM components, resulting in an altered composition and assembly of the BM and tubular dysmorphogenesis. The defect(s) could be transcriptional, translational or post-translational. Further attention should be directed to possible enzymatic defects in the biosynthesis/degradation of BM components and to tubular cell BM interactions in the pathogenesis of PKD.

Acknowledgments. Supported by NIH DK42304, DK28492, and Baxter Extramural Grants.

References

1. Grantham JJ (1983) A predominance of giant nephrons. Am J Physiol 224:F3–F10
2. Ishikawa I, Yuri T, Kitada H, Shinoda A (1983) Regression of acquired cystic disease of the kidney after successful renal transplantation. Am J Nephrol 3:310–314
3. Kanwar YS, Carone FA (1984) Reversible tubular cell and basement membrane changes in drug-induced renal cystic disease. Kidney Int 26:35–43
4. Baert L (1978) Hereditary polycystic kidney disease (adult form): A microdissection study of two cases at an early stage of the disease. Kidney Int 13:519–525
5. Hay ED (1984) Cell-matrix interaction in the embryo: Cell surface, cell skeletons and their role in differentiation. In: The role of extracellular matrix in development. A.R. Liss, New York, pp 1–31
6. Martinez-Hernandez A, Amenta PS (1983) The basement membrane in pathology. Lab Invest 48:656–677
7. Carone FA, Rowland RG, Perlman SG, Ganote CE (1974) The pathogenesis of drug-induced renal cystic disease. Kidney Int 5:411–421
8. Carone FA, Hollenberg PF, Nakamura S, Punyarit P, Glogowski W, Fluoret G (1989) Tubular basement membrane change occurs pari passu with the development of cyst formation. Kidney Int 35:1034–1040
9. Carone FA, Nakamura S, Schumacher BS, Punyarit P, Bauer K (1989) Cyst-derived cells do not exhibit accelerated growth or features of transformed cells in vitro. Kidney Int 35:1351–1357
10. Lelongt B, Carone FA, Kanwar YS (1988) Decreased de novo synthesis of proteoglycans in drug-induced renal cystic disease. Proc Natl Acad Sci USA 85:9047–9051
11. Carone FA, Makino H, Kanwar YS (1988) Basement membrane antigens in renal polycystic disease. Am J Pathol 130:466–471
12. Carone FA, Kanwar YS, Butkowski RJ (1987) Tubular cell and basement membrane changes in polycystic kidney. In: Hudson B, Price R (eds) Third International Symposium on Renal Basement Membrane. Academic, London, pp 413–423
13. Grantham JJ, Donoso VS, Evan AP, Carone FA, Gardner KD (1987) Viscoelastic properties of tubule basement membranes in experimental renal cystic disease. Kidney Int 32:187–197
14. Ebihara I, Killen PD, Laurie GW, Huang T, Yamada Y, Martin GR, Brown KS (1988) Altered mRNA expression of basement membrane components, in a murine model of polycystic kidney disease. Lab Invest 58:262
15. Bernstein J, Evan AP, Gardner KD (1987) Epithelia hyperplasia in human polycystic kidney diseases. Am J Pathol 129:92–101
16. Cowley BD, Smando FS Jr, Grantham JJ, Calvet JP (1987) Elevated c-myc proto-oncogene expression in autosomal recessive polycystic kidney disease. Proc Natl Acad Sci USA

17. Trundel M, D'Agati V, Costantini F (1989) The c-myc oncogene induces kidney cysts (KC) in transgenic mice. Kidney Int 35:364
18. Carone FA, Ozono S, Samma S, Kanwar YS, Oyasu R (1987) Renal functional changes in experimental cystic disease are tubular in origin. Kidney Int 33:1–6
19. Gattone VH II, Calvet JP, Cowley BD Jr (1988) Autosomal recessive polycystic kidney disease in a murine model. Lab Invest 59:231–238